52 Surgeries

What They Don't Tell You Before You Go Under

Linda Arbizu

LFA Publishing

Book Cover designed by Linda Arbizu with Claude

1st edition 2024

Dedication

I dedicate this book to my phenomenal surgeons, nurses, physical therapists, and hospital personnel who put my body back together and helped me heal. In addition, I dedicate it to my five extraordinary children, Joshua, Benjamin, Miriam, Hannah, and Eve, who survived my recovery process and supported me through all fifty-two surgeries. Also, to anyone preparing for the daunting task of their own surgery, my heart is with you. You are the reason I wrote this book.

Contents

1. Your Amazing Body Needs Surgery Sometimes 1
2. Research, Second Opinions, and Potential Conflicts of Interest 10
3. Managing Finances and Logistics 19
4. Pre- and Post Operative Nutrition, Fasting, Exercise, and Sleep 26
5. Mental Preparation For Surgery 34
6. Activating Your Energy Centers for Healing 42
7. Preparing Your Home and What to Take to the Hospital 50
8. The Big Day of Surgery 58
9. The First Twenty-Four Hours and Possible Complications 65
10. Follow Up Appointments and Physical Therapy 74
11. Revolutionizing Surgical Procedures 83
12. Glossary of Medical Terms Used in Surgical Procedures 93
13. Quick Recap of the 11SecretsFor You 96
14. Works Cited: 98

Chapter 1
Your Amazing Body Needs Surgery Sometimes

I Am Awed

Alex expressed his admiration after anatomy class: "Whenever I look at my hands or see my upright body in a mirror, I am awed by the resilience and fragility of the human body. For example, one baby falls out a window three stories up and gets scratched, while another baby falls off a bed and dies." "I know," I responded, "I love learning about the organ systems and how they all work together magnificently and yet are still so vulnerable to unexpected forces."

Resilience and Fragility

Resilience and fragility in one physical form provide the vehicle for the experiences of a lifetime in this three-dimensional world: your body. At sixty-one years old, my body has been through six pregnancies, two major automobile accidents, fifty-two surgeries, and procedures under general anesthesia, and it miraculously healed so I can talk, walk, hold my loved ones, massage my clients, clean my home, and write books. Now, look in the mirror at yourself. Recognize that your body is a fantastic wonder and has given you all the incredible experiences of your lifetime!

Intricate Workings of the Body

And yet, you know how quickly health can change and how arbitrary life can be. Whether you have had a parent, child, life partner, friend, or colleague become ill or die, you know first-hand how intricate the workings of the human body are, and your doctor might advise you to have surgery. The first secret for you is that no matter what type of surgery your doctor recommends, weighing its potential risks and benefits in collaboration with your healthcare team, making informed decisions, and adequately preparing for the procedure will provide the best outcome.

Eleven Organ Systems

Eleven organ systems make up your body. According to med.libretexts.org, "An **organ** is a group of tissues that work together for the overall function of the organ, and an **organ system** is a group of organs that work together to perform a specific function. The human organism consists of eleven organ systems. They are the Integumentary (skin) System, Skeletal System (bones), Muscular System (muscles), Nervous System (brain, spinal cord, and nerves), Endocrine System (glands making hormones), Cardiovascular System (heart and blood vessels), Lymphatic System (immune system- bone marrow, spleen, thymus, lymph nodes and vessels carrying white blood cells), Respiratory System (oxygenates lungs and dispels carbon dioxide), Digestive System (breaks down food through mouth, esophagus, stomach, small and large intestines- other major organs also involved), Urinary System (filter blood and create urine as a waste by-product- kidneys, bladder, ureters, urethra), and Reproductive System (Female and Male- tissues, glands, and organs involved in producing offspring)." https://med.libretexts.org/Bookshelves/Anatomy_and_Physiology/Human_Anatomy_and_Physiology_Preparatory_Course_(Liachovitzky)/05%3A_Higher_Levels_of_Complexity-_Organs_and_Systems/5.01%3A_Organs_and_Systems_of_the_Human_Organism#:~:text=The%20human%20organism%20consists%20of

Malfunctions Occasionally Require Surgery

You visit a doctor when organ systems malfunction and cease to maintain homeostasis (internal stability or equilibrium). Sometimes, medications, physical therapy, chiropractic, massage therapy, acupuncture, or changing a lifestyle habit can remedy the situation. Occasionally, doctors prescribe surgery. Suppose your doctor has recommended an operation to repair a malfunction in your body. In that case, it's more complex than going to a mechanic to fix your car because you know you can get a new automobile if the worst should happen. However, you can't get a new body if something goes wrong. We have yet to create the technology for that, so it's still exciting science fiction speculation.

Preparing For Surgery

So, what do you do right now? Adequate preparation can significantly affect your recovery and overall experience, whether you're undergoing a routine or a more complex operation. In this book, "Surgery Prep Vitals," we will dive into the fundamental aspects of preparing physically and mentally for your procedure and equip you with the knowledge and tools to navigate this challenging period with confidence and peace of mind.

Optimizing Your Body to Withstand the Stress

Preparation is not merely a logistical checklist but a holistic approach encompassing physical, mental, and emotional readiness. It involves optimizing your body's condition to withstand the stress of the operation and facilitate a smooth recovery, which includes adhering to preoperative dietary guidelines, engaging in appropriate exercise routines, and addressing underlying health issues. By prioritizing your physical well-being, you can enhance your body's ability to heal and reduce the risk of complications during and after surgery.

Mental Preparation

Mental preparation is equally indispensable, as undergoing surgery can evoke feelings of anxiety, fear, and uncertainty. Learning coping strategies, such as relaxation techniques and mindfulness practices, can help alleviate preoperative stress and promote a sense of calmness. Building a support network of friends, family, and healthcare professionals can also provide invaluable emotional support throughout the surgical process.

Knowledgeable, Empowered Decision-Making

Also, your preparation includes figuring out logistics and making knowledgeable decisions. Researching your surgical procedure, understanding the potential risks and benefits, and discussing concerns with your healthcare team are integral steps in the preparation process. Being well-educated and proactive empowers you along your healthcare journey. By investing time and effort into your physical, mental, and emotional preparations, you can approach surgery confidently, bounce back quickly, and feel agency over your health and well-being. Throughout this book, we will explore various aspects of surgical preparation, equipping you with the knowledge and tools necessary to manage this transformative experience with grace and resilience.

Types of Surgeries

Surgery encompasses many procedures tailored to address specific medical conditions and objectives. From minor interventions to life-saving operations, the type of procedure you undergo can have profound ramifications for your health and quality of life. This section will explore the different types of surgeries and their respective effects. There are various classifications of surgery based on factors such as the body systems involved, the purpose of the procedure, and the degree of invasiveness. Ordinary types of surgeries include:

Elective Surgery- Planned procedures to address non-life-threatening conditions or improve quality of life. Examples include cosmetic surgery, joint replacements, and corrective eye surgery. I have had several right knee surgeries, from open to minimally invasive joint replacement surgery, which reduced the length of my suffering significantly. Still, the shortened rehabilitation period was harrowing.

- Researching your specific surgical procedure and the materials used gives you a better idea about your expected recovery times. I saw a documentary about the toxic nature of cobalt in joint replacements and some dangerous female contraceptive implants called "The Bleeding Edge" on Netflix, so beware. FDA approval for medical devices is easier to get than it seems. Here is a link to the trailer on YouTube. https://www.youtube.com/watch?v=slmilObZl28

Emergency Surgery- Urgent interventions performed to treat life-threatening conditions or sudden medical emergencies. Examples include appendectomies, trauma surgery, and emergency cesarean sections. I have had twenty-six of these trauma and emergency interventions because of two major automobile accidents. I was told it mostly involved orthopedic procedures, but I was in a coma for eleven days, so I don't know for sure. I also had three emergency bowel volvuli and blockage procedures.

Major vs. Minor Surgery- Major surgeries involve significant anatomical alterations or organ removal and typically require hospitalization and a more extended recovery period. I was in the medical facility for two weeks after one collision, two months after my second car accident and for a week each with several internal surgeries. However, most of my surgeries were only twenty-four hours in the hospital or outpatient procedures, where I left within a couple of hours after waking up from the general anesthesia. Minor surgeries are less invasive, and surgeons may perform them on an outpatient basis with minimal disruption to your daily activities.

Open vs. Minimally Invasive Surgery- Open surgery involves large incisions to access the surgical site. In contrast, minimally invasive techniques utilize smaller incisions and specialized instruments, leading to faster recovery and reduced scarring. I had my first operation at sixteen, and throughout my forty-four years and fifty-two surgeries and procedures done under general anesthesia, there have been many changes. Laparoscopy, endoscopy, and arthroscopy involve inserting an endoscope through small incisions to see and repair the damaged tissues within the eleven organ systems of the human body. Open surgeries, which carry a greater risk of infection and a more extended recovery period, are less prevalent than endoscopic procedures.

Surgical Implications

Each type of surgery carries its own implications, including potential risks, benefits, and postoperative considerations. Factors such as the complexity of the procedure, your overall health status, and the expertise of your surgical team can influence the outcomes and recovery process, so you must thoroughly comprehend the type of procedure you will undergo and its potential effects on your health and well-being.

Risks of Surgery

While surgery can offer significant therapeutic benefits and improve quality of life, it also carries inherent risks and uncertainties. Learning the potential risks and benefits associated with your surgical procedure helps provide information you may need to analyze to make your best choice.

Anesthesia Complications- Adverse reactions to anesthesia medications, including allergic reactions, respiratory problems, and anesthesia awareness (consciousness during surgery).

Infection- Surgical site infections can occur following any surgical procedure, leading to prolonged recovery, antibiotic therapy, or additional interventions.

Bleeding- Excessive bleeding during or after surgery can necessitate blood transfusions, surgical interventions, or prolonged hospitalization.

Organ Damage- Surgery risks unintentional damage to nearby organs or structures, leading to complications such as hemorrhage (profuse bleeding), infection, or impaired organ function.

Blood Clots- Prolonged immobility during surgery and recovery can increase the risk of blood clots, which may travel to vital organs and cause life-threatening complications such as pulmonary embolism or stroke. That is why hospital staff want to get you up and moving as soon as possible after surgery.

While these risks are inherent to any surgical procedure, careful preoperative assessment, adherence to best practices in surgical technique, and diligent postoperative monitoring and care can mitigate them.

Benefits of Surgery

On the other hand, surgery also offers a myriad of potential benefits, including:

Disease Management or Cure- Surgery can be curative for specific medical conditions, such as cancerous tumors, obstructive lesions, or structural abnormalities.

Symptom Relief- Surgery may alleviate symptoms associated with underlying medical conditions, such as pain, dysfunction, or impaired mobility.

Improved Quality of Life- Certain surgical procedures, such as joint replacements or reconstructive surgeries, can significantly enhance a patient's quality of life and functional capacity.

Preventative Measures- Some surgeries reduce the risk of future complications or disease progression through preventive measures. Examples include prophylactic mastectomies for individuals with a high risk of breast cancer or bariatric surgery for morbid obesity.

Informed Consent is a Cornerstone

Informed consent is a cornerstone of ethical medical practice and patient autonomy, ensuring that patients are adequately familiar with the risks, benefits, and alternatives of a proposed treatment or procedure before consent. In surgery, obtaining informed consent is a legal requirement and an ethical imperative that respects patients' rights to self-determination and bodily integrity. It requires three components:

Disclosure of Information—Your healthcare provider should explain the nature of the planned operation, including its purpose and anticipated outcomes, potential risks and complications, alternative treatment options, and expected recovery process. They should present this information clearly and understandably, allowing you to make wise decisions about your care.

Understanding and Competence—You must have the legal capacity to understand the information provided and the consequences of your decision. If you have questions or concerns about the proposed procedure, please don't hesitate to ask for clarification or a second opinion.

Voluntary Agreement—You must consent voluntarily without being under duress for any medical procedure.

The first secret for you is that no matter what type of surgery your doctor recommends, weighing its potential risks and benefits in collaboration with your healthcare team, making informed decisions, and adequately preparing for the procedure will provide the best outcome. You can actively advocate for the nuts and bolts that align with your health goals and preferences.

Conversation With Alex Continued

"What was your first surgery?" Alex asked. "My first surgery was an arthroscopic partial meniscectomy of a bucket-handle tear when I was seventeen, and then they did an oral procedure taking out my impacted wisdom teeth a week later," I responded, "but I wasn't under general anesthesia for the second one. What was yours, Alex?" I inquired. "Gosh, I had a tonsillectomy and adenoidectomy (T&A) when I was nine. As a kid, I remember I was terrified of the IV they put in because I did not like needles, but the red-haired nurse who put in the IV was really gentle and kind. I remember my throat was sore, and my mom brought me my favorite chocolate ice cream from Snelgrove's when I could first eat," Alex replied. "Wow, I didn't have a T&A until I was almost eighteen, twice your age," I said.

Chapter 2
Research, Second Opinions, and Potential Conflicts of Interest

Ischemic Bowel Volvulus

"Dr. Nelson (name changed), you said I had an ischemic bowel volvulus. What went wrong, and what exactly did you repair? Isn't this in the same place you operated a few years ago? Why did I need this surgery?" I asked. "All you need to know is that I fixed it, Linda," he replied.

The second secret for you is to do your research, understand the diagnosis, ask questions, seek second opinions if necessary, investigate your doctor's ties to pharmaceutical or medical device companies, and insist on transparency as much as possible. Unfortunately, Dr. Nelson didn't answer my questions, so I have always wondered what he did to my intestines.

Do Your Research

Determining whether surgery is necessary and who you want to perform it involves gathering information from various sources to make a well-informed decision. In other words, do your research. Here's a step-by-step guide on how to approach this:

1. **Understand the Diagnosis-** Ask your doctor to explain your condition in detail. Please don't hesitate to ask questions or ask for clarification about any aspect of your diagnosis, treatment plan, or prognosis. Comprehending the rationale behind recommended treatments and potential alternatives empowers you to advocate for your health. Examine the possible risks and benefits associated with your procedure. Be sure you understand the implications of not having the surgery versus undergoing it.

2. **You can explore Non-Surgical Options-** Inquire about alternative treatments or therapies that might help your condition without surgery. Options could include medication, physical therapy, lifestyle changes, or other interventions.

3. **Review Scientific Literature-** Look for peer-reviewed studies or clinical trials related to your condition and the proposed procedure. Pay attention to success rates, potential complications, and long-term outcomes associated with the surgery—research reputable medical institutions and specialists specializing in treating your condition or medical issue. Seek recommendations from trusted sources, such as friends, family members, or support groups, and ask your primary healthcare provider for referrals to qualified specialists.

4. **Seek Second Opinions-** Following medical advice and treatment is often complicated, especially when facing significant health concerns or difficult treatment decisions. While many people trust their primary healthcare provider's expertise, there are instances where seeking a second opinion becomes necessary, so don't hesitate to consult other medical professionals, preferably specialists in the relevant field, for their views. Provide access to your complete medical history and any diagnostic tests you've undergone. They may offer different perspectives or suggest alternative treatment approaches.

Signs that a Second Opinion May be Necessary

- Uncertainty or Lack of Clarity—If you feel uncertain about your diagnosis, treatment plan, or prognosis, it may be a sign that you should seek a second opinion. A different perspective from another qualified medical professional can provide clarity and peace of mind.
- Complex or Serious Medical Conditions—For severe or complex medical conditions, such as cancer, heart disease, or neurological disorders, obtaining multiple opinions from specialists with expertise in the relevant field can help provide a thorough evaluation and comprehensive treatment planning.
- Conflicting Recommendations— If you receive contradictory treatment recommendations from different healthcare providers, seeking additional opinions to understand the available options and make informed decisions about your care is wise.
- Lack of Improvement or Worsening Symptoms- If your symptoms persist despite following the recommended treatment plan or if your condition worsens over time, it may be beneficial to consult with another medical expert to explore other possible approaches or potentially overlooked underlying issues.
- Personal Preference or Peace of Mind- Ultimately, seeking a second opinion is an individual decision, and it's entirely valid to do so for peace of mind, reassurance, or to explore alternative treatment options that align better with your preferences and values.

How to Approach Requesting a Second Opinion

- Open Communication- Discuss your concerns with your current healthcare provider openly and respectfully. Express your desire to seek a second opinion and explain your reasons. A good healthcare provider will respect your autonomy and support your decision to seek additional input.

- Prepare Your Medical Records- Gather copies of your medical records, including test results, imaging scans, and treatment history, for the healthcare provider conducting the second opinion evaluation. Comprehensive medical records enable the second opinion provider to assess your case well.
- Schedule Consultations- You can contact the healthcare provider or medical institution of your choice to schedule a consultation for a second opinion. Be prepared to discuss your medical history, current symptoms, previous treatments, and any questions or concerns you may have about your condition or treatment options.
- Evaluate the Second Opinion- After receiving the second opinion, carefully evaluate the recommendations and insights provided by the healthcare provider. Compare them with your initial diagnosis and treatment plan, and consider factors such as the provider's expertise, communication style, and comprehensiveness of their evaluation.

Not an Indication of Distrust or Disrespect

Knowing when to seek a second opinion is imperative to advocate for your health and well-being. By recognizing the signs indicating the need for additional input, approaching the process of requesting a second opinion thoughtfully, and making informed decisions about your care, you can confirm that you receive the most comprehensive evaluation and treatment possible. Remember that seeking a second opinion does not indicate distrust or disrespect towards your current healthcare provider but rather a proactive step towards obtaining the best care for your unique needs and circumstances.

5. Consider the Risks and Benefits- Evaluate the potential risks and benefits of the surgery based on your circumstances, including your overall health, age, and lifestyle factors. Assess whether the potential benefits outweigh the risks. After obtaining multiple opinions, consider all available treatment options and their potential risks, benefits, and outcomes. Consult with your primary healthcare provider, specialists, and trusted loved ones to weigh the pros and cons of each option. Sometimes, an outside perspective can provide valuable insights. Finally, I'd like you to make an informed decision that aligns with your values and goals.

6. **Evaluate the Quality of Life Impact-** Consider how the surgery may impact your quality of life, including recovery time, potential side effects, and any changes to your daily activities or abilities.

7. **Ask Questions-** Don't hesitate to ask your healthcare provider any questions or express any concerns you may have about the necessity of the surgery. Make sure you fully understand the reasons behind their recommendation. Be proactive in your healthcare sojourn by advocating for yourself and discussing your treatment plan, goals, and preferences. Don't be afraid to assert your needs and preferences or to seek additional opinions or information when necessary.

8. **Trust Your Instincts-** Ultimately, the decision to undergo surgery is personal. Trust your instincts and intuition to make the right choice after thoroughly considering all available information. If something doesn't feel right or you're uncertain about a particular treatment approach, express your concerns openly to your healthcare provider and seek further clarification or alternative options. After all, it's your body and your health. They can provide valuable guidance and support, but it is still your decision.

Investigating Your Doctor's Ties to Pharmaceutical or Medical Device Companies

Unfortunately, in today's healthcare landscape, patients must inform themselves about their healthcare providers' potential conflicts of interest, particularly regarding financial relationships with pharmaceutical or medical device companies. We'll explore resources for checking financial relationships and how to advocate for transparent healthcare practices.

Understanding Potential Conflicts of Interest-

- **Definition-** A conflict of interest occurs when a healthcare provider's financial interests or affiliations with pharmaceutical or medical device companies may influence their clinical judgment or treatment recommendations. Such relationships have the potential to compromise patient care and undermine trust in the healthcare system.

- **Impact on Patient Care-** Financial relationships with pharmaceutical or medical device companies may lead healthcare providers to prioritize certain medications, treatments, or devices based on financial incentives rather than solely on their patient's best interests, which can result in overprescribing of medications, unnecessary procedures, or biased treatment recommendations. Again, I refer you to the documentary about dangerous female contraception implants and toxic cobalt joint replacements called "The Bleeding Edge" on Netflix, so beware and opt for titanium instead. Here is a link to the trailer on YouTube. https://www.youtube.com/watch?v=slmilObZl28

- **Transparency and Disclosure-** While many healthcare providers have legitimate collaborations with industry partners for research, education, or consulting purposes, they must disclose these relationships to patients for transparency, which fosters trust and allows patients to make informed decisions about their healthcare.

Resources for Checking Financial Relationships-

- **Open Payments Database-** The Open Payments database, maintained by the Centers for Medicare & Medicaid Services (CMS), provides information on financial relationships between healthcare providers and pharmaceutical or medical device companies. Patients can search this database to access data on payments, gifts, or other transfers of value made to individual healthcare providers. Here is the link. https://openpaymentsdata.cms.gov/

- **State Medical Boards-** State medical boards may require healthcare providers to disclose financial relationships with industry partners as part of their licensing or registration requirements. Patients can contact their state medical board or visit their website to inquire about relevant disclosure policies and procedures. Input your state name medical board to find out the state's information. From the Federation of State Medical Boards, here is a link to verify a doctor's license and professional background. https://www.docinfo.org/#!/search/query

Unfortunately, information from my state's medical board isn't as forthcoming as it could be. It may be the same in your state, but it's still an investigation worth your efforts. According to the azcentral.com website, https://www.azcentral.com/story/news/local/arizona-investigations/2023/12/13/how-to-check-doctor-background-in-arizona/71891724007/#:~:text=Patients%20also%20can%20try%20to"Arizona patients have few options to find out if their doctor has problems. They can look them up on the state medical board's website, but misconduct published on the state medical board's website is limited to the past five years, and the state hides advisory letters to doctors revealing misconduct as serious as sexual misconduct and violence. Patients can also try to search for them in decisions from the Office of Administrative Hearings (by entering names in the "full-text" field) and search for them in The Arizona Republic's database of doctor misconduct, which attempts to fill gaps in government oversight of doctors. But many gaps remain."

- **Academic Medical Centers-** Academic medical centers often have policies regarding financial relationships between faculty members and industry partners. Patients receiving care at academic medical centers can inquire about these policies and request information about their healthcare providers' financial disclosures. In case you are wondering what an academic medical center is, it is a teaching hospital like the one I went to after my second serious accident in 1997- Loyola University Medical Center.

- I was in a coma for eleven days and had many doctors, interns, and students working on my four limbs, performing twenty-two surgeries on me during the five weeks I was there until they moved me to a hospital in Michigan City, Indiana, for another 4 weeks. From the definitivehc.com website, this link shows the top twenty-five under the top largest academic medical centers. https://www.definitivehc.com/resources/healthcare-insights/top-largest-academic-medical-centers

- **Professional Organizations-** Professional medical associations, such as the American Medical Association (AMA) or the American College of Physicians (ACP), may provide guidance or resources on transparency in healthcare and ethical considerations related to financial relationships with industry partners. I looked these up but found little information except whether the doctors are members.

Advocating for Transparent Healthcare

- Patient Education- Empower yourself with knowledge about the importance of transparency in healthcare and potential conflicts of interest. Educate yourself about how financial relationships between healthcare providers and industry partners can impact patient care and outcomes.

- Ask Questions- Don't hesitate to ask your healthcare provider about their financial relationships with pharmaceutical or medical device companies. Request information about any relevant disclosures and how these relationships may influence your treatment options or recommendations.

- Support Transparency Initiatives- Advocate for policies and initiatives to promote transparency in healthcare, such as mandatory disclosure requirements for financial relationships between healthcare providers and industry partners. Support legislation or regulations that enhance transparency and accountability in the healthcare system.

- Seek Second Opinions- If you have concerns about potential conflicts of interest or are uncertain about your treatment options, consider seeking a second opinion from another healthcare provider who does not have financial ties to industry partners. A second opinion can provide an independent perspective and help reassure you that your healthcare decisions are based solely on your best interests.

Transparency

Investigating your doctor's ties to pharmaceutical or medical device companies helps to advocate for transparent and ethical healthcare practices. By understanding potential conflicts of interest, utilizing resources to check financial relationships, and advocating for transparency in healthcare, you can be more knowledgeable about your treatment options and insist on accountability within the healthcare system. Remember, the second secret for you is to do your research, understand the diagnosis, ask questions, seek second opinions if necessary, investigate your doctor's ties to pharmaceutical or medical device companies, and insist on transparency as much as possible.

Doctor Conversations Continued

"Well, Linda," Dr Huang began, "You have three hernias that we can repair with mesh to strengthen those tissues so they won't tear open again. I see you have an incision site below one of the hernias that showed up on your CAT (computed axial tomography) scan. What is that for?" asked the doctor. "That was where Dr. Nelson repaired an ischemic bowel volvulus. I tried to contact him last year after the surgery, but his office was closed down, and I couldn't find any forwarding information to locate him," I replied. "Strange," said Dr. Huang.

Chapter 3
Managing Finances and Logistics

$500,000 of Medical Bills

"Terry," I commented, "I was lucky when I woke up from my coma in 1997 and found that even though I had $500,000 worth of medical bills, Medicaid paid for my twenty-two surgeries and hospital stay for the eleven days in a coma in the Intensive Care Unit and rest of the two months in the hospital until the lawsuit settled. A nurse told me that if I didn't sue the trucking company, I would be responsible for half a million dollars of medical costs myself, even though they didn't know if I was going to be able to walk or function." "Wow," reacted Terry, "That's a hefty price tag, but I know medical costs can add up quickly."

I Didn't Want to Sue

Yeah," I said, "I didn't want to sue. I didn't blame the truck driver who crossed the double yellow line because I understood his choice was to rear-end another semi at seventy-five miles per hour, hit the bus full of people in the right lane, or take his chances with the oncoming traffic, which might be empty. I don't know what I would have chosen. Unfortunately, the oncoming traffic was me and my four children: nine, six, four, and three and a half weeks old." Terry responded, "That was an awful predicament. That is why it was called an accident."

Trucking Company Went Bankrupt

I kept going, "The trucking company strategized by declaring bankruptcy so they wouldn't have to pay me the four million dollars the lawyers assured me from the lawsuit. They reorganized with another letter in their name and were back open for business within three weeks. Fortunately, they had an insurance policy for one million dollars that paid my medical costs and the lawyers. I ended up with the smallest amount, but at least I didn't have medical bills looming over my head for decades."
"It's a good thing you didn't have to come up with the half million for the medical bills," added Terry, "You never would have been able to pay that off."

The third secret for you is to manage the surgery's financial and logistical aspects beforehand, like arranging time off work, childcare or pet care, transportation to and from the medical facility, and post-operative caregivers for peace of mind. Handling surgery's financial and logistical aspects can be overwhelming, but careful planning and preparation can lessen stress and create a more satisfying experience. This chapter will provide the groundwork for insurance and medical bills, your hospital stay and time off work plan, arranging your transportation, post-surgery care, and building a support network.

Understanding Insurance and Medical Bills

1. Review Your Insurance Coverage- Familiarize yourself with your health insurance plan, including coverage details, deductibles, copayments, and out-of-pocket expenses. Understand which medical services and procedures are covered by your insurance and which may require preauthorization or additional documentation. All of my surgeries required pre-authorization and referrals from my primary care physician, except for life-saving emergency surgeries.

2. Verify In-Network Providers- If possible, choose healthcare providers, hospitals, and facilities that are in-network with your insurance plan to minimize out-of-pocket costs. Contact your insurance company or visit their website to search for in-network

providers and verify coverage details for your planned surgery. Most providers have a number on the back of their card that you can call to clarify what is covered and what isn't if you can't find the information you require on their website.

3. Understand Your Financial Responsibility- Determine your financial responsibility for surgery-related expenses, including deductibles, copayments, coinsurance, and non-covered services. Request a cost estimate from your healthcare provider or hospital before you get admitted for the medical procedure to help budget for anticipated expenses and avoid surprises. If you know all out-of-pocket costs, you can estimate whether you can afford the surgery now or will need to save up for it later.

4. Ask About Financial Assistance Programs- Inquire about financial assistance programs or payment options available through your healthcare provider or hospital, such as payment plans, discounts, or charity care programs. These programs can help mitigate financial burdens and make healthcare more affordable for you if you are experiencing economic hardship.

Planning for Hospital Stay and Time Off Work

- **Arrange for Time Off Work-** Coordinate with your employer or human resources department to arrange for time off work for surgery and recovery. Understand your rights and responsibilities regarding medical leave, including eligibility for paid time off, sick leave, or short-term disability benefits.

- **Plan for Childcare and Household Responsibilities-** If you have dependents or household responsibilities, arrange for childcare, pet care, or assistance with household chores during your hospital stay and recovery period. Reach out to family members, friends, or community resources for support if needed. In retrospect, I should have taken advantage of this more when my girls were little, but I felt too ashamed. They had such a hard time with a mommy always recovering from surgery.

Arranging Transportation and Post-Surgery Care

1. Coordinate Transportation- Arrange transportation to and from the hospital for your surgery day and any follow-up appointments or medical visits during your recovery period. Consider asking a friend or family member to drive you or arranging for a ride-sharing service, like Uber or Lyft, if you cannot drive yourself. Some insurance providers also have transportation services to and from medical appointments, so check into that.

2. Plan for Post-Surgery Care- Arrange for post-surgery care and support to assist with activities of daily living, medication management, wound care, and transportation as needed. This may involve hiring a professional caregiver, enlisting the help of family members or friends, or utilizing home health services or rehabilitation facilities.

3. Communicate with Healthcare Providers- Keep open lines of communication with your healthcare providers before and after surgery to address any questions or concerns about your recovery plan, medication regimen, follow-up care, or discharge instructions. Don't hesitate to reach out if you need help or clarification about any aspect of your care.

Resources for Post-Surgical Care

Various resources and options are available to provide adequate care support to safeguard your recovery needs:

- **Home Health Services-** Many healthcare providers offer home health services, where trained professionals, such as nurses, physical therapists, or home health aides, visit patients in their homes to provide medical care, assist with activities of daily living, and monitor recovery progress. These services may be covered by insurance or through government-funded programs like Medicare or Medicaid. I had a home health nurse and one of my physical therapists who came to my home for a few months until I could travel to their offices.

- **Rehabilitation Facilities-** For individuals who require ongoing medical care and rehabilitation after surgery, rehabilitation facilities or skilled nursing facilities (SNFs) can provide short-term or long-term care in a supervised setting. These facilities offer various services, including physical therapy, occupational therapy, and medical monitoring, to support recovery and facilitate a safe return to independent living. I have been to countless rehabilitation facilities in several states for physical therapy. These professionals helped me learn to walk after both major accidents.

- **In-Home Caregivers-** Hiring a professional caregiver or home health aide to assist with daily living activities, medication management, and transportation can help individuals maintain independence and recovery at home. Caregivers can provide companionship, emotional support, and practical assistance with tasks such as meal preparation, personal hygiene, and mobility.

- **Volunteer Organizations-** Many volunteer organizations and community groups offer support services for individuals recovering from surgery, such as meal delivery programs, transportation assistance, and companionship visits. These organizations rely on volunteers to provide valuable help and support to individuals in need, free of charge or at a nominal cost.

- **Family and Friends-** Reach out to family members, friends, neighbors, or other trusted individuals in your social network for support during recovery. Loved ones can help with grocery shopping, household chores, transportation to medical appointments, and emotional support. Feel free to ask for help when needed, as many people are willing to lend a helping hand. I relied on my mother after many of my surgeries and then Terry while he was alive.

- **Telemedicine and Remote Monitoring-** Take advantage of telemedicine and remote monitoring technologies to stay connected with healthcare providers and receive virtual medical care from home. Telemedicine platforms allow patients to consult with healthcare professionals, receive medical advice, and monitor vital signs remotely, reducing the need for in-person appointments and facilitating access to care. This has become more popular since the pandemic but wasn't available before then.
- **Community Resources-** Explore local community resources and support services available in your area, such as senior centers, community centers, religious organizations, or social service agencies. These organizations may offer programs, support groups, or assistance programs for individuals recovering from surgery or facing temporary or long-term caregiving needs.

Building a Support Network

A strong support network is invaluable during the surgical process, providing emotional reassurance, practical assistance, and encouragement when needed. Here are three tips for building and utilizing a support network:

1. Reach Out to Loved Ones- Share your feelings and concerns about surgery with trusted friends and family members. Even if they can't be there physically, stay connected virtually. In today's digital age, staying connected with loved ones has never been easier. Use video calls, social media, and messaging apps to keep in touch with friends and family. Allow yourself to be vulnerable and accept their support and encouragement. Knowing you're not alone in this medical process can provide immense comfort and strength.
2. Join Support Groups- Consider joining a support group for individuals undergoing similar surgical procedures or facing similar health challenges. Connecting with others who understand what

you're going through can provide validation, empathy, and valuable insights.

3. Please be clear and specific about your needs and preferences for your support network. Whether it's practical assistance with household chores, transportation to medical appointments, or simply a listening ear, don't hesitate to ask for help when needed.

The third secret for you is to manage the surgery's financial and logistical aspects beforehand, like arranging time off work, childcare or pet care, transportation to and from the medical facility, and post-operative caregivers for peace of mind. By proactively managing finances and logistics before surgery, you can minimize stress and focus on your recovery with more assurance. Feel free to seek support from healthcare professionals, financial counselors, or trusted individuals in your support network if you need assistance navigating the complexities of surgery-related planning and preparation.

Continued Conversation With Terry

"Hey, honey," Terry declared, "Come look at the shower seat I built so close to the ground so you can keep the surgical site from the artificial knee replacement surgery dry, as the doctor suggested for next week. I also have large garbage bags and duct tape to keep it covered while you use the handheld shower nozzle to wash." "Awww, sweetie," I replied, "You are so thoughtful and capable. Thank you so much!" "Well, I am going to take great care of you after your surgery because I love you!" said Terry.

Chapter 4
Pre- and Post Operative Nutrition, Fasting, Exercise, and Sleep

Want Some Steak?

"Hey, honey, do you want a bite of my steak?" Terry queried. "No, I don't want to eat any red meat tonight before my surgery. I am just going to have salad and fish tonight. I will drink some honey lavender tea later, but then I have to stop eating and drinking by midnight, NPO, nothing by mouth," I replied. "Yeah, but one bite of steak isn't going to hurt," Terry responded. "Maybe not, but I don't want ever to experience the kind of constipation I have had after many of my surgeries. The anesthesia and post-op pain relievers do that by themselves. It's like they paralyze your intestines, and red meat doesn't exactly digest quickly," I said. "Suit yourself," Terry countered.

Preparing is More Than Mentally Readying

The fourth secret for you is to eat foods that will help you heal, avoid ones that don't, exercise, sleep adequately, and quit habits that will slow your recovery in advance. Preparing for your surgery involves more than just mentally readying yourself; it involves what you do with your body to enhance healing and recovery. This chapter reviews various aspects of physical preparation, including pre and postoperative nutrition (what foods to eat and what foods NOT to eat), exercise, the compelling need for sleep in the preoperative period, and quitting habits for better healing outcomes.

Pre and Postoperative Nutrition, Fasting, and Exercise

Proper nutrition and exercise are primary components of preparing for your operation. A well-nourished body is better equipped to handle the stress of your procedure, heal efficiently, and facilitate your quickest recovery. Certain foods can hinder or support healing, so it's essential to be mindful of your diet before and after surgery. Here's a list of foods to avoid before surgery and foods that may aid in recovery:

Foods to Avoid

1. Fatty Foods- Avoid consuming high-fat foods, such as fried foods, fatty cuts of meat, and rich sauces, before surgery. These foods can delay gastric emptying and increase the risk of postoperative complications such as nausea, vomiting, and indigestion.

2. Spicy Foods- Spicy foods can irritate the stomach lining and exacerbate gastrointestinal symptoms, such as acid reflux or heartburn. Before your operation, it is best to avoid spicy foods, including hot sauces, chili peppers, and hot, zesty seasonings.

3. Carbonated Beverages- Carbonated beverages, such as soda, sparkling water, and carbonated energy drinks, can cause bloating and gas buildup in the stomach, leading to discomfort and potential complications during and after surgery. Try plain water or herbal teas instead.

4. Caffeine—Before your procedure, limit your intake of caffeinated beverages, including coffee, tea, and energy drinks. Caffeine can interfere with anesthesia and contribute to dehydration, which can prolong recovery time and increase the risk of postoperative complications.

5. Alcohol- Avoid consuming alcohol in the days leading up to surgery, as it can interfere with anesthesia, impair liver function, and increase the risk of bleeding during and after your operation. Alcohol can also dehydrate the body, which is counterproductive to healing.

Foods That May Aid in Recovery

1. Lean Proteins- Incorporate an increase in lean protein sources into your diet to support muscle maintenance, tissue repair, and wound healing after surgery. Choose lean meats, poultry, fish, eggs, tofu, legumes (beans, lentils), and low-fat dairy products to meet your protein needs.

2. Fruits and Vegetables- Consume various fruits and vegetables rich in vitamins, minerals, and antioxidants to promote immune function and reduce inflammation. Include colorful options such as berries, citrus fruits, leafy greens, carrots, and bell peppers in your meals and snacks.

3. Whole Grains- Choose whole grains such as brown rice, quinoa, oats, barley, and whole wheat bread to provide sustained energy and promote digestive health. Whole grains are fiber-rich, which helps regulate bowel movements and prevent constipation, a typical postoperative issue.

4. Healthy Fats- Incorporate sources of healthy fats, such as avocados, nuts, seeds, and olive oil, into your diet to support cardiovascular health and reduce inflammation. Omega-3 fatty acids in fatty fish like salmon and sardines are anti-inflammatory and may also aid healing.

5. Hydration- Drink plenty of water throughout the day before surgery until they direct you to fast. When you come out of general anesthesia, you must continue to drink plenty of water to flush out the anesthesia and support optimal recovery. In addition, adequate hydration is essential for maintaining blood

volume and circulation, regulating body temperature, and facilitating the transport of nutrients and oxygen to mending tissues.

6. Probiotic Foods- Consider consuming probiotic-rich foods such as yogurt, kefir, sauerkraut, and kimchi to promote gut health and support immune function. Probiotics can help maintain a healthy balance of beneficial bacteria in the digestive tract, which is essential for overall well-being and recovery.
7. Supplements- Consult with your healthcare provider about necessary supplements, such as iron or vitamin D, to address any deficiencies that could impact healing. According to the National Library of Medicine, vitamins B12, C, D, and E may promote wound healing. https://pubmed.ncbi.nlm.nih.gov/33242075/

Being mindful of your dietary choices before and after surgery can improve your nutritional status and support the body's healing process. Adequate intake of vitamins and minerals supports the immune system and aids tissue repair. Be sure to follow any specific dietary guidelines provided by your healthcare provider and consult with a registered dietitian or nutritionist if you have any questions or concerns about your diet during the perioperative period.

Fasting

Please follow any fasting instructions your surgeon or anesthesiologist gives. Typically, the pre-admission personnel will ask you to refrain from eating or drinking for a certain period before your procedure (NPO-Nothing by mouth after midnight is typical) to reduce the risk of complications during the procedure and to safeguard the effectiveness of anesthesia. Here are some key reasons why pre-surgical fasting is required:

- **Prevention of Aspiration-** When undergoing an operation, an anesthesiologist typically administers anesthesia to induce unconsciousness and prevent pain. Anesthesia can reduce the protective reflexes in the throat, making it easier for stomach contents to enter the lungs if vomiting occurs during surgery. This is known as aspiration, and it can lead to severe complications such as pneumonia or lung damage. Fasting before the medical process empties the stomach, reducing the risk of aspiration if vomiting occurs under anesthesia.

- **Minimization of Gastric Volume-** Fasting helps minimize the volume of gastric contents in the stomach, including food and liquids. An empty stomach reduces the likelihood of regurgitation or reflux during anesthesia induction and intubation, which could lead to aspiration. It also provides a more apparent surgical field for the surgeon and minimizes the risk of abdominal distension or discomfort during the procedure.

- **Improved Anesthetic Safety-** Anesthesia medications can affect physiological functions, including breathing and cardiovascular stability. Fasting before surgery helps maximize the safety and effectiveness of anesthesia by reducing the risk of complications such as aspiration pneumonia, pulmonary aspiration, or cardiovascular events. By following fasting guidelines, anesthesiologists can administer anesthesia more safely and accurately, minimizing the risk of adverse reactions or complications.

- **Enhanced Recovery-** Fasting before an operation can make your recovery smoother and more comfortable. After surgery, the body may experience temporary changes in gastrointestinal function, including reduced appetite, nausea, or vomiting. Fasting beforehand helps prepare your body for these changes and minimizes the risk of postoperative complications such as delayed gastric emptying or ileus (intestinal paralysis). Additionally, fasting can help reduce the likelihood of postoperative nausea and vomiting, which are common side effects of anesthesia.

Fasting before surgery is a standard practice to optimize your safety and surgical outcomes. It helps reduce the risk of anesthesia-related complications and ensures the surgical team can perform the procedure safely and effectively. You should follow your healthcare provider's instructions regarding fasting guidelines, including specific timeframes for abstaining from food and liquids before the procedure, to minimize the risk of adverse events and support a successful surgical outcome. (NPO, nothing by mouth after midnight the day before the procedure is typical).

Exercise- Engage in regular, moderate exercise leading up to surgery. Exercise improves circulation, strengthens muscles, and enhances overall fitness, facilitating a smoother recovery.

Sleep in Preoperative Preparation- Adequate sleep is paramount for mentally and physically preparing for surgery. Quality sleep supports your body's immune function, reduces stress, and promotes optimal healing. Consider the following tips to guarantee you get enough rest before your procedure:

- Establish a Routine- Aim for a consistent sleep schedule in the weeks before surgery. Going to bed and waking up at the same time each day helps regulate your body's internal clock and promotes better sleep quality. Also, getting twenty minutes of sunlight exposure earlier in the day helps balance the circadian rhythm.

- Create a Relaxing Environment- Keep your bedroom dark, quiet, and cool to facilitate sleep. Minimize exposure to screens (such as smartphones and computers) before bedtime, as the blue light emitted can interfere with melatonin production and disrupt sleep.

- Practice Relaxation Techniques- Engage in relaxation techniques such as deep breathing, meditation, or gentle yoga to help alleviate preoperative anxiety and promote relaxation before bedtime.

- Limit Stimulants- Avoid consuming caffeine or other stimulants in the hours leading up to bedtime, as they can interfere with your ability to fall asleep and stay asleep.

Quitting Habits That Can Impair Healing- Certain habits can impair healing and increase the risk of complications after surgery. Quitting or minimizing these habits before your operation can significantly improve outcomes. Consider the following:

1. **Smoking-** Smoking impairs blood flow and oxygen delivery to tissues, slowing down the healing process and increasing the risk of infections and difficulties. Quitting smoking before surgery can improve wound healing and reduce the risk of postoperative complications.

2. **Alcohol Consumption-** Excessive alcohol consumption can interfere with the body's ability to heal and metabolize medications properly. It's advisable to limit alcohol intake or abstain from it entirely in the days leading up to surgery.

3. **Recreational Drugs-** Avoid recreational drugs, as they can have unpredictable effects on the body and interact negatively with anesthesia and other medications used during surgery.

4. **Medication Review-** Review all medications with your healthcare provider, including over-the-counter drugs and supplements. Some medicines may need to be adjusted or discontinued before surgery to minimize the risk of complications.

The fourth secret for you is to eat foods that will help you heal, avoid ones that don't, exercise, sleep adequately, and quit habits that will slow your recovery in advance. Preparing physically for surgery involves more than just mentally readying yourself; it involves physical preparation to enhance healing and recovery, including pre and postoperative nutrition (what foods to eat and what foods NOT to eat), exercise, adequate sleep during the preoperative period, and quitting detrimental habits for better healing outcomes. By paying attention to these aspects of preoperative preparation, you can enhance your body's ability to undergo surgery and promote a smoother recovery process. In addition, you can consult your healthcare provider for personalized recommendations tailored to your needs and medical history.

Red Meat

"Yeah," Terry commented, "After this last surgery, I get why you said red meat wasn't a good idea before the procedure. I feel like I have cement sitting in my stomach, and trying to go feels like I have to crap a brick sideways." "Oh, baby, I am so sorry, but we all have to learn for ourselves," I commiserated. "If I ever have to have another surgery, I will definitely eat lighter foods the day before," Terry said, "Experience is the best teacher."

Chapter 5
Mental Preparation For Surgery

Meditation

"Hey honey, do you mind if I put on my headphones and do my hour-long Centerpointe binaural beat meditation?" I asked. "What in the world is that binaural stuff?" responded Terry with another question. "Well, the current popular thinking is that it is supposed to help you get into a meditative state faster," I replied. "Okay, whatever works for you," reacted Terry. "Go ahead and meditate. I'll let you know when we get close to the doctor's office because it's a two-hour trip from our place to Northwest Phoenix."

Effectively Managing Pre-procedure Emotions

Preparing for surgery goes beyond the physical aspect; it also involves mental readiness to handle the challenges and uncertainties of a medical procedure. The fifth secret for you is effectively managing anxiety and fear, utilizing meditation, visualization and relaxation techniques, calling upon your faith community, and using therapeutic music for inner peace and confidence. These practices will provide more emotional stability, inner peace, and better pain management throughout the medical process.

Managing Anxiety and Fear

Facing surgery can evoke a range of emotions, including anxiety and fear. However, effectively managing these emotions is vital for maintaining mental well-being and promoting a positive surgical experience. Consider the following methods:

1. Education and Information- We already talked about doing your research. It doesn't hurt to Google the intended procedure and see how others have felt about having the procedure you are contemplating. I believe in researching first because I didn't do it sometimes, and I wish I had. After all, my parents' generation trusted their doctors implicitly. And when I had automobile accidents, I didn't know enough to question my doctors. I figured they did all that schooling so they could rebuild me. They were like Gods who performed miracles for me so I could walk. Unfortunately, I found out firsthand that they are human and make mistakes, like the doctor who performed some intestinal work but wouldn't tell me what he "fixed," so I had to have another surgery a few years later in the same spot.

2. Open Communication- Maintain open and honest communication with your healthcare providers. Express any concerns or anxieties you may have, and seek clarification on any aspects of the operation that are unclear to you. Feeling heard and supported by your medical team can reassure and ease anxiety. After my second auto accident, I had no bladder control because the pelvic floor lost its innervation. The car crash disrupted the nerves in the brain or the spinal cord, and the organs supported by the pelvic floor began to fall out.

- For seven years, I had urinary incontinence (I peed my pants) and never left the house because I was ashamed and never spoke of it to my doctors. Finally, I mentioned it because I wanted to go back to work. The doctor implanted an InterStim device that delivers a mild electrical shock to the muscle area via a lead to the sacral nerve through the S3 foramen every 20 seconds, and now I have urinary control. Later, I wrote a letter to a subsequent doctor about the device negatively affecting my vaginal area and showed up for an appointment when the lady at the front desk informed me I "was no longer a patient of doctor ___." He would not talk to me, and they would not give me any information except that I was "no longer his patient."

- I suppose he must have been offended by something I wrote in the letter. I had difficulty finding another doctor who would deal with a device previously implanted by another doctor because they didn't want to be sued for someone else's mistake. After calling fifteen doctors, I finally found a female doctor who would listen, accept me as a patient, and fix the problem. It's funny because she was in the same medical group as the male doctor who would not communicate with me. Open communication needed to be improved.

3. Mindfulness and Relaxation Techniques- To soothe yourself and reduce anxiety, Practice mindfulness-based techniques such as deep breathing exercises, meditation, and progressive muscle relaxation. These techniques can help calm the mind and alleviate physical tension, fostering a sense of inner peace and tranquility. After every surgery, I listened to guided meditations and meditative music instead of watching television. It helped me recover more quickly.

- I started Transcendental Meditation when I was twenty-three. Unfortunately, my first husband banned me from the "evil practice" of meditation, so it took me until I was forty to trust the world enough to begin again. Fortunately, for the last twenty years, I have tried many types of meditation and find that all of them have served me well for a time. Peacefully observing without judgment is the most incredible gift meditation offers.

4. Positive Self-Talk- Dispute negative thoughts and beliefs related to your procedure by replacing them with positive affirmations and statements. Please remember your strengths, resilience, and ability to deal with obstacles effectively. Tony Robbins says, "Positive thinking without action is delusional." In other words, if you are trying to change a belief, you have to DO something to prove that new belief to yourself.

- For instance, if you believe you will be a professional baseball player when you grow up, you must stop playing video games long enough to practice baseball as a child. If you believe you are strong, healthy, and recover quickly, you must eat nutritious food, exercise, and quit smoking so you can honestly believe your body can recover quickly. So, keeping a positive mindset means you will do your best to mentally and physically prepare for an optimistic result.

5. Distraction Techniques- Engage in activities that distract your mind from worrying thoughts about surgery. Whether reading a book, listening to music, or spending time with loved ones, finding enjoyable distractions can temporarily relieve anxiety and promote a sense of normalcy. When I was young, I heard about Norman Cousins, who cured himself of cancer by laughing and receiving massive intravenous doses of vitamin C. He watched comedy after comedy, including "Candid Camera."

- I did laughter yoga with an intimate group several years ago and enjoyed it immensely. It helped me cope with a difficult time by distracting me from the severity of my living situation. Anything that makes you laugh, as long as it's not at someone else's expense, is good for your body because it releases feel-good endorphins and benefits healing.

6. Call Upon Your Faith Community- If you subscribe to a religious or faith group, ask them to pray, fast, or meditate for your healing and quick recovery. This spiritual support pulls the love of the Universe/God/Quantum Field down on your behalf because so many extend their love and well wishes to you. Love is powerful energy! I felt the force of the love and prayers of those exerting their efforts to petition the deity's favors for me, and it healed me more quickly. Love is the power that creates worlds!

Visualization and Relaxation Techniques

Visualization and relaxation techniques can be potent tools in preparing mentally for your operation. Esther Hicks, who channels Abraham, has made a whole career about the law of attraction by visualizing and focusing on what you want, not what you don't want. By harnessing the mind-body connection, these techniques help you feel more confident and peaceful so you can be more assured and poised in preparing for the big day. Here's how to incorporate visualization and relaxation into your preoperative preparation:

- **Guided Imagery-** Close your eyes and imagine yourself in a peaceful and serene setting, such as a beach, meadow or forest. Visualize every detail of the environment, including the sights, sounds, and sensations. Allow yourself to immerse fully in the experience, letting go of any tension or worries, says the hopkinsmedicine.org website. https://www.hopkinsmedicine.org/health/
- **Progressive Muscle Relaxation-** According to the psychologytoday.com website, Dr. Marilyn Mitchell gives Herbert Benson's "steps to elicit the Relaxation Response: Sit quietly in a comfortable position. (That might be lying on your side or back.) Close your eyes. Deeply relax all your muscles, beginning at your feet and progressing up to your face. Keep them relaxed. [Relax your tongue—and thoughts will cease.] Breathe through your nose. Become aware of your breathing.
    - As you breathe out, say the word "one"* silently to yourself. For example, breathe in and then out, and say "one"*, in and out, and repeat "one."* Breathe easily and naturally. Continue for 10 to 20 minutes. You may open your eyes to check the time but do not use an alarm. When you finish, sit quietly for several minutes, first with your eyes closed and later with your eyes opened. Do not stand up for a few minutes.
    - Do not worry about whether you successfully achieve a deep level of relaxation. Maintain a passive attitude and permit relaxation to occur at its own pace. When distracting thoughts occur, try to ignore them by not dwelling upon them

and return to repeating "one."* With practice, the response should come with little effort. Practice the technique once or twice daily, but not within two hours after any meal, since the digestive processes seem to interfere with the elicitation of the Relaxation Response." https://www.psychologytoday.com/us/blog/heart-and-soul-healing/201303/dr-herbert-benson-s-relaxation-response

- **Visualization of Successful Outcomes-** Visualize the surgical procedure going smoothly and successfully. Picture yourself recovering quickly and effortlessly, feeling strong, healthy, and vibrant. The key here is allowing the emotional charge to flow through you. Visualizing positive conclusions can instill confidence and optimism, reduce anxiety, and provide inner peace.
    - Tony Robbins offers a free fifteen-minute guided visualization tapping into your grateful, happy, successful emotions from the past and the future and stacking these positive feelings to prime yourself for success. You can use this priming before visualizing your happy outcome to make it more impactful. https://www.youtube.com/watch?v=faTGTgid8Uc
- **Deep Breathing Exercises-** According to the my.cleavelandclinic.org website, diaphragmatic breathing, also called abdominal breathing or belly breathing, can help you relax, increase blood oxygen, and reduce blood pressure and heart rate. https://my.clevelandclinic.org/health/articles/9445-diaphragmatic-breathing Practice deep breathing exercises to calm the nervous system and promote relaxation.
    - Breathe slowly and deeply through your nose, allowing your abdomen to expand fully, and then exhale gradually through your mouth. Focus on the rhythm of your breath, letting go of any tension or stress with each exhalation. Authorities recommend this deep abdominal breathing when labor begins for an expectant mother. I used it during labor for each of my

five children.

Using Music Therapy

Integrating soothing music into pre and post-operative care can profoundly benefit you in pain management and relaxation as you undergo your medical procedure. According to the harmonyandhealing.org website, "Music therapy is an evidence-based practice that involves using music interventions to address individual needs and improve well-being. The power of music in therapy lies in its ability to bypass verbal barriers and tap into our emotions directly. Music reaches deep within us, connecting with experiences and feelings that are sometimes difficult to express verbally."

1. The Healing Power of Music- Music has been used for centuries as a therapeutic tool for promoting relaxation, reducing stress, and alleviating pain. Research has shown that listening to music can profoundly impact the body and mind, influencing heart rate, blood pressure, and stress hormone levels. Again, according to the harmonyandhealing.org website, "Listening to calming or soothing music has been shown to lower cortisol levels, the hormone associated with stress. Additionally, engaging in musical activities such as playing an instrument or singing releases endorphins, the body's natural feel-good chemicals, which can improve mood and reduce stress." https://www.harmonyandhealing.org/how-music-can-reduce-stress/#:~:text=Absolutely!,a%2061%25%20reduction%20in%20anxiety

2. Creating a Healing Playlist- Curate soothing and uplifting music to support your recovery journey. Choose songs that resonate with your emotions, evoke positive memories, or align with your intentions for healing. Experiment with different genres, tempos, and musical styles to find what resonates with you. And sing along because nitric oxide increases by 15x when humming, according to the National Library of Medicine's pubmed.ncbi.nlm.

nih.gov website https://pubmed.ncbi.nlm.nih.gov/12119224/and the www.buteykobreathing.nz website https://www.buteykobreathing.nz/ Nitric oxide is antifungal, antiviral, and antibacterial, so humming helps you heal!

Remember that it's normal to experience a range of emotions before surgery. Mental preparation is just as necessary as physical preparation, if not more so, to ensure a positive surgical experience and successful recovery. Employ the fifth secret for you, effectively managing anxiety and fear, utilizing meditation, visualization and relaxation techniques, calling upon your faith community, and using therapeutic music for inner peace and confidence. These holistic practices will provide more emotional stability, inner peace, and better pain management throughout the medical process.

Conversation With Terry Continued

"Hey, baby," said Terry, "We are at the doctor's office, and you will want to start stretching your ankle and foot to walk inside the building." "Thanks, Terry," I replied. "Thank you for letting me do my meditations while you drove. I know dealing with all the Phoenix traffic is demanding, and I appreciate your sacrifice. It makes me very anxious when I drive! By the way, I wonder if the doctor will schedule my surgery today." "Yeah," said Terry, "I don't enjoy the traffic much, but I do enjoy long drives in the country. Besides, I am glad you are arriving refreshed and calm. You are very welcome!"

Chapter 6

Activating Your Energy Centers for Healing

Transcendental Meditation

"So, Jim," I commented, "When did you start doing Transcendental Meditation?" "Well," replied Jim, "I began practicing Transcendental Meditation in 1976, about forty-five years ago. Yeah, I actually attended the Maharishi University in Fairfield, Iowa, and got a great education in business. They have a fantastic organic, vegetarian food program and grow all the food there. I also taught TM for about twenty years in Washington State in the Seattle area."

Other Meditation Practices

"Wow," I responded, "You practiced it much longer than I did. I only did it for two years before my first husband banned me from the practice and kind of scared me away from meditation for a decade because he had a bad experience once. It made me doubt myself and my decision to begin meditation. I think he has some undiagnosed mental or personality disorder, so I shouldn't have let him dissuade me. However, for the last twenty years, I have practiced many meditation types, and it has helped me quiet the 'monkey mind' so my energy can be more emotionally calm and present. My son, Josh, taught me Vipassana about five years ago, which was also really good."

Intentionally Directing Your Body's Energy Wheels to Accelerate Your Recovery

"Energy can not be created nor destroyed," according to the first law of thermodynamics. So, how can you work with your body's inherent energy to accelerate your recovery? You may not be able to create or destroy it, but you can certainly strengthen the energy by understanding how it works and directing it intentionally. "Chakra (cakra in Sanskrit) means 'wheel' and refers to energy points in your body. They are thought to be spinning disks of energy that should stay 'open' and aligned, as they correspond to bundles of nerves, major organs, and areas of our energetic body that affect our emotional and physical well-being." https://www.healthline.com/health/fitness-exercise/7-chakras#Chakra-101

The sixth secret for you is that you can intentionally activate your chakras through elemental nature, meditations, affirmations, and solfeggio frequency chakra music for pain relief, healing, and renewal. By activating your chakras, the energy centers of your body, you can regenerate your body before and after surgery. These subtle energy centers pulsate with life force energy, governing your experiences, emotions, and consciousness. They are not abstract concepts but tangible sources of consciousness and vitality, influencing your physical, emotional, and spiritual well-being.

Chakras Regulate the Energetic Flow

From Vedic ancient Indian philosophy and spiritual traditions, chakras are the energy centers positioned along the spine, each associated with specific qualities, emotions, and aspects of human consciousness. There are seven primary chakras, each corresponding to different body parts and aspects of life. Chakras create coherent contentment by regulating the energy flow throughout the body. When your chakras are balanced and aligned, you feel inner harmony, vitality, and overall health. However, imbalances or blockages in the chakras can manifest as physical ailments, emotional turmoil or spiritual disconnection. Meditation, yoga, and Reiki will help realign all the chakras, but before surgery, you may not feel able to do the more physical aspects of these disciplines.

Chakras and Surgery Prep

Instead, while preparing for surgery, you can focus on balancing all the chakras or those specifically related to your procedure with elemental connection and meditation. For example, if you are having a heart operation, specifically do the balancing exercises and music related to the heart chakra. Wear green or eat green food, connect with the air element (breathing exercises), meditate on the heart with a green ball of light, and repeat the love affirmations.

Pain or Discomfort After Surgery

Another example is if you're experiencing physical pain or discomfort after surgery, focus on meditations that target the root chakra for grounding and stability or the sacral chakra for emotional healing and release. Below, I list the seven chakras, their locations, colors, elements, sounds, body parts, and awareness words. I show how you will feel when this chakra is unbalanced or balanced and what you can do or say to bring your chakra back into balance, according to yourblissfulself.com website, under the chakra cheat sheet pdf:

1. Root Chakra- located at the base of the spine- is associated with red, the earth element, the seed sound Lam, the adrenal glands, and "I am." When unbalanced, you feel insecure, anxious, depressed, and fearful. When balanced, you feel safe, secure, grounded, and centered. Spend time in nature before your operation, even walking barefoot on grass or sand, feeling gratitude for the sun on your face or the wind in your hair, and smelling the earth's fragrances. Then massage your feet when you finish.

    - Consider using a grounding sheet or earthing pad on your bare skin for relaxation, sleep, and pain relief. These are readily available through a Google search. For five minutes, sit with your spine straight, do a minute or two of deep diaphragmatic breathing, breathing in by the count of four through your nose as your abdomen expands, and breathe out your mouth by the count of six as your abdomen sinks in. Then close your eyes and imagine a red energy ball at the base of the spine as you repeat: I am centered and grounded; I am safe in my body; the Universe protects me; I trust more and fear less; I love my body.

2. Sacral Chakra- located below the navel- is associated with orange, the water element, the seed sound Vam, the gonads, and "I feel." When unbalanced, you feel guilty, overly sensitive, and lack creativity. When balanced, you feel creative, passionate, and energetic. Drink water before and after surgery and notice how refreshing it is. Days before your procedure, enjoy a luxurious bath or shower with your favorite soaps and lotions or swim. Of course, use the surgical soap (antibacterial) the medical staff gives you for the night before and on the day of your procedure.
   - Do something that feels fun and creative! Close your eyes. Slowly take ten deep breaths, focus on your breath, and relax. Imagine gentle ocean waves in your sacral area. Now, picture a ball of shining orange light immersed in the water, allowing it to sway softly as the waves become orange, covering you with incredible tranquility and warmth. Repeat: My creativity flows effortlessly; I am an empowered sexual being; I am free to express my emotions healthily; I am passionate about my life; It is my birthright to receive pleasure.
3. Solar Plexus- located in the upper abdomen above the navel- is associated with yellow, the fire element, the seed sound Ram, the pancreas, and "I do." When unbalanced, you feel doubtful and insecure and seek continuous approval. When balanced, you feel empowered, confident, and courageous. Spend time outdoors in the sun and increase your Vitamin D levels. Walk, relax in the sun (ensure your UV filters are on if you use them), and admire the sunset.
   - Break boring, predictable patterns and do something differ-

ent. If you are talkative, stay silent; If inactive, get moving; Challenge yourself. Overcoming challenges will help to increase your confidence and motivation. You can light and meditate on a candle until you picture the yellow fireball in your solar plexus. As the ball expands and gets warmer, notice how it dissolves all energy blockages within you.

- Feel the power of fire inside your body. Now close your eyes and visualize yourself achieving your goals, like healing from a successful surgery and enjoying the activity made possible by the operation. Repeat: I radiate confidence and can achieve anything I set my mind to; I have everything I need to succeed; I am enough! I love and accept myself. Smile with gratitude.

4. Heart Chakra- located in the center of your chest- is associated with the color green, the air element, the seed sound Yam, the thymus, and "I love." When unbalanced, you feel jealous, bitter, lonely, and needy. When balanced, you feel loving, kind, and compassionate. Feel thankful for your shower, your food, the sun, your body and all of the experiences of your life. Do something you love, sing, dance and feel joy.

    - Do deep breathing exercises like three long deep breaths, three short breaths, six long breaths, six short breaths, nine long breaths, nine short breaths and on the last ninth short breath, hold it for as long as you can. Then, repeat the process two more times. Meditate on your heart area, visualizing a green ball of love expanding to your family, friends, those you don't know and even your enemies. Repeat: I am love; I am worthy of love; I choose kindness and compassion over judgment; I forgive myself; I am grateful for loving people around me; I love all people.

5. Throat Chakra- located in your throat area- is associated with the color light blue, ether space, the seed sound Ham, the thyroid, and "I speak." When unbalanced, you feel shy, dishonest, critical,

and unauthentic. When balanced, you feel truthful, outspoken, authentic, and assertive. Do neck stretches and massage your neck. Sing, hum, make noise, journal, and speak your truth.

- Meditate, focusing on your breath with your eyes closed. When thoughts or distractions arise, simply observe them and let them pass. Let your muscles relax, and imagine a ball of sparkling blue light in the center of your throat expancing with honesty, peace and relaxation. Focus on feeling blissful and give thanks for your throat chakra opening as you smile. Repeat: My words are powerful; I speak my inner truth; I express myself clearly and effortlessly; When I talk, others listen; I value others' words.

6. Third-Eye Chakra- located in the center of your forehead- is associated with the color indigo, the light element, the seed sound OM, the pineal gland, and "I see." When unbalanced, you feel fearful, uncertain, indecisive, and have memory problems. When balanced, you feel intuitive, open to change, and imaginative. Meditation is a handy way to balance and open any of your chakras.

   - Visualize a ball of indigo light between your eyes, and focus your attention on your third eye center in your forehead. As you breathe deeply, imagine the ball of light getting bigger and brighter, cleansing any negativity from your mind. Repeat: I trust and follow my intuition; I see the more profound truth and surrender to the divine; I have a brilliant mind; I am open to inspiration; I feel bliss in everything I do.

7. The Crown Chakra- located on the top of your head where you would wear a crown- is associated with the color violet, the thought element, the seed sound Ah, the pituitary gland, and "I know." When unbalanced, you feel lost or without purpose. When balanced, you trust the Divine and feel the Oneness.

- Meditate on a violet, bright light illuminating the top of your head that helps you feel connected with pure consciousness. Feel thankful to be your true self on your path to enlightenment and the bliss of meeting the divine within. Repeat: I am a unique point of awareness connected to the Universe; I release doubt and have faith that the Divine will guide me; I am more than my body; I live in the present moment. https://yourblissfulself.com/chakra-cheat-sheet-pdfs-free-printables/

Conversation With Jim Continued

"Linda," Jim asked, "Why did you try other forms of meditation when you knew how to do TM? Why didn't you go back to it?" "Well," I replied, "When I tried TM again after fifteen years, it wasn't the same, so I felt like I must be doing it incorrectly. That's why I went for a refresher one-on-one with a teacher in Phoenix.

Binaural Beat Meditations

After that, I purchased a Holosync program from the Centerpointe Research Institute, founded by Bill Harris. It uses binaural beats to quickly get your brainwave patterns into the Alpha state. I did that for about nine years. There are many binaural beat meditations on the Internet now. However, when I meditate now, I focus on my third eye, breathe deep abdominal breaths and exhale slowly while trying to tune in to the frequencies of the Higher-Level beings I encountered when I had my near-death experience.

Chakra Activation

Often, I envision activating each chakra to different vibrations by mentally communicating with each one. I put my awareness on them, imagine the color and spin, and request they come to "coherence, harmony, and balance," opening to understanding and wisdom for the crown, intuition and inspiration for the third eye, speaking my truth for the throat, love, forgiveness, and appreciation for the heart, claiming my personal power for the solar plexus, healing the sacred, sexual and creative energies of the sacral, and connecting to Mother Earth for the root. Then I ask that all incoherent frequencies and negative energies regarding whatever comes into my mind be released and leave me. I finish by remembering joyful past and future times with loved ones, feeling their happiness, and sending gratitude to the Creator for it all."

Chapter 7

Preparing Your Home and What to Take to the Hospital

No Phone Charger

"Hello, nurse Jessica," I said as I squinted to read her name tag. "I hate to ask this, but I didn't get to prepare anything to bring with me since I was brought in by ambulance, and I can't even contact my children to pick me up with a dead phone battery. Do you happen to have a charger that could charge my old phone? It's a Samsung Galaxy s7." "Yeah," Jessica said, "I think we have some chargers at the nurse's station. I will check and see if any of them fit your phone. Also, we have a comb, toothbrush, toothpaste, soap, shampoo, lip balm, and lotion whenever you feel ready to shower." "Oh, that's wonderful!" I exclaimed, "Thank you!"

Prepare Your Home and What to Take to the Hospital

Now that you have focused on nutrition, exercise, and sleep and have managed your fear and anxiety using meditation, visualization, chakra restoration, and music to bolster your body and mind, it's time to prepare your home environment and gather the things you will need to take to the hospital, depending on whether it is an outpatient surgery, a twenty-four-hour stay, or several days to a week in a hospital room.

The seventh secret for you is to take proactive steps to prepare your home for post-surgery recovery, prioritize safety and accessibility, and decide what to take to the hospital for your comfort while minimizing clutter so you can reduce stress, enhance comfort, and promote a faster, uneventful healing process. Preparing your home for post-surgery recovery is vital to ensure a safe, comfortable, and supportive environment for healing. Here are nine steps to help you organize your home for a smooth recovery after surgery:

1. Create a Recovery Space- Designate a comfortable and accessible area in your home where you can rest and recuperate after surgery. Choose a bedroom or living area on the main level of your home to minimize stairs and reduce your risk of falls. Arrange essential items within arm's reach, including pillows, blankets, medications, water, and entertainment options.
    - Depending on your surgery, you may need a medical reacher/grabber if you can't strain your abdominal muscles or arms to reach for supplies. Practice rolling over or getting out of bed differently without straining the proposed surgical site so you know what movements you need to modify. You may also need a lift chair, commode, or overnight pads. Keep hand sanitizer readily available, and remember to have chargers and headphones nearby so your phone will be ready for guided meditation or relaxing music.
2. Clear Pathways- Remove clutter, obstacles, and tripping hazards from your hallways, doorways, and pathways to create a safe and accessible environment for mobility aids, such as crutches, canes, walkers, or wheelchairs. Ensure your pathways are well-lit and free of rugs or loose carpeting that could cause you to misstep or fall. When my mom was caring for me after my twenty-two surgeries in two months, she often humorously said, "Rule number one is don't fall. Rule number two refers back to rule number one: don't fall." Then we'd giggle.
3. Modify Furniture Layout- Rearrange your furniture to accommodate your post-surgery needs and maximize comfort and acces-

sibility. Consider placing a bedside table or tray within easy reach to hold essential items such as medications, tissues, and snacks. Use chairs with sturdy armrests and firm cushions to facilitate sitting and standing with minimal strain.

- You must remember that you don't want to pull open stitches or staples, so the body part that will undergo the proposed surgical procedure can't be stressed or pressured at all. If you have hip, foot, or leg surgery or won't make the distance to your toilet, you must place a bedside commode near your bed. Even though it is hard to let others take care of this job for you, it is better than the alternative. I have used bedpans, bedside commodes, walkers, crutches, canes, wheelchairs, and reachers to grab things. I was always grateful I had them when I needed them.

4. Install Safety Equipment- If necessary, install grab bars, handrails, or other safety equipment in critical areas of your home, such as bathrooms, showers, and stairways, to provide stability and support during mobility. Use non-slip mats or adhesive strips in the bathtub and shower to prevent slips and spills. In addition, if you have a cast or wound site that can't get wet, you may need garbage bags and duct tape to cover the wound or cast. Also, shower chairs or some other accommodation may help.

   - Your doctor may prescribe bed baths at first to prevent incision sites from getting wet. Keeping the wound dry until the skin closes is vital to avoid infection. I didn't get a shower for three months after my second accident and the twenty-two surgeries necessary to put me back together during my two months in the hospital. Of course, I was in a coma for the first eleven days, so I wasn't aware I needed a bath.

5. Arrange Assistance- Please be sure to enlist the help of family members, friends, or professional caregivers to help with your household chores, meal preparation, pet care, and transporta-

tion during your recovery period. Communicate your needs and preferences with your support network to guarantee a coordinated and effective caregiving plan. If you don't have family, friends, or neighbors, many insurance providers can direct you to home health services available through their network. Call the number on the back of your insurance card for information.

6. Stock Up on Supplies- Stock up on essential supplies and groceries before surgery to minimize the need for trips to the store during your recovery. Purchase non-perishable foods, toiletries, medications, wound care supplies (band-aids, gauze, medical tape, nonstick stérile bandages and roller gauze in assorted sizes), and other household necessities to be sure you have everything you need on hand.

7. Plan for Medication Management- Organize medications in advance and establish a system for managing your medication regimen during recovery. Use pill organizers, medication schedules, or smartphone apps to track doses, refill prescriptions, and ensure timely administration of medications as prescribed by your healthcare provider. I set alarms on my smartphone to alert me when my next medication was due.

8. Create a Restful Environment- Create a calm and restful environment in your home to promote relaxation and healing. Use soft lighting, soothing colors, and comfortable bedding to create a peaceful atmosphere conducive to restorative sleep and recovery. Have sheets, washcloths, and towels easily accessible for caregivers attending to your post-surgical needs. Your doctors may prescribe disposable bed bath wipes or chucks that caregivers can easily change to prevent infection. Remember that the part of your body that has been cut open needs a clean environment and a vacation to rest and heal.

9. Stay Connected- Stay connected with loved ones, friends, and healthcare providers during your recovery period to maintain

emotional support and receive assistance as needed. Keep significant phone numbers like your doctor's, hospital's, or home health nurse's contact information and family emergency contacts readily accessible in case of unexpected complications or emergencies.

- Prioritize safety, accessibility, and support to create an environment that facilitates optimal recovery and well-being. Don't hesitate to contact healthcare professionals, family members, or community resources for assistance and guidance as you handle the challenges of post-surgery recovery at home.

What to Take to the Hospital and What to Leave at Home

Now that your home is ready, you need to figure out what to take to the hospital and what to leave home. What you need to bring depends on how long the doctor projects you will stay in the medical facility after the procedure. You must carefully consider what basic necessities and conveniences to carry to ensure your comfort while minimizing clutter and unnecessary items.

What to Take

- **Personal Identification and Insurance Information—** Bring your driver's license or other form of identification, your insurance card and any relevant medical documents or paperwork.
- **Comfortable Clothing—** Pack loose-fitting, comfortable clothing, such as pajamas, sweatpants, and T-shirts, to wear during your hospital stay. Choose items that are easy to put on and take off and appropriate for the weather.
- **Footwear**— Wear non-slip, closed-toe shoes or slippers with rubber soles when walking around the hospital. Avoid wearing socks with slippery surfaces to reduce the risk of falls.

- **Toiletries—** Pack travel-sized toiletries if you want to choose the brand, including toothpaste, toothbrush, shampoo, conditioner, soap or body wash, and deodorant. Remember items like a hairbrush or comb, lip balm, and moisturizer to keep yourself feeling fresh and comfortable.

- **Medications—** Please bring any prescription medications you're currently taking, along with a list of their names, dosages, and instructions. You must include regular and specific medications your healthcare provider has instructed you to take during your hospital stay.

- **Personal Electronics—** Consider bringing a smartphone, tablet, or laptop to stay connected with loved ones, access entertainment, or work remotely if necessary. Please bring chargers for your electronic devices and take them home when you leave the hospital. I forgot and left chargers still in the electrical sockets at the hospitals where I stayed on several occasions.

- **Comfort Items—** Bring comfort items from home, such as a favorite pillow, blanket, or stuffed animal, to provide familiarity and emotional support during your hospital stay. In addition, books, magazines, or hobby supplies like knitting can also help pass the time.

- **Snacks—** Pack some non-perishable snacks, such as granola bars, crackers, or nuts, to have on hand in case you get hungry between meals. Of course, check with your healthcare provider or the hospital staff to certify that outside food is allowed after your surgery.

What to Leave at Home

1. Valuables- Avoid bringing valuable items to the hospital, such as jewelry, expensive electronics, or large sums of cash. While most hospitals have safeguards for securing personal belongings, leaving valuables at home is best to minimize the risk of loss

or theft. I had one hospital lose the clothing and shoes I came in with. They searched for hours but to no avail, so I went home in the hospital gown and non-slip socks they provided.

2. Large Bags or Luggage- Limit the amount of luggage or bags you bring to the hospital, as space may be limited in your hospital room. Opt for a small, lightweight bag or suitcase that can easily fit in your hospital room and be stored out of the way. There are usually some cupboards, but the space varies depending on the medical facility. Regardless, there's not enough space for your clothing closet.

3. Strong Fragrances- Avoid bringing items with strong fragrances, such as perfumes, colognes, or scented lotions, as these can be bothersome to other patients and healthcare staff, especially those with sensitivities or allergies. I can't stress this enough. Nausea, difficulty breathing, or swelling can happen to you or someone nearby if the aroma irritates air passages. Even if you have never had previous problems, combining general anesthesia or pain medications with scented personal care products can cause temporary reactions, so leave the hair spray and perfume at home.

4. Excessive Clothing or Accessories- While hospitals recommend comfortable clothing and footwear, avoid overpacking or bringing unnecessary items that will only clutter your hospital room. Stick to primary clothing items and accessories to help you feel cozy during your stay.

5. Alcohol or Recreational Drugs- Refrain from bringing alcohol, recreational drugs, or any other substances prohibited by the hospital's policies. These items can interfere with your treatment and recovery process and may not be allowed on hospital premises.

The seventh secret for you is to take proactive steps to prepare your home for post-surgery recovery, prioritize safety and accessibility, and decide what to take to the hospital for your comfort while minimizing clutter so you can reduce stress, enhance comfort, and promote a faster, uneventful healing process. Preparing your home for post-surgery recovery is necessary to ensure a safe, comfortable, and supportive environment for healing. Also, by carefully selecting what to take to the hospital and what to leave at home, you can ensure an uneventful and satisfying experience during your hospital stay while lessening stress and clutter. Be sure to check with your healthcare provider or the hospital staff for any specific guidelines or recommendations regarding anything else to bring with you.

Conversation With Nurse Jessica Continued

"You are in luck. We had a charger plug that fits your phone. If you had an iPhone, we couldn't have helped you. We have chargers that other patients have left behind, and there is no budget to buy more of them, so people need to bring chargers with them," said nurse Ashley, since the shift change had already happened and I had a new nurse. "Well, I do feel lucky," I replied, "I couldn't even call my kids to come pick me up when the doctor discharges me tomorrow because I don't know their numbers without looking them up on the phone."

Chapter 8
The Big Day of Surgery

Surgery Forty-Seven

"Honey," Terry announced in his deeper voice, "I can stay here if you need me. The doctor said the surgery would take about one hour, and then you would be in recovery for another hour to two hours before I pick you up for the two-hour drive home." "No, babe," I responded, "You go enjoy your hot wings with Murray and JT. You don't see them as often now that we have moved up north, and I would feel better knowing you are enjoying your friends. Besides, I have done this many times before, forty-six, in fact, and I don't want you just sitting around waiting while I have another surgery. This one isn't a biggie, or else they wouldn't be doing it outpatient. We did bring my pillows for the ride home, though, didn't we?" "Yeah, they are in the car," Terry finished, "I'll be back soon."

The Big Day

The eighth secret for you is that even though you may be anxious on the big day of surgery, you can have greater confidence and resilience by effectively interacting with hospital staff, knowing what to expect, and employing coping strategies for managing pre-surgery nerves. The actual day of your operation is a significant milestone in your healthcare journey, marking the culmination of careful preparation and anticipation. While feeling anxiety, fear, or apprehension about the upcoming procedure is natural, understanding what to expect and handling interactions with hospital staff can help ease your concerns and give you a calm, steady experience.

Hospital Nurse Call

About four or five days before the surgery, I usually had a telephone call from a nurse at the hospital or medical facility where the scheduled procedure would occur. They had already taken my vitals (blood pressure, heart rate, oxygen saturation, respiratory rate, the number of breaths I take in one minute) and done blood tests to see if my liver and kidneys could metabolize and expel the general anesthesia.

Antibacterial Soap

They instructed me on what antibacterial soap to use or the surgical soap the medical staff gave me at the doctor's office for the night before and on the day of the operation. The nurses always told me not to use deodorant, lotion, cream, perfume, or anything else on my skin to prevent infection. In addition, they directed me to be NPO (nothing by mouth) after midnight the night before, not even gum or water. When you get the call, it will be your first contact with the hospital staff. Make sure you ask any questions now.

What to Expect on the Day of Surgery

1. Arrival and Check-In- Upon arrival at the hospital or surgical center, you'll be greeted by the admissions staff and guided through the check-in process. This process may involve providing personal information, signing consent forms, and completing necessary paperwork. I remember the first time I signed the paperwork. I was only sixteen, and the legal jargon sounded like they took no responsibility for what might happen, even my death; however, by the time the fifty-second surgery rolled around, I wasn't afraid to sign on the line anymore.

2. Preoperative Preparation- An aide or hospital volunteer will escort you to a preoperative area, where nurses and medical staff will prepare you for surgery. Preparation will include changing into a hospital gown (it always amazes me that they have the same fashion designer- hee hee), monitoring your vital signs, and receiving any preoperative medications or interventions as

directed by your healthcare provider.

   - At some point, the nurse will insert the IV cannula, most commonly in your hand, arm, or foot, for the Intravenous medications. When I was young, it was never a problem. As I matured, I had "rolling veins" or "blood vessel valve" issues. If you suspect you have these issues, be sure to tell them so they will get the most experienced staff person or use a machine to place the IV. I have had to be stuck five or six times (that makes a lot of arm or hand bruises) when I was dehydrated because I couldn't have water after midnight.

3. Consultation with Anesthesiologist- Before surgery, you'll meet with the anesthesiologist responsible for administering anesthesia and monitoring your vital signs throughout the procedure. They will review your medical history, discuss anesthesia options, and address any questions or concerns you may have. Usually, it was the only time I ever saw the anesthesiologist because they do not handle any postoperative steps with you. Even though it was brief, I have always had a pleasant experience with the anesthesiologists.

4. Surgical Team Briefing- The surgical team, including your surgeon, nurses, and other healthcare professionals, will conduct a preoperative briefing to review the surgical plan, confirm patient information, and secure all necessary equipment and supplies for your procedure. It might seem repetitive because every person looks at your ID bracelet and verbally asks you your name, if this is the correct birthdate on your bracelet, and what procedure you are there for; however, I feel comforted knowing this is how they prevent mistakes. You don't want the doctor taking out the wrong organ or operating on the healthy leg.

5. Transfer to Operating Room- When it's time for surgery, you'll be transferred to the operating room in the pre-op hospital bed, on a stretcher or in a wheelchair. Hospital staff will accompany

you and provide support as needed to ensure your comfort and safety. For some of my earlier surgeries, they took me in a wheelchair to the Operating Room and asked me to hop up onto the operating table there.

- I think that has changed, though, because, in recent procedures, they usually took me to the OR in the hospital bed from Pre-Op and sometimes transferred me there onto the operating table or moved me into a position more convenient for the surgery. They usually knocked me out before they moved me, but I remember, on one occasion, telling jokes and being in the middle of a laugh when I succumbed to the general anesthesia.

Interacting with Hospital Staff and Understanding Your Role

- **Communication-** Open and honest communication with hospital staff ensures a positive surgical experience. Please feel free to ask questions, express concerns, or request clarification about any aspect of your care. I only remember positive experiences with the pre-op staff.

- **Active Participation-** Take an active role in your healthcare by advocating for your needs and preferences. Please inform the surgical team about any allergies, medications, or medical conditions and participate in talks about the surgical plan and postoperative care. Yes, make sure each attending nurse and doctor notes drug allergies. Reminding them keeps it fresh in their minds.

- **Follow Instructions-** Follow preoperative instructions provided by your healthcare provider, such as fasting guidelines or medication protocols, to minimize the risk of complications and ensure the procedure's success. I already stressed the importance of fasting the night before the procedure.

- **Trust the Team-** Trust in the expertise and experience of the surgical team, including your surgeon, anesthesiologist, and nursing staff. They are dedicated to providing safe, high-quality care and will work collaboratively to ensure the best possible outcomes for you.

Coping Skills for Pre-Surgery Nerves

1. Deep Breathing Exercises— Practice deep breathing exercises to promote relaxation and reduce anxiety before surgery. Take a slow, deep, abdominal breath through your nose, hold for a few seconds, and exhale slowly through your mouth. I often breathe in for the count of four, hold for the count of four, and exhale for the count of four because that's all I can remember when I get too nervous. Repeat this process several times to calm your nerves.

2. Visualization Techniques— Close your eyes and visualize a peaceful, serene scene, such as a tranquil beach or lush forest, to distract your mind from pre-surgery worries. Focus on this imagined environment's sights, sounds, smells, and sensations to promote relaxation and reduce stress. Doing this has helped me, too.

    - I have a meadow with many flowers in the forest, a stream that runs through it, and two mountains behind. I feel the warm sunshine and a cool breeze as deer, rabbits, squirrels, and other cute forest creatures drink from the stream. You may select a beach with surfers, sand and sunshine. It's wherever you feel safe.

3. Positive Affirmations— Repeat positive affirmations or mantras to bolster your confidence and alleviate pre-surgery nerves. Affirmations such as "I trust in my medical team's expertise," "I am calm, confident, and prepared for surgery," or "All is well, my higher power directs the doctor's hands, and I heal quickly" can help shift your mindset from fear to empowerment.

4. Seek Support— Lean on friends, family members, or a trusted support person for emotional support and encouragement on the day of surgery. A supportive presence by your side can provide comfort and reassurance during this challenging time. My mom was there when I was young, and Terry was there until he passed, and then my children, but I have had many surgeries alone, with my children coming to pick me up afterward.

    - It is ideal to have friends, family, or a prayer group. But even alone, you can do it! Someone must take you home and care for you post-op for twenty-four hours, so you may need to get aides through your insurance provider. The hospital won't release you by yourself. I tried it, but it didn't work. I had to call a friend to pick me up and say they would be there to watch me for twenty-four hours.

5. Engage in Distractions— Engage in activities that distract your mind from pre-surgery worries, such as reading a book, listening to music, or practicing a hobby you enjoy. You may still be on your electronic devices until the medical staff removes them with your clothes. There are usually many people in and out before the surgery; however, I often meditate when I am alone. Keeping your mind occupied can help alleviate anxiety and promote a sense of normalcy.

The eighth secret for you is that even though you may be anxious on the big day of surgery, you can have greater confidence and resilience by effectively interacting with hospital staff, knowing what to expect, and employing coping strategies for managing pre-surgery nerves. Remember that you actively participate in your healthcare journey, and your voice matters. Trust in the expertise of your surgical team, lean on your support network for encouragement, and focus on staying calm, positive, and prepared for the road ahead. You can do it!

Pre-surgical Conversation Continued

"My name is Jennifer, and I am the nurse who will be prepping you for surgery. Denise over there will be helping me too because we have a full house this morning," reported the lovely blond nurse. Denise piped in, "We have to get your IV placed now. I will use this elastic band to pump up your veins to find a juicy one," she said as she firmly tapped the vein on the inside of my elbow. "Here's one. It's going to pinch a little. Are you an easy stick, or do you have rolling veins?" asked Denise as she shoved the IV cannula into a vein on the inside of my elbow and chased it about as it rolled away.

Rolling Veins and Blood Vessel Valve Issues

"Well," I replied, "When I am dehydrated, my veins roll, and I have been NPO since last night at eight pm. I used to be an easy stick, but the older I get, the more difficult it seems to be," I replied. "Sometimes there have even been issues with blood vessel valves that won't allow the needle to advance." "Yeah, I see what you mean," said Denise as hospital staff bustled about her. I will try the other arm, and if it doesn't work this time, I will get Jennifer." "Cool," I replied.

Chapter 9
The First Twenty-Four Hours and Possible Complications

Breathe, Linda

"Linda, can you hear me?" asked the recovery nurse, "You have got to take another breath, sweetie. She stops breathing sometimes, so you must watch her and remind her to keep breathing," I heard her say to someone nearby. "Should we get the doctor?" they said. "No, I think she is just having a little trouble wanting to come back," stated the nurse. "She responds to me when I prompt her to breathe again. Just keep reminding her to breathe, and she should be fine. Her vitals are fine, the incision site looks good, and she isn't vomiting, so we just have to wait for the anesthesia to wear off and keep prodding her to breathe."

The first 24 hours after surgery are a critical period of recovery, marked by a combination of physical discomfort, emotional adjustment, and ongoing medical care. The ninth secret is understanding what to expect immediately post-op, managing pain effectively, dealing with common post-surgical complications and how to handle setbacks, and remembering that productive communication with healthcare professionals about your care is crucial to a smooth, successful recovery.

Immediate Post-Op Recovery

In the post-op recovery room, you will experience three things:

1. Monitoring— In the recovery room, you'll be connected to monitoring equipment to track your heart rate, blood pressure, oxygen saturation, and other vital signs. This continuous monitoring allows healthcare providers to identify and address potential complications early in recovery.

2. Waking Up— As the effects of anesthesia wear off, you'll gradually regain consciousness and become more alert. You may experience grogginess, confusion, or nausea during this normalizing transition period, which typically resolves with time. It's weird to be blacked out for an hour or many hours and not remember, but soon you'll return to your old self.

3. Assessing Pain and Comfort— Healthcare providers will frequently assess your pain levels and comfort in the recovery room, using a pain scale to determine the intensity of your discomfort. Please communicate openly and honestly about your pain experience, as this information guides pain management strategies and ensures your comfort during the recovery process.

Pain Management and Monitoring

- **Medications-** Pain management after surgery often involves a combination of medications, including opioids, nonsteroidal anti-inflammatory drugs (NSAIDs), and local anesthetics. Doctors may dictate administering these medications orally, intravenously, or via other routes to relieve pain and minimize side effects. I recommend using whatever pain management the doctor prescribes at first, but wean off as quickly as possible, not just to avoid addiction but to avoid opioid constipation.
    - The constipation became more painful for me than some of the recovering body parts, so I quit taking them as soon as possible. Unfortunately, after my second major accident, an eleven-day coma, and twenty-two surgeries in two months, I tried to cold-turkey off my pain meds a month after getting

home, and my blood pressure skyrocketed to 183/132. My home health nurse explained that I was liable to have a stroke or heart attack because my body was still registering pain, causing high blood pressure, even though I was trying to "tough it out."

- She said, "Slowly weaning off any medication is best." I took her advice after that scare and resumed retaking the regular dose until my blood pressure normalized, but then smaller doses over time, so it took three weeks. I did not take any more opioids until the subsequent surgery. However, I continued taking NSAIDS for a decade after that.

- **Patient-Controlled Analgesia (PCA)-** In some cases, you may be given a PCA pump, which allows you to self-administer prescribed doses of pain medication by pressing a button. PCA pumps empower patients to manage their pain more effectively and can improve overall comfort during the recovery period. I had this after my first auto accident when the crash posteriorly dislocated my legs at the knees. The system won't let you overdose because it stops dispensing after you have reached the maximum dosage in a period, so you don't have to worry about that.
- **Alternative Therapies-** Besides medication, alternative pain management therapies such as ice packs, heat therapy, elevation, compression therapy, relaxation techniques, and guided imagery may complement conventional approaches and promote comfort and relaxation. Remember that elevating your affected limb can reduce inflammation and pain, so prepare your pillows and ice packs.
  - Compression therapy is typical in hospitals, but Thrombo-Embolic Deterrant stockings (TED hose) at home use the same idea- to keep the blood flowing in the legs where it might pool and form a clot. The nurses and aides had ice packs on me 24/7 after the first accident. It helped substantially, but having

such cold legs and trying to keep my core warm was a strange sensation.

- After every surgery as an adult, I always used some form of meditation as soon as I got out of the recovery room, either going home or going to a hospital room. Often, music mentioned in Chapter 6 on Activating Your Energy Centers helps quicken recovery, like the chakra restoration and cleansing music on YouTube, using all nine Solfeggio frequencies for restoring and cleansing all the chakras because it helps you relax and rest. Check out https://www.youtube.com/watch?v=NHUS_5vhi90 or this Solfeggio instrumental on YouTube for the deepest healing and pain-relieving sound bath. https://www.youtube.com/watch?v=MK9PMr71ty4

- **Monitoring for Complications-** While pain management is a large part of post-operative care, you must check for potential post-surgery complications that can arise for you during recovery. You can become aware of the common complications and learn how to handle them. Knowing when to seek medical attention (sometimes it's okay to bug your nurse or doctor) and dealing with the emotional and psychological facets of recovery setbacks are indispensable for a successful recovery.

Common Post-Surgery Complications and How to Handle Them

1. Infection— Surgical site infections can occur after surgery and may present with symptoms such as redness, swelling, warmth, pain, or drainage from the incision site. Especially in the first few days, look at your surgical incision and notice how it appears. If it might be infected, keep the wound clean and dry, follow any prescribed wound care instructions, and contact your healthcare provider for evaluation and possible antibiotic treatment.

2. Blood Clots— Blood clots, such as deep vein thrombosis (DVT) or pulmonary embolism (PE), can develop after surgery, particu-

larly in the legs or lungs. Symptoms may include swelling, pain, warmth, redness in the affected limb, chest pain, shortness of breath, or coughing up blood. If you suspect you have a blood clot, seek immediate medical attention, as it can be life-threatening.

3. Bleeding— Excessive bleeding or hemorrhage can occur after surgery, both internally or from your surgical site. Apply direct pressure to your wound if bleeding is external, elevate your affected limb if possible, and seek emergency medical care if bleeding is severe or persistent.

4. Adverse Reactions to Anesthesia— Some individuals may experience adverse reactions or side effects to anesthesia, such as nausea, vomiting, confusion, or allergic reactions. If you encounter any concerning symptoms after your surgery, please let your healthcare provider know immediately for evaluation and management.

5. Respiratory Complications— Respiratory complications, such as pneumonia or atelectasis (partial lung collapse), can occur after surgery, particularly if you have underlying lung conditions or undergo procedures involving general anesthesia. Practice deep breathing exercises, use incentive spirometry as directed, and seek medical attention if you experience difficulty breathing or chest pain.

    - An incentive spirometer is used for ribcage injuries, bed rest (you can't get out of bed yet), asthma, pneumonia, chronic obstructive pulmonary disease (COPD), cystic fibrosis, sickle cell anemia, and atelectasis, according to the myclevelandclinic.org website. https://my.clevelandclinic.org/health/drugs/4302-incentive-spirometer

    - I used an incentive spirometer after any surgery where I could not get out of bed immediately. Ten times an hour, I held the plastic tube that had a blue BB-looking thing that rose when I sealed my mouth over the breathing tube and took the deepest breath I could. Then I held my breath there for at least five seconds and breathed out slowly, working to keep the BB stable. The more modern ones have a yellow piston that rises and falls. Thankfully, I didn't need to use it once I could walk around.

When to Seek Medical Attention

- **Fever-** Contact your healthcare provider if you develop a fever (temperature above 100.4°F or 38°C) after surgery. An elevated temperature may indicate an infection or other underlying issue that requires evaluation and treatment.
- **Worsening Pain-** If you experience increasing or uncontrolled pain after surgery despite taking prescribed pain medications, notify your healthcare provider for further assessment and management.
- **Swelling or Redness-** Report any significant swelling, redness, warmth, or drainage from the surgical site, as these may be signs of infection or other complications requiring medical attention.
- **Difficulty Breathing-** Seek immediate medical attention if you experience difficulty breathing, shortness of breath, chest pain, or coughing up blood, as these symptoms may indicate a severe respiratory complication or blood clot.
- **Changes in Mental Status-** If you experience confusion, disorientation, extreme fatigue, or changes in mental status after surgery, notify your healthcare provider immediately. These symptoms may indicate complications such as anesthesia-related delirium or electrolyte imbalances.

Productively Communicating with Healthcare Professionals

1. Clear Communication— Productive communication with healthcare professionals safeguards addressing your post-operative needs quickly and appropriately. Be honest and specific when describing your symptoms, pain levels, and concerns, and don't hesitate to ask questions or seek clarification about your care plan.

2. Advocating for Yourself— As a patient, you have the right to advocate for your needs and preferences regarding pain management, mobility, and other aspects of your care. If you feel your current medicine is not adequately controlling your pain, or if you have concerns about your treatment plan, please let your healthcare team know.

3. Follow-Up Care— Before you leave the hospital or surgical center, please be sure that you understand your discharge instructions, including medication dosages, activity restrictions, and follow-up appointments. Ask for clarification if anything is unclear, and confirm arrangements for any necessary post-operative care or support services.

4. Emergency Contact Information— Guarantee you can access emergency contact information for your healthcare provider or surgical team if you experience unexpected complications or have urgent questions or concerns after discharge.

Emotional and Psychological Facets of Recovery Setbacks

- **Acknowledge Your Feelings-** It's normal to experience a range of emotions, including frustration, anxiety, sadness, or disappointment, in response to setbacks or complications during recovery. Acknowledge and validate your feelings, and don't hesitate to seek support from loved ones, friends, or mental health professionals if needed.

- **Practice Self-Care-** Prioritize self-care activities that promote emotional and psychological well-being, such as mindfulness, relaxation techniques, journaling, or engaging in activities you enjoy. Taking care of your mental health is as important as caring for your physical health during recovery.

- **Set Realistic Expectations-** Recovery from surgery can be challenging and unpredictable, with ups and downs, so set realistic expectations for your recovery. Be patient and compassionate with yourself as you deal with setbacks and obstacles.

- **Stay Connected-** Stay connected with your support network of family, friends, and healthcare providers for encouragement, guidance, and reassurance during difficult times. Don't hesitate to seek help or companionship, as social support can be crucial in coping with emotional challenges during recovery.

- **Seek Professional Help-** If you're struggling to cope with emotional or psychological issues related to your recovery setbacks, consider seeking professional help from a therapist, counselor, or psychologist who specializes in working with individuals undergoing medical trauma or surgery. Therapy can provide valuable support, coping strategies, and resources to help you handle emotional stumbling blocks, promoting healing and resilience.

Again, the first 24 hours after surgery are a critical period of recovery, marked by a combination of physical discomfort, emotional adjustment, and ongoing medical care. The ninth secret is understanding what to expect immediately post-op, managing pain effectively, dealing with common post-surgical complications and how to handle setbacks, and remembering that productive communication with healthcare professionals about your care is crucial to a smooth, successful recovery.

Recovery Nurse Conversation Continued

"There she is," said the recovery nurse as I opened my eyes, "You gave us a scare because I had to keep reminding you to breathe, or you wouldn't do it. What was going on?" she queried. "Oh my," I answered, "I was just meditating, and sometimes my breathing slows down when I do it."

"Well, maybe you shouldn't meditate right after surgery," said the nurse. How is your pain level from one to five? Do you need to urinate yet?"

Not Much Pain, But Nausea

"I am not in much pain... still waking up. No, I don't need to pee yet," I replied, "But I do feel a bit nauseous, so I could use an emesis basin, and I am so thirsty. Can I get some water?" "Not yet," she explained, "But I can get you some ice chips for now. We must ensure you are fully alert before we try water." "Okay," I said, "I'll take the ice chips. Has someone called Terry to come pick me up yet?" "Sara is doing that right now," stated the nurse as she smiled, "You'll be home soon."

Chapter 10
Follow Up Appointments and Physical Therapy

Dr. Bromley

"Dr. Bromley will see you now, Linda," Lana, the medical assistant, said, "Wow! You have both legs in casts. Can we take a picture? I haven't seen both legs in casts at the same time. That must be rough. What happened?" "I was in an automobile accident on University Parkway on my way to work as a janitor in the Harmon Building on the BYU campus at 5 am," I explained, "They said I t-boned an elderly couple on their way to the temple because the light wasn't working, but I was on the main road, and he thought he saw a green light because he saw the next intersection up the hill.

I Don't Remember

I just feel so bad because I don't remember the accident; maybe I could have done something differently. Anyway, Dr. Bromley put my legs back together, so that's why I am here today." "Well, you will probably never know what happened. The mind has a way of protecting us from too traumatic things. I am glad he could put them back together for you. Now you need to focus on getting better. " said Lana, "Here is room three. Have a seat, and Dr. Bromley will be there soon."

The tenth secret for you is to optimize your healing and recovery by attending follow-up appointments, assessing your progress, and consistently engaging in physical therapy. These are foundational components of post-surgical rehabilitation, promising you the proper medical care and support to regain health and well-being. Here are some tips to keep you on track:

Periodically Reacquaint yourself with Post-Surgery Instructions

When you are in pain and one day melts into another, sometimes you forget what the medical professionals advised you to do. Look at the post-surgery instructions once or twice a day to be sure you are still following the recommended protocol. Keep the list of possible complications the hospital staff provides near you, telling you what to do and when to contact your healthcare provider because things may still appear unexpectedly. Also, faithfully do wound care because infection can slow down your progress.

Infection Two Months Later

When I had an external fixator on my crushed right wrist and forearm, the doctor instructed me to dilute the hydrogen peroxide with sterile, distilled water and Q-tip the long screws going down into my bones that were attached to the fixator every other hour I was awake. It had been over two months since the accident, and the flesh would stick to the screws whenever I tried to move my thumb or do physical therapy, so the skin tore open, bled and oozed fluid.

Neosporin Plugged the Drainage Holes

My home health nurse thought Neosporin would be good to keep the flesh movable on the screws but provide the antibiotic needed. She meant well. Unfortunately, the holes couldn't drain, so puss started bubbling up out of the holes and almost infected my bones. I had to have another round of oral antibiotics, and we went back to the diluted hydrogen peroxide. The story's moral is to keep up the recommended post-op protocol, even if it seems burdensome.

1. Track Symptoms and Progress— Keep a journal or record of your symptoms, progress, and any notable changes in your condition during recovery. It's good to have a thermometer or blood pressure device to take your vitals in the morning and early evening to safeguard against infection creeping in. Also, as I previously mentioned, your body may be registering pain even if you try to tough it out.
    - Assess whether your pain medication is keeping your blood pressure low enough to sleep and heal optimally. Note improvements in your pain levels so you can wean off the constipating opioids as quickly as possible without jeopardizing your recovery. It's a delicate balance. Also, pay attention to your increasing mobility, overall well-being, and any concerns or adverse reactions to medications or treatments. Monitoring your progress can help you and your doctor assess the effectiveness of your recovery plan and make adjustments as needed.
2. Adhere to Activity Guidelines— Follow the activity guidelines provided by your healthcare provider to resume normal activities while avoiding overexertion or strain gradually. Start with light activities such as walking or gentle stretching and slowly increase intensity and duration as tolerated. Notice changes in any pain, swelling, or discomfort during activities and adjust your level of exertion accordingly. Go easy, but be diligent.
    - Unfortunately, five days after having a hysterectomy, I mowed the lawn because someone needed to do it, and I was a single mom of two young girls. There was no one else. My doctor said nothing about it beforehand, so I thought it would be okay. I began having severe pain and hemorrhaging. When I called the doctor, he wanted to see me immediately. At his office, he started laughing when he found out I had mowed the lawn and said he would have to add that one to his list of things NOT to do after surgery for six weeks. Oops.

3. Attend Follow-Up Appointments— Attend all scheduled follow-up appointments with your healthcare provider or surgical team to see your progress, address any concerns or questions, and receive personalized guidance and recommendations for ongoing care, even if it is difficult to get to their office. After my head-on collision with the semi, being in an eleven-day coma, and not being able to sit up long enough to travel to the doctor in Chicago, I rode by ambulance for a couple of months, even after they released me from the hospital, but I still got to the appointments.
    - Your follow-up appointments may include physical exams, imaging, or laboratory tests to evaluate your rehabilitation and healing process. I had a couple of tests where the technician had to leave the room after placing a radioactive substance in my IV because it was so toxic, and yet it was being pumped throughout my body. It disturbed me, but I did it because the doctor recommended the test.

4. Communicate with Your Healthcare Provider— I have mentioned this repeatedly, but it's essential. I probably drove the medical professionals crazy because I asked about everything. I just wanted to understand what was happening with my body and what I could do to help it heal. I took Human Anatomy and Physiology in college, which allowed me to understand some medical jargon. You don't have to take anatomy, but be sure to discuss any changes in your symptoms, concerns, or challenges you may be experiencing and ask questions about your treatment plan, medications, or recovery milestones. Your healthcare provider is there to support you and help you navigate the challenges of post-surgery recovery.

5. Advocate for Your Needs— Be proactive in advocating for your needs and preferences during follow-up appointments and interactions with healthcare providers. If you have questions or concerns about your treatment plan, recovery goals, or

post-surgery care, don't hesitate to speak up and express your concerns. Your input and feedback guarantee you receive the best care and support throughout your recovery. I changed doctors a few times because some were not open to listening to me.

6. Follow Long-Term Care Plans— Work with your healthcare provider to develop a long-term care plan that supports your ongoing health and well-being beyond the immediate post-surgery recovery period. This plan may include recommendations for lifestyle modifications, preventive screenings, physical therapy, or additional follow-up appointments to monitor your progress and address any lingering issues or concerns.

Physical Therapy Benefits

Physical therapy can be painful and laborious because muscles atrophy quickly. Before my first accident, I jogged five miles daily and attended modern dance and ballet classes three times a week. My muscles were strong and toned. Two weeks later, when they went to change the casts, my leg muscles had atrophied so much that I didn't recognize them because they had no shape and were like draping flaps of skin. It took me nearly a year the first time, but I walked again because of physical therapy.

- **Enhancing Recovery-** Physical therapy is essential for rehabilitation after surgery because it promotes healing, prevents complications such as muscle atrophy and joint stiffness, and restores flexibility and functional abilities. You have to keep moving to be able to keep moving.

- **Restoring Mobility and Function-** Surgery can often result in temporary or permanent limitations in mobility and function. Physical therapy helps you regain strength, flexibility, and range of motion, allowing you to perform daily activities and resume your everyday lifestyle. Also, scar tissue forms at the incision site but can also form internally. Physical therapy stretches the internal scar tissue and prevents more from forming so you can have more flexibility and less pain.

- **Pain Management-** Employ physical therapy techniques, such as manual therapy (massage), therapeutic exercises (like leg lifts, riding a stationary bicycle, or lifting weights in specific movements), and modalities like heat and cold therapy. These can help alleviate pain, inflammation, and discomfort associated with surgery, reducing pain medications and promoting a faster recovery.

- **Preventing Secondary Complications-** Being bedridden or a couch potato means you are inactive. Being immobile after your surgery can increase your risk of secondary complications such as blood clots, pressure ulcers, and respiratory problems. Movement keeps the blood flowing, and deep breathing keeps the lungs pumping life-giving oxygen throughout your body. Physical therapy interventions like moving your arms and legs for mobility, stretching, and breathing exercises help mitigate these risks and promote overall health and well-being.

Setting Realistic Expectations for Physical Therapy

1. Gradual Progression— Recognize that surgical recovery takes time, and your progress in physical therapy may be frustratingly gradual. You should set realistic expectations about your rehabilitative pace because setbacks or plateaus may occur, but you must maintain your motivation. When I pushed myself too hard, I got injured and had to wait to heal again. When I didn't push hard enough, I felt like it took too long. It's another delicate balance.

2. Individualized Treatment Plans— Physical therapists tailor programs to meet each patient's specific needs, goals, and abilities. Communicate your goals and concerns to your physical therapist, who will work with you to develop a personalized treatment plan

that aligns with your skills and expectations. I was motivated when I wanted to walk and hold my baby again.

3. Patience and Persistence— Recovery from surgery and rehabilitation through physical therapy require patience and persistence. It's normal to experience challenges and setbacks along the way. Still, consistent effort and commitment to the treatment plan can significantly improve mobility, function, and quality of life.
    - For example, at one point, my "big goal" was to rock back and forth enough with my hip abduction triangle between my legs to slip a bedpan underneath my bottom. I made progress inch by inch until I reached the fulcrum point, which took two weeks. I celebrated because I didn't have to wait long periods anymore for an aide to come so I could relieve my bladder.
4. Gradual Return to Activities— While physical therapy aims to restore mobility and function, you should understand that returning to your pre-surgery activity level may take time. It's essential to follow the physical therapist's guidance and gradually reintroduce activities and exercises to prevent re-injury or overexertion.

Maximize Your Physical Therapy

Actively participate in physical therapy sessions and follow home exercise programs prescribed by the physical therapist. Put your heart and soul into it. Be consistent and adhere to your treatment plan. Maintain open communication with the physical therapist regarding any changes in your symptoms, progress, or concerns during rehabilitation. Your physical therapist can adjust your treatment plan as your needs and goals evolve, so if you want to do some yoga, ask them what exercises will get you there quickly.

Focus On Functional Movements

Focus on functional movements for your daily activities: walk, climb stairs, and lift objects to show yourself the gains in real life. Finally, adopt healthy lifestyle habits, such as maintaining a balanced diet, staying hydrated, getting adequate rest, and avoiding smoking and excessive alcohol consumption to continue your body's healing process.

The tenth secret for you is to optimize your healing and recovery by attending follow-up appointments, assessing your progress, and consistently engaging in physical therapy. Follow-up appointments with your doctor and physical therapy are integral to your progress following surgery, facilitating healing, restoring mobility and function, and promoting overall well-being. You can achieve your goals and reclaim your life by understanding the importance of rehabilitation, setting realistic expectations, and maximizing the benefits of physical therapy.

Progress May Vary

Remember that your progress may vary depending on the type of surgery you had, your pre-existing health conditions, and your adherence to the treatment plan. Don't get discouraged. With your dedication, patience, and collaboration with skilled physical therapists, you can improve your bodily function and quality of life after surgery. You can do it!

Conversation At Dr. Bromley's Office Continued

"Hello, Linda," greeted Dr. Bromley, "How are you doing today?" "Pretty good, considering what happened to my legs. What did you call it? A posterior dislocation at the knees?" "Yes," replied Dr. Bromley. It was pretty bad. Luckily, both legs' main nerves and arteries were okay, but everything around them was like spaghetti. I would recommend a bilateral knee replacement, but you are only nineteen, and we don't like to do joint replacements until patients are sixty or older. We want you to keep walking as long as you can." "So you think I'll be able to walk again?" I asked nervously.

Laxity in Both Knees

"Well, that's what we hope," he said, "You see, most knee joints work like a hinge and only bend. Unfortunately, with not much support from the surrounding ligaments, the bottom half of your legs slops around every time you put your leg out for a step, so it will depend on how you respond to physical therapy. You have significant laxity in both knees, so it will be important to strengthen your quads."

Experimental Gore-Tex Ligaments

He reported, "Cutting-edge surgeons are experimenting with Gore-Tex replacing ligaments to stabilize the joints, but that is still a few years away. We will keep in touch and see what we can do then. For now, I'll write orders for a physical therapist on the BYU campus, and we'll see what happens." I exclaimed, "Thank you so much, Dr. Bromley! I am so grateful to you! You were able to do the surgery. Now, I will do my part in physical therapy because I want to walk again!

Chapter 11
Revolutionizing Surgical Procedures

Horses and Buggies to Rockets

"Terry, I remember conversing with my grandmother when I was fifteen. I was interviewing her for my United States history class, and when I asked what technologies had changed throughout her lifetime, I remember being astonished by her answer. She said she had been alive while most people used horses and buggies to get around. Then she saw cars become popular, and later, she watched on television while a man landed on the moon. She couldn't have imagined that when she was young. Then there were the simple things like she was even overwhelmed by the choices of soaps at the store because they only had lye or non-lye soap in her day. That was it," I said.

Newspapers Popularity Diminished

"Well, Linda," Terry responded, "I watched my dad, a big executive at a newspaper in Phoenix, lose his job because of how things modified when the newspaper's popularity diminished because of television and computers taking over the communications industry. When I was young, you had to crank the phones on the wall and ask the operator to connect you to the number, and now we have an entire computer in our hands. In addition, wars were fought on the other side of the world until TV brought the Vietnam War into our living rooms, where we saw friends and loved ones die in front of our faces. I remember being absolutely spellbound when I saw a man land on the moon, and now Elon Musk wants to take us to Mars."

The Only Constant is Change

"I know what you mean, Terry," I acknowledged, "The only constant is change. With what is happening in the medical field, I feel like I lived in the Stone Age of medicine with my fifty-two surgeries and procedures under general anesthesia. It has changed so much since my first surgeries. Innovators replaced open surgeries with minimally invasive arthroscopic or laparoscopic procedures so the body would have less exposure to infection and heal faster. I always tell the kids that when they get old, there probably won't even be surgery anymore because if you have a bad heart, they'll just inject nanobots into you to grow you a new one."

The eleventh secret for you is that surgery is getting more precise and customized, and in a few years, it may be replaced altogether with AI analysis, nanotechnology, mRNA, virtual and augmented reality, neurotechnology, 3D printing, and stem cells focusing on restorative and regenerative medicine. Surgical procedures may be one of the most dynamic and rapidly evolving areas in the vast healthcare landscape. From ancient times, when healers used crude tools for invasive interventions, to the modern era of minimally invasive techniques, surgery has undergone remarkable transformations. However, the future promises even more radical changes, driven by technological advances, artificial intelligence (AI), and innovative medical techniques.

Surgical Robotics: Precision and Automation

One of the most striking developments in recent years has been the integration of robotics into surgical procedures. Robotic-assisted surgery offers surgeons unparalleled precision and control, allowing for more delicate maneuvers and enhanced outcomes. Miniaturized robotic instruments, guided by skilled surgeons through a console, can perform intricate tasks with minimal tissue damage and faster recovery times.

According to vanderbilt.edu, under the future of robotic surgery tab, "Over the next few years, surgical procedures that are driven by artificial intelligence, machine learning, natural language processing and computer vision are predicted to grow and will greatly aid in the future of robotics and AI in surgery." https://blog.engineering.vanderbilt.edu/the-future-of-robotic-surgery.

AI Algorithms and Haptic Feedback

In the future, surgical robots will become even more sophisticated, incorporating AI algorithms for real-time decision-making and autonomous actions. These robots will be capable of analyzing vast amounts of patient data, imaging scans, and surgical histories to customize procedures and optimize outcomes. Additionally, advancements in haptic feedback technology, according to wikipedia.org, will enable surgeons to perceive tactile sensations remotely, enhancing their dexterity and sense of touch during robotic procedures. https://en.wikipedia.org/wiki/Haptic_techn ology

Nanotechnology: Targeted Therapy at the Molecular Level

According to cdc.gov/niosh/topics/nanotech, "Nanotechnology is the manipulation of matter on a near-atomic scale to produce new structures, materials, and devices." https://www.cdc.gov/niosh/nano/about/?CDC_AAref_Val=htt ps%3A%2F%2Fwww.cdc.gov%2Fniosh%2Ftopics%2Fnanotech%2F The National Institute for Occupational Safety and Health (NIOSH), through its Nanotechnology Research Center, is researching how to use this technology safely, developing partnerships, and strategic plans to implement nanotechnology into medicine.

One Thousand Times Smaller Than a Sheet of Paper

To give you a picture of how microscopic nanodevices are, according to the builtin.com/hardware/nanotechnology website, "These devices typically have a scale of fewer than 100 nanometers (nm). A nanometer is a very small unit of measurement equal to one billionth of a meter.

For reference, a sheet of paper is about 100,000 nanometers thick." https://builtin.com/hardware/nanotechnologyThat means nanodevices are one thousand times smaller than a sheet of paper.

Precisely Targeted Therapy

Nanotechnology holds immense promise for revolutionizing surgical interventions by enabling targeted therapy at the molecular level. Nanoparticles, engineered to deliver drugs, genes, or therapeutic agents directly to diseased tissues, offer unprecedented precision and efficacy in treatment. In the future, surgeons may utilize nanorobots - microscopic machines capable of navigating through the bloodstream to specific sites of pathology - to perform precise surgical tasks at a cellular level. According to https://www.cdc.gov/niosh/nano/about/?CDC_AAref_Val=https%3A%2F%2Fwww.cdc.gov%2Fniosh%2Ftopics%2Fnanotech%2F , "These applications include fluorescent biological labels, drug and gene delivery, bio-detection of pathogens, detection of protein, probing of DNA structure, tissue engineering, tumor detection, separation and purification of biological molecules and cells, MRI contrast enhancement and phagokinetic studies."

Nanotechnology Spares Healthy Tissue

Imagine a scenario where nanorobots are deployed to repair damaged cardiac tissue following a heart attack or eradicate cancerous cells with pinpoint accuracy, sparing healthy surrounding tissue. Such advancements in nanotechnology will not only transform surgical procedures but also redefine the boundaries of medical intervention, ushering in an era of personalized and targeted therapy. This personalized, targeted therapy is some exciting news!

Virtual and Augmented Reality: Immersive Surgical Training and Planning

Virtual and augmented reality (VR/AR) technologies are poised to revolutionize surgical education, training, and preoperative planning. Surgeons can immerse themselves in realistic virtual environments, simulating complex surgical procedures and practicing intricate maneuvers before entering the operating room. "Virtual reality in surgery training provides students with immersive experiences that reduce the risk of injury for their patients — and lack nothing compared to traditional learning experiences," according to https://ventionteams.com/healthtech/virtual-reality/surgery-trainingThis immersive training experience enhances surgical proficiency, reduces the learning curve, and improves patient safety.

MRIs Create VR Practice Specific to Patients

According to the National Center for Biotechnology Information, MRIs can create VR practice and instruction individualized to the patient: "All the images and 3D models contained in the aforementioned simulators are based on magnetic resonance imaging (MRI) and recordings of in vivo procedures... To create realistic 3D models of internal organs, a collection of computed tomography scans and MRIs are required.... recreating 3D reconstructions based on medical imaging." https://www.ncbi.nlm.nih.gov/pmc/articles/PMC9993190/

Remarkable Clarity

In other words, virtual reality helps train surgical personnel before and assist during the procedure. AR overlays can provide surgeons with real-time guidance and anatomical insights during operations, enhancing their situational awareness and decision-making capabilities. By integrating patient-specific imaging data into AR platforms, surgeons can visualize internal structures with remarkable clarity, allowing for more precise surgical navigation and optimal outcomes.

Gene Editing and Regenerative Medicine: Transforming Surgical Paradigms

The advent of gene editing technologies, such as CRISPR-Cas9, has opened new frontiers in surgical interventions by offering the potential to correct genetic defects and treat hereditary diseases at their root cause. According to proclinical.com's top 10 medical technologies, "Clustered Regularly Interspaced Short Palindromic Repeats (CRISPR) is the most advanced gene-editing technology yet. It works by harnessing the natural mechanisms of the immune systems of bacterium cells of invading viruses, which... (can) 'cut out' infected DNA strands. This cutting of DNA is what has the power to transform the way we treat disease potentially. By modifying genes, some of the biggest threats to our health, like cancer and HIV, could potentially be overcome in a matter of years." https://www.proclinical.com/blogs/2022-4/top-10-new-medical-technologies-2022

In the future, surgeons may employ gene editing techniques to modify patient's own cells ex vivo, correcting genetic abnormalities before reintroducing them back into the body. This approach holds immense promise for treating various genetic disorders, from cystic fibrosis to sickle cell anemia, with unprecedented precision and efficacy. "CRISPR has many potential applications, including correcting genetic defects, treating and preventing the spread of diseases, and improving the growth and resilience of crops. However, despite its promise, the technology also raises ethical concerns, mostly over humanity's right to 'play God' and worries over gene editing being used to produce designer babies." https://www.proclinical.com/blogs/2022-4/top-10-new-medical-technologies-2022

Messenger RNA: Using the Body to Produce Medicine

"mRNA technology has been put under the spotlight recently as the new vaccines for Covid-19 use this science. With their high effectiveness, capacity for rapid development, and potential for low production costs, mRNA vaccines offer an alternative to the traditional vaccine approach... derived from DNA..., they produce viral proteins so the body can then produce an immune response... getting the body to produce a drug-like response... by using mRNA technology, development times and costs could be cut by setting the human body to work on manufacturing the proteins instead," says proclinical.com. https://www.proclinical.com/blogs/2022-4/top-10-new-medical-technologies-2022

Neurotechnology: Electrical Stimulation Cures

"In healthcare, neurotechnology is currently being used in brain imaging by recording magnetic fields produced by electrical activity within the brain, neurostimulation, stimulating the brain and nervous system to influence brain activity; and in neurodevices, an emerging technology that monitors or regulates brain activity using an implant. Neurodevices are still mostly in the research phase but hold major potential for treating brain disorders. An example of this is Neuralink, pioneered by Elon Musk. Neuralink is developing a device that would be embedded into the human brain… to record brain activity and transmit this data wirelessly to a computer. Researchers would then be able to analyze these findings and use them to electrically stimulate brain activity. If successful, it can possibly be used to cure brain diseases like Alzheimer's and Parkinson's. Neuralink has been tested on animals so far, but Elon Musk has said the company hopes to start implanting its chips in humans in 2022." https://www.proclinical.com/blogs/2022-4/top-10-new-medical-technologies-2022

3D Printing: New Organs and Body Parts

"3D printers can create implants and even joints… for surgery. 3D-printed prosthetics are increasingly popular because they are entirely bespoke, with digital functionalities enabling them to match an individual's measurements down to the millimeter. This allows for unprecedented levels of comfort and mobility. Using 3D printing for presurgical planning is also gaining momentum. Using a realistic replica of an actual patient's anatomy allows surgeons to attempt procedures they wouldn't have previously been able to do. The ability to plan a complex surgery and train prior to the procedure by using 3D-printed models has the potential to… increase success rates and reduce time in the operating room and recovery time…

...While it was initially ground-breaking to be able to regenerate skin cells for skin draughts for burn victims, this has slowly given way to even more exciting possibilities. Scientists have been able to create blood vessels, synthetic ovaries and even a pancreas. These artificial organs then grow within the patient's body to replace the original faulty one. The ability to supply artificial organs that are not rejected by the body's immune system could be revolutionary, saving millions of patients who depend on lifesaving transplants every year." https://www.proclinical.com/blogs/2022-4/top-10-new-medical-technologies-2022

Stem Cells: Replacement Beta Cells for Insulin

According to time.com's top health innovations, Harvard biologist Doug Melton is "using stem cells to create replacement beta cells that produce insulin (to cure diabetes). He started the work over ten years ago when stem-cell research was raising hopes and controversy. In 2014, he co-founded Semma Therapeutics—the name is derived from Sam and Emma (his children)—to develop the technology, and this summer, it was acquired by Vertex Pharmaceuticals for $950 million. The company has created a small, implantable device that holds millions of replacement beta cells, letting glucose and insulin through but keeping immune cells out. https://time.com/5710295/top-health-innovations/This device will cure diabetes.

Restorative and Regenerative Medicine

Furthermore, regenerative medicine techniques, such as tissue engineering and stem cell therapy, will enable surgeons to regenerate damaged tissues and organs, offering novel solutions for patients with debilitating injuries or degenerative diseases. From 3D-printed organs to bioengineered tissues, the future of surgical procedures will be characterized by a paradigm shift towards restorative and regenerative approaches, heralding a new era of personalized medicine.

Other Disrupting Innovations

Drone-delivered medical supplies, health wearables providing heart rate, sleeping patterns, and other information, implantable devices dispensing medicine, pocket-size ultrasound devices costing 50 times less, in-home testing devices, telemedicine, wristbands that read your mind by CTRL-Labs to help stroke recovery and amputees... All these other innovations will also disrupt healthcare, reducing the need for surgery. Even mental healthcare uses AI for intake workups and initial diagnoses, chatbots to help practice cognitive behavioral therapy on smartphone apps, software like Ellipsis to recognize emotional distress in how a patient speaks, and video games like EndeavorRx to improve ADHD attention spans. The only constant is change.

Ethical and Societal Implications

As we embark on this journey toward the future of surgical procedures, we must consider these advancements' ethical and societal implications. We must carefully address questions surrounding patient consent, privacy, equity of access, database breaches, and potential unintended consequences to ensure medical innovators deploy these transformative technologies responsibly and ethically. Moreover, the increasing reliance on automation, AI, and advanced technologies raises concerns about surgeons' roles in the operating room and the potential for dehumanization of healthcare. While these technologies offer unparalleled precision and efficiency, they must complement, rather than replace, the expertise and empathy of skilled surgical teams.

The eleventh secret for you is that surgery is getting more precise and customized, and in a few years, it may be replaced altogether with AI analysis, nanotechnology, mRNA, virtual and augmented reality, neurotechnology, 3D printing, and stem cells focusing on restorative and regenerative medicine. Even though you may be preparing for your stone-age surgery today, the future of surgical procedures holds immense promise for improving your outcomes, enhancing surgical precision, and expanding the boundaries of medical intervention. Your kids and grandkids may never need surgery when they get older. By embracing these technological innovations, fostering interdisciplinary collaboration, and upholding ethical principles, we are ushering in a new era of healthcare where surgical procedures are safer, more effective, and more personalized than ever before.

Conversation With Terry Continued

"Linda," said Terry, "While the future medical field is mind-blowing, it's a great idea to anticipate and adapt to what is coming. I like to start working on solutions from where I am, not where I want to be. If I don't deal with what is right in front of me exactly as it presents itself right now, I will miss what needs to be done. You are having this incredible knee pain, which significantly curtails your quality of life. Your doctor has suggested a knee replacement.

They Can't Grow You a New One Yet

They can't grow you a new one today but they can replace the joint this month. It is your choice. Do you want to wait a few more years in pain, or do you want to go ahead with the surgery?" "Gosh, Terry," I replied, "I have had so many surgeries. I am not looking forward to having another one, but everyone I have talked to says it helped them, and I have thoroughly researched it. I think I am ready to have the surgery if you will help me with recovery." "Of course, my dear," Terry responded, "You are the love of my life, and I will always be here for you."

Chapter 12

Glossary of Medical Terms Used in Surgical Procedures

Here's a glossary of medical terms dealing with surgical procedures:

1. **Amputation**: Surgical removal of a limb or part of a limb.
2. **Anastomosis**: The surgical joining of two structures, such as blood vessels or bowel segments.
3. **Anesthesia**: The administration of medications to prevent pain and discomfort during surgery.
4. **Arthroscopy**: A minimally invasive surgical procedure used to visualize, diagnose, and treat problems inside a joint.
5. **Biopsy**: The removal of a small sample of tissue for examination under a microscope to diagnose disease.
6. **Catheterization**: The insertion of a thin tube (catheter) into a body cavity or vessel, usually to drain fluid or administer medication.
7. **Cautery**: Using heat or electricity to burn or destroy tissue, often used to stop bleeding.
8. **Craniotomy**: Surgical opening of the skull.

9. **Debridement**: Remove dead, damaged, or infected tissue to promote healing.
10. **Graft**: A tissue or organ is transplanted into a patient to replace damaged or missing tissue.
11. **Hemorrhage:** bleeding, especially when profuse.
12. **Hemorrhoidectomy**: Surgical removal of hemorrhoids, swollen blood vessels in the rectum or anus.
13. **Hemostasis**: The process of stopping bleeding during surgery.
14. **Incision**: A surgical cut made into the body tissues during an operation.
15. **Laparoscopy**: A minimally invasive surgical procedure performed through small incisions with the aid of a camera.
16. **Ligation**: The surgical tying off or closing of a blood vessel or duct.
17. **Mastectomy**: Surgical removal of one or both breasts.
18. **Ostomy**: Surgical creation of an artificial opening (stoma) between a hollow organ and the body surface.
19. **Prosthesis**: An artificial device used to replace a missing body part or to support a damaged body part.
20. **Resection**: The surgical removal of part or all of an organ, tissue, or structure.
21. **Scalpel**: A small, sharp knife used for making incisions during surgery.
22. **Staples**: Metal clips or fasteners used to close surgical incisions.
23. **Surgical drain**: A tube used to remove excess fluid or air from a surgical site.

24. **Suture**: A stitch or series of stitches used to close a wound or incision.

25. **Thoracotomy**: Surgical incision into the chest cavity.

26. **Tracheostomy**: Surgical creation of an opening in the neck to access the trachea (windpipe) for breathing.

Chapter 13
Quick Recap of the 11SecretsFor You

The first secret for you is that no matter what type of surgery your doctor recommends, weighing its potential risks and benefits in collaboration with your healthcare team, making informed decisions, and adequately preparing for the procedure will provide the best outcome.

The second secret for you is to do your research, understand the diagnosis, ask questions, seek second opinions if necessary, investigate your doctor's ties to pharmaceutical or medical device companies, and insist on transparency as much as possible.

The third secret for you is to manage the surgery's financial and logistical aspects beforehand, like arranging time off work, childcare or pet care, transportation to and from the medical facility, and post-operative caregivers for peace of mind.

The fourth secret for you is to eat foods that will help you heal, avoid ones that don't, exercise, sleep adequately, and quit habits that will slow your recovery in advance.

The fifth secret for you is effectively managing anxiety and fear, utilizing meditation, visualization and relaxation techniques, calling upon your faith community, and using therapeutic music for inner peace and confidence.

The eighth secret for you is that even though you may be anxious on the big day of surgery, you can have greater confidence and resilience by effectively interacting with hospital staff, knowing what to expect, and employing coping strategies for managing pre-surgery nerves.

The ninth secret is understanding what to expect immediately post-op, managing pain effectively, dealing with common post-surgical complications and how to handle setbacks, and remembering that productive communication with healthcare professionals about your care is crucial to a smooth, successful recovery.

The tenth secret is to optimize your healing and recovery by attending follow-up appointments, assessing your progress, and consistently engaging in physical therapy.

The eleventh secret for you is that surgery is getting more precise and customized, and in a few years, it may be replaced altogether with AI analysis, nanotechnology, mRNA, virtual and augmented reality, neurotechnology, 3D printing, and stem cells focusing on restorative and regenerative medicine.

Chapter 14
Works Cited:

Arizona Office of Administrative Hearings. (2024). OAH Decision Search. Portal.azoah.com, Retrieved (March 12, 2024) from https://portal.azoah.com/search1400/

AZCentral.com. (2024). How to check your doctor's history and other options for better health care in Arizona. The Arizona Republic, Retrieved (March 12, 2024) from https://www.azcentral.com/story/news/local/arizona-investigations/2023/12/13/how-to-check-doctor-background-in-arizona/71891724007/#:~:text=Patients%20also%20can%20try%20to

Burke, H. (2022, April 14). Top 10 new medical technologies 2022 | Proclinical blogs. Proclinical, Retrieved (March 12, 2024) from https://www.proclinical.com/blogs/2022-4/top-10-new-medical-technologies-2022

Center For Disease Control and Prevention. NIOSH. (2026, March 3). Nanotechnology| National Institute for Occupational Safety and Health. Centers for Disease Control and Prevention, Retrieved (May 36, 2024) from https://www.cdc.gov/niosh/nano/about/?CDC_AAref_Val=https%3A%2F%2Fwww.cdc.gov%2Fniosh%2Ftopics%2Fnanotech%2F

Cleveland Clinic. (2022, August 31). Incentive spirometer: Purpose, goals & how to use. Cleveland Clinic, Retrieved (March 12, 2024) from https://my.clevelandclinic.org/health/drugs/4302-incentive-spirometer

Definitive Healthcare. (2024). Largest academic medical centers | Academic medical institutions. Www.definitivehc.com, Retrieved (March 12,

2024) from https://www.definitivehc.com/resources/healthcare-insights/top-largest-academic-medical-centers

DocInfo.org. (2024). Verify a doctor's license and professional background information. Docinfo.org, Retrieved (March 12, 2024) from https://www.docinfo.org/#

Georgios Ntakakis, Plomariti, C., Frantzidis, C. A., Antoniou, P. E., Bamidis, P. D., & Georgios Tsoulfas. (2023). Exploring the use of virtual reality in surgical education. World Journal of Transplantation, 13(2), 36–43, Retrieved (March 12, 2024) from https://doi.org/10.5500/wjt.v13.i2.36

LibreTexts. (2019, February 18). 5.1: Organs and systems of the human organism. Medicine LibreTexts, Retrieved (March 12, 2024) from https://med.libretexts.org/Bookshelves/Anatomy_and_Physiology/Human_Anatomy_and_Physiology_Preparatory_Course_(Liachovitzky)/05%3A_Higher_Levels_of_Complexity-_Organs_and_Systems/5.01%3A_Organs_and_Systems_of_the_Human_Organism#:~:text=The%20human%20organism%20consists%20of

Meditative Mind. (2023). All 9 SOLFEGGIOS | [No Ads] | FULL Body Restoration & Aura Cleanse. Www.youtube.com, Retrieved (March 12, 2024) from https://www.youtube.com/watch?v=NHUS_5vhi90

Netflix. (2018). The Bleeding Edge | Trailer [HD] | Netflix. In YouTube, Retrieved (March 12, 2024) from https://www.youtube.com/watch?v=slmilObZl28

OpenPaymentsData.cms.gov. (2018). Open Payments Data - CMS | CMS Open Payments Data. OpenPaymentsData.CMS.gov, Retrieved (March 12, 2024) from https://openpaymentsdata.cms.gov/

Oppermann, A. (2023, February 13). What Is Nanotechnology? (Definition, Examples, Risks) | Built In. Builtin.com, Retrieved (March 12, 2024) from https://builtin.com/hardware/nanotechnology

Rask, D. M. G., Puntel, M. R., Patzkowski, J. C., & Patzkowski, M. S. (2021). Multivitamin Use in Enhanced Recovery After Surgery Protocols: A Cost Analysis. Military Medicine, 186(9-10), e1024–e1028, Retrieved (March 12, 2024) from https://doi.org/10.1093/milmed/usaa505

Robbins, Tony. "This Daily Habit Will Prime Your Brain to Be Its Best | Tony Robbins." YouTube, 20 Apr. 2020, https://www.youtube.com/watch?v=faTGTgid8Uc

Saini, R., Saini, S., & Sharma, S. (2010). Nanotechnology: The future medicine. Journal of Cutaneous and Aesthetic Surgery, 3(1), 32, Retrieved (March 12, 2024) from https://doi.org/10.4103/0974-2077.63301

Stelter, G. (2016, October 4). Chakras: A Beginner's Guide to the 7 Chakras. Healthline. https://www.healthline.com/health/fitness-exercise/7-chakras#Chakra-101

TIME Staff. (2019, October 25). 12 innovations that will change health care and medicine in the 2020s. Time; Time, Retrieved (March 12, 2024) from https://time.com/5710295/top-health-innovations/

Vanderbilt School of Engineering. (2024). The Future of Robotic Surgery: 3 Trends to Look For. Blog.engineering.vanderbilt.edu, Retrieved (March 12, 2024) from https://blog.engineering.vanderbilt.edu/the-future-of-robotic-surgery-3-trends-to-look-for#:~:text=That

Vention. (2024). Virtual Reality for surgery training. Ventionteams.com, Retrieved (March 12, 2024) from https://ventionteams.com/healthtech/virtual-reality/surgery-training

Victor, D. (2023, November 21). How music can reduce stress and improve mental health - harmony & healing. Harmony & Healing. https://www.harmonyandhealing.org/how-music-can-reduce-stress/

Wikipedia Contributors. (2019, March 13). Haptic technology. Wikipedia; Wikimedia Foundation, Retrieved (March 12, 2024) from https://en.wikipedia.org/wiki/Haptic_technology

www.ingramcontent.com/pod-product-compliance
Lightning Source LLC
Chambersburg PA
CBHW031352230926
51848CB00002B/496
9781964694252

Geriatrics 3

Gynecology · Orthopaedics · Anesthesiology
Surgery · Otorhinolaryngology · Ophthalmology
Dermatology

Contributors

E. A. Balazs A. Basso C. Beck L. J. Benedek-Jaszmann
J. L. Denlinger M. Devas B. A. Gilchrest K. Green
H. Hockwin C. Lauritzen E. Lütjen-Drecoll
F. H. Meythaler H. C. Nohl-Oser C. Ohrloff M. Paneth
M. Reim J. W. Rohen E. Rügheimer P. F. Schofield
D. E. F. Tweedle R. A. Weale J. K. Webb

Edited by Dieter Platt

With 150 Figures

Springer-Verlag
Berlin Heidelberg New York Tokyo 1984

Professor Dr. med. DIETER PLATT
Direktor des Instituts für Gerontologie
der Universität Erlangen-Nürnberg
und der 2. Medizinischen Klinik
Klinikum Nürnberg, Flurstraße 17
D-8500 Nürnberg, FRG

ISBN-13: 978-3-642-68978-9 e-ISBN-13: 978-3-642-68976-5
DOI: 10.1007/978-3-642-68976-5

Library of Congress Cataloging in Publication Data. (Revised for volume 3) Main entry under title: Geriatrics. Includes bibliographies and indexes. Contents: v. 1. Cardiology and vascular system. Central nervous system – v. 2. Digestive system. Endocrine system. Kidney and urogenital system. Haematological system. Respiratory system. Rehabilitation. Nutrition. Drug treatment – v. 3. Gynecology. Orthopaedics. Anesthesiology. Surgery. Otorhinolaryngology. Ophthalmology. Dermatology. 1. Geriatrics – Collected works. I. Baldinger, A. II. Platt, Dieter. [DNLM: 1. Cardiovascular diseases – In old age. 2. Central nervous system diseases – In old age. WG 100 G369] RC952.5.G4435 1982 618,97'61 81-18481
ISBN-13: 978-3-642-68978-9

Softcover reprint of the hardcover 1st edition 1984

Typesetting, printing, and bookbinding: Brühlsche Universitätsdruckerei, Giessen
2122/3130-543210

List of Contributors

BALAZS, E. A., M.D.
Department of Ophthalmology, College of Physicians and Surgeons, Columbia University, New York, NY 10032, USA

BASSO, A., M.D.
Professor of Urology, Winchester Urology Clinic, 130 Peyton Street, Winchester, VA 22601, USA

BECK, C., Professor Dr.
Ärztlicher Direktor, Abteilung Allgemeine HNO-Heilkunde mit Poliklinik, Universitäts Hals-, Nasen- und Ohrenklinik, Klinikum der Albert-Ludwigs-Universität, Killianstr. 5, D-7800 Freiburg, FRG

BENEDEK-JASZMANN, L. J., Dr.
Head, Department of Obstetrics and Gynaecology, Regional Protestant Hospital, Edeseweg 118, NL-6720 GA Bennekom, The Netherlands

DENLINGER, JANET L., M.D.
Department of Ophthalmology, College of Physicians and Surgeons, Columbia University, New York, NY 10032, USA

DEVAS, M., M. Chir., F.R.C.S.
Professor of Orthopedics, Stamford House, Chipping Campden, Gloucestershire GL55 6AD, Great Britain

GILCHREST, BARBARA A., M.D.
Scientist I, Northeastern Region Human Nutrition Research Center on Aging at Tufts University, 711 Washington Street, Boston, Massachusetts 02111, USA

GREEN, K., Ph.D.
Regents' Professor of Ophthalmology, Professor of Physiology, Department of Ophthalmology, Box 3059 School of Medicine, Medical College of Georgia, Augusta, GA 30912, USA

HOCKWIN, H., Professor Dr.
Leiter der Abteilung für Experimentelle Ophthalmologie, Medizinische Einrichtungen der Universität Bonn, Augenklinik, Sigmund-Freund-Str. 25, D-5300 Bonn 1, FRG

LAURITZEN, C., Professor Dr.
Ärztlicher Leiter der Frauenklinik der Universität Ulm, Prittwitzstr. 43, D-7900 Ulm/Donau, FRG

LÜTJEN-DRECOLL, ELKE, Professor Dr.
Anatomisches Institut der Universität Erlangen-Nürnberg, Krankenhausstr. 9, D-8520 Erlangen, FRG

MEYTHALER, F. H., Professor Dr.
Augenklinik mit Poliklinik der Universität Erlangen-Nürnberg, Schwabachanlage 6 (Kopfklinikum), D-8520 Erlangen, FRG

NOHL-OSER, H. C., M.D.
23, Bracknell Gate, Frognal Lane, London NW3 7AE, Great Britain

OHRLOFF, C., Professor Dr.
Oberarzt, Universitäts-Augenklinik Bonn, Sigmund-Freud-Str. 25, D-5300 Bonn 1, FRG

PANETH, M., M.D., F.R.C.S.
Consultant Cardiothoracic Surgeon, Brompton Hospital, Fulham Road, London SW3 6HP, Great Britain

REIM, M., Professor Dr.
Vorstand der Abteilung für Augenheilkunde der Medizinischen Fakultät an der Rhein.-Westf. Technischen Hochschule Aachen, Goethestr. 27/29, D-5100 Aachen, FRG

ROHEN, J.W., Professor Dr. Dr.
Vorstand des Anatomischen Instituts der Universität Erlangen-Nürnberg, Krankenhausstr. 9, D-8520 Erlangen, FRG

RÜGHEIMER, E., Professor Dr.
Direktor des Instituts für Anaesthesiologie der Universität Erlangen-Nürnberg, Maximiliansplatz, D-8520 Erlangen

SCHOFIELD, P. F., M.D., F.R.C.S.
Consultant Surgeon, Withington Hospital, University Hospital of South Manchester, West Didsbury, Manchester M20 8LR, Great Britain

TWEEDLE, D.E.F., M.D., Ch.M., F.R.C.S.
Honorary Consultant Surgeon, Withington Hospital,
University Hospital of South Manchester, West Didsbury,
Manchester M20 8LR, Great Britain

WEALE, R.A., Professor, Ph.D.
Director, Department of Visual Science, Institute of Ophthalmology,
University of London, Judd Street, London WC1H 9QS,
Great Britain

WEBB, J.K., M.D., F.R.C.S.
Consultant Orthopaedic Surgeon, Department of Orthopaedics,
Queen's Medical Centre, University Hospital,
Nottingham NG7 2UH, Great Britain

Preface

Volume 3 of this series is concerned with geriatric aspects of surgical specialties: gynecology, orthopedics, general surgery, otorhinolaryngology, and ophthalmology. Closely associated with these specialties is anesthesiology. Dermatology has an intermediate position between surgical and nonsurgical fields.

The peculiarities of physiological and pathological aging of organs and the consequences for diagnosis and therapy – presented in the first two volumes – are of great significance, especially for surgical specialties. There are a large number of pre-, intra-, and postoperative problems in multimorbid geriatric patients, e.g., coronary insufficiency, bradyarrhythmias, hypertonia, and hypotonia. While as recently as the turn of the century the age of 65 years was viewed as a contraindication for surgery, today even older patients undergo operations on aortic aneurysms, bypass operations for coronary sclerosis, pulmonary resections, and abdominosacral resections of rectal carcinomas, for example. Prerequisite for successful surgery at an advanced age is good pre- and postoperative care of multimorbid patients. Physiological changes of the lungs with aging, the increased frequency in pneumonia and pulmonary embolisms with age, and the decrease in receptors, to give just a few examples, confront anesthetists with difficulties. The maxim "in old age a little less" is also applicable in this field. Only improved experimental gerontological research, possibly reaching even into anesthesia, will provide objective data for anesthesia in elderly patients.

The skin is an organ that experiences characteristic qualitative and quantitative changes in old age. It is obvious even to a layman that the taut elastic skin of an infant is transformed by a loss of fluid, a reduction in the number of elastic fibers, and an increase in collageneous fibers into a loose structure which can be grasped in folds. Thus in the elderly the following quote from Goethe is probably not applicable: "Most difficult of all is what you would think to be easiest, to see with your eyes what lies in front of your eyes."

I would like to take the opportunity to express my sincere gratitude to everyone who contributed to the three-volume series. I would also like to thank Springer-Verlag for making it possible to publish in English this study covering the special problems of multimorbid geriatric patients from the entire field of medicine. Mrs. Herion and Mr. Bergstedt of Springer-Verlag deserve a special word of thanks for their always positive and friendly cooperation, patience, and assistance.

Erlangen-Nürnberg DIETER PLATT

Contents

Gynecology

Pre- and Postmenopause. C. LAURITZEN. With 14 Figures

A. The Premenopause 2
B. The Menopause 2
I. Causes of the Climacteric 2
II. Consequences of Estrogen Decrease 3
III. Treatment 4
1. Indications 4
2. Contraindications 4
3. Preparations 6
4. Therapeutic Effectiveness 6
5. Dose 6
a) Genital Atrophy 7
b) Psychotropic Effects 8
c) Osteoporosis 9
d) The Skin 11
6. Side Effects 11
7. Costs 13
8. Risks 13
a) Vascular Complications 13
b) Mortality 14
9. Risk: Benefit Ratio 15
10. Controls 15
11. Duration of Treatment 16
12. Summary of Treatment Recommendations 16
C. Cancers 16
I. Cancer of the Vulva 16
1. Symptoms 18
2. Diagnosis 18
3. Staging 18
4. Treatment and Prognosis 19
II. Cancer of the Vagina 19
1. Premalignant Lesions 19
2. Malignant Lesions 20
a) Symptoms and Diagnosis 20

b) Treatment 20
3. Secondary Cancer of the Vagina 21
III. Cancer of the Cervix Uteri 21
1. Symptoms 22
2. Diagnosis 23
3. Staging 23
4. Treatment 23
5. Radiation Therapy 25
6. Cervical Stump Carcinoma 26
7. Results of Treatment 26
8. Recurrence 27
IV. Cancer of the Corpus Uteri 27
1. Premalignant Changes in the Endometrium 27
2. Dysplasia of the Endometrium 27
a) Treatment 28
3. Malignant Neoplasms of the Endometrium 28
a) Signs 29
b) Diagnosis 29
c) Staging 30
d) Recurrence 30
e) Results of Treatment 31
4. Sarcoma of the Uterus 31
V. Cancer of the Fallopian Tubes 31
1. Symptoms and Diagnosis 31
2. Treatment 31
3. Prognosis 32
VI. Malignant Tumors of the Ovaries 32
1. Estrogen-Producing Ovarian Tumors 33
2. Arrhenoblastoma 34
3. Primary Malignant Ovarian Tumors 45
4. Metastatic Ovarian Carcinomas 35
5. Clinical Aspects 36
a) Symptomatology 36
b) Differential Diagnosis 38
c) Treatment 39
d) Prognosis 40
e) Follow-up 40
VII. Cancer of the Mammary Glands 41
1. Etiology 41
2. Morphology 41
3. Symptoms 42
4. Diagnosis 42
5. Therapy 42
6. Hormones 42
7. Cytostatic Therapy 43
8. Prognosis 43
References 44

Epidemiology: Some Aspects of the Climacteric Woman.
L.J. BENEDEK-JASZMANN. With 6 Figures

A. Introduction 46
B. International Definitions of the Climacteric Period 47
C. Age at Menopause 49
D. Epidemiology: Duration of the Reproductive Stage (Climacteric menstrual patterns) 52
E. Genital Changes in the Postmenopausal Period 56
F. Extragenital Symptoms and Complaints 57
I. Influences on the Incidence of Complaints 61
References 62

Orthopaedics

Orthopaedics in the Elderly. M. DEVAS. With 7 Figures

A. Introduction 66
B. Fractures Near the Hip: the Problem 67
I. Social Status of the Patient 68
II. The Clinical Manager 68
III. Treatment 69
IV. The Geriatric Orthopaedic Team 69
V. Admission Procedures 72
VI. Anaesthesia 73
VII. Operation 74
1. Femoral Neck Fractures 74
2. Trochanteric Fractures 76
3. Sepsis 76
4. Bleeding and Haemostasis 77
5. Length of Operation 77
6. Transfusion 77
VIII. Bedsores 78
IX. The Bladder 78
X. The Rectum 79
XI. Acetabular Erosion 79
XII. Medical Complications 84
C. Fractures in General 85
I. The Lower Limb 85
1. Fractures of the Femoral Shaft 85
2. Fractures of the Patella 86
3. Fractures of the Tibia 86
4. Fractures of the Ankle and Foot 86
II. The Pelvis and Trunk 87
1. Pelvis 87
2. Spine 87

III. The Arm 87
1. Neck of Humerus 87
2. Dislocation of the Shoulder 87
3. The Elbow 88
4. The Colles' Fracture 88
D. Outpatient Management of Fractures in Elderly Patients . . 88
E. Pathological Fractures and Metastatic Paraplegia 88
F. Radiculography 89
G. Scintigraphy 89
I. Metastatic Deposits 89
II. The Loose Prostesis 90
III. Stress Fractures 90
H. Computer Assisted Tomography 90
J. Spinal Stenosis 90
K. The Practical Management of Arthroplasties in the Elderly . 91
I. The Programme 92
II. The Assessment Clinic 93
III. Admission 95
IV. Skin Preparation 96
V. The Clean Air Theatre 96
VI. The Operation 97
VII. Physiotherapy in the Recovery Room 98
VIII. Infection 98
IX. Care After Operation 98
L. Conclusion 99
References 99

Anesthesiology

Anesthesia. E. RÜGHEIMER. With 16 Figures

A. Introductory Remarks 102
B. Changes of Aging: Anesthesiologic Aspects 106
I. Cardiovascular System 106
II. Respiratory System 108
III. Brain 113
IV. Other Organs 114
V. Pharmacology 114
1. Pharmacokinetics 114
2. Pharmacodynamics 115
C. Hazards of Anesthesia and Surgery 117
I. Preoperative Status 117
1. Quantification of the Anestetic Risk 117
2. Prediction of Cardiovascular and Pulmonary Risks . 118

II. Surgical Procedure . . . 120
1. Nature of the Operation . . . 120
2. Repeat Operations . . . 121
3. Duration of Anesthesia and Surgery . . . 121
4. Elective vs Emergency Surgery . . . 121
III. Anesthesia . . . 122
D. Preoperative Management . . . 123
I. Diagnosis and Treatment of Preexisting Disease . . . 123
1. Cardiovascular System . . . 124
2. Preoperative Cardiac Therapy . . . 124
3. Respiratory System . . . 126
4. Fluid and Electrolyte Balance . . . 127
II. Premedication . . . 128
E. Anesthetic Management . . . 129
I. Regional Anesthesia . . . 130
II. General Anesthesia . . . 131
III. Monitoring . . . 134
F. Postoperative Care . . . 135
I. Circulatory Complications . . . 136
II. Respiratory Disorders . . . 137
References . . . 141

Surgery

Gastrointestinal Surgery in the Elderly.
D.E.F. TWEEDLE and P.F. SCHOFIELD

A. Introduction . . . 152
B. Hiatus Hernia and Reflux Oesophagitis . . . 152
C. Carcinoma of the Oesophagus . . . 153
D. Carcinoma of the Stomach . . . 155
E. Peptic Ulceration . . . 156
I. Gastric Ulceration . . . 157
II. Duodenal Ulceration . . . 158
F. Gallstones . . . 159
I. Cholelithiasis . . . 159
II. Choledocholithiasis . . . 160
III. Cholelithiasis and Choledocholithiasis . . . 161
IV. Complications of Gallstones . . . 161
1. Acute Pancreatitis . . . 161
2. Carcinoma of the Gallbladder . . . 162
G. Carcinoma of the Pancreas . . . 162
H. Carcinoma of the Periampullary Region . . . 163
J. Carcinoma of the Large Intestine . . . 163

I. Colonic Adenomas 165
1. Treatment 165
II. Large Bowel Carcinoma 166
1. Prophylaxis 166
2. Treatment of Carcinoma of the Colon 166
3. Treatment of Rectal Carcinoma 166
4. Other Methods 167
5. Supplementary Treatment 167
K. Anal Tumors 168
L. Diverticular Disease 168
I. Infective Complications 169
II. Fistulas 170
III. Massive Bleeding 170
M. Colitis in the Eldery 171
N. Rectal Prolapse and Incontinence 172
References 173

Surgery in Old Age – Fractures. J.K. WEBB. With 7 Figures

A. Introduction 177
B. Osteoporosis 178
C. Osteomalacia 181
D. Paget's Disease 181
E. Fractures 182
I. Femoral Neck 182
II. Trochanteric Fractures 186
III. Diaphyseal Fractures 186
IV. Supracondylar Fractures 188
V. Tibial Plateau Fractures 189
VI. Tibial Fracture 190
VII. Ankle Fracture 190
VIII. Upper Limb Fractures 190
F. Conclusion 190
References 191

The Prostate in the Elderly. A. BASSO. With 8 Figures

A. Introduction 193
B. Hormonal Control of Prostatic Growth 193
C. Benign Prostatic Hyperplasia 194
D. Prostatitis 199
I. Acute Bacterial Prostatitis 200
II. Chronic Bacterial Prostatitis 200
III. Nonbacterial Prostatitis 201
IV. Prostatodynia 201
E. Prostatic Adenocarcinoma 201
I. Surgical Treatment 205

II. Radiation Therapy 206
III. Hormonal Therapy 207
IV. Chemotherapy 208
V. Conclusions 208
References 209

Thoracic Surgery in the Elderly: Heart and Vessels.
M. PANETH

A. Definition 213
B. Principles of Cardiac Surgery 213
I. Support of the Whole Patient 213
II. Protection of the Heart 214
1. Coronary Perfusion 214
2. Intermittent Ischaemia 214
3. Cold Cardioplegia 215
III. Correction of Lesion 216
IV. Haemostasis 216
C. Technique 217
I. Exposure 217
II. Cannulation 217
1. Aorta 217
2. Right Atrium and Cavae 218
3. Left Ventricular Decompression 218
D. The Lesions 218
I. Congenital 218
1. Atrial Septal Defect 219
2. Persistent Ductus Arteriosus 219
3. Coarctation 220
II. Acquired 221
1. Ischaemia 221
a) Angina 221
b) Left Ventricular Aneurysm 221
c) Ventricular Septal Defect 222
d) Mitral Regurgitation 223
2. Degenerative 224
a) Valve Defects 224
α) The Aortic Valve 224
β) The Mitral Valve 225
γ) Ruptured Chordae 225
b) Aorta 226
α) Annuloaortic Ectasia and Aneurysms 226
β) Dissections of the Aorta 226
E. Postoperative Support 227
I. Intraaortic Balloon Counterpulsation 227
II. Left Ventricular Assist Devices 228

Pulmonary and Oesophageal Surgery in the Elderly.
H.C. NOHL-OSER. With 3 Figures

A. Pulmonary Surgery . . . 229
I. Introduction . . . 229
II. Carcinoma of the Bronchus . . . 230
1. Pathology . . . 230
2. Staging . . . 232
3. Presentation . . . 232
a) Symptoms . . . 232
b) Febrile Chest Illness . . . 232
c) Unusual Manifestations . . . 233
d) Asymptomatic Lesions Discovered on Routine Chest Radiography . . . 233
4. Diagnostic Investigations . . . 233
a) Radiology . . . 234
b) Cytology . . . 234
c) Bronchoscopy . . . 234
d) Mediastinoscopy . . . 235
e) Percutaneous Lung Biopsy . . . 235
f) Pleural Biopsy . . . 235
g) Exploratory Thoracotomy . . . 236
5. Assessment . . . 236
a) General Condition . . . 236
b) Heart and Circulation . . . 237
c) Respiratory System . . . 237
d) Kidney . . . 238
e) Liver . . . 239
f) Metabolism . . . 239
g) Summary . . . 239
6. Preoperative Treatment . . . 240
7. Choice of Operation . . . 240
8. Postoperative Management . . . 241
9. Palliative Treatment . . . 242
10. Summary . . . 242
III. Empyema . . . 242
1. Treatment . . . 243
2. Acute Empyema . . . 243
3. Intercostal Drainage . . . 244
4. Rib Resection and Drainage . . . 244
IV. Spontaneous Pneumothorax . . . 245
V. Emphysematous Cysts . . . 246
VI. Retrosternal Goitre . . . 246
VII. Chest Trauma . . . 247
B. Oesophageal Surgery . . . 248
I. Introduction . . . 248
1. Assessment . . . 248

2. Radiographic Examination 248
3. Endoscopy 249
4. Manometry and pH Studies 249
II. Carcinoma of the Oesophagus 250
1. Pathology 250
2. Symptoms 251
3. Clinical Assessment 251
4. Preoperative Management 251
5. Treatment by Resection 252
a) Carcinoma of the Cardia 253
b) Carcinoma of the Lower Third of the Oesophagus 254
c) Carcinoma of the Middle Third of the Oesophagus 254
d) Carcinoma Above the Aortic Arch 254
e) Transhiatal Oesophagectomy Without Thoractomy 255
6. Postcricoid Carcinoma 255
7. Postoperative Management 256
8. Nonresectable Carcinoma 257
9. Radiotherapy 257
III. Hiatus Hernia and Gastro-Oesophageal Reflux 258
1. Management 259
2. Antireflux Fundoplication Operation 260
IV. Strictures 260
V. Neuromuscular Disorders of the Oesophagus 261
VI. Pharyngeal Diverticulum 262
1. Operation 262
VII. Intrathoracic Oesophageal Pulsion Diverticulum . . . 262
VIII. Achalasia of the Oesophagus 263
1. Preoperative Oesophagoscopy 263
2. Treatment 264
3. Preoperative Treatment 264
IX. Diffuse Oesophageal Spasm 265
X. Scleroderma 265
References 266

Otorhinolaryngology

Otolaryngology in the Elderly. C. BECK. With 10 Figures

A. Introduction 270
B. Ear 270
I. Inner Ear 270
1. Presbycusis 270
a) Morphological Findings 271
b) Impairment of Function 272
c) Contributory Factors 274

d) Consequences of Presbycusis 275
e) Treatment 275
2. Vertigo in the Elderly 277
II. External and Middle Ear 277
C. Nose and Paranasal Sinuses 278
I. External Nose 278
II. Mucosa of Nose and Paranasal Sinuses 278
III. Olfactory Impairment 280
IV. Epistaxis 280
D. Pharynx and Salivary Glands 280
I. Mucosal Changes 280
II. Loss of Taste 281
III. Salivary Glands 281
E. Larynx 283
I. Morphological Findings 283
1. Macroscopic Changes 283
2. Histologic Findings 283
a) Laryngeal Cartilages 283
b) Mucosa 284
c) Vocal Folds 284
II. The Voice in Old Age 285
F. Therapeutic Aspects 287
I. Conservative Treatment 287
II. Ear, Nose, and Throat Operations in the Elderly 287
1. General Aspects 287
2. Specialized Aspects 288
G. Malignant Ear, Nose, and Throat Conditions in the Elderly . 289
H. Concluding Remarks 290
References 290

Ophthalmology

Aging of the Eyelids. H. MEYTHALER. With 13 Figures

A. Significance of the Lid in Vision 298
B. Lid Changes Caused by Aging 298
I. Senile Atrophy 298
II. Senile Pigment Abnormalities 299
III. Blepharochalasis 299
IV. Bags Under the Eyes 300
V. Fat Hernia 300
VI. Senile Blepharophimosis 300
VII. Seborrheic Dermatitis 301
C. Anomalies in the Position of the Lids Caused by Aging . . . 301
I. Senile Ectropion 301
II. Senile Entropion 301

D. Motor Disorders of Lid Function Caused by Aging 302
I. Senile Ptosis 302
E. Tumors of the Lid 302
I. Pseudocancerous Lesions 303
II. Precancerous Lesions 304
III. Squamous Cell Carcinoma 305
IV. Sebaceous Gland Carcinoma 305
V. Basal Cell Carcinoma 305
References 308

The Eye in the Aging Patient: Cornea. M. Reim. With 11 Figures

A. Structure of the Cornea 310
I. Epithelium 310
II. Stroma 310
III. Endothelium 310
IV. Metabolism 311
V. Physiology 311
B. Senile Changes of the Cornea 311
I. Clinically Visible Signs of Aging 311
1. Arcus Senilis 311
2. Increased Shagreen of the Aged Cornea 312
3. Line of Stähli 312
4. White Limbus Girdle of Vogt 312
5. Cornea Guttata 312
II. Clinical Changes Detectable by Special Techniques . . . 313
1. Thickness of the Cornea 313
2. Sensitivity of the Cornea 314
3. Specular Microscopy of the Endothelium 314
a) Number of Cells 314
b) Cell Distribution 315
4. Swelling Properties of the Stroma 316
5. Regenerative Power of the Epithelium 316
6. The Endothelium in Old Donors 318
III. Microscopic Changes in Old Age 318
1. Descemet's Membrane 318
2. Basement Membrane of the Epithelium 319
3. Collagen Fibrils 319
IV. Biochemical Changes in Old Age 319
1. Collagen 319
2. Glycosaminoglycans 320
3. Lipids, Physical and Chemical Explanation of Arcus Senilis 321
a) Lipid Spectra 321
b) Precipitation of Lipoproteins 322
c) Arcus Senilis and the Blood Level of Lipoproteins 322

4. Metabolism 323
V. Diseases of the Cornea Not Specific for Old Age 323
References 323

Age-Related Changes in the Anterior Segment of the Eye.
J.W. ROHEN and E. LÜTJEN-DRECOLL. With 12 Figures

A. Introduction 326
B. Cornea 326
I. Stroma 327
II. Descemet's Membrane 328
III. Corneal Endothelium 330
C. Trabecular Meshwork 331
I. Trabecular Beams 333
II. Cribriform Layer 336
III. Trabecular Cells 337
D. Ciliary Body 338
I. Ciliary Muscle 338
II. Ciliary Processes 340
III. Ciliary Epithelium 341
IV. Zonular Apparatus and Internal Limiting Membrane . . 344
E. Iris 345
I. Anterior Border Layer 347
II. Pigment Epithelium 347
References 347

Aqueous Humor and Vitreous Production. K. GREEN, E.A. BALAZS, and J.L. DENLINGER. With 1 Figure

A. Aqueous Humor 352
I. Volume 352
II. Composition 353
III. Intraocular Pressure 354
IV. Formation 356
V. Outflow 358
VI. Summary 359
B. Vitreous 360
I. Structure 360
II. Composition 362
1. Sodium Hyaluronate 363
2. Collagen 363
III. Basement Membranes 364
IV. Posterior Vitreous Detachment 364
V. Summary 366
References 367

The Eye in the Elderly: Lens. O. HOCKWIN and C. OHRLOFF. With 36 Figures

A. Introduction 373
B. Lens Structure 375
I. History of Development 375
II. Anatomy of the Lens 377
III. Histology and Fine Structure of the Lens 378
C. Growth of the Lens 379
I. Lens Weight 380
II. Lens Weight and Volume in Relation to Age 380
III. Specific Weight of the Lens 380
IV. Diameter of Equator: Lens Thickness 381
V. Lens Volume/Eye Volume 381
VI. Lens Biometry with Respect to Accommodation 382
D. Nutritional Supply of the Lens 382
I. Aqueous Humor Composition 382
II. Changes of Aqueous Humor Composition by the Lens . 382
III. Changes of Lens Properties by Aqueous Humor 383
IV. Aqueous Composition in Aphakic Eyes 383
V. Aqueous Composition and Age 383
VI. The Lens as Part of an Open Biologic System 383
E. Light Transmission of the Lens 385
I. Transparency for Visible and Ultraviolet Light 385
II. Disturbances of Transparency 385
III. Lens Fluorescence 386
IV. Applications of Scheimpflug Photography 386
1. Lens Photography 386
2. Densitometric Image Analysis 387
3. Calculation of the Methodological Error 391
F. The Lens and Aging 394
I. Presbyopia 394
II. Age Changes of Lens Transparency, Development of Lens Opacities 396
III. Age Changes of Biochemical Lens Properties 399
1. Protein Metabolism 402
a) Deamidation and Degradation 406
b) Disulfide Bridges and Other Covalent Cross-Links 406
c) Racemization of Aspartic Acid 406
d) Nonenzymatic Glycosylation 406
2. Enzymes and Energy Metabolism 407
IV. Age Changes of Lens Morphology 412
G. Senile Cataract as a Result of Multifactorial Origin 413
I. Surgical Therapy 415
II. Drug Treatment of Lens Opacities 415
References 417

The Aging Retina. R.A. WEALE. With 12 Figures

A. Introduction . . . 425
B. A Dilemma . . . 425
C. Structural Changes in Homo sapiens . . . 426
I. Vasculature . . . 428
II. Changes in the Pigment Epithelium . . . 431
III. Outer Nuclear Layer and Photoreceptors . . . 436
D. Objective Indices of Retinal Function . . . 440
I. The Electro-retinogram . . . 440
II. The Electro-oculogram . . . 441
III. The Early Receptor Potential . . . 441
E. Subjective Information on the Senescent Retina . . . 441
I. Visual Resolution . . . 442
II. Dark Adaptation . . . 444
Appendix . . . 447
References . . . 447

Dermatology

Physiologic and Pathologic Alterations in Old Skin.
BARBARA A. GILCHREST. With 1 Figure

A. Overview . . . 452
B. Age-Associated Changes in Normal Skin . . . 452
I. Morphologic and Histologic Changes . . . 452
II. Physiologic Changes . . . 454
III. Biochemical and Biophysical Changes . . . 456
C. Age-Associated Pathologic Processes in the Skin . . . 456
I. Decubitus Ulcers . . . 456
II. Xerosis . . . 458
III. Pruritus . . . 458
IV. Herpes Zoster . . . 458
V. Bullous Pemphigoid . . . 460
VI. Skin Cancer . . . 460
1. Epidemiology . . . 460
2. Possible Age-Associated Risk Factors . . . 461
3. Prevention and Treatment of Skin Cancer in the Elderly . . . 461
VII. Dermatoheliosis (Sun-Induced Aging) . . . 462
References . . . 463

Subject Index . . . 465

Gynecology

Pre- and Postmenopause

C. Lauritzen

A. The Premenopause

In the premenopause a significant decrease of the mean ovarian estrogen production of plasma and tissue values occurs. Follicle-stimulating hormone (FSH) rises more than luteinizing hormone (LH) and accordingly the LH : FSH ratio falls. The incidence of ovulations diminishes, luteal insufficiency or absence of corpus luteum is frequent (monophasic cycle). As a consequence, endometrial hyperproliferation, anomalies of the cycle, and of menstrual bleeding may occur. Myomas become symptomatic. The incidence of curettage and hysterectomy rises. Premenstrual syndrome, mastopathy, and migraine are more common. Benign and malignant genital and breast tumors are more often found. Typical climacteric complaints (mostly of low to medium severity) occur in about 20% during the premenopause while they occur in 60%–84% during the postmenopausal period. Hot flushes are relatively rare, while irritability, nervousness, and depression are relatively more frequent. Neuroses and psychotic reactions show up more often in this age period.

The treatment consists in a correction of the cycle anomalies by progestogen administration during the second phase of the cycle or with a sequential estrogen–progestogen from day 5 to day 25. Also, low doses of estriol may be adequate. There is moreover a place for diverse psychotropic measures.

B. The Menopause

The menopause is the moment of the last menstrual bleeding still governed by ovarian hormonal function. It occurs at about 52 ± 3 years (see chapter by Benedek-Jaszmann). Thereafter the postmenopause begins. The period of pre- and postmenopause is called the perimenopause or climacteric. It ends, when the senium begins (60–65 years).

I. Causes of the Climacteric

The climacteric is the consequence of an ovarian primary insufficiency which occurs physiologically during the fifth and sixth decade of life. It results from an aging of the female reproductive glands which occurs earlier then aging of the other endocrine glands. As the ovarian reproductive and endocrine structures regress,

Table 1. Incidence of climacteric complaints in the different stages of the climacteric in outpatients of the Department of Gynecology, University of Ulm

Complaints (%)	Premenopause	Menopause	Postmenopause	
			1–3 years	>3 years
Hot flushes	36	69	74	42
Sweating	28	58	67	31
Dizziness	14	33	41	25
Tingling	8	20	28	11
Depression	26	72	76	58
Nervousness	67	51	48	22
Irritability	65	49	46	17
Tension	44	40	33	25
Headache	41	31	24	19
Sleeplessness	53	56	63	41
Anxiety	33	44	26	12

their estrogen production and secretion declines. Accordingly, the estrogen concentration in blood, target organs, and target cells decreases and the conditions of estrogen deficiency arise.

II. Consequences of Estrogen Decrease

As for the hypothalamopituitary–ovarian feedback system, the ovarian failure creates an open-loop defect. Gonadotrophin-releasing hormones and gonadotrophins are secreted in increased amounts. However, this gonadotrophic hypersecretion is futile as the ovaries no longer respond. The gonadotrophin rise lasts for 10–15 years, then decreases in the senium. Estrogens in the plasma fall off below 40 pg estrone and 20 pg estradiol; total estrogens in 24-h urine samples decrease to less than 10 μg. These estrogens are mainly of adrenal origin from androgens such as androstenedione, testosterone, and dehydroepiandrosterone. The ovaries no longer contribute estrogens; however, in some cases they still secrete small amounts of androgens. These androgens are converted in to estrone by the subcutaneous fat tissue to the extent of 1%–3%.

The decrease of estrogens also disturbs the balance of the autonomic nervous system. The brain is a target organ for estrogens. These influence brain hormones and are metabolized in the brain tissue. Because of the withdrawal of the parasympathomimetic stabilizing effect of the estrogens on the hypothalamic centers, hypersympathotonic attacks occur, which are mediated to the periphery by the cervical sympathicus and manifest themselves as hot flushes and sweating. These typical climacteric complaints occur in about 70% of all climacteric patients. They may begin 1–2 years before menopause, have their maximum 2–3 years after menopause, and usually diminish in the following years (Table 1). Estrogens exert psychotropic effects. They regulate the production and metabolism of biogenic amines and enzymes in the brain, which influence the state of mind. Estrogen withdrawal therefore often creates a state of decreased mental well-being, depression, nervousness, and irritability, which adversely affects the quality of life. Affective symptoms can be registered in about 60% of all climacteric patients (see chapter by KOPERA).

It is later, namely 5–10 years after the menopause, that atrophic changes become evident in the urogenital tract. The epithelia of the outer genitalia, of the inner genital tract, and of the urethra and bladder show a thinning of the epithelial and tissue layers and a decrease of proliferation. Also, the blood perfusion and water-binding capacity are decreased. The elasticity and the turgor of the supporting tissues diminishes. The consequence is an atrophy of the vulva and of the vagina, urethra, and bladder with many different complaints such as: pruritus, discharge, dyspareunia, descensus of vagina and uterus, as well as urinary urge and stress incontinence. The skin becomes atrophic, dry, inelastic, and wrinkled and estrogen withdrawal apparently plays a significant part in this process.

The metabolism of female bone is partly dependent on estrogen. Estrogen deficiency causes a loss of bone mass by an increase of osteoclast activity and thus may lead to postmenopausal osteoporosis, which occurs in a high proportion of postmenopausal women. Fractures of radius, hip, ribs, and spine may occur and the morbidity and mortality of postmenopausal osteoporosis is a grave sociomedical problem.

In summary, estrogen deficiency may cause a lot of very unpleasant neurologic, psychotropic, atrophic, and metabolic symptoms, some of which are on the borderline of severe disturbance of body homeostasis or even overt disease.

III. Treatment

1. Indications

In most of the cases with severe complaints, genital, or metabolic alterations, there is a clear indication for hormone substitution according to the rules of endocrinology as in the case of hormonal insufficiency of any other endocrine gland. The need for hormone replacement therapy can be determined by the answer to two questions:

1. Will the fall in estrogen cause severe subjective or objective deficiency syndromes which adversely affect the quality of life?
2. Will the hormonal insufficiency have a negative effect on the health, physical, and mental fitness, ability to work, self-reliance, and self-fulfilment of the individual? Will it disturb social well-being? Will it even provoke diseases which might reduce life expectancy?

If the answer is yes or probably yes, the indication for treatment is clear.

2. Contraindications

Before the treatment is begun, the patient has to be thoroughly informed as to the possibilities and risks of the therapy. Contraindications and risk factors have to be controlled and accordingly the most suitable preparation and mode of administration has to be selected. A gynecologic checkup is performed, a Pa-

Table 2. Contraindications to estrogen therapy in the climacteric

Absolute contraindications	
Severe liver diseases	
Cholestasis	
Porphyria	
Estrogen-dependent tumors	
Untreated mammary and endometrial cancer	
Malignant melanoma	
Hypertension	
Cerebral apoplexy	
Cerebral and retinal vascular diseases	
Severe therapy-resistant migraine	
Deep venous thrombosis and emboly	
Sickle cell anemia	
Relative contraindications (individual decision):	
Strict supervision, low estrogen doses	Mastopathia fibrosa cystica
Estriol?	Severe diabetes with hypertension and vascular disease
Consider combination with progestogen or androgen	Hyperlipidemia
Additional medical therapy	Cardiac and nephrogenic edema
	Severe migraine
	Severe epilepsy
	Pancreatitis
	Cholecystitis
	Cholelithiasis
	High cancer risk
Withdrawal of estrogen necessary	Allergic reaction
	Aggravation of migraine and headache
	Permanent nausea
	Icterus
	Gall bladder complaints
	Pancreatitis
	Deep venous thrombosis
	Impending operation
	Impending endocrine investigation
	Newly detected endometrial and mammary cancer
Dose reduction	Breast complaints
Consider addition of a progestogen	Cervical discharge
Change preparation (estriol?)	Endometrial hyperplasia
	Uterine bleeding
	Weight increase
	Hypertension
	Edema
	Hyperpigmentation

panicolaou smear test is done; in cases with endometrial risk, an office aspiration curettage is to be considered. The contraindications to treatment with estrogens are listed in Table 2.

In treatment with estrogen–progestogen, there is so far no mode of administration which is completely satisfactory according the pharmacokinetic criteria and which really mimics the normal process of estrogen–progesterone secretion of the ovaries. Oral medication is certainly the method which allows the best individualization and modulation of daily dose. However direct resorption from the stomach to the liver causes some unwanted supraphysiologic stimulatory reactions such as changes in lipids and coagulation factors, which account for some unpleasant or even dangerous side effects at higher doses. Injections are indicated when the patient has stomach complaints or is an unreliable pill taker. After passage through the intestine, estradiol changes mostly to estrone. The drawback with injections and implants is that the individual dose is less variable, resorption is unpredictable, the application is irreversible, and the dose released is not subjected to normal feedback regulation. Percutaneous administration of estrogens is a new and promising possibility.

3. Preparations

Oral estrone sulfate, micronized estradiol, conjugated estrogens, and estradiol valerate are about equally effective. At ages 45–45 years, the estrogen should be given in sequence with a progestogen during the second phase of treatment for at least 12 days. Estriol is, on a weight basis, less effective in the treatment of climacteric complaints and psychotropic effects. It influences the metabolism of lipids and coagulation factors only in very high doses. It does not prevent osteoporosis. Estriol also has a very low endometriotropic effect. However estriol is as effective as the other natural estrogens in its proliferating action on the vagina, urethra, and trigonum urethrae.

Injections of estradiol valerate, combined with androgens such as dehydroepiandrosterone enanthate and testosterone valerate are very effective and well tolerated. They have beneficial effects especially against climacteric complaints and depression. Dehydroepiandrosterone is not a virilizing agent. However, testosterone may cause deepening of the voice, hirsutism, and stimulation of libido. Therefore, it should be given with caution and the patient should be made aware of these side effects.

4. Therapeutic Effectiveness

The therapeutic effects of oral estrogens on typical climacteric complaints (and also on other subjective symptoms: nervousness, irritability, depression, and others) have been proven beyond doubt. In open investigations as well as in double-blind studies in comparison with placebos and in crossover studies, a highly significant success rate of more than 90% has been achieved (Tables 3 and 4).

5. Dose

The usual dose of oral estrogens is: 10–25 μg ethinylestradiol; 1–2 mg estrone sulfate; 2–4 mg micronized estradiol; 0.6–1.25 mg conjugated estrogens; 1–2 mg estradiol valerate; and 2–6 mg estriol or estriol succinate. Higher doses of estrogens should not be given. If estrogens are not sufficient, small doses of androgens or, in the case of special psychotropic complaints, tranquilizers or even antidepressants should be added.

Table 3. Results of the treatment of climacteric hot flushes with estrogens

Preparation	No. of patients	Dose (mg/day)	Complaints (%)	Improved (%)	Unchanged (%)
Oral	68	1.0	79	17	4
Estradiol valerate	117	2.0	89	11	0
Estradiol (micronized)	50	2.0	80	18	2
	20	4.0	86	14	0
Estriol	112	2.0	68	22	10
	57	4.0	73	19	8
	31	6.0	80	16	4
Estriol succinate	78	4.0	71	20	9
	50	6.0	80	16	4
Injection: intramuscular depot polyestriolphosphate	89	80 mg/month	81	16	3
Estradiol valerate + dehydroepiandrosterone enanthate (Prasteron)	59	4 mg +200 mg/month	79	21	0
Estradiol valerate + testosterone enanthate	51	4 mg +90.3 mg/month	96	4	0

Table 4. Double-blind crossover-study with conjugated estrogens, estriol, and placebo (126 cases)

Complaints	No. of patients with complaints before therapy (=100%)	Remaining complaints[a] after 8 weeks therapy (%)			
		Conjugated estrogens 1.25 mg/day	Placebo (milk, sugar)	Estriol	
				2.0 mg/day	4.0 mg/day
Hot flushes	122	3	87	12	2
Sweating	120	4	90	8	4
Vertigo	103	3	94	6	5
Palpitation	94	10	92	14	7
Irritability	87	6	88	8	4
Anxiety	63	8	97	10	6
Insomnia	56	14	90	13	10
Depression	46	6	95	9	5
Headaches	33	13	97	17	8

[a] Estriol 2 mg versus placebo; all complaints $P<0.001$
Estriol 4 mg versus placebo; all complaints $P<0.001$
Conjugated estrogens 1.25 mg versus placebo; all complaints $P<0.001$

a) Genital Atrophy

In atrophic changes of the urogenital system, equally good results have been reported as regards findings and symptoms (Table 5). A thickening of the atrophic vaginal epithelium occus within 2 weeks; the atrophic vaginal smear shows pro-

Table 5. Estrogen treatment of atrophic changes in the urogenital system (563 patients; conjugated estrogens 1.25 mg/day 3 months; LAURITZEN 1975)

	Result of treatment (%)		
	Cured	Improved	Unchanged
Atrophic colpitis	84	16	
Kraurosis vaginae with intercourse problems	69	22	9
Kraurosis vulvae with dyspareunia	62	27	11
Atrophic urethrocystitis	57	39	4

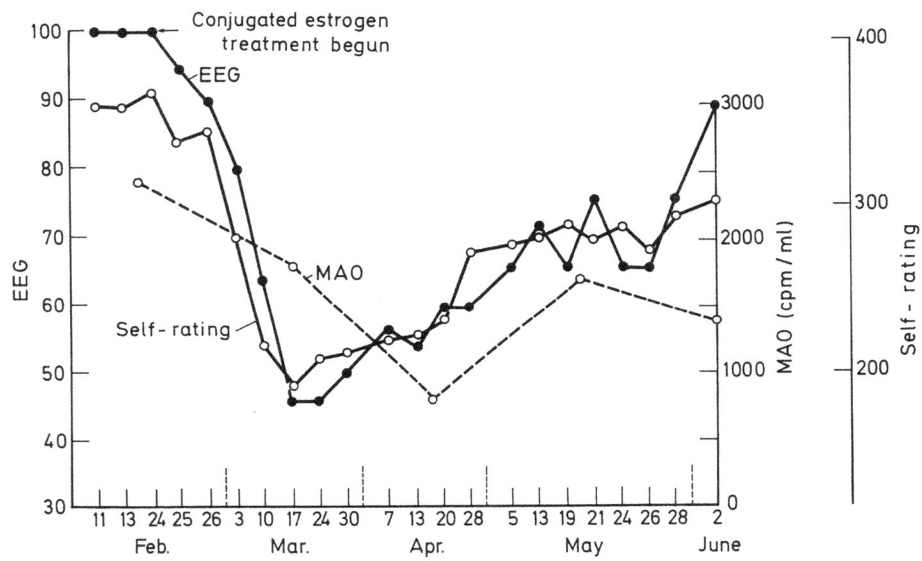

Fig. 1. Improvement of self-rating, EEG curves, and normalization of monoamine oxidase (MAO) levels in plasma following conjugated estrogen treatment (ITIL et al. 1976)

liferation. Sexual reaction and vaginal transudation is restored, atrophic colpitis, discharge, and dyspareunia may disappear. Kraurosis vulvae (lichen sclerosus et atrophicus) with pruritus requires long-term treatment with local estradiol or estriol and parenteral estrogens; urinary frequency, dysuria, and urethral burning as well as ectropium urethrae are readily improved by estrogens if atrophy is the cause. Also first-degree stress incontinence will be ameliorated to continence in more than 90% of the cases by estradiol, estrone, and estriol preparations in the usual doses within 2 weeks.

b) Psychotropic Effects

The many psychic symptoms of estrogen deficiency are equilibrated by estrogen substitution. Estrogens produce a specific feeling of well-being. Anxiety, worry, nervousness, irritability, sleeplessnes, and depression disappear in a very high

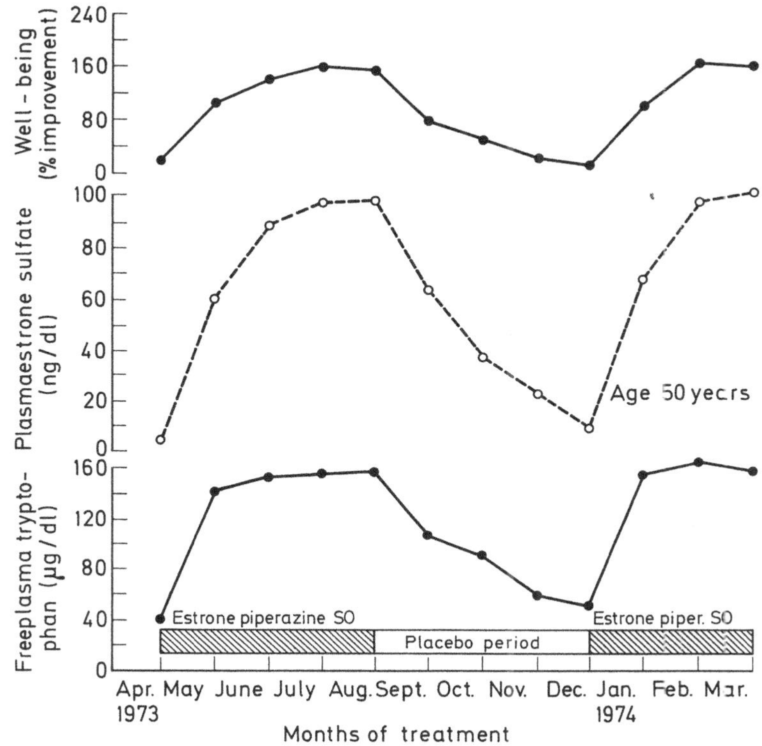

Fig. 2. Increase of well-being (Hamilton rating scale) and of free plasma tryptophan occurring simultaneously with the increase of estrone sulfate following oral estrogen medication (AYLWARD 1976)

proportion of cases. Concentration, alertness, and psychomotor efficiency as well as readiness for social contact improve. In self-rating scale scores, there is a normalization of feeling, well-being, and quality of life. The pathologic α-waves in depressive patients disappear (Fig. 1). There is also a biochemical correlate. The concentration of the enzyme monoamine oxidase (MAO) which is increased in blood and tissues in depressive patients, decreases to normal values (Fig. 1). Another mechanism of the antidepressive effect of estrogens is the increase of free plasma tryptophan (Fig. 2). Estrogens displace tryptophan from its plasma binding and the free amino acid is then biologically available for passage into the brain, where it is used as a precursor for the biosynthesis of serotonin, which regulates psychic processes.

c) Osteoporosis

This bone disease, which is mainly found in older postmenopausal women, is characterized by thinning of the bone cortex by increased osteoclast activity, decrease in plasma calcium, and increased loss of calcium and hydroxyproline in morning urine and feces. Spontaneous or slight trauma bone fractures of radius,

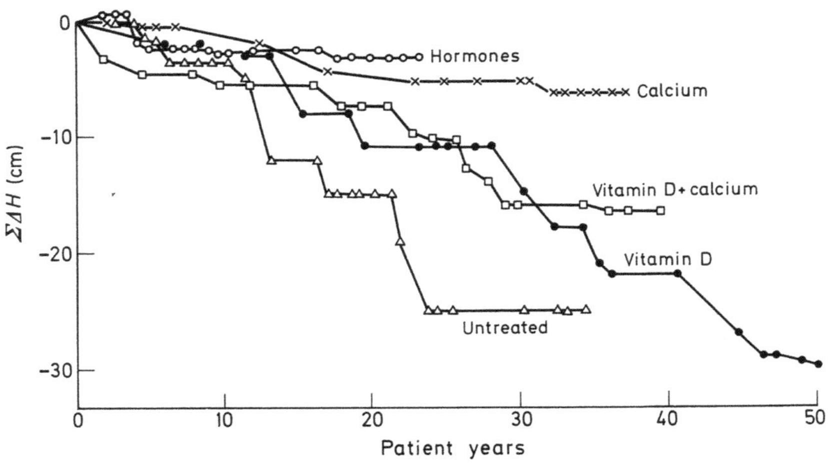

Fig. 3. Cumulative plot of changes in height $\Sigma \Delta H$ during estrogen therapy, compared with other treatments and untreated patients (MARSHALL et al. 1973)

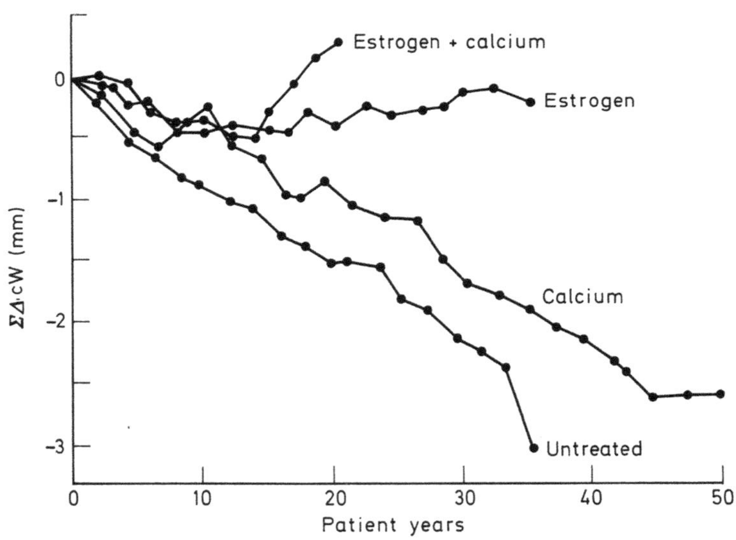

Fig. 4. Cumulative changes in mean metacarpal cortical width $\Sigma \Delta cW$ in four groups of normal postmenopausal women: untreated, calcium-treated, estrogen-treated, and treated with calcium + estrogen (MARSHALL et al. 1977)

hip, and ribs, and infractions of the vertebra occur with all their sequelae of hospitalization, morbidity, and mortality and at high cost to the community. Women in the postmenopause usually show a loss in their body height as a consequence of vertebral spine osteoporosis and kyphosis of the vertebral column. This can be prevented and, when already present, stopped by estrogens (Fig. 3). In prospective double-blind studies with patients receiving estrogens in comparison with a

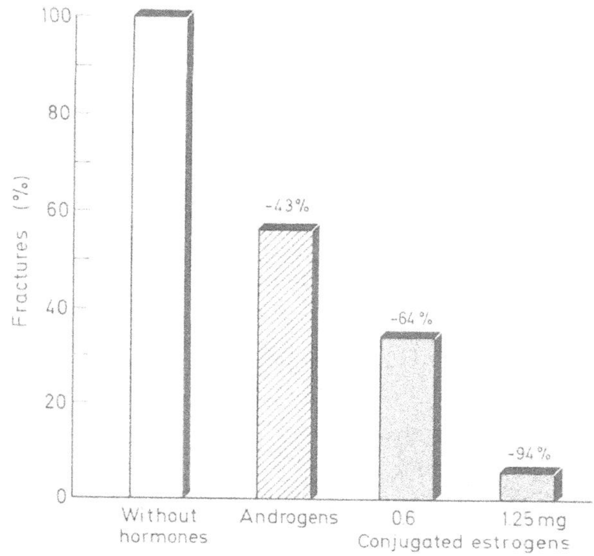

Fig. 5. Incidence of bone fractures in cases of androgen and estrogen prophylaxis against osteoporosis; 1,507 patient years (GORDON 1977)

placebo, it could be demonstrated that estrogen-substituted patients experienced no loss of metacarpal cortical width while controls, or patients treated with calcium only, did (Fig. 4).

In clinical retrospective studies, it was shown that androgens and conjugated estrogens in prophylactic long-term medication reduced the incidence of bone fractures dramatically to very low rates (Fig. 5). Thus, this effect of estrogens is one of the main arguments in favor of long-term treatment with estrogens.

d) The Skin

After castration and following natural menopause, a thinning of the epidermis occurs. In vitro, the incorporation of labeled amino acids such as valine and thymidine is decreased (Table 6). Estrogen medication reverses skin atrophy and stimulates mitosis, proliferation, and thickening of the epidermis. Water binding and elasticity are increased by extracellular sodium–water retention and stimulation of hyaluronic acid. Blood perfusion, skin temperature, and conduction are improved. In clinical studies, the profile of skin wrinkles is lessened.

6. Side Effects

The subjective side effects of oral and parenteral estrogen medication are remarkably slight. All natural estrogens are well tolerated. Exceptions occur mostly in placebo reactors or neurotics. Gastrointestinal symptoms dissappear when the estrogens are given after meals with large amounts of fluid. Leg cramps, water retention, hyperpigmentation, mastopathia, mastodynia, and cervical hypersecretion are seen only when excessively high estrogen doses are given. Nausea, ten-

Table 6. Influence of oophorectomy and estrogen treatment on epidermal thickness and thymidine incorporation in epidermal nuclei (RAURAMO and PUNNONEN 1973)

Thickness of epidermis (μm)			
Before castration	After castration		
	1 month	4 months	7 months
48.9 ± 0.5		44.6 ± 0.5	42.0 ± 0.4
	After estriol succinate 2 mg/day		
41.8 ± 0.5		50.0 ± 0.5	50.0 ± 0.4
	After estradiol valerate 2 mg/day		
43.3 ± 0.4		48.9 ± 0.6	46.5 ± 0.4
Incorporation of thymidine ^3H			
Thymidine ^3H index			
Before castration	After castration		
25.7 ± 2.7	13.1 ± 3.4	14.3 ± 3.4	18.6 ± 3.3
	After estriol succinate 2 mg/day		
17.0 ± 3.9		26.1 ± 3.2	30.9 ± 2.3
	After estradiol valerate 2 mg/day		
9.2 ± 3.1		31.9 ± 2.5	28.5 ± 3.2

Table 7. Frequency of uterine bleeding during cyclic medication with different oral estrogens in postmenopausal women

Estrogen	Dose (mg/day)	Uterine bleeding	
		(% of women)	(% of cycles)
Conjugated estrogens	1.25	8	0.3
	0.6	3	0.1
Estradiol valerate	2.0	10	0.3
	1.0	4	0.1
Micronized estradiol	2.0	16	0.7
Estriol and estriol succinate	4.0	1.0	0.05
	2.0	0.8	0.03

sion, headache, hypertension, cholestasis, and an increase of liver enzymes are rarely found and disappear soon after dose reduction or withdrawal of the medication. Between the ages of 45 and 56 years, estrogen–progestogen sequential therapy is usually given, which leads to regular and normal uterine bleeding. When bleeding is undesired, estriol can be given, which is not endometriotropic and will therefore not have a proliferative effect on the endometrium; it has no withdrawal effect. When estrogens like estradiol, estrone, or conjugated estrogens are used in a cyclic dose distribution, uterine bleeding from proliferated or even hyperplastic endometrium may occur. The frequency of such bleeding is given in Table 7. Fractional curettage is then necessary.

Table 8. Statistics of estrogen intake in patients with the symptom menopausal and postmenopausal uterine bleeding, classified according to the histologic findings; Department of Gynecology, University of Ulm 1968–1977 (LAURITZEN et al. 1977)

No. of patients	Total	Endometrial cancer	Proliferated or hyperplastic[a] endometrium	Atrophic endometrium
	756	245	243	268
Estrogens taken	82 (10.8)[b]	11 (4.5)	39 (16.05)	32 (11.9)
Duration of intake				
≦6 months	11 (13.5)	3 (27.3)	4 (10.3)	4 (12.5)
6 month–2 years	44 (53.5)	6 (54.4)	22 (56.4)	16 (50.0)
>2 years	27 (33.0)	2 (18.2)	13 (33.3)	12 (33.5)

[a] Three cases of atypical hyperplasia
[b] Numbers in parentheses are percentages

7. Costs

The costs of estrogen treatment are relatively low and in any case no more expensive than, for instance, long-term therapy with antihypertensive drugs. Treatment for 1 month costs about DM 10 (U.S. $ 5) for conjugated estrogens or estradiol valerate. Estriol costs about DM 12–30 dependent on dose; injections estrogen–androgen cost about DM 15 per month.

8. Risks

a) Vascular Complications

While the frequency of thrombosis, pulmonary embolism, myocardial infarction, and cerebrovascular complications is increased in patients who are taking pills, this is not the case in perimenopausal patients, who recieve natural estrogens in usually lower equivalent doses. In retrospective studies, it has been shown that there is even an apparent protective effect of estrogens (Table 8). This effect may be mediated by the lowering of the lipids by estrogens. In particular, the low and very low density lipoproteins are decreased. The high density lipoprotein fraction, which seems to act as an antiatherosclerotic agent, is increased by estrogens, which is considered to be advantageous. Also, procoagulatory effects (as in the pill takers) are not seen in patients receiving natural estrogens in low therapeutic doses. Accordingly, the risk of severe vascular complications is low, even lower than in controls. Nevertheless, the risk factors have to be respected and, in patients who are at risk, the indications and contraindications must be considered.

As for the possible increase risk of endometrial cancer in estrogen takers, suggested by American investigations, it is worth mentioning that in all European retrospective studies, including our own (Table 9), no correlation of estrogen intake and incidence of endometrial cancer could be found. Recent American studies, where the estrogen was sequentially combined with a progestogen, noted no

Table 9. Relative risk of long-term estrogen-treated patients for endometrial cancer; retrospective case control study N = 458 patients compared with controls; Department of Gynecology, University of Ulm 1968–1978

	Duration of treatment (years)			
	Total	1–3	5–10	> 10 years
Conjugated estrogens	0.78	0.60	0.81	0.93
Estradiol valerate	0.73	0.71	0.79	0.86
Estriol A. succinate	0.34	0.27	0.39	0.35
Estradiol valerate + progestogen	0.21	0.20	0.24	0.22
Estradiol + androgen	0.55	0.56	0.47	0.60

Table 10. Adenocarcinoma of the endometrium; Wilford Hall U.S.A.F. Medical Center 1975–1976 (GAMBRELL 1978)

	Estrogen[a]	Estrogen – progestogen	Other hormones[b]	Untreated	Total
Postmenopausal women	1,694	2,391	364	864	5,313
Endometrial carcinoma	6	1	1	3	11
Incidence of cancer per 1,000 patient years	3.5	0.4	2.7	3.5	2.5

[a] Duration of treatment 1–30 years (mean 4.27 ± 3.61 years); 577 patients treated for more than 5 years (2 cases of cancer); 202 patients treated for more than 10 years (2 cases of cancer); 23 patients treated for more than 20 years (0 cases of cancer)

[b] Treatment with: estrogen vaginal ointment (217 patients): progestogens only (75 patients), androgens only (18 patients)

increase, but actually a reduction, in the risk of endometrial cancer (Tables 9 and 10). It seems significant that, in Europe, estrogen therapy was always given cyclically and that, whenever possible, progestogens inhibiting hyperproliferation were added in the second half of the medication. Estriol, which does not usually stimulate the endometrium, was given in a high proportion of our cases. Also, contraindications were better observed in Europe than in America. So, in my opinion, the American results may show what may happen at worst, when the basic rules of estrogen therapy have been neglected for many years. An increase in the risk of mammary cancer in estrogen-treated patients has not been seen so far.

b) Mortality

Morbidity and mortality are good parameters for assessing the value of a long-term treatment regimen. The studies so far presented show that long-term estrogen medication does not increase morbidity and mortality, but actually decreases them (Fig. 6; BURCH et al. 1975).

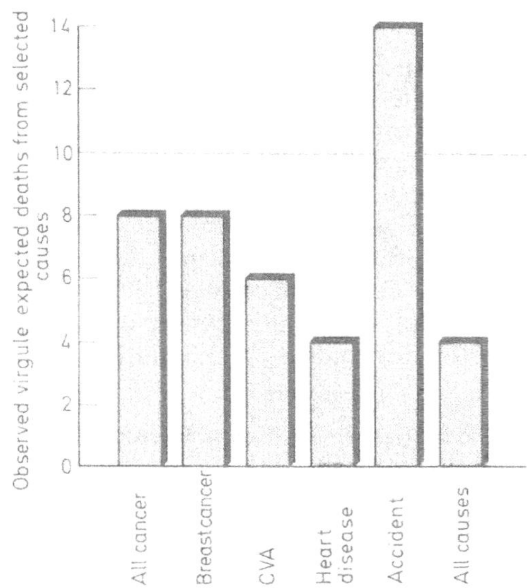

Fig. 6. Mortality of long-term estrogen-treated patients (BURCH et al. 1975)

9. Risk: Benefit Ratio

It is very difficult at present to establish a risk : benefit ratio or a cost : benefit ratio for estrogen–progestogen therapy in the climacteric. The evidence available suggests that the benefits, especially in terms of freedom from complaints, amelioration of the quality of life, and prophylaxis of postmenopausal osteoporosis with its consequences on morbidity, mortality, and sociomedical costs by far outweigh the possible risks of estrogen therapy. The basis of proper, successful, and safe therapy is a good indication, selection of the right preparation, observation of contraindications, exact controls, and optimal cooperation between therapist and patient. Estrogen therapy is a valuable tool for the treatment of climacteric complaints and has few adverse organic and metabolic sequelae in the hands of a wise therapist. However, much has still to be done in experimental and therapeutic research. I am quite sure that estrogen treatment can become still more effective, adequate, and safe by the use of new preparations and new modes of pharmacodynamic treatment, e.g., by the use of percutaneous, vaginal, or rectal administration.

10. Controls

Under estrogen–progestogen treatment, the patient has to be seen and checked every half year. Breasts and genitals have to be investigated, including a vaginal smear. If necessary, especially in cancer risk patients, mammography–thermography and suction curettage of the endometrium can be performed. Blood pressure and urinary status are controlled. The preparation can be changed and the dose adjusted, if necessary. Liver tests are only done if a special indication is found.

11. Duration of Treatment

The duration of treatment depends on the aim of the therapy. In women castrated early in life, the substitution lasts up to their fifties or even longer. When only climacteric complaints are treated, the medication will be given as long as the complaints occur, i.e., mostly for 2–3 years. When prophylaxis of osteoporosis is aimed at, the administration continues up to old age. On the whole, the treatment is given as long as is sensible and as long as no contraindications, severe side effects, or other grave problems occur. In our patients, the mean duration of treatment is 3.5 years. More than 30% maintain estrogen intake for more than 10 years. Most of the patients drop out of the treatment, mostly because they no longer have any complaints or because they fear side effects.

12. Summary of Treatment Recommendations

The selection of the preparation according to the wishes and needs of the patient is important and influences the rate of side effects. I propose the following recommendations for estrogen therapy in pre- and postmenopause.

1. Use the minimal effective doses. The treatment should be individualized.
2. Medication should always be cyclic with 1 week of interruption or dose reduction in week 4, except when estriol is given.
3. Sequential estrogen–progestogen therapy is recommended between the ages of 45 and 55 years. In patients who are at risk, the use of oral locally applied estriol should be considered if possible and sufficient.
4. The patients should be carefully supervised. A checkup is necessary every 6 months, when indication, mode of application, and dose should be scrutinized.
5. Risk factors and contraindications are to be observed.
6. When atypical bleeding occurs, curettage is necessary. In patients who are at risk, it is worth considering mammography and aspiration curettage once a year.
7. The treatment in the postmenopause should usually not last much longer than 5 years, except when special reasons exist.

C. Cancers

In older patients, the incidence of benign and malignant tumors increases greatly with a maximum at about 50–60 years of age. The most frequent tumor of the female primary and secondary sexual organs is mammary cancer. The second most frequent genital tumor is cervical, then endometrial, ovarian, vulvar, vaginal, and fallopian tube cancer. The age distribution of genital tumors is shown in Fig. 7.

I. Cancer of the Vulva

Primary cancer of the vulva accounts for approximately 5% of all cancers of the genitalia. In most cases, the lesion is a squamous cell carcinoma. Adenocar-

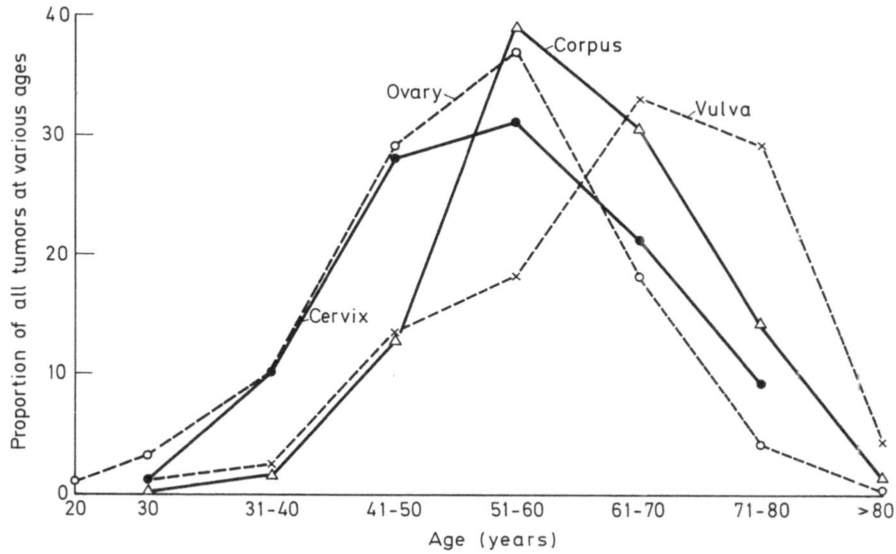

Fig. 7. Age-dependent frequency distribution of malignant tumors of the female genitalia, based on the total number of cases. The peak incidences of carcinoma of the vulva and corpus occur later than those of the cervix and ovary (BELLER et al. 1974)

cinoma of the Bartholin or sebaceous glands is rare, namely 0.2% of all genital carcinomas. Squamous cell carcinoma arises from a premalignant lesion in 30%–40% of cases, i.e., in 60%–70% the carcinomatous transformation appears without an antecedent premalignant stage. Cancer of the vulva ist most common in patients between the ages of 60 and 70 years. Epidemiologic studies suggest that poor hygiene and chronic infections, atrophy, and skin diseases are predisposing factors.

The clinical picture in the early stages shows localized, not infrequently multiple, small nodules with eroded surfaces. The labia majora are the most frequent location (40%), followed by the posterior commissure (28%), the clitoris (17%), and the labia minora (15%). Extension of the tumor occurs by exophytic papillomatous growth. Another form of spread is endophytic. Large parts of the labia majora, the perineum, or the clitoral area may be involved in later stages. The margin of the carcinomatous area may be marked by an inflammatory reaction. Localization of the tumor inside the introitus can be associated with a lesion on the opposite side.

One reason that cancer of the vulva has a poor prognosis is the rich lymphatic supply of the vulva. The main lymphatic drainage involves the inguinal lymph nodes, the lymph nodes at the femoral ring, and the external iliac lymph nodes. The cancer finally spreads through the lymph nodes below the inguinal ligament, extending to the deep inguinal, hypogastric, and iliac lymph nodes. Thus, cancer of the vulva metastasizes early to the adjacent lymph nodes in the groin, which not infrequently undergo ulceration (Fig. 8).

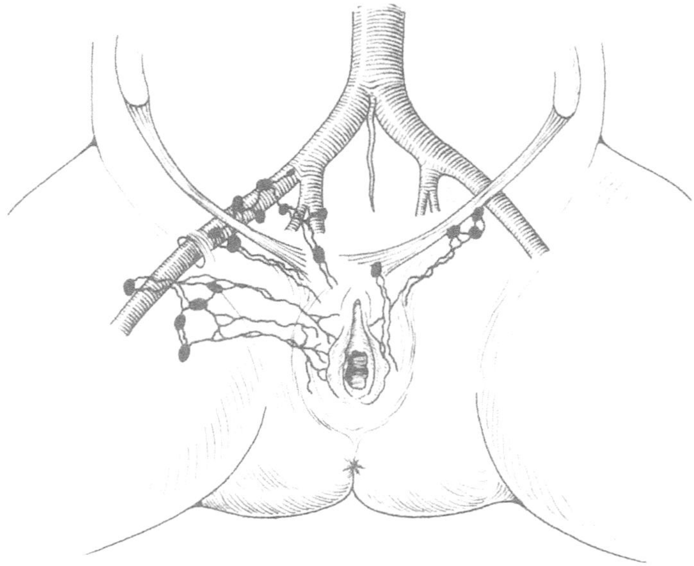

Fig. 8. Regional lymphatics and lymph nodes of the vulva. The lymph channels of the vulva drain into the superficial deep inguinal lymph nodes, to Cloquet's node in the femoral ring, and to the hypogastric and iliac lymph nodes (BELLER et al. 1974)

1. Symptoms

Vulval cancer often causes no signs or symptoms. Pruritus and pain on urination or defecation are related to ulcerations. Foul-smelling, and bloody, watery secretions are present in later stages. Loss of weight is a fairly constant sign.

2. Diagnosis

Single or multiple firm ulcerations with sharp edges and infiltration of the adjacent tissue are seen. Exophytic cauliflower-like ulcerations are common. The tumor may involve part or all of the vulva, perineum, and rectum. Palpable lymph nodes fixed to the skin suggest metastases. Proctoscopy may reveal involvement of adjacent rectum. Prolapse of the urethra or a paraurethral cyst is occasionally mistaken for vulval cancer. A primary luetic lesion in older women or lymphopathia venereum may also simulate vulval carcinoma. Biopsy provides the diagnosis in these case.

3. Staging

The Cancer Committee of the International Federation of Gynecology and Obstetrics (FIGO) proposed a classification according to the TNM system, where T stands for primary tumor, N for lymph nodes, and M for metastases. This sys-

Table 11. Stages of vulva cancer

T_1	Tumor of the vulva less than 2 cm diameter
T_2	Tumor more than 2 cm diameter
T_3	Tumor of any size that involves surrounding structures such as urethra, vagina, anus, or rectum
T_4	Tumor of any size with infiltration of the bladder mucosa, the upper part of the urethral mucosa, or the rectal mucosa, or extension to bones
N	Inguinal nodules
M	Metastases

tem allows a classification of the size of the tumor, relation of the tumor to adjacent organs, lymph node involvement, and distant metastates (Table 11).

4. Treatment and Prognosis

In approximately 50% of cases, the inguinal lymph nodes are involved when the patient is seen for the first time. The treatment of choice is radical vulvectomy. Statistical evaluation is difficult because the number of cases in one medical center often does not allow evaluation of different types of treatment and the patients treated are rarely comparable. Radical surgery involves vulvectomy with resection of skin and fatty tissues, including lymphatics and lymph nodes down to the external aponeurosis and fascia lata, with dissection of lymph nodes of the femoral and inguinal canals. Whether resection of the deep iliac lymph nodes improves the 5-year survival and, therefore, whether this additional extensive dissection in older women is justified, is under discussion. The deep iliac lymph nodes are, with rare exceptions, involved only in the presence of positive nodes in the groin or femoral canal. Postoperative complications are frequent. In more than 50%, the large skin defect breaks down and secondary healing requires prolonged hospitalization.

In stages I and II, the 5-year survival is 50%–80%, with an average of 75%. The figures decrease in stage II (lymph node involvement) to 20%–50% with an average of 41%, and in stage IV it is close to zero. In some centers, radiation therapy with high energy electrons has been used with success in vulval carcinoma. Betatron external irradiation is not an effective therapy, however, and the main treatment of carcinoma of the vulva remains operation.

II. Cancer of the Vagina

1. Premalignant Lesions

Premalignant lesions of the squamous epithelium of the vagina are similar to those of the cervix. A suspicious or positive cytologic smear suggests a lesion of the vagina if cervical cancer is excluded. The entire vagina is then painted with Lugol's solution. The unstained areas are examined by colposcopy and subjected to biopsy. A simple excision of the premalignant lesions is sufficient, provided that the margins of the specimen are free of atypical cells. Frequent follow-up is required.

2. Malignant Lesions

Primary carcinoma of the vagina accounts for only 1.5%–2% of all female genital cancers. Vaginal cancer is more common after the menopause. Predisposing factors are not clear, but prolonged use of pessaries may be etiologically related to carcinoma. In most cases, the lesion is a squamous cell cancer.

Squamous cell vaginal cancer is located most commonly on the posterior wall of the upper third of the vagina. The primary lesion bleeds easily on touch. The tumors grow either exophytically, filling the vagina with a cauliflower-like tumor, or endophytically, progressing like a cuff along the vaginal vault. Local growth into the paravaginal and parametrial tissues results in a firm, fixed vaginal tube. Involvement of the adjacent bladder and rectum and lymphatic metastasis occur early. When the upper part of the vagina is involved, lymph node metastasis is similar to that in cancer of the cervix. Involvement of the lower third of the vagina results in an extension similar to that in cancer of the vulva. Not infrequently, both modes of spread occur simultaneously. Local extension finally causes obstruction of the ureters, and uremia is the most frequent cause of death. Hematogenous metastases to distant organs are rare.

a) Symptoms and Diagnosis

The symptomatology is nearly identical with that of cancer of the cervix. Diagnosis is provided by speculum examination and biopsy. It is occasionally quite difficult to identify the vagina as the primary organ involved if the cancer extends into the cervix or the vulva. In case of doubt, the lesion is best regarded as a cervical or vulval carcinoma with extension to the vagina.

Primary cancer of the vagina is staged in a manner similar to that employed for cancer of the cervix: stage 0: carcinoma in situ; stage I: carcinoma limited to the vaginal wall; stage II: carcinoma involves paravaginal connective tissue, but has not reached the pelvic wall; stage III: carcinoma has reached the pelvic wall; stage IV: carcinoma has penetrated the mucosa of the bladder or rectum, or has extended beyond the pelvis.

b) Treatment

Neither surgical nor radiation therapy has resulted in entirely satisfactory results. Radical surgical treatment requires careful selection of patients. The type of operation depends on the extent of the lesion. Colpectomy in addition to radical hysterectomy is often required. For some carcinomas of the lower vagina, a vaginal radical hysterectomy (Schauta's operation), combined with radical vulvectomy may be necessary. Occasionally, an anterior or posterior exenteration is required to remove the lesion. Radiation therapy requires local treatment with radium by vaginal applicator or radium needles with additional external irradiation. The 5-year survival rate for primary operation is 40%, for irradiation approximately 32%, and for the combined approach 38%. Sarcomas of the vagina are rare. The prognosis is very poor, even after ultraradical surgical procedures.

3. Secondary Cancer of the Vagina

The vagina may be involved in cervical cancer stages II, III, and IV by local extension of the tumor. Less frequently, vaginal cancer represents metastasis from a primary cancer of the ovary, fallopian tube, or chorioncarcinoma. Rarely, the vagina is involved by distant metastasis from mammary cancer or hypernephromas. Involvement of the vagina occurs by metastasis, direct extension, or recurrence in approximately 10% of adenocarcinomas of the endometrium. Treatment is discussed in relation to that of the primary tumor.

III. Cancer of the Cervix Uteri

Cancer of the cervix is the most common malignant tumor of the female genitalia (50%). The success in treatment during the last decade is more the result of early detection of lesions by cytologic means than of improvements in treatment of advanced lesions. The need for routine cytologic examination of the adult cervix is thus obvious. At least 95% of all cases of cervical cancer begin in the area of the squamocolumnar junction. In the menopause, as a result of involution, the squamocolumnar junction moves up into the cervical canal.

More than 50% of all cancers of the female genitalia arise in the cervix. Only breast cancer is more common in women. The highest incidence of invasive cervical cancer is between the fifth and sixth decades. Of cervical cancers, 95% are squamous cell carcinomas; 5% are adenocarcinomas. Only rarely does a cervical cancer arise from remnants of Gartner's ducts.

The cause of development of cervical cancer is unkown. Evidence is mounting to suggest an association with infection by herpesvirus type 2. Local inflammatory changes may also be predisposing factors. In general, cercival carcinoma is more common in women with multiple sex partners, those who marry and have children early, and those with poor genital hygiene. It is associated with low socioeconomic status, multiparity, and promiscuity. Poor penile hygiene of the sexual partner has also been implicated. Whether smegma and lack of circumcision of the male partner cause cervical carcinoma is doubtful except insofar as they predispose to poor genital hygiene. Familial factors may also be important.

Microscopically invasive squamous cell cancer is composed of cell nests in the cervical tissue below the basement membrane. The cells are undifferentiated, with loss of polarity, dyskaryosis with nuclear hyperchromatism, and numerous atypical mitotic figures. Squamous cell cancer is often graded histologically with respect to differentiation. However, 5-year survival is not well correlated with histologic grade.

Lesions that have penetrated the basement membrane minimally are called microinvasive. This is included in stage Ia of the FIGO classification. In patients of menopausal age, early cervical cancer may begin in the cervical canal. The cervix is distended without macroscopic changes on the portio, but necrosis and deep craters develop as a result of endophytic growth. Later, the surface becomes irregular and bleeds easily on touch. The edges and the surrounding tissue are firm and fixed. The tumor may extend by continous growth into the parametrial tissues or

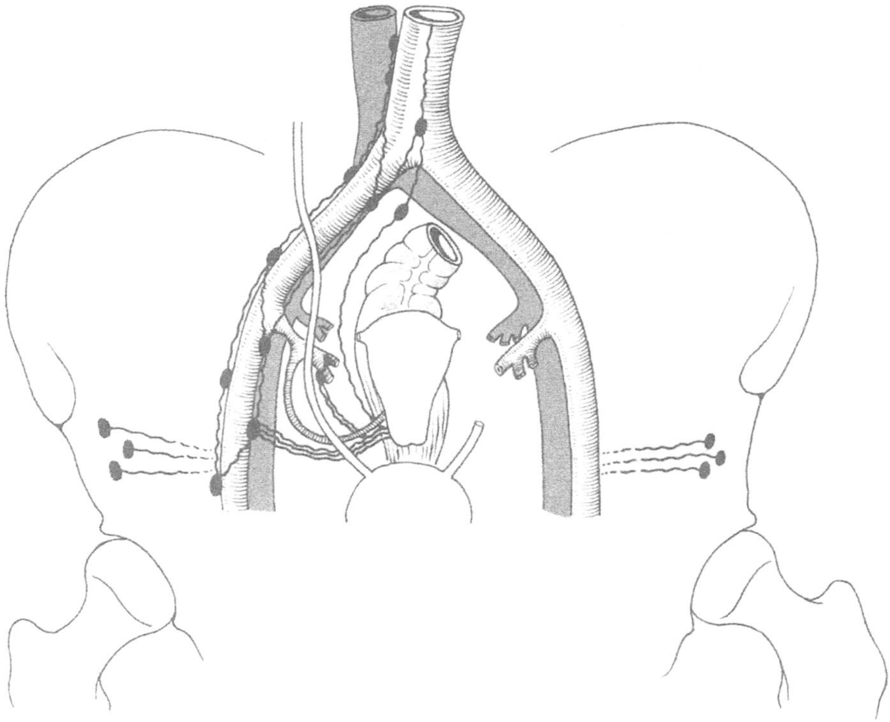

Fig. 9. Main lymphatics and regional lymph nodes of the cervix in the region of the parametria and the pelvic wall. The common iliac, obturator, external iliac, and hypogastric lymph nodes are the principal sites of lymphatic metastasis from cervical carcinoma (BELLER et al. 1974)

the vaginal wall, or both. Finally, the bladder or rectum is invaded with the formation of rectovaginal and vesicovaginal fistulas.

As a result of the rich lymphatic supply of the parametrial tissues, cervical cancer spreads rapidly. Lymph nodes in the parametrial tissues may be involved. The obturator and deep iliac nodes may contain cancer, even though the parametrial nodes are free of cancer. In the terminal stages, the entire pelvis may be filled with malignant tissue (Fig. 9). The ureters are invaded by cancer, or obstructed by cancer or scar tissue, with resulting hydronephrosis and uremia, the most common cause of death of patients with cervical cancer. Hematogenous metastasis to the liver, lungs, and skeletal system is a late development.

1. Symptoms

The earliest stages are asymptomatic. Only when the tumor begins to ulcerate is a brown-yellow discharge seen, especially after intercourse. Physical signs thus indicate a lesion beyond the early stages. Pain in the pelvis and difficulty with urination and defecation are late symptoms. Edema of the lower extremities indicates extensive involvement of lymphatics and is a late manifestation.

Table 12. Stages of cervical cancer

T_0	Carcinoma in situ (intraepithelial cancer, preinvasive carcinoma); this group is not included in the international annual report
T_1	The carcinoma is strictly confined to the cervix; extension to the corpus is disregarded
T_{1a}	Cases with microscopic invasion; all other cases of stage T_1
T_2	The carcinoma has extended beyond the cervix into one or both parametria, but has not reached the pelvic wall; the carcinoma has involved the vagina, but not the lower third
T_{2a}	Involvement of the vagina, but not the parametria
T_{2b}	Involvement of parametria, or parametria and vagina
T_3	The carcinoma has extended onto the pelvic wall; on rectal examination, there is no cancer-free space between the tumor and the pelvic wall; the carcinoma involves the lower third of the vagina
T_4	The carcinoma has extended beyond the true pelvis (lymphatic or hematogenous distant metastasis) or has invaded the mucosa of the bladder or rectum; bullous edema ist not sufficient to classify a lesion as stage T_4

2. Diagnosis

Early lesions are recognized only by cytology or colposcopy. Ulcerating lesions can be seen macroscopically. Endocervical lesions are identified by cytology and cervival curettage or conization. Rectovaginal examination identifies parametrial involvement, which must be distinguished from an inflammatory reaction (parametritis). Lymphography, to identify involved lymph nodes by dorsopedal injection of a contrast medium, has been popular in some centers. We consider this procedure of little value in either diagnosis or planning of therapy.

3. Staging

Cervical cancer is staged according to internationally established conventions. A TNM classification can also be made (Table 12). The principal deficiency of the FIGO classification is its dependence on the results of pelvic examination. Stages T_0 (carcinoma in situ) and T_{1a} (microinvasion), however, are histologic diagnoses. During pelvic examination, inflammatory involvement is frequently confused with spread of tumor. The only reliable staging, in addition to T_0 and T_1, is in stage T_4, where cystoscopy and proctoscopy, with histologic confirmation of the lesion, prove the involvement of adjacent organs (Fig. 10).

4. Treatment

The treatment of severe dysplasia and carcinoma in situ depends primarily on the age and parity of the patient. In patients beyond the age of 35 years, especially those with children, vaginal or abdominal hysterectomy is the treatment of choice rather than conization and follow-up.

Treatment in stage I is modified by the fact that the deep pelvic lymph nodes are involved in 15%–20% of patients. Radical treatment in stage I is therefore required to cure lesions with lymphatic involvement; 80%–85% of patients with stage I are overtreated by radical surgical or radiation therapy. To reduce the in-

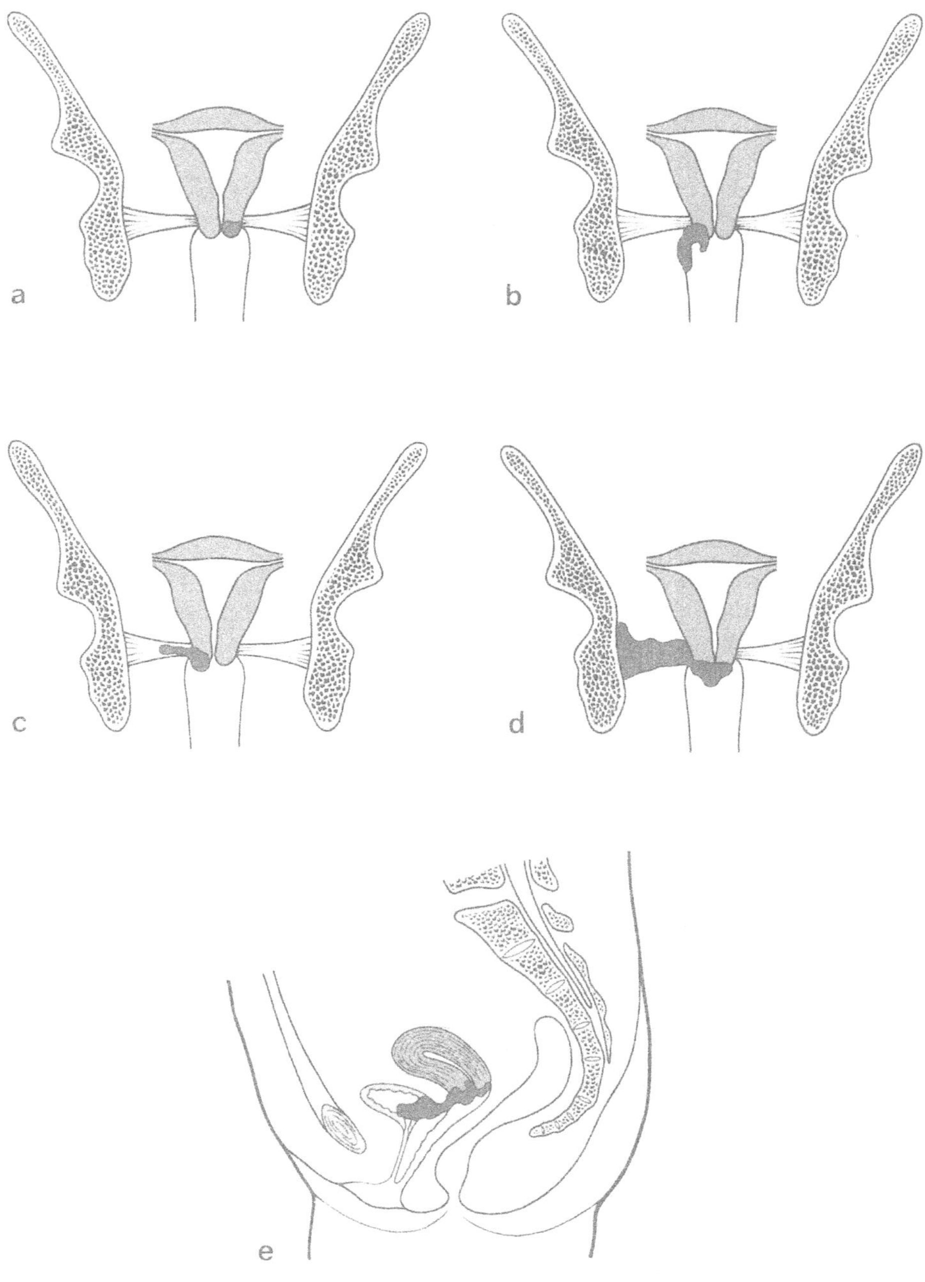

Fig. 10 a–e. Cervical carcinoma. **a** stage Ib, the carcinoma is limited to the cervix; **b** stage IIb, the left parametrium is involved adjacent to the cervix; **c** stage IIa, the upper third of the vagina is involved; **d** stage III, the right parametrium is involved throughout its extent up to the pelvic side wall; **e** stage IV, the carcinoma involves the anterior vaginal wall and has penetrated into the bladder (BELLER et al. 1974)

cidence of radical treatment, with its attendant mortality and morbidity, simple total abdominal hysterectomy is often now performed for some stage Ia lesions. In stage Ia (microinvasion) the lymph node involvement is less than 2%.

Stages Ib, IIa, and IIb may be treated by radical surgery, primary irradiation, or a combination of both. A properly performed radical hysterectomy entails removal of the uterus with an extended vaginal cuff (about one-third of the vagina), the parametria, and deep lymph node dissection.

5. Radiation Therapy

This form of treatment involves the insertion of radium. According to the inverse square law, the radiation effect will decline very rapidly with distance from the inserted radium. Therefore, additional external radiation is required, mostly in the form of $_{60}Co$ irridation. Numerous applicators have been developed for the insertion of radium into the cervical canal and uterine cavity. The unit of radiation absorbed dose is the rad; 1 mg radium in equilibrium with a 0.5-mm platinum filter gives 8.25 rad/h at a distance of 1 cm. In this terminology, a total tumor dose of 7,000–8,000 rad is administered in treatment of cervical carcinoma (including radium and external radiation). The rectum and the bladder my be irradiated beyond their tolerance during therapy, which is approximately 6,000 rad (Fig. 11). The amount of radium multiplied by the time it remains in place is the dose (mg h). A total of approximately 6,000 mg h is applied, usually delivered in two or three applications about 2 weeks apart. Cesium in the afterloading system requires much less radiation time.

Preoperative insertion of radium, for reduction of the size of the tumor and prevention of spread, is occasionally performed. Postoperative irradiation after radical surgical procedures for treatment of stage I is also performed in some centers when lymph node involvement is detected. The choice between surgery and irradiation is often difficult because the 5-year survivals are nearly identical. The choice depends more or less on preference and availability. Irradiation has the disadvantage of adverse effects on bladder, rectum, and sexual function because of stenosis of the vagina. Radical operations, because they involve removal of pelvic lymph nodes, provide prognostic information. Surgical treatment, however, is associated with a slightly higher mortality and a considerably higher morbidity. The incidence of ureterovaginal fistulas is 2%–10%. Thus, it seems that both forms of treatment are logical in selected situations and that neither surgical nor radiation therapy is preferable in all cases.

In stage II, both radical surgery and irradiation are used: Although most cases with more than minimal parametrial extension are probably better treated by radiation. In stage III, because it is illogical to cut through malignant tissue, primary irradiation is the only sensible treatment for lesions that have reached the pelvic wall or the lower third of the vagina. In stage IV, irradiation is usually not effective, and ultraradical procedures such as anterior, posterior, or total exenteration are performed if the tumor has not metastasized beyond the pelvis, and can be removed without cutting through malignant tissue. Treatment of the less common adenocarcinoma of the cervix is identical with that of squamous cell carcinoma.

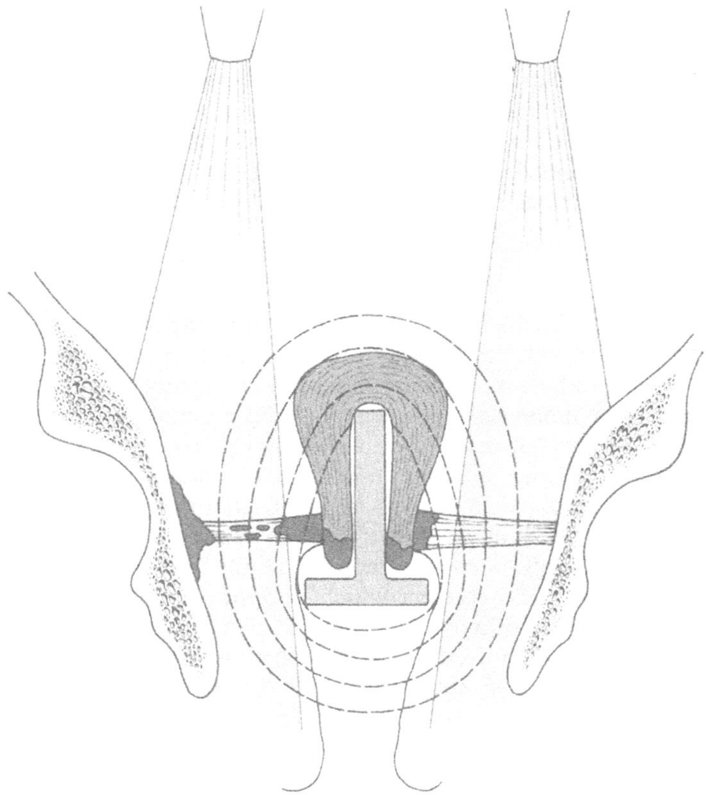

Fig. 11. Radiotherapy of cervical carcinoma. Schematic representation of local and external radiation. The local treatment permits the irradiation of the primary tumor and the immediately adjacent area. In this illustration the radium is applied with an intrauterine tandem attached to a colpostat. The infiltrate on the pelvic wall is reached by external radiation sources (BELLER et al. 1974)

6. Cervical Stump Carcinoma

This lesion should virtually disappear as the operation of supracervical hysterectomy becomes an unusual event. Many women, however, have had a supracervical hysterectomy 20–30 years ago and are now at risk. The incidence of cervical stump carcinoma is 4%–8%. Staging and treatment are the same as with cervical cancer in an intact uterus.

7. Results of Treatment

By international agreement, a cervical cancer is considered to have been cured if the patient is free of recurrence or mestastasis 5 years after inital treatment. The cure rates for cervical cancer according to staging are shown in Table 13.

Table 13. The 5-year survival in carcinoma of cervix by stage

Stage	5-year survival (%)
0 (Carcinoma in situ)	100
I a	95
I b	75–85
II	55–70
III	30
IV	0–8

8. Recurrence

Recurrence is said to exist when a lesion is recognized after a period between 6 months and 5 years in which the patient is apparently free of disease. Many lesions develop as recurrences on the pelvic wall, resulting from involvement of lymph nodes. They occur most frequently in the first year, and less frequently in the second year, after the original treatment. Recurrences 5 years or more after treatment are called late recurrences. The diagnosis can be very difficult since recurrences on the pelvic wall are often confused with scarring. If the original treatment was surgical, recurrences can be treated by radiation. Further radiation after primary irradiation is limited by the tolerance of the tissues. A second course, when possible, requires a considerable reduction in dose of radium and percutaneous irradiation. Since a recurrence after radiation often indicates a low radiosensitivity, recurrence may be cured by ultraradical surgery. The care of patients with incurable cancer requires considerable psychological skill. The patient is dependent on analgesics, often in extremely high doses, in the final stages. These women usually die from uremia, caused by obstruction of the ureters, and less often from hemorrhage or distant metastases.

IV. Cancer of the Corpus Uteri

1. Premalignant Changes in the Endometrium

Adenomatous hyperplasia is histologically characterized by hypertrophy and hyperplasia of glands and a reduction in stroma. The glands are crowded, back to back. The epithelial cells are regular and may be stratified. Mitoses are common. There are occasional areas of benign squamous metaplasia. In 1–10 years, 6%–12% of adenomatous hyperplasias develop into carcinoma of the endometrium. The lesion must therefore be considered precancerous.

2. Dysplasia of the Endometrium

Premalignant atypias of the endometrial epithelium are termed dysplasias. They are a stage between adenomatous hyperplasia and adenocarcinoma of the endometrium. Proliferation of cells into the glandular lumina is characteristic. The glands may be completely filled with cells. Individual cells may be poorly differentiated (polymorphic nuclei, abnormal mitoses, and edematous cytoplasm). The stroma is considerably reduced, but the basement membranes of the glands are intact. The basic difference between adenomatous hyperplasia and dysplasia is the cellular atypia. Some pathologists use the term adenocarcinoma in situ for this lesion. More than 50% of such lesions progress to adenocarcinoma of the endometrium within 1–3 years. The change is considered irreversible and therefore precancerous. Similar patterns may be found in polyps of the endometrium.

a) Treatment

Adenomatous hyperplasia is responsive to progesterone and progestins and may be shed by so-called medical curettage, as may some dysplastic lesions. In general, prophylactic hysterectomy should be considered.

3. Malignant Neoplasms of the Endometrium

Adenocarcinoma of the endometrium is, after mammary and cervical cancer, the third most frequent carcinoma of the reproductive organs in women. The age distribution has its peak at the menopause and in the postmenopausal years. Generally, as longevity increases, the prevalence of endometrial cancer increases. The ratio of frequency of cervical cancer to endometrial cancer was 10:1 a few decades ago, but it has decreased to 3:1 or less in the last decade. This change results in part from the reduction of cervical cancer by early cytologic detection. Endometrial cancer is more common in patients in higher socioeconomic groups. According to some investigators, there is a relation to unopposed estrogenic stimulation. The history frequently includes dysfunctional bleeding. Patients with estrogen-producing ovarian tumors and patients with Stein–Leventhal and Turner's Syndrome show a higher incidence of endometrial cancer than do patients in a normal control group with biphasic menstrual patterns. Endometrial cancer also appears to be associated with obesity, hypertension, and diabetes. Until two decades ago, an accepted treatment for preclimacteric, abnormal uterine bleeding was intrauterine radium to destroy the endometrium. These patients are now completing the 10- to 20-year lag period required for the development of cancer; endometrial carcinoma seems to be increased in that group. Radiation may therefore be an additional etiologic factor.

The main location for adenocarcinoma of the endometrium is the fundus and the area of insertion of the fallopian tubes (80%). The tumor spreads by superficial growth in the endometrium, polypoid extension, or exophytic growth into the uterine cavity. It may fill the entire endometrial cavity, extend downward into the cervical canal (1%–20%), and be seen in the external orifice of the cervical canal. Another pattern of growth occurs when the fallopian tubes are involved. Infiltration of the myometrium is a later development. Lymphatic spread occurs through the mesosalpinx and the infundibulopelvic ligament to the periaortic lymph nodes. Metastasis to the ovaries occurs in 5%–12% of cases. Occasionally, metastasis occurs via the round ligaments (Fig. 12). Once the adenocarcinoma has penetrated into the cervix, the lymphatic spread is identical with that of cervical cancer; the inguinal lymph nodes are involved in approximately 28% of cases. Since the fundus is richly vascularized, hematogenous metastasis is more frequent

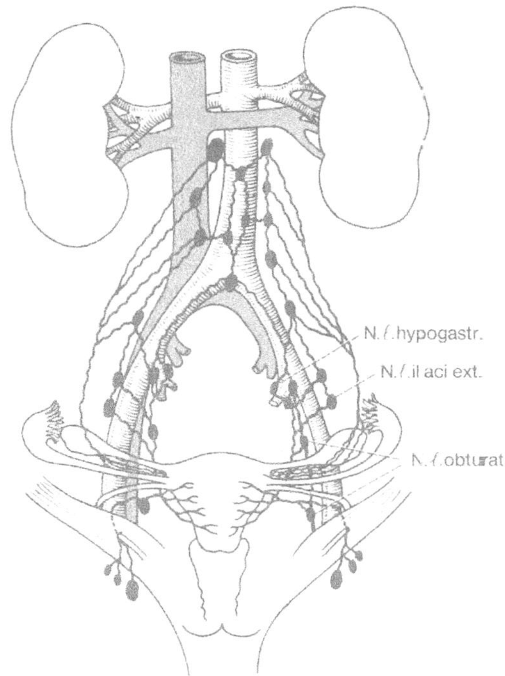

Fig. 12. Lymphatics and regional lymph nodes of the corpus. Carcinoma confined to the fundus spreads primarily by means of the lymphatics of the infundibulopelvic ligament to the periaortic lymph nodes. When endometrial carcinoma involves the lower uterine segment and cervix, the hypogastric, iliac, and obturator nodes may also be involved (BELLER et al. 1974)

than in cervical cancer. Distant metastasis occurs to the lungs, liver, skeletal system, and brain. Pyometra may result from infection of necrotic tumor masses when the cervical canal is stenotic. Various degrees of histologic differentiation may be seen, including the most undifferentiated patterns. Polymorphism and hyperchromasia of nuclei and abnormal mitoses are common. Stromal invasion or complete loss of stroma may be seen. In 15%–20% of adenocarcinomas of the endometrium, squamous metaplasia may be identified. Such a tumor is termed an adenoacanthoma. Rarely, a clear cell carcinoma that resembles hypernephroma is found. In general, the more undifferentiated the pattern, the worse is the prognosis.

a) Signs

Endometrial cancer produces metrorrhagia in younger women and postmenopausal bleeding later in life. The discharge is frequently serosanguineous. Endometrial cancer accounts for up to 40% of cases of postmenopausal bleeding.

b) Diagnosis

Cytology is an unreliable method of diagnosis for endometrial carcinoma. Cancer cells from the endometrium are identified in less than 40% of cases in the vaginal pool. Endometrial biopsies obtained with an aspiration curette improve the accuracy of diagnosis. Palpation of the uterus in the later stages may reveal a slight

Table 14. Classification of endometrial cancer

Stage 0:	Histologically suspected intraepithelial lesion, not malignant, no infiltration through basal membrane
Stage I:	Endometrial cancer with infiltration of the uterine corpus (less than 3 mm)
Stage II:	Endometrial cancer also affecting the uterine cervix
Stage III:	The endometrial cancer is deeply invading the uterus, but not the small pelvis
Stage IV:	The endometrial cancer has invaded the small pelvis, including the vesical or rectal mucosa

increase in size and softness of the organ. Pyometra is usually associated with a tender, cystic enlarged uterus. The diagnosis is confirmed by fractional curettage, in which the cervical canal is scraped by a small curette before dilatation. After dilatation, the endometrial cavity is scraped separately with a medium-sized curette. The specimens from the cervix and corpus are submitted to the pathologist in separate containers. Perforation may readily occur in advanced stages of the disease when the myometrium in infiltrated by the tumor. In case of pyometra, the cervical canal is dilated and the endometrial cavity drained. The uterus is scraped a few days later.

c) Staging

The staging (Table 14) proposed by the FIGO in 1962 is generally accepted and allows comparison of results on an international basis. The treatment consists of: (a) surgery; (b) radiation; and (c) a combination of radiation and surgery. The treatment of choice in stage I is total abdominal hysterectomy with bilateral salpingo-oophorectomy and resection or a large vaginal cuff. The operation is usually performed by the abdominal route, but vaginal hysterectomy may be performed as well. The adnexa must be removed since the most common mode of spread is along the lymphatics of the ovarian vessels. Preoperative cobalt or radium is used by some medical centers to shrink the tumor. Some investigators believe that preoperative radium reduces the likelihood of recurrences in the vaginal vault. Primary irradiation without hysterectomy is used only in patients presenting a very great operative risk. The treatment of stage II is simple total hysterectomy with a full course of external radiation. Radiation and various extensive surgical procedures are tried in stages III and IV, but the therapeutic results are poor.

d) Recurrence

The definition is the same as that for cervical carcinoma. Diagnosis is made by curettage, palpation, cytology, lymphangiography, venography, and roentgenography. Recurrences are observed in approximately one-fifth of patients in the vagina, parametria, uterus, and ovaries, in that order of frequency. Treatment is similar to that of recurrent carcinoma of the cervix. Recurrence and distant metastases may be suppressed by treatment with high doses of progestational agents such as 17α-hydroxyprogesterone caproate or medroxyprogesterone acetate. Progestational drugs and other chemotherapeutic agents, in general, provide only temporary remission.

e) Results of Treatment

The total 5-year survival of all stages is at present 62.6% (see the Annual Reports of the Results of Treatment in Carcinoma of the Uterus and Vagina). The 5-year survival depends on the size of the uterus and histologic grade of the tumor, among other factors. For stage I, the 5-year survival is 75%–85%, for stage II, 20%–40%, for stage III less than 20%, and for stage IV less than 5%.

4. Sarcoma of the Uterus

Approximately 2% of malignant neoplasms of the uterus are sarcomas. They may be derived from the myometrium or from myomas (leiomyosarcoma) or, less frequently, from the stroma of the endometrium. They occur in all age grups. Leiomyosarcomas may grow rapidly. Endometrial sarcomas may occur in polypoid form projecting as far as the external orifice. Sarcomas may cause pain in the lower abdomen and are often recognized by apparently rapid growth of "myomas". Irregular uterine bleeding is more commonly found with sarcomas of the endometrium. Diagnosis is made by histologic examination. The treatment of choice is abdominal hysterectomy with bilateral salpingo-oophorectomy and possibly postoperative irradiation. The prognosis is poor if any spread has occurred.

V. Cancer of the Fallopian Tubes

Primary carcinomas of the fallopian tubes are the least common genital carcinomas (0.1%–0.8%). They usually occur between the ages of 40 and 60 years. These are adenocarcinomas and unilateral in 80% of cases. Primary carcinomas are more common in the ampullary than in the isthmic part of the tube. Carcinoma of the fallopian tube is characterized by early involvement of the peritoneum. Metastasis occurs by lymphatics or by local spread to the uterus, ovaries, vagina, bladder, and rectum. Hematogenous metastasis is a late development. Histologically, the differentiated papillary or alveolar adenocarcinomas are more common than poorly differentiated medullary forms.

1. Symptoms and Diagnosis

Since there are no pathognomonic signs, carcinomas of the fallopian tubes are in most instances accidentally found at laparotomy. Hydrorrhea occasionally provides as clue to diagnosis, but correct preoperative diagnosis is made only infrequently. Rarely, malignant cells have been identified in vaginal cytologic smears. The tumor is frequently mistaken for a hydrosalpinx or an ovarian mass. Since tubal carcinomas spread rapidly, peritoneal signs occur early. At laparotomy, brown-red papillary tumor masses are seen to have penetrated the wall of the fallopian tube.

2. Treatment

This is identical with that of ovarian tumors. Radical surgery plays little role in treatment, but irradiation and chemotherapy may be tried for advanced lesions.

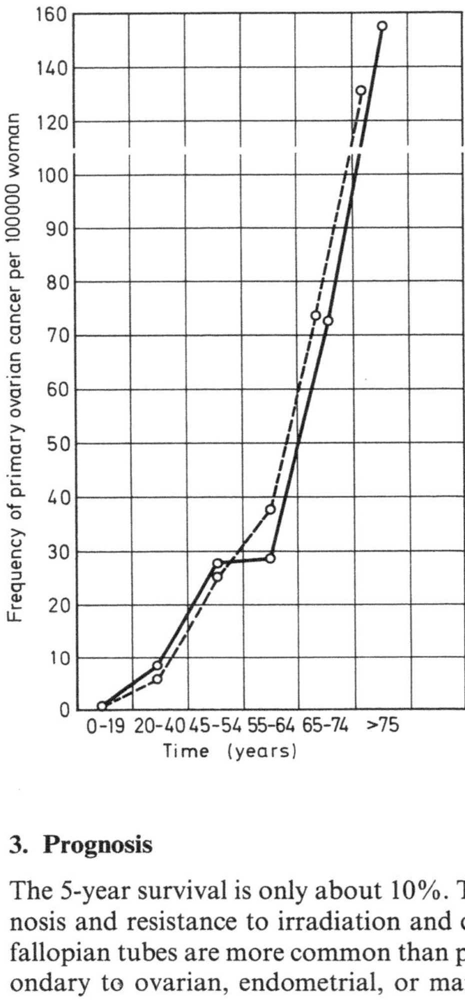

Fig. 13. Frequency of primary ovarian carcinoma in relation to age, based on 100,000 women. *Circles* data of BENNINGTON et al. (1969); *crosses* data of GERBER et al. (1962)

3. Prognosis

The 5-year survival is only about 10%. The poor prognosis reflects delayed diagnosis and resistance to irradiation and chemotherapy. Metastatic tumors of the fallopian tubes are more common than primary cancers. They are most often secondary to ovarian, endometrial, or mammary carcinoma, in that order or frequency.

VI. Malignant Tumors of the Ovaries

Malignant ovarian tumors account for 15%–20% of all genital tumors; their frequency is shown in Fig. 13. They are surpassed only be carcinomas of the cervix and endometrium. Approximately one-third of all ovarian tumors show malignant change. As a result of incomplete knowledge and various interpretations of ovarian embryology, a generally accepted classification is not yet available. Even the differentiation between benign and malignant tumors is often difficult, for many of the benign tumors must be considered potentially malignant. Among ovarian tumors, the greatest likelihood of malignant change occurs in papillary cystadenomas. About half of all papillary serous cystadenomas are actually or potentially malignant (Table 15). Penetration of the cyst wall by papillary growth

Table 15. Incidence of different ovarian tumors, of bilaterality, and of malignant transformation

Type of tumor	All ovarian tumors (%)	Bilaterality (%)	Malignant change (%)
Serous cystadenoma	20–25	20 in benign, 50 in malignant forms	50
Mucinous cystadenoma	10–18	5 in benign, 23 in malignant forms	12–15
Dermoid cyst	15	25	1–3
Struma ovarii	1–3 (of benign dermoids)	Rare	5–10
Brenner tumor	1–7	Very rare	Very rare
Fibroma	1–5	10	< 1 Fibrosarcoma
Granulosa cell tumor	1–3	5	10–30
Theca cell tumor	1–2	Rare	1
Arrhenoblastoma	0.1	5	20–25
Hilar cell tumor	Very rare	Rare	1
Dysgerminoma	Very rare	17	Always at least potentially malignant
Malignant teratoma	0.015	Rare	Malignant
Primary ovarian carcinoma	15	33	Malignant

Table 16. Symptomatology of ovarian carcinoma stages I a and I b (SPECHTER, from BELLER et al. 1974)

Symptoms	Incidence (%)
Nonspecific lower abdominal pain	34
Increase in abdominal girth	27
Bleeding abnormalities and dysmenorrhea	21.5
Vaginal discharge	3
Weight loss	1.5
Uncommon: fever, nausea, vomiting, fullness, urinary tract	5
Complaints, no complaints	7

is particularly suggestive of malignancy. Bilateral cystadenomas should always arouse the suspiction of malignancy. The general symptomatology is described in Table 16.

1. Estrogen-Producing Ovarian Tumors

Granulosa cell tumors are estrogen-producing ovarian neoplasms that account for 1%–3% of all ovarian tumors and are mainly unilateral (95%). Granulosa and theca cell tumors rarely reach large size. They may remain as small nodules inside the ovary, which maintains its normal size and shape. Larger tumors may be palpated as solid firm masses with a smooth or slightly irregular surface. The cells resemble granulosa cells and are arranged in either rosettes or columns supported by a connective tissue network. Local pressure symptoms are rare and the clinical picture is more often related to the excessive production of estrogen. Granulosa cell tumors may be found in all age groups, but mainly during the postmenopausal years. Irregular menstrual bleeding is the predominant sign in premenopausal women, and postmenopausal bleeding in older women. The bleeding is related to endometrial hyperplasia. Early diagnosis and treatment are important because of the possible relation of granulosa cell tumors to endometrial carcinoma. The frequency of malignant transformation of the tumor itself varies between 10% and 30%. In addition, there is often a discrepancy between a histologically benign appearance and clinically malignant behavior. A primary malignant form is occasionally found. These tumors are generally resistant to radiation therapy. Regular periodic gynecologic examinations and measurements of estrogen are required to detect reccurences. In older women who have completed their families, total hysterectomy with bilateral salpingo-oophorectomy is the procedure of choice.

2. Arrhenoblastoma

The arrhenoblastoma is unilateral in 95% of cases and is variable in size. It seldom occurs in older women. Histologically, tubular formations similar to those in the testis are found. The degree of differentiation varies considerably. They may arise from residual elements of the originally undifferentiated embryonic gonad. Malignant change occurs in 20%–25% of cases. Malignant ovarian tumors are classified as primary and secondary, or metastatic.

3. Primary Malignant Ovarian Tumors

Primary ovarian carcinoma accounts for about 15%–20% of all gynecologic cancer and approximately 5% of all malignant tumors in women. Recent statistics indicate a relative increase in incidence of ovarian carcinomas, compared with those of the cervix and endometrium. Mortality statistics indicate that death from ovarian cancer is exceeded only by that from cervical cancer. Of all women with this lesion, 76% are older than 45 years. The peak incidence occurs in the sixth and seventh decades. Epidemiologic factors are poorly understood. The estimated mortality rate for Europe is 7–8 per 100,000 women. In Japan it is only 1.69 per 100,000. Socioeconomic studies reveal a higher incidence among unmarried women of a higher social status.

The majority of malignant ovarian tumors are of epithelial origin. They arise from "germinal" or surface epithelium of the ovary of inclusions of coelomic epithelium acquired during embryonic development. There is some dispute about the origin of the mesonephroid ovarian tumors (mesonephromas) that look like clear cell carcinomas. Rare forms include the malignant teratoma and, in some classifications, the dysgerminoma. Primary adenocarcinomas of the ovary are predominantly solid or cystic structures of variable size and consistency, with smooth and irregular surfaces and multiple morphological patterns. Well-differentiated glands and papillary epithelial structures may be interspersed with areas of rather poorly differentiated adenocarcinoma. The stroma varies from fibrotic (scirrhous type) to sparse (medullary type). Serous and mucinous cystadenocarcinomas differ from benign cystomas in their exuberant proliferation of epithelium, marked polymorphism of nuclei, and invasion of neighboring tissues and organs. The endometrioid carcinoma of the ovary develops either from a benign variant or without apparent antecedent benign stages. Histologically, it resembles adenocarcinoma of the endometrium. Endometrioid carcinoma of the ovary may be derived from embryonic coelomic epithelium or from malignant transformation of an endometrioma of the ovary. Diagnosis of a primary ovarian endometrioid carcinoma requires the exclusion of a primary carcinoma of the endometrium. This differential diagnosis is sometimes difficult. Ovarian cancer tends to spread quickly to the endometrium and, conversely, the ovaries are involved at an early stage by metastases from endometrial cancer. One-third of epithelial ovarian carcinomas are bilateral. The size varies considerably. The tumor grows rapidly and infiltrates the pelvis, predominantly the posterior cul-de-sac. Early spread to neighboring organs and the other ovary is common. The tumor then spreads to the surfaces of the fallopian tube, uterus, bladder, vagina, and rectum. At the same time, malignant cells may reach the uterus via the oviducts. Large fixed tumors results from extensive adhesions and infiltrating growth. Early spread to the peritoneum is common, with implantation on the omentum and development of ascites. Spread occurs via the lumbar lymph nodes and the lymphatics of the diaphragm, whence the tumor involves the pleural cavity. Liver, lungs, and bones may be involved by hematogenous spread. The multiple pathways of metastasis and rapid proliferation result in generalized carcinomatosis.

Malignant ovarian teratoma is a rare tumor (0.015% of all ovarian tumors); 75% of patients are below the age of 25 years. These tumors appear as small, firm, solid masses that penetrate the capsule early and spread widely in the pelvis. Malignant teratomas are thought to arise from primordial germ cells and contain derivatives of all three germ layers. Since the mesodermal elements often predominate, teratomas histologically and clinically resemble sarcomas such as rhabdomyosarcoma or chondrosarcoma. In contrast to the components of well-differentiated benign teratomas (dermoid cysts), the cells and tissues of the malignant variants are poorly differentiated and embryonal. Rapid proliferation and infiltration lead to early lymphatic and hematogenous spread. Treatment is the same as that of carcinoma of the ovary. Some malignant teratomas are moderately sensitive to radiation.

4. Metastatic Ovarian Carcinomas

Of all malignant ovarian tumors, 25%–30% are metastatic (Table 17). Since the ovarian metastasis is often larger than the primary tumor, it may first call attention to cancer in other organs. Spread to the ovary is usually by hematogenous or lymphatic routes and less frequently by direct spread. Metastatic ovarian tumors are seen predominantly before the menopause, 40% occurring over the age of 50 years. In general, they are bilateral. Shape, size, and consistency vary considerably. They may consist of solid structures with cystic areas. Pedunculated

Table 17. Frequency of metastases of extragenital primary tumors in the ovary (GOMPEL and SILVERBERG 1969; KNÖRR et al. 1982)

Primary tumor	Frequency of metastasis (%)	
Mammary cancer	41	Mostly bilateral
Gastrointestinal cancer	37	Krukenberg tumor
Genital cancer	22	Mostly endometrial cancer

metastatic ovarian tumors are occasionally seen. Breast carcinoma commonly metastasizes to the ovary, as indicated by examination of tissue removed at the time of prophylactic bilateral oophorectomy. Malignant tumors of the stomach, bowel, and occasionally gallbladder are the next most frequent extragenital sites of primary cancers that metastasize to the ovary. Ovarian metastases may proliferate rapidly and reach large sizes in a very short time. The term Krukenberg tumor was originally used in reference to an ovarian metastasis from the gastrointestinal tract with "signet ring" cells. Tumors of the same histologic appearance may be seen occasionally as primary lesions. Among genital cancers, endometrial carcinoma and the rare carcinomas of the fallopian tubes spread to the ovaries, as does cancer from one ovary to the other. Surgical management is hysterectomy and bilateral salpingo-oophorectomy, together with the appropriate treatment of the primary tumor.

5. Clinical Aspects

a) Symptomatology

Since only very large ovarian tumors cause pain and other symptoms, cancer of the ovary is often found accidentally, as a sequence of complaints in ovarian carcinoma stages Ia and Ib. It is obvious that the signs and symptoms of localized ovarian carcinoma are nonspecific. Among these complaints, only postmenopausal vaginal bleeding is of diagnostic significance. In 7% of cases it is caused by benign tumors and in 3%–4% of cases by malignant ovarian tumors. Regardless of the patient's age, irregular bleeding occurs in about one-third of all women with ovarian tumors. Uterine bleeding is a major sign of hormonally active tumors. Diffuse lower abdominal discomfort may occasionally be caused by pressure on neighboring organs. Malignant tumors often spread to the peritoneal cavity, the serosa of the intestine, and the omentum before a change in the patient's general condition becomes apparent. The staging of ovarian cancer is shown in Table 18.

Symptoms of unilateral pressure occur early when the tumor develops within the broad ligament. Extremely large tumors may affect the patient's general condition, whether they are benign or malignant, and may cause a feeling of generalized weakness. Progressive anorexia, cachexia, increase in abdominal girth with or without ascites, a feeling of fullness, and constipation are typical of a malignant tumor. These signs and symptoms indicate an advanced stage of the disease.

Table 18.

A. Stages of ovarian cancer	
Stage I:	Tumor limited to the ovaries
Stage I a:	Only one ovary involved; no ascites
Stage I b:	Both ovaries involved; no ascites
Stage I c:	Both ovaries involved; ascites with tumor cells
Stage II:	Tumor in one or both ovaries with spread elsewhere in pelvis, with or without ascites
Stage II a:	Direct spread or metastasis only to the uterus, tubes, or both
Stage II b:	Spread to other pelvic organs
Stage III:	Tumor in one or both ovaries with extensive intraperitoneal metastasis (omentum, intestine, mesentery) with or without ascites
Stage IV:	Tumor in one or both ovaries with distant metastasis outside the peritoneal cavity, with or without ascites

B. Stages of metastasis of ovarian cancer	
Distant metastasis M	
Stage 0:	No metastasis observed
Stage I a:	Infiltrated lymph nodes palpable in the small pelvis
Stage I b:	Any distant metastases palpable; from this classification any combination can be derived, as given in the scheme
Stage I:	T_1, N_0, M_0
	T_1, N_1, M_0
Stage II:	T_2, N_0, M_0
	T_2, N_1, M_0
Stage III:	T_3, N_0, M_0
	T_3, N_1, M_0
	T_3, N_2, M_0
	T_1, N_3, M_0
	T_2, N_3, M_0
	T_1, N_2, M_0
	T_2, N_2, M_0
Stage IV:	T_3, N_3, M_0
	T_4, N_0, M_0
	T_4, N_1, N_0
	T_4, N_2, M_0, and all cases with M_{1a} or M_{1b}
	T_4, N_3, M_0

The lack of early symptoms explains why, in 50%–80% of all cases, ovarian tumors at the time of laparotomy have already spread beyond the ovaries. Every ovarian tumor must therefore be considered potentially malignant until proved otherwise by histologic examination.

Acute signs and symptoms may result from the following complications of an ovarian tumor: (a) torsion of the pedicle; (b) rupture; (c) hemorrhage; (d) incarceration; and (e) infection. Torsion of the pedicle leads to sudden onset of severe abdominal pain, rebound tenderness, nausea, vomiting, ileus, and sometimes shock. The temperature is slighly elevated; in general leukocytosis is moderate. Elevation of the erythrocyte sedimentation rate may occur. Complete torsion with obstruction of the arterial blood supply may lead to gangrene of the tumor. Extensive infarction and necrosis increase the risk of rupture, which may occur spontaneously or during examination or laparotomy. When torsion is incomplete, the signs and symptoms are less striking. Obstruction of venous return may result in a decreased blood flow, with edema and extravasation of blood into the cyst. The tumor may then appear to grow rapidly in size. At the time of laparotomy, it is usually edematous and cyanotic. Spontaneous rupture of a benign or malignant ovarian tumor is a rare event. It may occur, however, during pelvic examination under anesthesia or when the tumor is delivered from the abdomen at laparotomy. Thin-walled cysts are more likely to rupture; the contents of the cysts produce a chemical peritonitis. Rupture of a mucinous cystoma may result in pseudomyxoma peritonei. How often spillage of malignant cells, after rupture of an ovarian carcinoma, results in implantation of cancer is not clear. Hemorrhage into the tumor occurs rather frequently, even without previous torsion or trauma. Rarely is the bleeding extensive enough to cause acute signs or symptoms. Incarceration of a mobile ovarian tumor in the posterior cul-de-sac is a rare complication. The signs it characteristically produces are acute urinary retention, caused by impingement on the bladder, and pressure on the urethra by the anteriorly displaced cervix. The rectum may also be compressed. Infection of an ovarian tumor is an unusual complication. A cystoma may become infected by spread from an acute salpingitis. Spread may also occur from local inflammation of neighboring organs such as appendicitis or diverticulitis. Symptoms are related to the primary disease and the accompanying peritonitis.

Irregular firm or cystic masses filling the cul-de-sac are suggestive of a malignant ovarian tumor. The suspicion is strengthened by the presence of ascites and nodular masses in the abdomen. Doubtful findings on palpation require examination under anesthesia and laparoscopy. Carcinoma of the ovary is ruled out by laparotomy. Histologic diagnosis by frozen section, obtained during laparotomy, provides the basis for treatment. In the presence of ascites or hydrothorax, an attempt should be made to demonstrate malignant cells in the fluid preoperatively.

b) Differential Diagnosis

Differential diagnosis includes enlargement or displacement of normal organs. Large ovarian tumors extending beyond the true pelvis may be mistaken for tumors originating from abdominal organs. Occasionally a retroverted uterus may be mistaken for a solid ovarian tumor.

Firm fixed masses in the pelvis in any woman over 50 years old may be caused by an ovarian carcinoma or a malignant tumor of the lower intestinal tract. History, signs, and symptoms such as constipation, diarrhea, colicky pain, and rectal bleeding suggest intestinal disease. Carcinoma of the rectum is palpable on rectal examination as a firm tumor extending over the surface of the mucosa or as an ulcer with indurated edges. The examining finger may be stained with blood. Proctoscopy and barium enema confirm the diagnosis. It is difficult to differentiate an ovarian carcinoma fixed to the pelvic side wall from a carcinoma of the sigmoid. Diverticulosis of the sigmoid must also be considered. A posterior ill-defined mass of doughy consistency located high in the pelvis suggests diverticulosis. Ileocecal tumors are located high in the abdomen and can hardly be reached by rectal or vaginal examination. Gurgling bowel sounds may be heard after displacing the mass with the palpating hand. Acute appendicitis and appendiceal absesses are seldom confused with ovarian tumors. Ruptured or twisted ovarian cysts may occasionally be mistaken for a perforated appendix, however, and vice versa. Retroperitoneal tumors may extend into the pelvis. An immobile, firm resistant mass near the posterior wall of the pelvis is easily differentiated from an ovarian tumor as long as the genital organs can be palpated separately. Questionable findings at palpation may be clarified by laparoscopy. A pelvic kidney appears as a rather doughy, egg-shaped mass. An intravenous pyelogramm confirms this diagnosis. Differentiation between ovarian cysts and ascites is made on the basis of the findings on abdominal percussion before and after change of position, and by ultrasonography.

c) Treatment

In general, all ovarian tumors should be removed surgically. Because of the malignant potential of many benign neoplasms of the ovary, surgical treatment is also an effective prophylaxis. The extent of the operation depends on whether the tumor is benign or malignant, the age of the patient and her reproductive history, and the malignant potential of the tumor. In menopausal women, bilateral oophorectomy with hysterectomy is performed, even if the neoplasm involves only one ovary. Treatment and prognosis of carcinoma of the ovary depend mainly on the extent of spread at the initiation of treatment. To compare different methods of treatment and their respective cure rates, the internationally accepted classification should be used for the staging of primary ovarian carcinomas. Treatment is: (a) surgical; (b) radiotherapeutic; and (c) chemotherapeutic. There is general agreement about the prime role of surgical treatment. The value of radiation and chemotherapy is somewhat less clearly defined. Cure of ovarian carcinoma is possible only after total removal the tumor. If the operation is incomplete, that is, if any of the tumor is left behind, the prognosis becomes much worse. Removal of the uterus and adnexa is preferable to removal of the adnexa only. The primary objective of surgical exploration is to ascertain the extent of the tumor. The decision as to whether the tumor can be removed completely can be made only during laparotomy. In most instances, it is not known definitely whether the tumor is benign or malignant before laparotomy. Frozen sections, cytology, and inspection and biopsy of the other ovary provide the basis for deciding the best procedure. The opposite ovary was found to be microscopically involved in 12% of carcinomas. Malignant tumors always require hysterectomy and bilateral salpingo-oophorectomy. Spillage of contents of the cyst into the abdominal cavity may not be so dangerous as previously thought, since the capacity of these cells to implant is questionable.

If it is not possible to deliver a large cystic tumor through the abdomen, it may be necessary to reduce its size by aspiration. Prophylactic partial or total removal of the omentum is advised in ovarian cancer since microscopic metastases are frequently found there. If total removal of the tumor is not possible because of adhesions formed, complete extirpation may be successful in a so-called second look operation after a trial of chemotherapy. The objective of the adjunctive methods of treatment is to transform an inoperable into an operable tumor by isolating

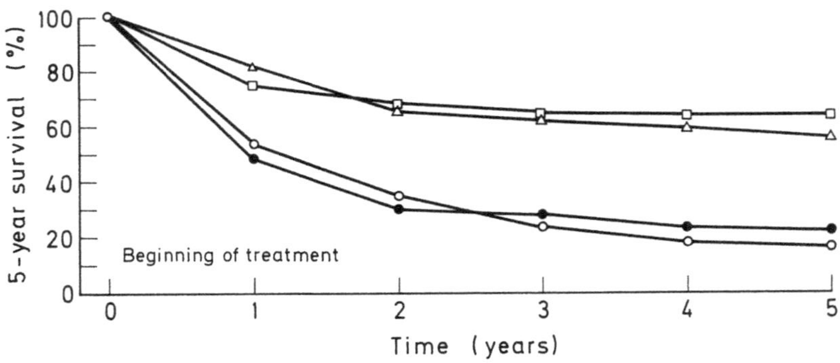

Fig. 14. Prognosis of ovarian carcinoma in relation to histologic type. *Triangles* endometrioid carcinoma; *squares* mucinous carcinoma; *open circles* serous carcinoma; *full circles* unclassified carcinoma. (After KOTTMEIER 1969)

the tumor from the surrounding tissues. The simultaneous use of several chemotherapeutic agents that interfere with different steps in cell metabolism is the treatment of choice. The effect is somewhat independent of the histologic type and degree of differentiation of the tumor. Possible side effects of chemotherapy include leukopenia, thrombocytopenia, anemia, nausea, and vomiting. Patients receiving chemotherapeutic agents require constant supervision because of depression of bone marrow. Chemotherapy often prolongs life and provides symptomatic relief although it is not curative. With few exceptions, most ovarian tumors are fairly resistant to radiation. Because of the extent of the tumor, an effective dose usually cannot be administered without seriously damaging abdominal organs.

d) Prognosis

Although significant progress in treatment has been achieved, the prognosis of ovarian carcinoma is still poor (Fig. 14). The 5-year survival rates for all malignant neoplasms is 30%. This low survival rate is explained mainly by the fact that in 50%–80% of women, the tumor has already spread beyond the ovary at the onset of therapy. Prognosis is closely related to the stage of the disease at the beginning of therapy. Survival drops from 62.2% in stage I (when only one ovary is involved) to 38.8% in stage II (when tumors are found in both ovaries). In addition to the extent of tumor spread, the histologic type is also important for the prognosis. The less differentiated the carcinoma, the worse is the prognosis. The 5-year survival rates of the mucinous and endometrioid carcinomas are definitely better (51.3%) than those of the serous cystadenocarcinomas (20.6%).

e) Follow-Up

Examinations at regular intervals are required because of the high incidence of recurrence. During long-term chemotherapy, platelet, and leukocyte counts are important methods of monitoring the patient. If therapy is unsuccessful, as indicated by further spread of the tumor, palliative measures are employed: narcotics for pain and repeated peritoneal taps to reduce accumulations of ascitic fluid.

VII. Cancer of the Mammary Glands

Mammary cancer will develop in 4%–5% of all women. Thus, this neoplasm shows the highest incidence of all cancer localizations in women. Most patients are between 45 and 55 years old when the diagnosis is made. However, the relative frequency increases further with age.

1. Etiology

The reasons why breast cancer develops are unknown. Endogenous factors play an important role. Familial disposition increases the risk. Higher social classes show a higher incidence of breast cancer. In western countries, the proportion of cases is higher than in eastern countries like Japan. Long-lasting anovulation, sterility, nulliparity, oligoparity, and late first pregnancy result in an increased risk of mammary cancer. Proliferating mastopathy also increases the risk of cancer development (four- to tenfold).

2. Morphology

Breast cancer can develop in the ducts or in the lobules of the breast. The most frequent histologic forms are the following:

1. Milk duct cancer
   a) No infiltration (cancer in situ)
      Papillary (milk duct papilloma)
      Solid (comedo cancer)
   b) Infiltration
      Papillar
      Solid (comedo cancer)
      Productive fibrotic (scirrhus)
      Colloid cancer
      Medullary
      Circumscribed milk duct cancer with plasma cell infiltration
2. Lobular cancer
   a) Carcinoma in situ
   b) Infiltrating lobular cancer
3. Rare cancers (e.g., Paget's disease of the breast)

The different morphological types of breast cancer also show different clinical symptoms, course, and prognosis of the disease. The histology is connected with the malignity of the cancer. The prognosis of solid cancer is less favorable than medullary cancer. Women with untreated breast cancer may survive 5 years in 20%, 15 years in less than 5% of cases. The right and left mammary gland are affected with equal frequency. The localization is 48% in the right upper quadrant, 10% in the right lower, 18% in the left upper, 8% in the left lower quadrant, and 16% at the nipple and areola. When one breast has cancer, the chance of the other also developing a neoplasm is 16%. The papillary cancers are mostly situated in the middle of the breast.

The spread of mammary cancer is mostly via the lymph and leads to the axillary lymph nodes and the lymph ducts along the internal thoracic artery. When the tumor is more than 1–2 cm in diameter, there is a discontinous lymphogenous metastasis in 55% of cases. When the tumor is 6 cm, the local lymph nodes are already carcinomatous in 85% of cases and there are usually general metastases as well. Thus, mammary cancer is a general disease, even in its earlier stages.

3. Symptoms

The patients usually experience no pain. When the nodule is felt, early diagnosis has already been missed, the more so when axillary nodules are present and when the tumor is adherent to its basis or to the skin.

4. Diagnosis

Self-palpation is important for diagnosis. However palpation, even by an experienced doctor, will seldom provide really early diagnosis. This is only possible by regular mammography in women who are at risk (familial history, nulliparity, mastopathy). In all other cases, we propose a basis mammography at the age of 40 years, thereafter controls every 1–2 years. Thermography and ultrasonography are only additional methods. Nodules of doubtful malignity are subjected to micropuncture or diagnostic extirpation. Cysts are filled with air. Xerography or galactography are aids in special cases. The overall reliability of these methods is about 95% for early diagnosis. Before treatment is begun, a liver and bone scintiscan is performed.

5. Therapy

Ablation of the breast is the treatment of choice. Ultraradical methods such as that of Rotter and Halsted are no longer preferred. This method involves ablation "en bloc" with resection of the greater pectoral muscle, the parapectoral fat and lymph nodes, the fat and lymph tissue of the axilla and the infraclavicular fossa, facultatively also of the supraclavicular fossa and the mammary cord.

In the last few years, ablation with resection of the axillary fat and lymph nodes has become the preferred operation. In very advanced cases, mastectomy and radiation can be performed. Only in very early cases can breast preservation with lumbectomy be considered. In some centers radiation only is preferred with high voltage therapy and good, comparable results. Pre- or postoperative radiation produces no increase in cure rates.

6. Hormones

In all operated cases, the determination of estrogen and progesterone receptors should be performed. In the presence of such receptors, there is a much better prognosis than when receptors are missing. While hormonal treatment is effective in only 30% of all cases, it is effective in up to 90% of all receptor-positive cases.

Table 19. Stages (Steinthal and TNM) and 5- and 10-year survival rates in mammary cancer

Stage	Steinthal	TNM	Survival rate after treatment (%)	
			5 years	10 years
I	Tumor localized, no metastases	$T_1 N_0 M_0$	83 (40–88)	55 (45–70)
II	Tumor localized; skin and pectoral muscle affected; axillary lymph nodes	$T_{1-2} N_2 M_0$	57 (30–70)	31 (15–40)
III	Tumor 2 cm; axillary and supraclavicular lymph nodes	$T_{2-3} N_3 M_x$	25 (15–60)	5 (0–12)
IV	Hematogenous metastases	$T_{2-4} N_3 M_1$	7 (0–10)	0

The recurrence rate is then significantly less. When metastases are present, a remission is gained for months or years and the pain of bone metastases is reduced.

In women less than 5 years past the menopause, especially with bone metastases and when estrogen values are 40 pg estradiol per milliliter plasma, oophorectomy is performed. Adrenalectomy and hypophysectomy are obsolete. Instead of androgens, estrogens or progesterone in very high doses are preferred at present. The dose is two tablets of tamoxifen (Nolvadex) twice a day. Thrombocytes and calcium plasma levels have to be controlled every 14 days. The treatment is relatively well tolerated.

7. Cytostatic Therapy

An adjuvant treatment is tried at present in all probable cases of advanced mammary cancer and also when a spread has been found. A high dose short-lasting therapy once or twice a month is preferred to a long-lasting low or medium dose therapy. However the side effects are severe and in some cases the quality of life is badly reduced. The effect of cytostatic therapy on recurrence, cure, and remission is still doubtful.

8. Prognosis

The prognosis of the different stages of mammary cancer is given in Table 19.

References

Aylward M (1976) Estrogens, plasma tryptophan levels in perimenopausal patients. In: Campbell S (ed) The management of the menopause and postmenopausal years. MTP Press, Lancester, pp 135–147

Beller KF, Knörr K, Lauritzen C, Wynn MR (1974) Gynecology. A textbook for students. Springer, Berlin Heidelberg New York

Bennington M, James L, Benjamin R, Ferguson A, Haber L (1968) Incidence and relative frequency of benign and malignant ovarian neoplasms. Obstet Gynecol 32:672–632

Burch JC, Byrd BF, Vaughn WK (1975) The effects of long-term estrogen administration to women following hysterectomy. In: Van Keep PA, Lauritzen C (eds) Estrogens in the post-menopause. Karger, Basel, pp 208–211

Campbell S (ed) (1976) The management of the menopause and post-menopausal years. MTP Press, Lancaster

Cooke JD (ed) (1978) The role of estrogen/progestagen in the management of the menopause. MTP Press, Lancaster

Gambrell RD (1978) The role of hormones in endometrial cancer. South Med J 71:1280–1289

Gerber M, Walter C, Frick CH (1962) Cancer in New York State exclusive of New York City. Bureau of Cancer Control, New York Department of Health

Gompel C, Silverberg SG (1969) Pathology in gynecology and obstetrics. Lippincott, Philadelphia

Gordon GS (1977) Postmenopausal osteoporosis. Cause, prevention and treatment. Clin Obstet Gynecol 4:169–176

Greenblatt RB, Studd J (eds) (1977) The menopause. Clin Obstet Gynecol 4/1

Grimmer H (1974) Gut- und bösartige Erkrankungen der Vulva. Grosse, Berlin

Gusberg SB, Frick HC (1970) Corscaden's gynecologic cancer, 4th edn. Williams and Wilkins, Baltimore

Haspels AA, Musaph H (eds) (1979) Psychosomatics in peri-menopause. MTP Press, Lancaster

Itil TM, Laudahn G, Herrmann WM (1976) Psychotropic action of hormones. Spectrum, New York

Janowski NA (1979) Histologie und Einteilung der Ovarialtumoren. In: Döderlein G, Wulf KH (eds) Klinik der Frauenheilkunde und Geburtshilfe, vol 8. Urban and Schwarzenberg, Munich, pp 651–714

Jeffcoate TNA (1967) Principles of gynaecology, 3rd edn. Appelton-Century-Crofts, New York

Jern HH (1973) Hormone therapy of the menopause and ageing. Thomas, Springfield

Judmaier F (ed) (1980) Chirurgische Therapie des Mammakarzinoms. Karger, Basel

Knörr K, Knörr-Gärtner H, Beller F, Lauritzen C (1982) Lehrbuch der Geburtshilfe und Gynäkologie. Springer, Berlin Heidelberg New York

Kottmeier H (1969) Annual Report of Gynecologic Cancer. Almquist and Viksell, Stockholm

Lauritzen C (1975) The female climacteric syndrome: significance, problems, treatment. Acta Obstet Gynecol Scand Suppl 51:47–55

Lauritzen C (1978) Das Klimakterium. Z Allg Med 54:567–574

Lauritzen C (1982) Das Klimakterium. Schering, Berlin

Lauritzen C, Van Keep P (eds) (1978) Estrogen therapy. The benefits and risks. Karger, Basel

Lauritzen C, Wolf AS, Strabl M (1977) A retrospective study concerning postmenopausal estrogen therapy and endometrial cancer. In: Brush H, King J, Taylor C (eds) Endometrial Cancer. Baillière Tindall, London, pp 39–46

Lewis GA, Wentz WB, Jaffee RM (1966) New concepts in gynecologic oncology. Davis, Philadelphia

Marshall DH, Horsmann A, Nordin BEC (1977) The prevention and management of postmenopausal osteoporosis. Acta Obstet Gynecol Scand Suppl 65:49–56

Novak ER, Woodruff JD (1967) Novak's gynecologic and obstetric pathology, 6th edn. Saunders, Philadelphia

Pasetto N, Paoletti R, Ambrus JL (eds) (1980) The menopause and postmenopause. MTP Press, Lancaster

Rauramo L, Punnonen R (1973) Die Wirkung von Kastration und oraler Östrogentherapie auf die Haut der Frau. In: Van Keep PA, Lauritzen C (eds) Älter werden und Östrogene. Karger, Basel, pp 48–54

Te Linde RW, Mattingly RF (1970) Operative gynecology, 4th edn. Lippincott, Philadelphia
Teilum G (1971) Special tumors of the ovary and testis. Munksgaard, Copenhagen
TNM-Klassifikation der malignen Tumoren (1979) Der deutschsprachige TNM-Ausschuß (eds) Springer, Berlin Heidelberg New York
Committee on professional education of UICC (ed) (1973) UICC clinical oncology: A manual for students and doctors. Springer, Berlin Heidelberg New York
Van Keep P, Lauritzen C (eds) (1973) Ageing and estrogens. Karger, Basel
Van Keep P, Lauritzen C (eds) (1975) Estrogens in the post-menopause. Karger, Basel
Van Keep P, Greenblatt RB, Albeaux-Fernet M (1976) Consensus on menopause research. MTP Press, Lancaster
Van Keep P, Serr DM, Greenblatt RB (1979) Female and male climacteric. MTP Press, Lancaster

Epidemiology: Some Aspects of the Climacteric Woman

L. J. BENEDEK-JASZMANN

It is not enough for a great nation to have added new years to life. Our objective must be to add new life to those years.

John F. Kennedy

A. Introduction

Medical research is traditionally more concerned with pathology than normality. This certainly is true in case of the epidemiology of the climacteric and postclimacteric phases in a woman. The problems in the climacteric have recently been gaining increasing recognition as to their importance. This is particulary true of the last three decades and seems to be due to the fact that there has been a rapid increase in the number of women over 40 years old and to a growing interest in studying both health and fertility of different populations. Another contributing factor is the rapid development of hormone replacement therapy. This could be clearly seen in the attitude of WILSON (1965) who started his crusade by describing its object as "feminine forever" with the use of estrogens. However, he also stated rather apologetically that the climacteric years and the period following have to be regarded as a pathological condition. Epidemiological surveys of the normal development of the climacteric period and the years beyond show a big gap in our knowledge of the subject.

In the last decades because of changes in social structure, gerontology and its allied specialisations have received a great deal of attention. The important phase in a woman's life, the transition from the fertile period to the stage where geriatrics begins, has been largely disregarded. Chapters on this subject even in gynaecological handbooks were rather vague. Nomenclature, definitions of climacteric stages and common physiologically identifiable symptoms showed a wide variety of meanings, i.e. psychic, psychosomatic, neurovegetative, endocrine, and somatic. Opinions as to the exact relationship between these and the climacteric vary from one author to another. Climacteric symptoms or complaints are, therefore, somewhat arbitrary when not based on scientific study of the epidemiology.

There is another reason for the recent increase in epidemiological data for the climacteric and postclimacteric periods. Times have changed and continue to change; women have adopted different roles in society. The doctor is now consulted about many complaints which used to remain untreated or were treated by self-medication. There are not only medical but also psychosociological problems typical of the climacteric period such as cross-cultural factors and anthropoligical aspects. At the same time, the number of women in this transitional age group has increased and we have at last to realise that the climacteric period is the gateway to a new phase in life, to gerontology and its consequences.

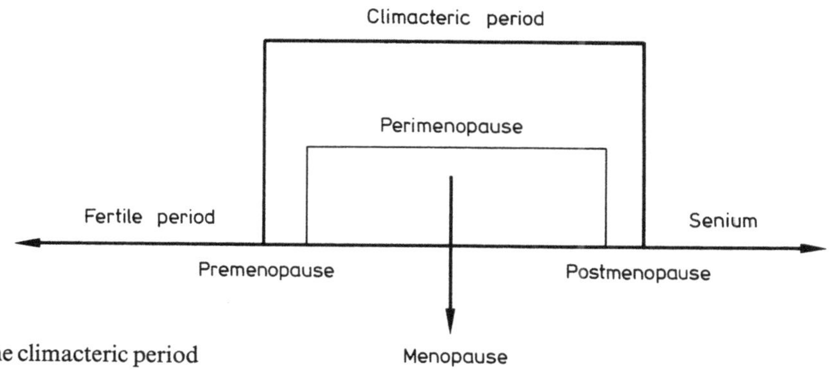

Fig. 1. The climacteric period

B. International Definitions of the Climacteric Period

First, I would like to draw attention to some definitions concerned with the menstrual periods of middle-aged women. According to the Nomenclature Committee of the International Federation of Obstetrics and Gynaecology, menopause means the last physiological bleeding from the uterus. The exact definition of menopause is important. Even in the present literature we often find this used as if it were synonymous with "climacteric". The term menopause is only a milestone, meaning the last bleeding from the uterus. This must be considered as the counterpart of the first blood loss from the uterus, called the menarche. It was KAISER and DAUME in 1965 who defined the terms menopause and climacteric. As a basis for a sound discussion of the definition of the climacteric and its phases, as well as the menopause, they analysed the entire period from full maturity to old age of a woman from various points of view.

The climacteric period (Fig. 1) is a phase of life when a woman changes, mentally and physically from sexual maturity to old age; and is thus a counterpart to puberty, and adolescence which lead to sexual maturity. For most clinical purposes we often use the term "perimenopausal" to describe a few years prior to and the last year following the menopause. The period preceding the menopause we call the premenopause not only from a theoretical, but also from practical point of view; the years following the menopause are the postmenopause. The various patterns of blood loss from the uterus in the premenopause are mostly caused by endocrine changes, but haemorrhage, bleeding from the uterus after 1 year, is however an arbitrary decision and could be considered as a pathological event. Clinical follow-up, diagnostic currettage, and/or cervical smear have to be done to exclude malignancy. In cases of blood loss one has to make a careful distinction between loss of blood from the cavity or from the cervix and portio vaginalis cervicis.

There is no sharp difference between the expressions postmenopausal or postclimacteric period, both definitions describe the period preceding the geriatric stage. Even the definitions of climacteric period and middle-aged woman must be differentiated. The climacteris is a physiological process with underlying hormonal changes and with a typical symptomatology. It is part of the picture of the middle-aged woman. We have to realise that symptoms and complaints in the climacteric period are not synonymous, although we usually make no distinction between these two definitions, but use the terms interchangeably. The normal symptoms of this phase can be divided into: (a) genital; (b) extragenital; and (c) psychosocial. The genital symptoms are very well known from normal menses via a changed pattern of menstruation, accompanied by infertility, cessation of uterine bleeding and postclimacteric genital atrophy. The cause of these changes is entirely hormonal and can be seen in every woman. In contrast, the extragenital symptoms of this phase of life do not neccesarily occur in all women and the causes are neurovegetative, psychosomatic and hormonal.Genital symptoms, changes in the menstrual pattern, are in general regarded by women as normal and are only mentioned as complaints when bleeding is abnormally heavy or frequent. Oral contraception with regulation of monthly bleeding is generally accepted. On the contrary, extragenital symptoms, although differing in intensity and frequency from one woman to another, are often regarded as unpleasant symptoms, and so they became complaints. The genital symptoms after the menopause are also well known to women, but many women ignore them and do not regard a blood loss 1 year after the menopause as a sign of possible malignancy.

It is well known that the middle age per se has its psychosocial aspects like the "empty nest syndrome", identity problems, attitude to sexual activity, changing patterns in the family, etc. The fact that psychosocial developments and behavior and the realisation of approaching old age are more important in this phase of life than the symptoms and problems of the climacteric itself is supported by the literature.

When speaking about climacteric and postclimacteric symptoms or complaints the question often arises: which symptoms belong to hormonal changes and which to psychosocial events? Sometimes we cannot exactly exlude the typical climacteric and postclimacteric symptoms or complaints without taking into account the complexity of the psychosocial aspects of the middle-aged woman. In no phase of life, however, is the line between what is normal, and therefore acceptable to the individual, and what is pathological, and therefore unacceptable, more vague than here. Climacteric symptoms, especially the extragenital ones, are very often reported by women who are neither in any distress from them nor looking for treatment. On the other hand, the same symptoms may develop into real complaints for psychosocial reasons, such as stress. Sometimes those symptoms accompany some somatic diseases and other pathological states.

Most of the studies of climacteric and postclimacteric women can be divided in two main groups:

1. Surveys concerning "genital events", like the age at menopause, menstrual patterns, including possible fertility, abnormal bleeding patterns during the premenopause, as well as in the postmenopause, and stimuli which may influence these events.

2. Epidemiology of extragenital symptoms and complaints of the climacteric and postclimacteric period, variables which may influence complaints and other

factors like cross-cultural, and anthropological considerations, and socioeconomic influences.

The investigation of these topics from an academic point of view is important, but they also have practical implications in terms of public health and prophylactic medicine. They can also be used as a guide in treatment. The history of the menopause and the female climacteric is well described in the thesis of WILBUSH (1980).

C. Age at Menopause

The fact that nowadays the menopause occurs later, and the menarche earlier, is an interesting evolutionary phenomenon. The reproductive period gets longer and life expectancy grows even faster. This discrepancy leads to a relative increase in the part of a woman's total life in which she is without estrogens. The average life expectancy of a woman of 50 years is about 27 years in western Europe. In countries in the third world it is about 15–17 years. The increase in life expectancy is not so much the result of people living to very great ages, but because fewer people are dying young. Last but not least, psychologically, the event of the menopause heralds for many the beginning of the geriatric period. In the past there have been quite a large number of descriptive surveys designed to estimate the mean age at menopause and the factors which may influence this age. However, many of these studies have suffered from methological defects which have created difficulties and interpretation. Bad selection of the sample under study and inappropriate statistical procedures are to blame.

There are different kinds of methods of study such as personal interviews, questionnaires and research into the literature. There are in fact three kinds of approach:

1. The retrospective method, which as been undertaken on predominantly postmenopausal subjects, asking their age at last blood loss or the age at which their periods ceased; of course this kind of approach is vulnerable to memory errors as older women have difficulty in recalling age at the last menses. Several surveys have used this method.

2. The most appropriate method is a longitudinal cohort survey as proposed by FLINT (1978) and carried out by TRELOAR (1974), but it also has its disadvantages, being is costly and time consuming.

3. The cross-sectional or status quo method is employed in most current studies of menopause age. Here the respondents are asked whether or not they are still menstruating. A simple "yes" or "no" answer to this question is then plotted against the respondent's current age, and by probit or logit curve fitting (FINNEY 1964) of the proportion of women who were postmenopausal at successive years of age, a median age of menopause can be obtained. This method is meant to be employed with a total population of women, in a specific geographical area, within a given age range, such as 40–60 years. By probit analysis, the median age of menopause arrived at is the age at which the last menstrual period appears, while with logit analysis, it is the age at which 50% of the population under study recognise that their periods have stopped. This event may be a few months later than their last period.

Although most of the recent epidemiological studies are based on the cross-sectional or status quo approach, we have to appreciate that it too has its limitations.

BRAND (1978) surveyed research on median ages at menopause; this review is concluded with a schematic representation of ten studies that were selected because they all used the status quo method (Table 1). The earlier data were collected by FROMMER (1964) and the latest were obtained in 1977 by BRAND.

Comparison of age at menopause determined from a literature survey is hampered by different methods of data acquisition, definition of age at menopause and the statistical analysis method. In England in 1933 the Council of the British Medical Women's Federation carried out a survey of healthy females, but they failed to mention the manner in which the data were collected; their data processing differed from that used by BRAND (1978).

FROMMER (1964) applied probit analysis, but his data originated from women in hospitals. The publications of HAUSER and WENNER and HAUSER et al. (1961, 1963) form no basis for comparison as they also obtained their data from hospitals and did not always clearly state their methods of statistical analysis. MCMAHON and WORCESTER (1966) in the United States also used a written questionnaire which had to be completed by the subjects: their statistical analysis (logit) was similar to that used in the "Ede study" (JASZMANN et al. 1969; probit). Their median value for the white population was 50.0 years and for the black population 49.3 years. BURCH and GUNZ (1967) presented an attempt to estimate with some precision the age at cessation of menstruation. This is one of the first reasonably reliable attempts to estimate the mean age at cessation of menstruation. The median and modal ages were estimated using a logarithmic transformation.

FRERE (1971) reported results in white women between the ages of 40 and 59 years black women of 40–55 years. Artificial menopause and gynaecological complaints were excluded. The ages at menopause were estimated as 50.4 years for white women, the black women reaching this point 9 months earlier with a median age of 49.7. MCKINLAY et al. (1972) collected their data from a sample of 736 women living in or near London, excluding those artificially castrated. The mean age at menopause was 50.78 years. The findings of THOMSON et al. (1973) reported a population survey in Aberdeen, Scotland; the mean age in this series being 50.1 years. The age at menopause in the Netherlands has been investigated three times within the last 15 years, using the same definitions and method of analysis. The sample of DE WAARD (1966) consisted of women of 45–55 years, who visited their general practitioners; most of the respondents lived in larger cities, fewer in the country. A mean age of 51.4 years was found. A population survey was done in 1967 in the community of Ede, Netherlands, a partly urbanised rural community, by JASZMANN et al. (1969 a); based on the data supplied by those subjects who had never undergone genital surgery the mean age at menopause was 51.4 years. BRAND's survey carried out 10 years later on the same population as that studied by JASZMANN et al. (1967) states a mean age at menopause of 51.5 years. The age at menopause appeared in the Netherlands studies to be independent of environmental factors, no effect could be demonstrated of age at menarche, number of pregnancies or age at last pregnancy. A significant difference was found by JASZMANN et al., between women who were married or had at

Table 1. Estimated median ages at menopause from selected studies that used the status quo method (BRAND 1978)

Reference	Year of study	Country	Population studied			Menopausal status	Analysis	Median age (years)
			Number	Origin	Age range (years)			
FROMMER (1964)	1951–1961	England	443	Hospital in-patients	40–55	9 months amenorrhoea	Probit	50.1
DE WAARD (1965)	1964	Netherlands	739	General practice patients	45–55	1 year amenorrhoea	Probit	51.2
MCMAHON and WORCESTER (1966)	1964	United States	3,108	General population	35–59	Cessation of menstruation	Logit	49.8
BURCH and GUNZ (1967)	1967	New Zealand	485	General practice patients	30–65	1 year amenorrhoea	Logarithms	50.7
JASZMANN et al. (1969a)	1967	Netherlands	3,548	General population	40–60	1 year amenorrhoea	Probit	51.4
FRERE (1971)	1964–1967	South Africa	744	Hospital out-patients	40–59	1 year amenorrhoea	Probit	50.4
MCKINLAY et al. (1972)	1965	England	736	General population	45–54	1 year amenorrhoea	Logit	50.8
THOMPSON et al. (1973)	1970	Scotland	226	General population	40–60	1 year amenorrhoea	Logit	50.1
FUCHS and PASKARBEIT (1976)	1974	East Germany	2,097	General population	40–59	1 year amenorrhoea	50% end points	51.1
BRAND (1978)	1977	Netherlands	3,777	General population	40–60	1 year amenorrhoea	Probit	51.5

one time been married and those who never married. The ages at menopause for those groups were respectively 51.4 and 50.3 years. The same conclusion was reached by BRAND: no significant relation was found between any of the environmental variables investigated and corresponding mean ages at menopause obtained by means of probit analysis. With segmentation analysis, mean age at menopause appeared to be most sensitive to the woman's occupation. However, marital status, which came second in importance, probably exerts a stronger influence on the menopausal age than occupation. Other environmental variables that were shown to have measurable, but not significant correlation with the age at menopause were present and past smoking habits, age at last pregnancy and height.

An excellent literature survey was given by MCKINLAY and MCKINLAY (1973) on "Selected studies of the menopause" in three sections, each preceded by a brief discussion; they presented not only studies on the menopausal age, but also other surveys on the climacteric woman.

There are few data on menopausal age in Germany. FUCHS and PASKARBEIT (1976) and PRILL and LAURITZEN (1970) made brief observations on age at menopause, mentioning mostly the surveys already mentioned as well as that by KÄSER et al. in the Handbook of Gynaecology (1969). In a short survey HOFMANN and SOERGEL (1972) tabulated the previous investigations and in their summary mentioned that the age at menopause in Germany has shown a steady increase in the last 100 years and is at present approximately 50 years.

D. Epidemiology: Duration of the Reproductive Stage (Climacteric menstrual patterns)

The menstrual span of a woman is understood to denote the period between menarche and menopause. The years from the first to the last menstrual flow are not representative of the reproductive stage of woman as both puberty and the climacteric period are characterized by anovular cycles. So we have to differentiate between sexual maturity and fecundity on fertility. Fecundity is diminished in the first years after menarche and the last years before menopause. Postmenopausal conception has been reported (SNAITH and WILLIAMSON 1947), but these reports have become even more rare with the advent of objective documentation and the establishment of compulsory population registers and hospital records. True postmenopausal conception, if it exists, must be very uncommon indeed. Pregnancy is also known to occur occasionally before the first menstrual flow.

The capacity for fecundity was demonstrated by TIETZE (1957) in his study of reproduction span and the rate of pregnancies among Hutterite women. The menopause marks the completion of a gradual physiological process of declining fertility that has been developing during the course of a variable number of years. This progressive reduction in reproductive potential from middle age is evidenced by increasing intervals between confinements and increased incidence of miscarriages (HENRY 1961), increased perinatal mortality (BUTLER and BONHAM 1963) and increase in the proportion of anovular cycles (DÖRING 1969). In industrialised

Table 2. Frequency distribution of age at last pregnancy

Age at last pregnancy (years)	Frequency (%)
21–25	4
26–30	16
31–35	27
36–40	35
41–45	15
>45	3
Total number 2,860	100

Table 3. Frequency distribution of age at last pregnancy in the postmenopausal group

Age at last pregnancy (years)	Frequency (%)
≦25	5
26–30	10
31–35	22
36–40	39
41–45	21
>45	3
Total number 1,056	100

societies in particular, sociocultural factors, such as contraceptive pratice, recourse to termination of pregnancy, decreased frequency of intercourse and sexual abstinence, have also caused marked reduction in fertility among the older age group (GRAY 1976).

Changes in the pattern of menstruation can only be established by a longitudinal investigation as was done by TRELOAR (1974, 1981). In his survey the frequency distribution of age at menarche and menopause was given for 324 women whose menstrual histories had been recorded from their university student days until natural menopause terminated their potential for reproduction.

He stated an average length of menstrual life of 35.9 years. In our survey on duration of the reproductive stage (fecundity) and age at final pregnancy of women in their forties and fifties (JASZMANN et al. 1969a) we obtained data supplied by 3,916 women who had never undergone surgery of the ovaries and/or uterus. Table 2 which gives the frequency distribution of the age at the last pregnancy shows that 18% of the 2,860 women taking part in the survey had their last pregnancy over the age of 40 years. Nearly 3% were older than 45 years.

It should be noted that Table 2 is likely to underestimate the age at pregnancy because a number of women in the youngest age group (born between 1920 and 1925) certainly did not report their final pregnancy. Table 3 shows the frequency distribution for the postmenopausal group of age at last pregnancy. For this group it can be assumed that the last pregnancy reported is indeed their final one. The frequency distribution for this group (1,956 women) is given in Table 3 and shows a mean duration of 35.4 years; a similar period was stated by TRELOAR

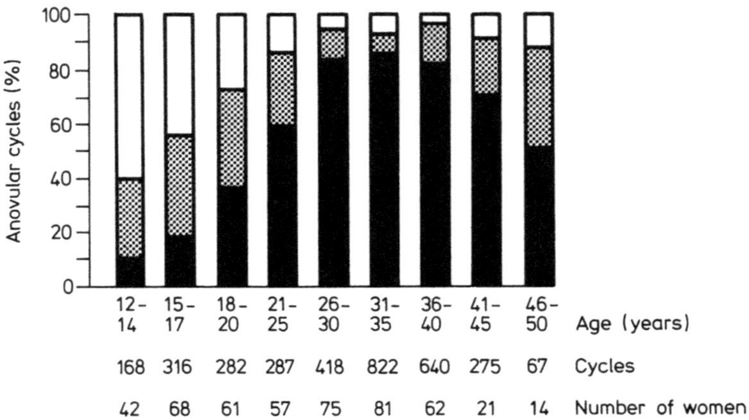

Fig. 2. Percentage of anovular cycles (*open bars*), shortened luteal phase (*stippled bars*) and normal cycles (*full bars*). (DÖRING 1963)

(1974). An average value of the length of the menstrual period for the total of 3,916 women investigated was 37 years.

In conclusion we have found a positive trend towards a prolongation of the menstrual period, indicating the further possibility of a longer fecundity in the late forties. A comparison of the distribution of the age at last pregnancy of these subjects (i.e. the fertility pattern of contemporary women in their forties) with the data from the younger generation indicates a shift to a lower age at last pregnancy. The report of the Netherlands Institute of Preventive Medicine for 1968 showed a clear decrease in married fertility (reproductive frequency) of women over 30 years of age; this shift was noticeable as far back as 1950 (see VAN WIERINGEN et al. 1968). From a practical point of view it would be interesting to see whether the prolonged menstrual period could influence the actual fertile span (fecundity) of a woman. The years of puberty and menopause are characterized by a large number of anovular cycles, i.e. a considerably reduced fertility. The mean age of menarche in the Netherlands has been reported as 13 years 5 months; there has been a shift of 3 months to an earlier age in one decade (VAN WIERINGEN et al. 1968). It may suffice here to quote the data of DÖRING (1963) concerning 1,440 very young mothers. It appears that in spite of regular coitus the first conception took place only during the second year after menarche. Figure 2 shows the precentage of anovular cycles, shortened luteal phase and normal cycles according to DÖRING (1963). According to him the age of women who still have ovular menses seemed to be between the ages 40 and 45 years (approximately 70%). At ages between 46 and 50 years the probable ovulation rate is 50%.

It seems likely that the manner in which the change in the menstrual pattern during this stage of life occurs from regular (ovular) menses to cessation (anovular bleeding), is also subject to secular changes, mostly in western societies. However, no concrete evidence exists to back up this hypothesis.

Some useful data emerged from our survey, although these represent only a momentary cross-section and not a longitudinal research result. For each year of

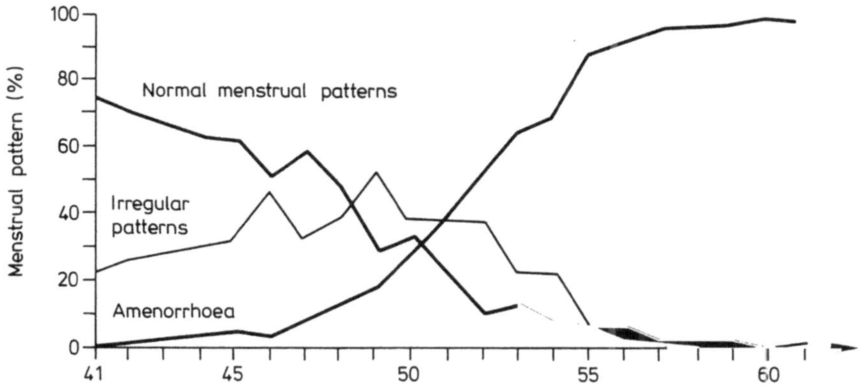

Fig. 3. Menstrual pattern in women who had not undergone surgical treatment. (JASZMANN et al. 1967)

birth (calendar age) the percentage of women who menstruated regularly or irregularly or whose menses had ceased during the past was determinated. The distribution (3,548 women) is given in Fig. 3. We found no important changes in the menstrual pattern in 50% of the patients between 46 and 48 years. It cannot be excluded that these menstrual patterns are also subject to a secular shift with an increase of ovulation cycles and pregnancy during the premenopause. The percentage of women with ovulation cycles seems to be about 70% between the age of 40 and 45 years (DÖRING 1963). This shows a decline of 50% between the ages of 45 and 50 years. Our findings support the same facts. The reproduction potential has also been presented by VOLLMANN (1966) in terms of the occurrence of monophasic basal-body temperature curves for each year of reproductive life. He concluded that 45% of all menstrual cycles in the first year of menstrual life are anovular. For each successive year he found the proportion of biphasic cycles to increase in an approximately direct manner until 97% of all menstrual cycles are biphasic at an average age of 23 years. The proportion of biphasic cycles thereafter remains reasonably constant until ages above 40 years are reached, when the proportion of biphasic cycles gradually decreases, to about 50% before menopause.

At the same time (vital statistics of the Unites States, 1967, quoted by TRELOAR 1974) the proportion of fertility among United States whites is estimated to have risen rapidly from 1% at the age of 15 years to a maximum level of 19% at age 23 years. Fertility fell slowly in the following 20 years untill the 1% level was reached again at the age of 43 years. TRELOAR (1974) pointed out that age at menarche has little value as a predictor of length of menstrual life, but it is highly dependent on the age at menopause. In his research, a longitudinal study of 324 women showed a 95% confidence interval for prediction of length of menstrual life which is almost ±6 years, or a total range of 12 years. Finally, we can now assume that with the secular trend of age at menopause (51.5 years), the menstrual period will show a longer regularity with the probable consequence of prolonged fecundity.

It cannot be excluded that the alterations in the menstrual pattern, that is a shift to older age, is also subject to secular change (the so-called biomorphosis of the endocrine; HAUSER 1963) with an increased possibility of pregnancy during the later phase in the middle-aged woman (TIETZE 1957; SOBERSON et al. 1966; ROBERTS 1964; HIGDON 1960; PARKS 1952; STANTON 1956; WHARTON 1964; JASZMANN 1971). With the knowledge of this fact, *contraceptive methods of different kinds are now generally assumed and taken into account in the climacteric period.* The age at menopause is an important determinant of the number of years of menstrual experience. All these findings, especially in western countries, are probably due to the evolution of socioeconomic conditions, better nutritional factors, medical care and treatment and also to a change of women's attitudes to this phase of life – a sign of the general welfare of our generation. The literature contains many data (KÄSER et al. 1969; PRILL and LAURITZEN 1970) of pathological menstrual disorders in the climacteric. We would like to mention a few other reports. GAVALLER-DEBREAU (1959) found that the maximum number of cases of climacteric haemorrhage required curettage between the ages of 41 and 45 years. KAISER and DAUME (1965) found this to be 45 to 50 years. In 80% of the cases histology showed the cause of blood loss to be dysfunctional, i.e. hormonal. More than 50% of these patients were already in their last premenstrual years as was revealed by a follow-up enquiry. Malignancy was found in 5.2% (fundal carcinoma); this was found in 5 of 615 cases of premenstrual bleeding. In 105 cases of postmenopausal blood loss there was a marked change in pathology. Fundal carcinoma was found in 47.6% cases. In all cases of haemorrhage there was an intact cervix.

In his study of 2,000 European women between the ages of 45 and 55 years, VAN KEEP (1970) specifically asked respondents if they had experienced metrorrhagia; 17% said that they had. One-third of these women had ignored this sign of possible danger and did not seek medical advice. In our survey 4,584 women were questioned whether they had ever undergone curettage; 3,965 replied. A positive answer was given by 25% of them. The reason for this treatment, abortion or metrorrhagia or different origin, could not be determinated by this survey. We found the highest proportion in the age group 41–45 years; this agrees with the findings of GAVALLER-DEBREAU (1959).

E. Genital Changes in the Postmenopausal Period

Considering the genital events of climacteric women, we generally find during the premenopause only the irregular pattern of uterine bleeding which is a typical symptom or complaint; there are not yet any marked changes in other target organs. The menopause is not only a milestone in a woman's life. In the postmenopausal period we find, besides the typical extragenital vasomotor symptoms, the first signs of geriatric systemic alterations of somatic origin. The most pronounced changes are atrophy of the target organs, namely the vulva, the vagina, the urethra, and the bladder, in particular its trigone. Maximum complaints usually occur 2–3 years after menopause. The atrophy of ovaries has already started in an earlier phase.

Simple vulval atrophy, sometimes accompanied by pruritus or burning sensations is a common sign. Atrophic vaginal epithelium may lead to a discharge sometimes with a feeling of dryness and itching or burning. The result will be dyspareunia. The male partner, not familiar with this normal change cannot understand the unexpected attitude of the woman to sexual relations. Libido decreases in a considerable proportion of cases in the postmenopausal years (KINSEY et al. 1955; PRILL and LAURITZEN 1970; VAN KEEP and GREGORY 1977). Urinary stress incontinence occurs sometimes with prolapse of the uterus, conditioned by many factors, such as constitution, number and mode of deliveries.

Estrogen deprivation is obviously an additional important cause, because in a large proportion it manifests itself at the period of the climacteric. These pathological conditions improve spontanously or can be cured in the majority of cases by local or systemic estrogen substitution therapy (LAURITZEN 1973). In the first degree of stress incontinence, urethral ectropion improvement can be obtained in 90%, and cure in about 80% of the cases. On the other hand, real stress–urge incontinence which is clearly due to anatomical insufficiency of the sphincter, responds better to surgery. Generally, administration of estrogens in mild cases of postmenopausal urinary tract conditions is to be recommended. BURCH et al. (1975) were interested in this problem and have reported their results in a group of women who had undergone hysterectomy and oophorectomy. The lack of epidemiological publications on this subject is still a hiatus in the postmenopausal literature. Atrophy of the breast is also a frequent occurrence in postmenopausal women. In about 60% of all women in this transitional phase there is a decrease in the volume and firmness of the breast (LIEPELT 1952).

F. Extragenital Symptoms and Complaints

There are many so-called extragenital symptoms and complaints of climacteric women, but these are very arbitrary. According to PRILL and LAURITZEN (1970) there are only hot flushes, with perspiration and dizziness, the typical extragenital climacteric symptom. The medical literature shows a wide variety of psychic, psychosomatic, neurovegetative, and endocrine extragenital symptoms which are regarded as climacteric symptoms or complaints. Opinions as to the exact relationship between these and the climacteric vary from one author to another, depending on their approach to climacteric problems. The Blatt Menopausal Index (BMI) devised in 1953 and modified by NEUGARTEN and KRAINES (1965) has been extremly useful in the past and, indeed, is often still used in its original form. Our survey (Jaszmann et al. 1969 a), (6,628 patients, response rate 71%) was stimulated by the opinion of WENNER and HAUSER (1957), who underlined the importance of the aging ovaries and their effect on the entire autonomic nervous system of the organism during the climacteric period. Our aim was mainly to test the validity and the significance index plotted against the underlying hormonal changes, i.e. cessation of estrogen production. In this investigation we used the population survey in the same community of Ede, Netherlands (1967) employed for the survey of the age at menopause. The analysis of symptoms and complaints of the cli-

Table 4. Frequency distribution of calendar age for each of the biological age groups

Groups		Calendar age (years)				Total	Mean calendar age (years)
		45	45–50	50–55	55		
		Frequency (%)					
Premenopausal	A	53	35	11	1	100	45.3
Menopausal	B	29	42	27	2	100	48.2
	C1	3	16	62	19	100	52.8
	C2	2	15	56	27	100	53.5
	C3	1	12	53	34	100	54.1
Postmenopausal	C4	1	8	35	56	100	55.4
	C5	0	3	18	79	100	57.7
	C6	0	4	22	74	100	58.2

Table 5. Criteria for biological (menstrual) age groups

Criterion	Group
Women menstruating regularly or with a menstrual pattern similar to that which they have had in the preceding years	A
Women menstruating during the last 12 months, but with a pattern different from that of the preceding years	B
Women whose LMP[a] occurred 12–24 months ago	C1
LMP 25–36 months ago	C2
LMP 37–48 months ago	C3
LMP 49–60 months ago	C4
LMP 5–10 years ago	C5

[a] LMP = last menstrual period

macteric were based on data supplied by subjects in the survey who had never undergone surgical treatment of the uterus and/or the ovaries.

Most studies into climacteric complaints describe the frequency of such symptoms in relation to the chronological age at which they occur. Table 4 shows the frequency distribution of calender age for each of the definied biological age groups. A much better insight is obtained when the symptoms or complaints are studied in relation to the so-called biological age. Our definition of the biological or menstrual age is dependent on the pattern of menstruation, the menopause, and the time which has elapsed since then.

Accordingly, the climacteric complaints of the respondents were studied when the women were grouped as shown in Table 5. It is obvious that typical climacteric symptoms or complaints are mentioned rarely by women in group A, relatively frequently by women in group B, (and to some degree in groups C1 and C2), but less often by women in groups C3, C4, and C5. In order to provide a basis for comparison with other studies, the 13 symptoms and complaints listed, were those of the BMI modified by NEUGARTEN and KRAINES (1965). Each of the

Table 6. Blatt's Menopausal Index modified by NEUGARTEN and KRAINES (1965)

Complaint	Factor[a]
Hot flushes	4
Perspiration	2
Paraesthesia	2
Insomnia	2
Muscle, joint, or bone pain	1
Fatigue	1
Headache	1
Irritability	1
Vertigo	1
Depression	1
Breath lessness	1
Palpitations	1
Mental imbalance	1

[a] Severity of complaints: 0 = no complaint; 1 = slight; 2 = moderate; 3 = marked or severe

various symptoms and complaints has been given a conversion factor, based on its severity score. The sum of these is the Menopausal Index. The unfortunate woman who suffers severely with all 13 complaints will have the maximum score of 57 (Table 6).

The rational underlying this survey was that in a woman with normal ovular menses the hormones and the autonomic hypothalamic centre functions (neurohormonal system) are at equilibrium, forming a functional entity. As soon as the menstrual pattern begins to deviate from the norm, disturbance of endocrine function may be expected to exist. This will be most pronounced after cessation of the menses, but in most cases nature will eventually restore a balance between the two functional systems (neurovegetative and hormonal). Our findings showed that the extragenital symptoms such as fatigue, headache, irritability, dizziness and to a lesser degree depression, showed their highest frequency in women in group B, i.e. women whose menstrual patterns had altered within the last year (Fig. 4). Such complaints could be regarded as psychosomatic manifestations of the beginning of disturbances in the balance between the neurovegetative and endocrine system. In these women, ovarian function, albeit to a lesser extent, is still present.

Hot flushes, perspiration, formication and pain in the muscles, joints, and bones were all most frequently experienced by women in the early postmenopause; in groups C1 and C2 (Fig. 5). These complaints could therefore be regarded as symptoms of disturbed hypothalamic regulation and lack of estrogen production by the ovaries; they are complaints related to endogenous estrogen production. The distribution of their frequency over the range of biological age is typical for a climacteric symptom or complaint.

Sleeplessness, breathlessness, palpitations, and mental imbalance (psycholability) did not show a peak in any one of the biological age groups (Fig. 6). These complaints of the BMI, therefore, are most probably not complaints which are

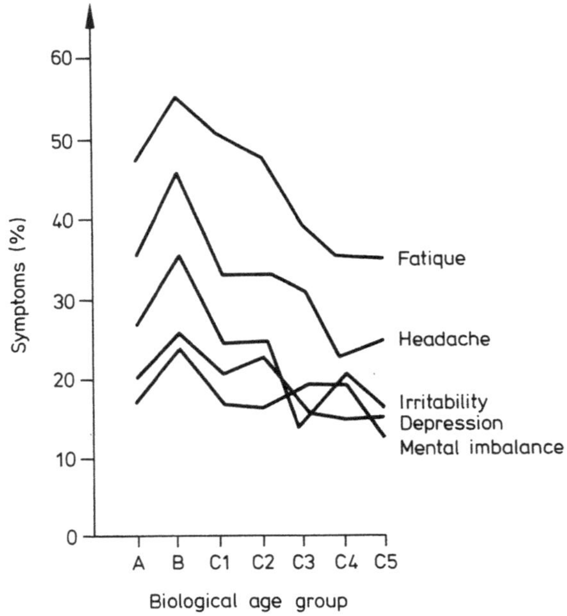

Fig. 4. Symptoms and complaints in women whose menstrual pattern had altered within 1 year

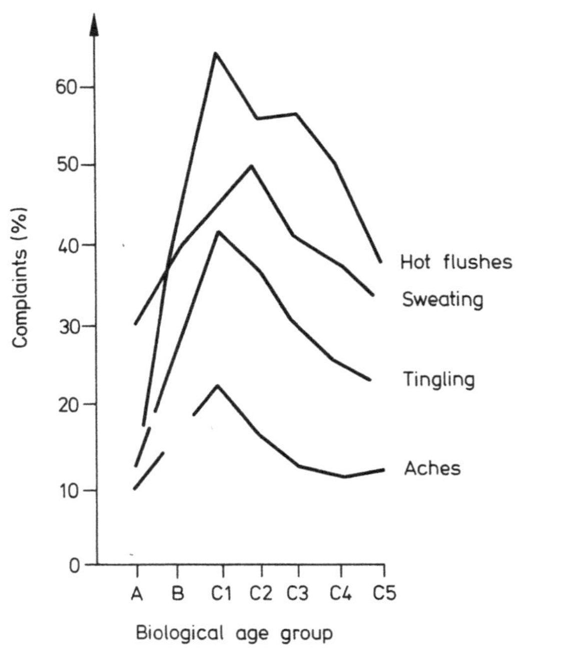

Fig. 5. Complaints during early menopause

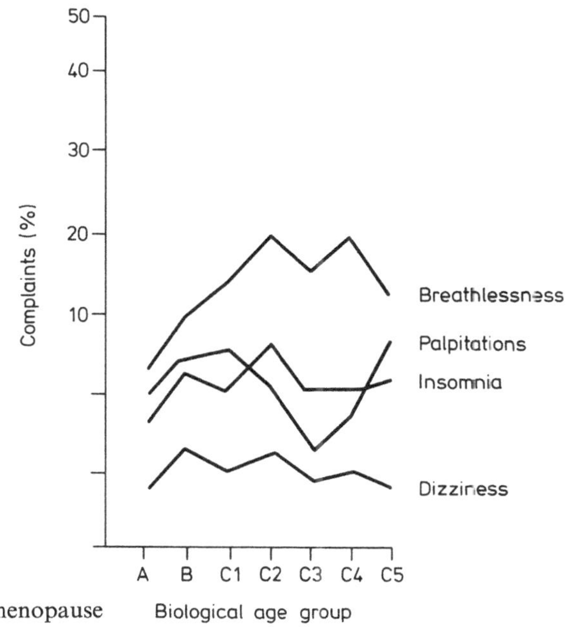

Fig. 6. Complaints during the postmenopause

peculiar to the climacteric age. It seems likely, therefore, that they are geriatric complaints rather than complaints of the climacteric or of the early postmenopause.

I. Influences on the Incidence of Complaints

It is well known that extragenital symptoms and complaints can be influenced by various factors. Minor symptoms may change to serious complaints. The variables tested in this study were age at menarche, number of pregnancies, age at last pregnancy, income level, education, marital status, and physical type. A summary of the conclusions gained is given here. More detailed data have been published by JASZMANN et al. (1969).

It was found that women who had a late menarche had fewer complaints than women whose menarche came early. Women who had never been pregnant had fewer complaints than women who had experienced one or more pregnancies. Women who had their last pregnancy after the age of 40 years fewer climacteric complaints than women whose last pregnancy occurred earlier. Women in the higher income groups had fewer complaints than women in the lower income groups. Women who had only a primary school education had more complaints than women of higher education. Physical type did not appear to be an influential factor. Unmarried women had fewer complaints than married women. The variables were analysed one-dimensionally. It is clear that some variables are highly correlated, therefore one and the same distinction may be found in several ways. The conclusion that fewer complaints were reported by women who had never been pregnant conveys to a large extent the same information as: married women appear to have more complaints than single, full-time working women.

Our research into extragenital symptoms and complaints suggests that the time has now come when this index should be revised by experienced epidemiologists from different disciplines to try to create a more suitable instrument which might be called the International Menopausal Index. Such an index could have different uses:

1. It would be of great use in helping one to be objective about subjective psychic, neurovegetative und psychosomatic symptoms of women and could also be a guide in therapy.
2. It could permit more exact registration of results and also comparison of different kinds of therapy.
3. It could serve as a basis for international studies in different disciplines, standardising basic research and providing treatment guidelines for women entering this new phase of life.

Interesting data were obtained in recent epidemiological research, carried out with the cooperation of a medical sociologist (Aakster and Jaszmann 1980). A sample of 1,500 Dutch women aged between 40 and 60 years were interviewed. The checklist we used consisted of 22 items; partly medical complaints due to the climacteric period (including menstrual patterns, menopause); partly psychosociological questions to assess positive and negative attitudes.

Two main patterns were found by different kinds of analytical methods:

1. Only hot flushes and perspiration showed significant correlations with biological (menstrual) age.
2. In 22 different kinds of analytical methods by a cross-table procedure, we found increasing age to be a significant factor in 20.

Briefly summarized: this medicopsychosociological study supports the view that the climacteric period is not only a medical problem due to the diminution of estrogen production, but that it belongs rather to the general physiological aging process often connected with different psychosocial variables. This chapter began with John F. Kennedy's statement of the prime objective of modern geriatric care; we should not forget that, for women, it is the menopause which marks the transition to geriatrics.

References

Aakster CW, Jaszmann LJB (1980) A medico-psychosociological epidemiologic survey of the middle-aged Dutch woman (in Dutch). Praeventiefonds Report. The Hague

Brand PC (1978) Age at menopause. Ph D thesis, Utrecht

Burch JC, Byrd BF, Vaughn WK (1975) The effect of "long-term" estrogen administration to women following hysterectomy. In: Van Keep PA, Lauritzen C (eds) Estrogens in the post-menopause. Karger, Basel, pp 208–212

Burch PRJ, Gunz FW (1967) The distribution of menopausal age in New Zealand. An exploratory study. NZ Med J 66:6–10

Butler N, Bonham D (1963) Perinatal mortality. Livingstone, London

De Waard F (1965) De menopause-leeftijd in Nederland. Huisarts en Wetenschap 8:325

De Waard F, Van Der Burgt AT (1966) The age at menopause (in Dutch). Ned Tijdschr Geneesk 110:289–291
Döring GK (1963) Über die relative Häufigkeit des anovulatorischen Zyklus im Leben der Frau. Arch Gynäk 199:115
Döring GK (1969) The incidence of anovular cycles in women. J Reprod Fertil [Suppl] 6:77–81
Finney DJ (1964) Probit analysis, a statistical treatment of the sigmoid response curve, 2nd edn. University Press, Cambridge
Flint M (1978) Is there a secular trend in age of menopause? Maturitas 1:133–139
Frere G (1971) Mean age at menopause and menarche in South Africa. S Afr J Med Sci 36:21–24
Frommer DJ (1964) Changing age of menopause, Br Med J ii:349–351
Fuchs M, Paskarbeit C (1976) Das Menopausealter in der DDR. Sante Publique (Bucur) 2:193–200
Gavaller-Debreau J (1959) Analyse der im Klimakterium auftretenden Blutungsstörungen. Arch Gynecol 193:33–36
Gray RH (1976) The menopause, epidemiological and demographical consideration. In: Beard RJ (ed) The menopause, a guide to current research and practice. MTP Press, Lancaster, pp 25–40
Hauser GA (1969) Rückbildung der Fortpflanzungsfunktionen im Klimakterium und in der Menopause. In: Käser O et al. (eds) Gynäkologie und Geburtshilfe, Vol 1. Thieme, Stuttgart, pp 784–810
Hauser GA, Wenner R (1961) Das Klimakterium der Frau. Ergeb Inn Med Kinderheilkd 152:126–197
Hauser GA, et al. (1963) Menarche und Menopause in Israel. Gynaecologia 155:39–47
Hauser GA, et al. (1971) Der Zusammenhang zwischen gynäkologischen Krankheiten und dem Menopausenalter. Gynaecologia 152:270–278
Henry L (1961) Some data on natural fertility. Eugen Q 8:81–83
Higdon AZ (1960) Pregnancy in women over forty. Am J Obst Gyn 80:38
Hofmann D, Soergel T (1972) Untersuchungen über das Menarche- und Menopausealter. Geburtshilfe Frauenheilkd 32:969–977
Jaszmann L (1971) A few data on the use of the pill by middle-aged women. Med Gyn Sociol 5:12
Jaszmann LJB (1976) Epidemiology of the climacteric syndrome. In: Campbell S (ed) The management of the menopause and post-menopausal years. MTP Press, Lancaster, pp 11–23
Jaszmann LJB, van Lith ND, Zaat JCA (1967) A survey on the problems, symptomatology of the contemporary Dutch woman (in Dutch). Praeventiefonds Report, The Hague
Jaszmann LJB, van Lith ND, Zaat JCA (1969 a) The age at menopause in the Netherlands: The statistical analysis of a survey. Int J Fertil 14:106–117
Jaszmann LJB, van Lith ND, Zaat JCA (1969 b) The duration of the reproductive stage at the age at final pregnancy of women in their fourties and fifties. Med Gynaecol/Androl Sociol 4:263–267
Kaiser R, Daume E (1965) Über eine einheitliche Nomenklatur für das Klimakterium und seine Begleitsymptome. Geburtshilfe Frauenheilkd 25:974–986
Käser O, Friedber V, Ober KG, Thomsen K, Zander J (1969) Gynäkologie und Geburtshilfe, vol 1. Thieme, Stuttgart, pp 784–810
Kinsey AC, Pomeroy WB, Martin CE, Gebhard PH (1953) Sexual behavior in the human female. Saunders, Philadelphia, Chap 9, p 303
Lauritzen C (1973) The management of the pre-menopausal and post-menopausal patient. In: Van Keep PA, Lauritzen C (eds) Ageing and estrogens. Karger, Basel, pp 2–21
McKinlay SM, McKinlay JB (1973) Selected studies of the menopause. J Biosoc Sci 5:533–555
McKinlay S, Jefferys M, Thompson B (1972) An investigation of the age at Menopause. J Biosoc Sci 4:161–173
McMahon B, Worcester J (1966) Age at menopause, United States 1960–1962. US vital and health statistics, ser 11, no 19. Washington DC

Neugarten BL, Kraines RJ (1965) Menopausal symptoms in women of various ages. Psychosom Med 27:266–270
Parks J (1952) Pregnancy after forty. Geriatrics 6:399
Prill HJ, Lauritzen C (1970) Das Klimakterium. In: Schwalm H, Döderlein G (eds) Klinik der Frauenheilkunde und Geburtshilfe, vol 8. Urban und Schwarzenberg, München, pp 341–432
Roberts DF (1964) Probability of spontaneous abortion in multiparae. J. Reprod Fert. 7:89
Snaith L, Williamson M (1947) Pregnancy after the menopause. J Obstet Gynaecol Br Emp 54:496–498
Soberson J, Calderon JJ, Goldzieher JW (1966) Relation of parity to age at menopause. Am J Obstet Gynecol 96:96–98
Stanton EF (1956) Pregnancy after forty-four. Am J Obstet Gynecol 71:270–272
Thompson B, Hart SA, Durno D (1973) Menopausal age and symptomatology in a general practice, J Biosoc Sci 5:71–82
Tietze C (1957) Reproductive span and rate of reproduction among Hutterite women. Fertil Steril 8:89–97
Treloar AE (1974) Menarche, menopause and interventing fecundability. Hum Biol 46:89–107
Treloar AE (1981) Menstrual cyclicity and the pre-menopause. Maturitas 3:249–264
Van Keep PA (1970) The menopause. International Health Foundation, Geneva
Van Keep PA, Gregory A (1977) Sexual relation in the ageing female. In: Money J. Musaph H (eds) Handbook of sexuology. Excerpta Medica, Amsterdam, pp 839–846
Van Wieringen JC, Wafelbakker F, Verbrugge HP, de Haas JH (1968) Groeidiagrammen (in Dutch). Wolters-Noordhoff, Groningen
Vollmann RF (1966) The length of the pre-menstrual phase by age of women. In: Westin JB, Wiqvist L (eds) In: Proceedings of the 5th world congress on fertility and sterility, ser 133. Excerpta Medica, Amsterdam
Wenderlein JM (1975) Sexualmedizinische Aspekte der Wechseljahre der Frau. Geburtshilfe Frauenheilkd 35:289–294
Wenner R, Hauser GA (1957) Die Biomorphose des Endokrinums im Klimakterium. Gynaekologia 144:300–303
Wharton LR (1964) Normal pregnancy with living children in women past the age of forty. Am J Obst Gynec 90:672
Wilbush J (1980) The female climacteric, Ph D thesis, Oxford
Wilson RA (1965) Feminine forever. Evans, New York

Orthopaedics

Orthopaedics in the Elderly

M. DEVAS

A. Introduction

The orthopaedic problems of the elderly cannot be solved in isolation because most of the conditions to be treated are inextricably involved with the medical ailments of old age which may be, and usually are, as important as the orthopaedic lesion if not indeed taking priority. Nevertheless, and particularly after a serious fracture, the physician is hampered in treating the patient until the orthopaedic surgeon has dealt with the problem, at best having obviated the fracture so that medical treatment can go ahead unimpeded by the restrictions of traction, splints, and ordained decubitus. Thus, the physician and orthopaedic surgeon must of necessity work together and, in order to achieve the best results for their patients, should form a unit specifically for dealing with such elderly patients who may need the combined care of each speciality.

It is necessary here to view the problems of the elderly from the surgeon's point of view; to point out certain differences in the application of the principles of orthopaedic surgery in the elderly and to emphasise that the present teaching of orthopaedics in the textbooks is almost invariably based on that for the healthy adult, with a few exceptions (DEVAS 1977a).

The main purpose of orthopaedics is to return the patient to full function. In the elderly full function is full independence. In dealing with the healthy young adult, time is on the side of the surgeon and a conservative approach is often the best. Time, the great healer, achieves results not necessarily obtainable by other methods; but this approach is reversed in the elderly. Time is against a patient with a short life expectancy. Time is not a healer in old age; it is treacherous and plays tricks with an old person who, separated from the customary activities of daily living and familiar household furniture, may well become unable to return to an independent and satisfactory life. Therefore, in geriatric orthopaedic care one principle is that the return to function, or independence, is quick. This can only be achieved by taking the whole patient into account, the operation being but an incident in the rehabilitation of the patient as a whole. It is because it is not possible for the surgeon to do this in isolation that the physician and the rest of the therapeutic team are necessary.

It is undoubtedly the heavy burden of geriatric patients with fractures near the hip that has necessitated the new approach to the problem (Fig. 1). Old people, poorly treated, lie in hospital beds with no hope of discharge back to independence because of bad management, and are then spoken of as "blocking beds" when it is the organisation that is at fault. Therefore, in order to understand the

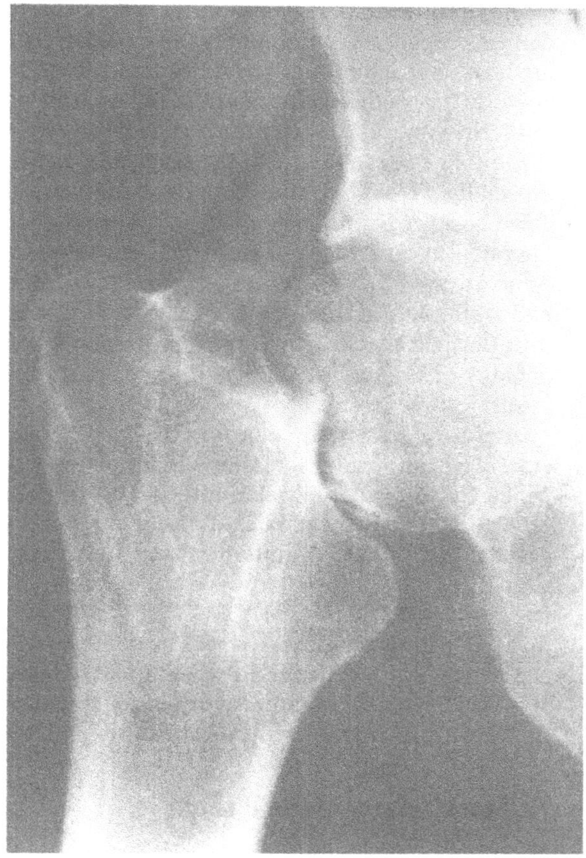

Fig. 1. It is the fracture of the neck of the femur that causes the main geriatric problem in orthopaedics. According to FENTON (1981) there is a real increase in its incidence, as well as an increase in the geriatric population

principles from the start, the proper management, treatment and general organisation for fractures near the hip will be given.

B. Fractures Near the Hip: the Problem

This condition is becoming more common. This is not merely because of an increase in old people; a higher proportion is suffering from fractures near the hip (FENTON 1981). The cause of this increase can at the moment only be deduced, but there is no doubt that of those elderly patients who enter hospital with a broken hip, at least 30% are very frail and in these the fracture is a symptom of impending dissolution. WILD et al. (1981) reported that, out of 100 old people who had a fall, 30 were dead within 1 year. Only 3% sustained fractures near the hip. As has been noted, about one-third of patients who present with a fractured hip are otherwise gravely ill and they fit well into the category of those in whom the fall precedes death within 1 year. Whatever the cause of the increase, fractures of the hip have reached epidemic proportions and cause great problems for the community, both financially and in the use of resources. The old person must not be denied proper treatment; but if this is incorrect and becomes long drawn out, using staff to an extent that prevents deployment for proper use elsewhere and keeps acute orthopaedic beds occupied for months at a time, then it is not surprising that criticism of such patients occurs. However, the criticism is totally misplaced. It should be of the failure of the surgeon to achieve a proper method of treatment, especially when the solution is easily and readily obtainable, by simple cooperation and proper management. It is not an uncommon practice for the hip to be operated upon and then the patient left to lie in bed for several weeks, with little or no attempt to preserve the function of the patient as a whole. If the patient had had a simple fracture of the wrist, the surgeon would have set the fracture, put it in plaster, checked the finger movements the next day, completed the plaster in a day or so, instituted physiotherapy and supervised the patient until there was return to function.

Before a description of any orthopaedic condition or treatment is given for the elderly it is important to understand the necessity for a proper organisation within which to do the actual rehabilitation, remembering that the operation may only take an hour but the medical treatment several weeks. At present there are many geriatric orthopaedic units designed to accept patients after the operation has been done, but the need now is for these units to be extended to take patients from the moment of admission. Only in this way will further inroads be made into the difficult problem of the proper care of the patient with the broken hip. If there is no such unit available then the patient will go into the acute orthopaedic ward. It is very important that all types of patient should be managed by a team, based on the geriatric orthopaedic unit (IRVINE et al. 1977).

I. Social Status of the Patient

The principles of geriatric orthopaedics will apply to any old person, but the need for many of the other services will vary with the income of the patient. Most of the methods of management are directed towards those social groups who are totally dependent on state pensions, living in municipal housing, with no private resources, and who, it not properly treated, are the most likely to become long-stay patients, blocking beds for no other reason than that they have nowhere to go. So the lower social or income groups are those to be considered throughout because they encounter the greatest problems in treatment and management.

II. The Clinical Manager

The main responsibility of the clinical manager is the well being of the patient and the manager is responsible to the clinician for this. In practice the clinical manager has administrative charge of the orthopaedic department so that all admissions and the workload in general are supervised and controlled. To the old in particular the manager has a very special duty, to provide total care, which starts with elective admissions from the outpatients department and ends only when the patient has died or left the neighbourhood; with emergency admissions total care should start as soon as the patient is brought to the accident department. The reason for following up geriatric orthopaedic patients indefinitely, and in many this is unfortunately only a few months, is because, having been through hospital for a serious illness, the patient may be expected to have more problems in the future. When they occur an early warning system will come into action to allow preventative treatment or at least to catch the condition in a state when it is easily amenable to treatment. The duties of the clinical manager will be discussed further when describing the geriatric orthopaedic team, and under the assessment of the elderly elective patient.

III. Treatment

The treatment of a fracture near the hip must allow the immediate rehabilitation of the patient so as to achieve independence by returning the patient to full function. The operation is, in one sense, an incident in the treatment of the patient, but in another it is the key to the successful medical rehabilitation thereafter.

There are two main types of fracture near the hip: fracture of the neck of the femur and the trochanteric fracture. No fractures of the femoral neck in the elderly merit internal fixation, all must be treated by replacement. The trochanteric fractures must be internally fixed. The technique must be such that, however osteoporotic the bone may be, the patient can get up and walk the following day (Fig. 2). There is no place for operating on old people and then leaving them in bed, for decubitus has its own complications without their having had an operation from which to recover. Therefore, once the fracture has been obviated, the patient must walk. This allows early, quick, and efficient rehabilitation, preferably in the geriatric orthopaedic unit, especially if the patient is one of those in whom the fracture was a symptom of underlying disease.

IV. The Geriatric Orthopaedic Team

We have seen that the medical conditions that beset an old person necessitate the combined approach of both the orthopaedic surgeon and the geriatric physician. Once a proper collaboration is forged it follows logically that, apart from the actual surgery, the general management of these patients should follow the same course as for any other geriatric patient. The reasons for this will become apparent later, and therefore a similar team is needed comprising the medical social worker, the occupational therapist, the physiotherapist, the clinical manager and a full nursing complement trained in geriatrics.

The social services vary from country to country, but in principle the medical social worker will maintain a constant liaison with relatives, housing authorities, local government, old people's homes and so on, as the patient may require. Further, the social worker will be responsible for assessing the financial aspects of the patient and will be instrumental in determining whether or not the patient could afford to contribute to the cost of care after discharge from hospital and whether or not a permanent paid help would be feasible. The social worker will also arrange for all the locally organised services to be available: home helps, health visitors, and so on, so that on return home the patient is expected and all the services will function including, of course, a home delivery meals service.

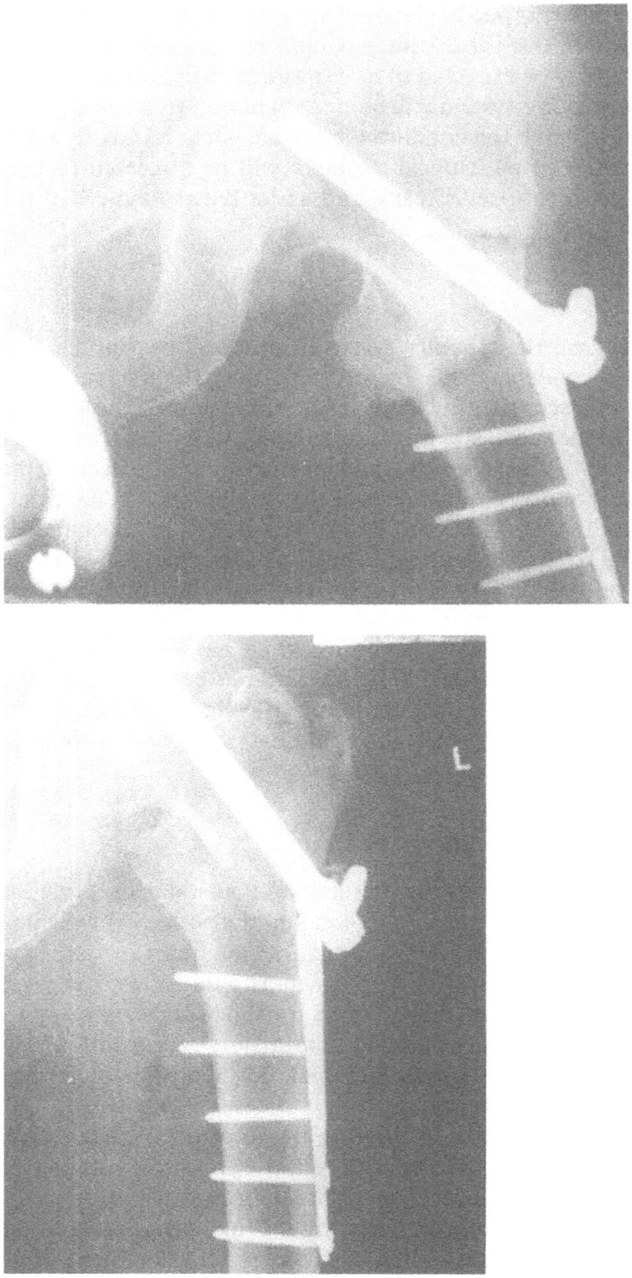

Fig. 2. a A trochanteric fracture treated (correctly) by the insertion of a pin and plate. **b** Although the proper method was chosen the technique was poor and because the pin was placed too high in the femoral head the osteoporotic bone gave way with the result shown. The nail has cut out of the top of the femoral head and lies in the joint itself, damaging the roof of the acetabulum

The physiotherapist is responsible for the general physical rehabilitation of the patient: making sure function returns to the injured part; exercising the patient as a whole; paying attention to the chest, deep breathing and coughing being so important. Isometric exercises will be given before the operation if the patient is sufficiently aware. The physiotherapist will be in the recovery room when the patient wakes and will there encourage isometric exercises again, proper breathing and as much activity as possible. The physiotherapist will be responsible for walking the patient after operation and will thereafter be the main coordinator of all walking exercises and in dealing with any problems that might arise from it.

Walking, being the most important physical sign in the elderly, is to be encouraged by the whole team and it is a large part of the activities of the occupational therapist, who will teach the patient to dress and to walk to the toilet and make sure the patient is properly capable of washing and of finding the way back to bed. As the patient progresses so greater distances and larger tasks are brought in, such as a kitchen assessment, in which a midday meal is cooked by the patient. This is a very important part of the rehabilitation. Finally, it may be that there is doubt about the patient going home and it will be the occupational therapist who will take the patient home for half a day or so to assess whether or not it would be possible to allow the permanent discharge of the patient. Perhaps a trial discharge will be arranged in which the patient is sent home at a time suitable to relatives or friends, but the bed in the geriatric orthopaedic unit is kept empty for a few nights in case the patient has not managed at home and needs to return to the hospital.

The nurse in charge of the wards has to perform, in part, all of the more specialised functions. During those hours when the team is not present it is the nurse in charge and the ward staff who must walk the patient, question relatives, take the patient to the toilet and do all those activities that are taught by the therapists, or seek information on behalf of the social worker.

The daily care of the patient is undertaken in the geriatric orthopaedic unit by the junior medical staff because it is at this period that the most intensive investigation and medical treatment will be needed. Therefore, the more ill the patient the more quickly should the complete care of the geriatric department come into play, leaving only a well-stitched wound to show for the surgical episode; the lesion now being so fixed that it can be totally disregarded.

Nevertheless, once a week the geriatric and orthopaedic consultants must do a grand round in the unit with the whole team present so that every aspect of every patient can be fully discussed, a full programme for the following week planned and any special tasks allotted to these whose responsibility it might be. At the end of the round there will be a programme for every patient and all members of the team will each know exactly what is happening. In this way, and only in this way can the team function properly.

There is no place for requests on slips of paper for one person to do this, for another to do that; all must know exactly what to do and what target to achieve in the coming week. At the ward round, every patient will be seen to walk; only in this way can the whole team be in complete agreement of this most important aspect of the progress towards home. This new approach to orthopaedics in the elderly makes it easier to decide, often after assessment by other members of the team, on the proper treatment and management of each particular patient.

Management is very important in geriatric orthopaedics. It must not be confused with treatment. By management is meant the total care of the patient including the planning of admission and discharges, organising help at home, rehabilitation before and after arthroplasty and fractures, assessment of capabilities, and so on. All members of the team participate, but the whole is brought together by the manager.

V. Admission Procedures

The investigation and preparation for an operation on a fracture near the hip is best done in a geriatric orthopaedic admission (or total care) unit, where the problems that beset the elderly are best understood. The old person who falls and breaks a hip has at least a 30% chance of the fracture having been caused directly or indirectly by a pre-existing condition which might or might not have responded to treatment. No better example of treatment and management can be given to emphasise the advantages of a properly organised geriatric orthopaedic service than that of the patient with a fracture near the hip. The multiple causes of such fractures, the medical complications and unsatisfactory results of treatment make it the most important emergency of the elderly and one which is still on the increase. The complacent manner in which patients are allowed by some surgeons to remain in bed. treated or untreated, is appalling, not only because this induces the blocking of beds, preventing their use by others, but the failure to treat satisfactorily because the patients is "too old or too ill" is a sad reflection on present-day methods. Further, the abysmal quality of existance for such untreated patients denies them hope and makes them long for death as a release, leaving them with no will to live or desire to return to the community. Proper management and correct treatment makes such methods obsolete.

Management is divided into three: first the admission, diagnosis and preparation of the patient for operation; second, the operation itself and recovery therefrom; and finally the medical rehabilitation. The organisation is based on a geriatric orthopaedic admission unit or ward into which all emergency admissions go with the least delay possible after entry into hospital. No old person who needs to be admitted because of an as yet unradiographed injury should be kept waiting in the accident department, but should be transferred within a few minutes to the unit so that all the resuscitative measures that may be necessary can be started at once.

Further, unnecessary waiting on trolleys, however well padded, predisposes the patient to bedsores. The sooner the patient is in bed in the care of nurses experienced in the necessary treatments the better. Here the injured part can be radiographed with good mobile machines which, in the hands of an experienced radiographer, can produce excellent pictures. The practice of transfer of ill, injured patients to a hard, cold X-ray table where each patient is kept until all the radiographs are processed is to be condemned.

Once the diagnosis of a fracture near the hip has been established, the patient is prepared for operation. However ill the patient may be, surgeon, physician and anaesthetist know that the best chance for the patient will lie in stabilising the fracture and then proceeding with medical rehabilitation. Perhaps the only exceptions to this are untreated heart failure or unstable diabetes. However neither of these should delay the patient for more than 24 hours.

While the patient is made ready for operation it is rarely necessary to apply traction or splints. If the fracture is painful sandbags judiciously placed will often relieve it. A urinary catheter will usually be indicated in both men and women, thus sparing the latter the sometimes painful use of the bedpan. The routine investigations are done to establish a baseline, but the haemoglobin content may be wrongly assessed because of haemoconcentration. Anaemia, in simple or serious form, is so common in the elderly that it is very important not to be misled by the laboratory findings. A trochanteric fracture can cause the loss of 1–2 litres of blood and the lower the fracture in the femoral neck the greater the blood loss; only those fractures totaly intracapsular will lose little blood, but then only if the capsule itself is not torn, when a haemarthrosis of the hip occurs which is self-limiting in volume.

The radiograph of the lung fields will be studied with interest by the anaesthetist, not so much for fear of anaesthetising a patient with bronchopneumonia, but to ascertain how to treat the lungs once the patient is unconscious. Waterlogged lungs may give rise to problems of oxygenation, but bronchopneumonia can be greatly improved by aspiration during and at the end of the operation. According to the condition of the patient 2–3 units of blood will be ordered. That operation should take place within 24 hours of admission is a rule of thumb: as yet there is no firm evidence to show that operation sooner than this is beneficial and certainly those units where the night time operating has to be done by those who work the following day are well advised to organise the operation during the normal working hours of the next day.

VI. Anaesthesia

Nowhere is a patient safer than on the operating theatre table in the hands of a competent anaesthetist and there should be no fear of a general anaesthetic in the elderly patient. However, there are certain points which must be borne in mind. One is that if cement is going to be used, as in a hip replacement, then there may be a sudden fall in blood pressure, the reasons for which are still unclear, and this fall may be alarmingly increased in the presence of halothane. However, the alert anaesthetist rarely has a problem in this respect. There is, perhaps, more of a problem from the tamponade of marrow fat when cement is forced down into the medulla of the bone and it may then flow into the general circulation and augment the fall in blood pressure. Here the anaesthetist may well criticise the surgeon for not venting the closed places where cement is to be inserted with a catheter, preferably attached to suction to draw the cement down and to remove the marrow fat at the same time.[1]

[1] A small added benefit is that it is easy to perforate an osteoporotic shaft of the femur while reaming it for the prosthesis; should this occur the suction will pull in soft tissue which will block the sucker and this indicates the cortex of the shaft has been broached

The anaesthetist who feels that a patient is suffering from broncho-pneumonia and therefore must not be anaesthetised is doing his patient a disservice because after the anaesthetic the bronchopneumonia will be in the suction bottle. Recurrent aspiration of secretions, particularly at the end of the operation after the tube has been removed, is one of the best treatments for the conditions; added to this will be the ability of the patient to sit out of bed, to walk and so to be very much better in general.

Heart failure can be treated very rapidly nowadays by the cardiologist or by the anaesthetist and need not delay operation unless there is considerable oedema which has to be got rid of by proper diuretic therapy before operation. This is indeed a proper indication for a short delay because to operate on an oedematous hip can cause complications and therefore the patient would be much better left for a further 24 hours until the oedema is dispersed. The anaesthetist will recognise that a patient who appears to be at death's door with a fracture near the hip will, if treated properly, be very much better after the fracture has been treated, when the pain and shock have been overcome. There is no place nowadays to defer operation because an old patient is "too ill", "too old", "too senile", and above all, "not worth doing" because some doctor in name only feels that the patient will die shortly. If this is true it is more than ever necessary to operate because the patient only has a very limited time left and does not wish to spend it suffering from the pain of a fracture.

Old people are particularly liable to the consequences of lack of oxygen and it is probable that cerebral confusion and even dementia can be increased by lack of oxygen at levels which would have little effect on a younger person. There is a body of opinion that prefers regional to general anaesthesia, but for the old person an epidural anaesthetic is time consuming and can be very distressing to the patient with a broken hip. Therefore, provided the anaesthetist keeps the patient saturated with oxygen throughout and provided the recovery ward staff watch the patient to prevent even a few seconds of anoxia, a general anaesthetic is preferred. This is a light anaesthetic, with paralysing drugs and a high dosage of analgesics. Finally, the patient should be awake and talking before leaving the theatre.

VII. Operation

The fracture of the femoral neck requires prosthetic replacement, but if the fracture is trochanteric then a form of pin and plate or nail plate must be used.

1. Femoral Neck Fractures

The description given here is for the Hastings hip prosthesis which appears to have advantages over the ordinary Austin Moore, Thompson and other prostheses for the reasons to be given. The patient is prepared for operation and the site cleansed with an organic iodine compound 1 hour or more before operation. Premedication is given at which time the antibiotic of choice is injected; the cephalosporins are favoured. The patient is anaesthetised and placed on the theatre table which has a lateral tilt on it, away from the injured side. The buttock of the

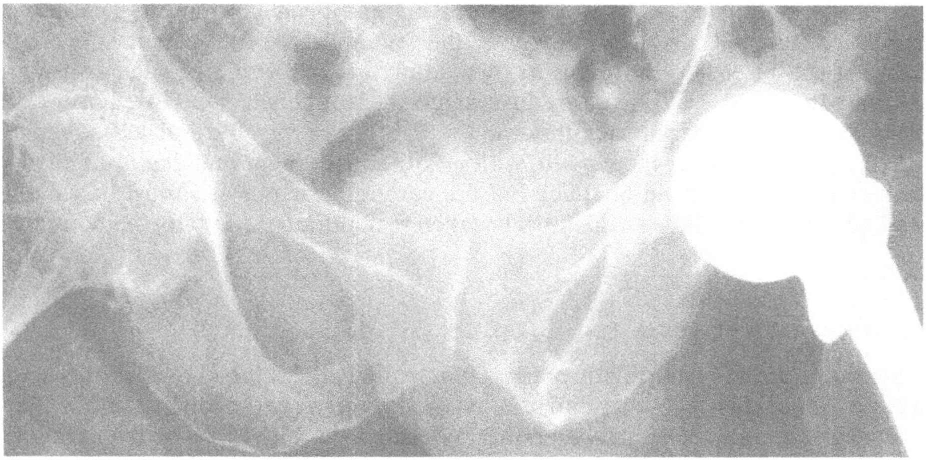

Fig. 3. The excellent results of femoral head replacement for a fracture are marred by acetabular erosion, as occurred in this octogenarian who was a keen cyclist. The prosthesis ultimately eroded into the pelvis

fractured hip is raised by a sandbag placed high up, so as to avoid pushing the sciatic nerve anteriorly.

The leg of the affected side must be carefully towelled to below the knee so that it may be held and moved during the operation. The flank is painted again with the cleansing compound and the patient towelled, an assistant meanwhile holding the affected leg. Great care must be taken with the perineum which is best sealed off with a plastic apron adhering at its top edge.

After the towels are in position, but before the large sheet with the operation space in its centre is put over the hip region, adhesive plastic, such as "Op-site" (Smith and Nephew, Welwyn Garden City, England) is stuck over the skin. The details of the surgical approach to the hip need not be given here, but once the capsule has been opened and the head and part of the broken neck removed, the former should be measured, a suitable sizer head attached to its handle and the measurements of the acetabulum assessed accurately. The remaining neck of the femur will need to be shortened to the correct length and the medulla reamed from neck to upper shaft of femur. A trial fit is done and, if felt necessary, a trial reduction.

The wound is cleansed including brushing and washing the femoral medulla. A small plastic plug is placed at the correct distance down the femur to stop cement going down to far; a catheter with suction is passed down the shaft to the plug and the cement both pushed and sucked down the medulla. The prosthesis is then pressed home firmly, but not hammered until its shoulder is seated on the femoral calcar when one or two taps are given with the mallet. The proper size of cup or outer head is taken (Fig. 5), firmly pushed onto the smaller head and tested for free rotation; then the whole is reduced into the acetabulum, which, because of the mobility of the outer on the inner head, is easier than with a solid prosthesis.

Antibiotic powder such as a streptomycin and penicillin mixture should be sprinkled into the medullary cavity of the femur before the cement is pressed home if the latter does not have its own admixture of antibiotic, such as gentamicin. More antibiotic powder is dusted into the wound which is closed over one deep and one superficial vacuum drain. A light air-permeable and self-adhesive dressing is placed over the wound, with no other padding or bandaging. The operative technique should be quick but not carefree; haemostasis must be secure; and above all, the greatest care must be taken to maintain sterility throughout.

2. Trochanteric Fractures

The procedure of preparing the patient is essentially the same as for the fractured neck of femur, but the patient must be positioned on an orthopaedic table so that the operation may be controlled either by ordinary radiographs or by an image intensifier. The direct lateral approach must be used and if the fracture did not reduce to a satisfactory position when placed on the table, the surgeon must be prepared to improve the position once the bone is exposed. When a satisfactory guide is in place, with its proximal end in the posterior inferior quadrant of the femoral head – no other position should be accepted because it will allow the pin to cut out of osteoporotic bone (see Fig. 2) by the force of the lateral rotator muscles of the hip – then the nail can be driven in and, with the nail introducer still firmly in place on the nail the upper fragment can be controlled while the femoral shaft, held by heavy bone forceps, has its position adjusted. The plate may then be attached and screwed to the femoral shaft. If the bone is very soft it pays very well to use Gallannaugh plates (GALLANNAUGH 1973; IRVINE et al. 1977) of high density polythene on the medial side of the femur; small holes are drilled into it where the screws will come which can then bite into the polythene and achieve a very firm fixation. It is to be remembered that the patient will walk the following day and the surgeon must not use osteoporotic bone as an excuse for prolonging decubitus because that merely enhances the loss of calcium from the skeleton and augments the problems of the patient as a whole. The wound is treated with antibiotic powder and drains as for the fracture of the femoral neck.

3. Sepsis

The elderly patient is perhaps less able to withstand infection than the younger person, and although physiologically there is no indication that age increases the risk of infection, there are other factors including diabetes or the prediabetic state and early vascular disease that can militate against the patient. There is no greater tragedy than to see a primary joint replacement become septic at any age, but in the old it may be impossible to do anything further, thus destroying the whole chance of an improved quality of life. Deep infection is not something that occurs spontaneously; it is the direct result of the surgeon failing in one or another aspect of technique. The old person has enough problems without sepsis being added to the terrible detriment of the surgical result. Superficial sepsis, skin deep, cannot always be prevented because often the confused patient will fiddle with the wound because it itches. But because the wound in both instances is lateral, it does not get contaminated by incontinence, nor by sweat in the inguinal region which may cause problems with the anterior approach, especially in fat patients with pendulous abdomens.

4. Bleeding and Haemostasis

An operation on an old person should be done with diathermy for haemostasis, but this must be done properly. The bleeding points are to be picked up on tiny forceps and no other tissue included as it would be by taking a large "bite" at the area of bleeding with large instruments. The vessel must be sought with care so as only to coagulate it and not the surrounding tissue. The more dead tissue in the wound the more likely is infection. Careful haemostasis supplemented by efficient vacuum drainage gives the geriatric patient a good start on the road to wound healing and a speedy recovery.

5. Length of Operation

The time taken to do the operation is important because the longer the wound is open the more likely is it to become infected then or thereafter because the tissues that are allowed to become dry form a film of dead cells which encourage the growth of bacteria. Therefore the surgeon must complete the procedure with proper celerity. A hip replacement should not take more than 1 hour.

6. Transfusion

The blood loss of an elderly patient with a fracture near the hip has already been mentioned as has the possibility of the haemoglobin estimation being misleading. Often fluid deprivation, because the old person has been lying for a long time on the floor before being found, has occurred. Therefore as soon as the patient arrives and the diagnosis is known an intravenous infusion of saline or Hartmann's solution (compound sodium lactate) is set up and blood cross-matched. Because there will be an operation, sufficient blood to cover the blood loss during surgery as well as to replace that lost by the fracture must be ordered; also the anaemia of so many old patients must be taken into account. It is very important that the patient has a high haemoglobin concentration, approaching normal, as soon as possible. A low haemoglobin concentration is detrimental to a speedy rehabilitation.

In some centres it is the practice to use up the blood on geriatric patients that is almost "time expired" in the blood bank: it must be noted that such blood, although satisfactory at the time of transfusion is soon denatured and the haemoglobin content will drop. Therefore weekly estimations are to be made. The intravenous infusion should be by means of a small intravenous catheter so that it will remain in situ until after the operation and it is only taken down when the patient is drinking well.

The amount of fluid replacement must be carefully monitored, as is routine, with full input and output charts. The cardiovascular system must also be considered so that it is not overloaded by excess fluid. The mouth is still a good clinical indicator of the state of the fluid balance: a wet tongue with normal saliva being good evidence that the patient is not dehydrated.

VIII. Bedsores

Irrespective of the immediate care given to the patients admitted there are some predestined to the developement of a sore because of the time they may have been lying on the floor with the blood supply occluded from the back of the heel or one cheek of the buttock. Apart from these, however, there should be no bedsores started after admission to hospital. Prevention starts when the patient is first put on to the ambulance stretcher which is supplied with a thick foam mattress, which is not removed when the patient is admitted to hospital to be returned to the ambulance, but another mattress is given in exchange. This eliminates extra movement of the patient. The speed with which the patient is seen and radiographed is important; portable machines give excellent results and again, if proper resuscitation trolleys are used the patient need not be disturbed in radiographing the injured hip: for the lateral view the opposite leg only need be moved. Thus the patient can remain well padded and comfortable without the added insult of having to lie on a cold X-ray table.

As soon as the patient is in bed, the nurses will assess the pain from the fracture and consider whether temporary foam traction (not adhesive strapping) is needed so that the skin can be properly attended to. It will then be treated very carefully and very frequently and this is adjusted to the mobility and activity of the patient. There should never be a rule that skin is only done so often; to prevent bedsores it must be done as often as the condition of the patient warrants it. The lotions, creams and ointments used must be bland: it is the application that is important and the rubbing and stimulation of the skin that goes with the medicament that is the main preventative.

Sheepskins, ripple beds, water beds, etc. are not essential in the first 24 hours before operation unless the patient is unconscious or otherwise severely ill, such as with a new stroke or paraplegia. They are, however, useful in the treatment of an established coma or for certain patients needing longer bed rest. Once the operation is over the patient not only becomes mobile, but is able to take the best of all precautions against bedsores, namely to be up.

IX. The Bladder

Many elderly patients have some form of partial incontinence as described in Sect. K. II, but when admitted with a fracture or for any other operation they are best treated with an indwelling catheter to allow free drainage until the operation is over, although spigotted off during the time in theatre. In this way the painful use of a bedpan is avoided and a true value of urinary output obtained. As a final benefit there will be no wet sheets, so conducive to bedsores. The catheter must be inserted with full aseptic precautions so that no infection is introduced into the bladder. Cystitis is common enough in the elderly without an iatrogenic cause being added. In men the decision whether or not to catheterise on admission, before operation or not at all must be made for each individual, although it is better to err on the side of introducing the catheter; should there be any indication of an enlarged prostate from the history or from the rectal examination it is indicated.

After the operation 48 hours should be allowed before withdrawing the catheter. This should be done early in the morning to give the patient a whole day in which to attempt to regain normal control of micturition. Should this not be successful the catheter is replaced. If problems continue cystoscopy is indicated.

X. The Rectum

The bowels need not be opened deliberately until after the operation in patients with fractures. Then patients will be allowed to sit out of bed on a commode by the bedside. Later, of course, the occupational therapist will make a point of walking the patient to the toilet and supervising the ability of the patient to manage unaided.

Rectal incontinence is almost invariably caused by impacted faeces and is easily diagnosed by rectal examination. There is usually no alternative to manual removal of the faeces and the sooner this is done, without going through several days of ill-advised, painful and debilitating enemas of more, or less, toxic contents, the better. If there is any further doubt as to the state of the rectum, it should be subjected to sigmoidoscopy at once; there is no necessity to wait, because the fracture has been dealt with and only a little extra gentleness is needed with the part that has been operated upon.

XI. Acetabular Erosion

There is no place for internal fixation of the femoral neck in the elderly, by whatever method or with however many different pins. All these fractures must be replaced and up to the present the Austin Moore or the cemented Thompson prostheses have been the usual choice. The rehabilitation after a replacement is far easier and quicker than after internal fixation.

The literature on the subject of fixation versus replacement is plentiful and it shows that surgically the results of replacement are marginally better. However these results would be greatly improved if the morbidity from acetabular erosion could be eliminated (Figs. 4 to 6; Devas 1977b). Medically the results of replacement allow much quicker return to function.

In 1976 Barnes et al. did a study of the pinned hips in 940 women and found that only 73% united and that of these 24% developed late segmental collapse of the femoral head. This means that little over half the patients, around 56%, where satisfactory. In another study in the same year D'Arcy and Devas (1976) reported on 361 subcapital fractures of the femoral neck all treated by replacement with a cemented Thompson prosthesis and were able to follow up 161 of whom 82% were good–excellent; 11% showed acetabular erosion and this was

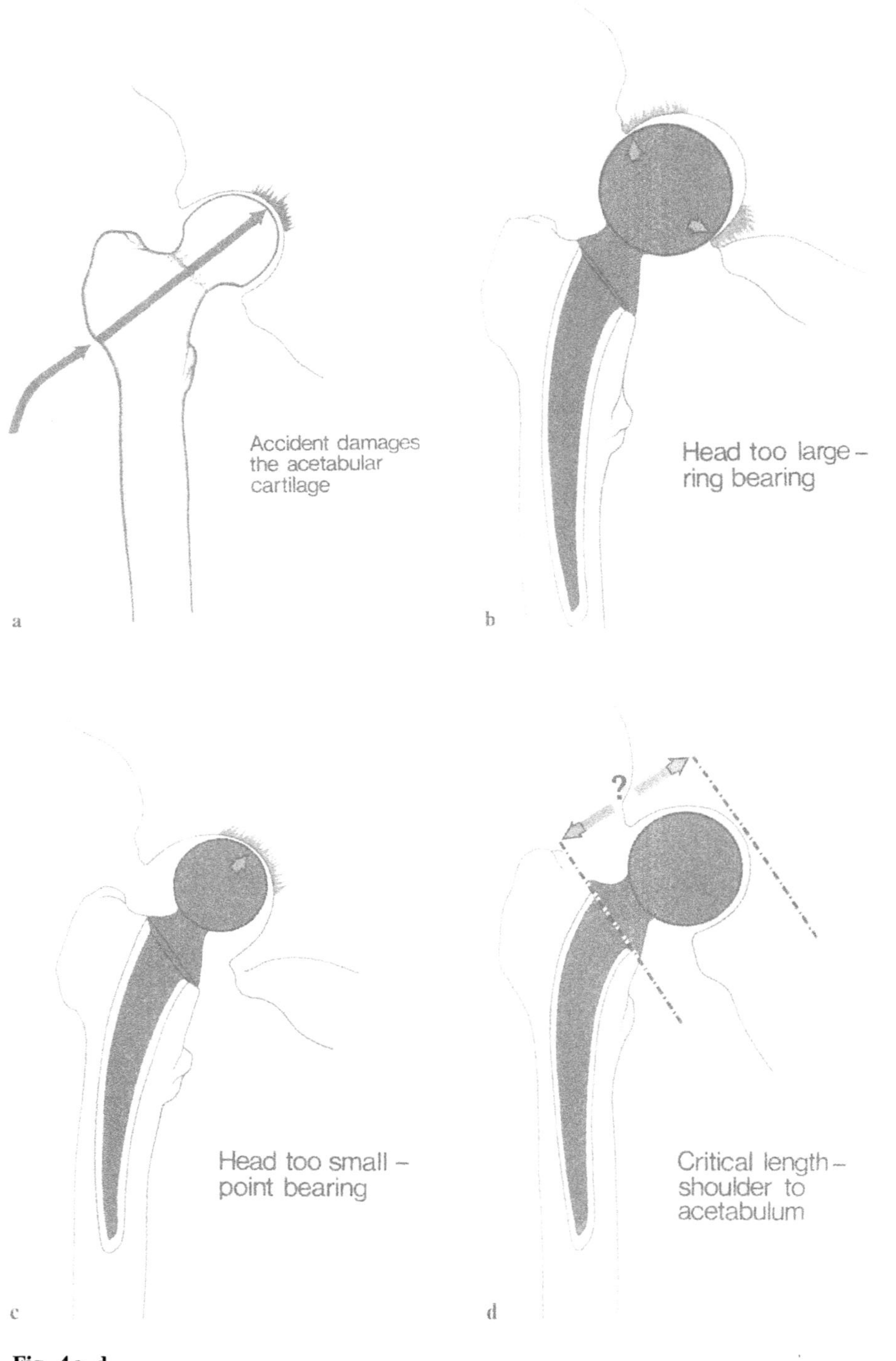
Accident damages
the acetabular
cartilage
a
Head too large -
ring bearing
b
Head too small -
point bearing
c
?
Critical length -
shoulder to
acetabulum
d

Fig. 4 a–d

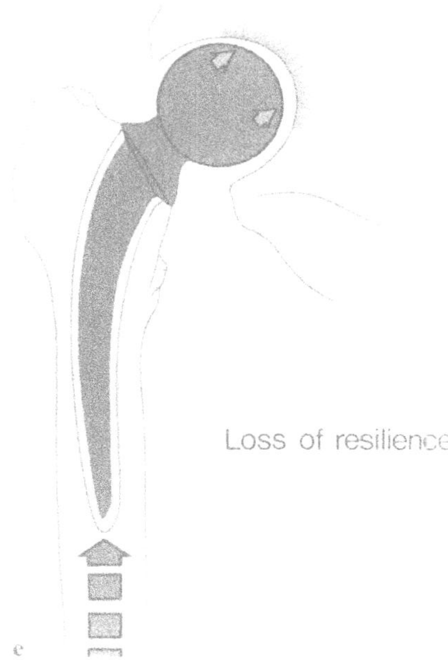

Fig. 4 a–e. Five possible causes of acetabular erosion after cemented Thompson replacement **a** damage to the acetabulum by the impact of the fall; **b** a prosthetic head that is too large, causing ring bearing; **c** one that is too small with point bearing (this is thought to be the most likely cause); **d** the shoulder may be the wrong length because it is of a different measurement for each size of Thompson prosthesis; **e** the loss of resilience allows the unbuffered impact of each footstep to be transmitted to the acetabulum

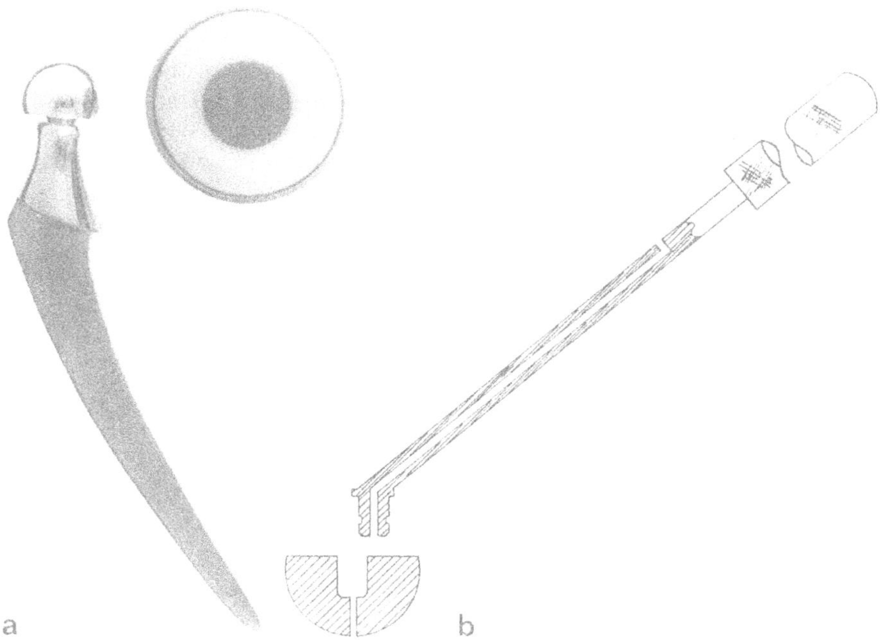

Fig. 5. a The Hastings hip has features that are designed to eliminate the causes of acetabular erosion including a constant apex of outer head to shoulder length, outer heads in 1-mm sizes, and buffering of impact by the high density polythene within the cup
b Accurate measurement of the acetabulum, which is essential, is achieved by the special sizer

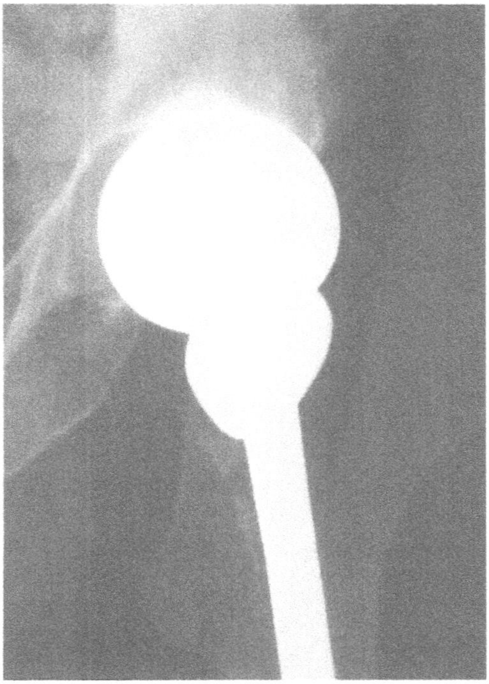

Fig. 6. A Thompson prostesis beginning to erode the top of the acetabulum; this is shown not only by the head of the prosthesis being above the joint line, but also by the condensation of the trabeculae at the apex of the head

more common in the younger and more active patients. If the problem of erosion could be overcome then the results of hemiarthroplasty for the fractured neck of femur would indeed be very much better than any form of internal fixation.

A new prosthesis specifically designed to prevent erosion was introduced at the Royal East Sussex Hospital, Hastings, England. This appears to have succeeded in preventing acetabular erosion; it has features to counter as many as possible (even if theoretical) causes of erosion (Fig. 4). The latter may include damage to the acetabulum at the time of the accident (most elderly people fracture the femoral neck by a direct fall on to the hip); by the prosthesis being too large or too small (the latter producing point bearing is considered to be the most likely cause of acetabular erosion); the neck of the prosthesis being too long or too short and, finally, the transmission of the impact of each footstep from the uppermost third of the femur to the acetabulum through the unyielding metal implant; the normal femur bends slightly with each walking step (DEVAS 1975; D'ARCY and DEVAS 1976).

The Hastings hip has millimetre head sizes and a constant apex of head to shoulder length, unlike the Thompson prosthesis which has a different length for every size. The Hastings prosthesis has an outer head, or cup, easily applied to the inner femoral component head which is the same size as the Charnley prosthesis (22.25 mm) so that the replacement can be converted into a total hip without removing the cemented femoral component.

The shape of the cup, or outer head, is such that it will move in the acetabulum and on the femoral component head to reorientate itself to the line of force pass-a b c

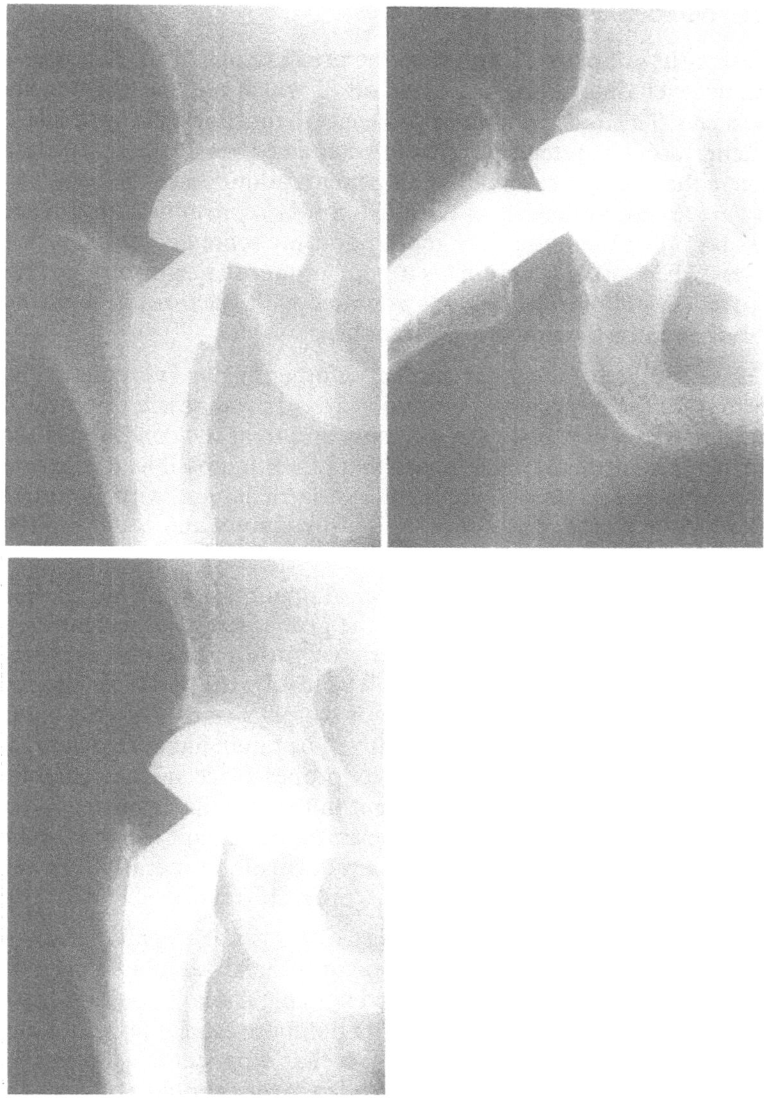

Fig. 7 a–c. The radiograph of the same hip as shown in Fig. 1 taken 2 years after replacement with a Hastings hip; **a** note the umbrella-like position of the outer head; **b** the same hip in abduction; **c** adduction without weight-bearing; note the altered position of the outer head, showing that it moves freely in the acetabulum. On weight-bearing the head took up the position shown in **a**

ing through the hip, thus taking the thrust in different parts of the acetabulum (Fig. 7). A special but simple device is used to ensure very accurate measurement of the acetabulum which is considered to be an essential part of the operation. There have been seen no cases of acetabular erosion with this prosthesis.

XII. Medical Complications

At least 30% of patients with this fracture have one or more serious medical conditions, excluding simple anaemia, all of which require urgent attention by the physician. The most common problems are those affecting the heart, lungs renal system, vascular system, and senile dementia or brain failure. The latter is so common, either mild or severe, that all patients admitted to the geriatric orthopaedic unit are tested for their mental state. If a 50% score at best improves over the next few days then the outlook is good, but if the score decreases, or is around 30% or less when tested, then this is a poor prognostic sign. It is not feasible to test the feebler and more ill patients admitted with fractures near the hip before operation because the results are unraliable.

It is because of the great number of other medical conditions that it is so important for the physician to be involved as early as possible because it is the medical team that will investigate, diagnose and treat the conditions that are present. Further, the medical team realises that, if not impossible, it is extremely difficult to investigate and properly to treat a geriatric patient with an untreated fracture or, which is worse, one badly treated by splints and traction as the definitive method.

Therefore both medical and surgical opinion is in favour of operation at the earliest possible time, allowing for the proper initial investigation and preparation. After the operation, if the geriatric orthopaedic unit is separate from the acute orthopaedic ward, no time will be lost by the geriatric department in starting medical treatment because one of the physicians will visit the patient in the orthopaedic ward and arrangements will be put in hand for a very quick transfer. In this way the fracture assumes its proper place in the rehabilitation of the patient as a whole and as an incident in the remainder of the investigations, diagnosis and treatment; but nevertheless an important incident and one to which full regard must be paid to ensure every detail of the operation, as well as the preparation and aftercare of the patient, is properly done.

However ill the patient the chance of survival can only be augmented by operation; only those who are at the point of death should be given suitable analgesia and left to the care of dedicated nursing; if death does not rapidly ensue the patient must be reviewed, that is, after not more than 2 days, and the whole problem carefully reviewed. Again, the fact that a patient is suffering from a disease which will inevitably be fatal within a few weeks should not deter the surgeon or the anaesthetist from operating; why, they should ask themselves, need this patient suffer from a broken hip for the last remaining period of life? The most important part of life to everyone is that which remains. Therefore the whole principle of geriatric orthopaedics in regard to the medical problems is, as usual, to obviate the fracture at the soonest possible moment so that the other ailments can be investigated, diagnosed, and treated.

It is appropriate to point out here that the surgeon is not operating, as some have said, to save the lives of elderly people who might wish to be left to die, but to restore a quality of life that is satisfactory to the patient. Should these efforts fail, directly or indirectly, the surgeon will not strive to maintain life to the great discomfort of the patient, but will accede to the inevitable and, with all necessary skills, ensure that the patient does not suffer.

It is quite usual to find, after the full medical investigation, the cause of the fall; this may range from a drop attack to postural hypotension, or a small stroke to previously undiagnosed parkinsonism.

C. Fractures in General

Provided the philosophy of treating the fracture near the hip is applied to other fractures there is little that need be said in regard to general management. There are some special techniques in the surgery of the elderly and certain special indications for operation that can differ from those of younger patients and it is only these that are considered here; but it must be remembered that if a fracture necessitates the admission of an elderly person for whatever reason, operation is indicated if it is possible to restore that patient to independence quickly and to allow an early discharge.

I. The Lower Limb

1. Fractures of the Femoral Shaft

Internal fixation is indicated using a Küntscher nail. This may inserted from the knee, the entry into the femur being in the intercondylar notch, a non-weight-bearing area. The patient lies supine on the operation table with the knee flexed over its end. It is easy to apply traction in this position by giving the table a head-down tilt, but if the fracture does not fully reduce a small midline incision anteriorly over the fracture will allow two fingers to pass through the vastus intermedius muscle and to remove the muscle tissue blocking reduction, which is usually the cause. The guide wire safely in place, the largest nail that will fit without reaming is passed up into position. Should the fixation in the bottom part of the femoral shaft not be satisfactory (and often the normal enlargement of the medullary canal is augmented by osteoporosis) a second nail can be stacked within the first, and this is possible because of the clover leaf design. The second nail need not be as long as the first.

After the fracture is fixed a small rebate is made above the entry hole in the intercondylar notch to grip the cement that is then put into the hole to prevent the nail slipping down. If cement is not available, the entry hole should be made rectangular, and the piece of cortex which has been removed is replaced transversely to prevent the downward migration of the nail. This approach is ideal for the prophylactic nailing of a femur about to sustain a pathological fracture, or, of course, if it has already occurred.

There need be no fear in allowing the geriatric patient to walk on the leg so fixed. At a younger age weight-bearing might well be restricted or guarded because of the fear of the nail bending (which can occur in the healthy young adult with free bed exercises only). But concomitant with old age comes a loss of muscle tone and this weakness allows early walking without fear, although, according to the physique of the patient, crutches or a walking frame may be advocated until callus is showing radiologically, which is usually at about 4–6 weeks.

It is tempting, when looking at the radiograph of a fracture of the upper third of the femoral shaft, to advise an intramedullary nail but often there is a hidden extension of the fracture running up to the trochanteric region so that, if this method is used, the whole upper fragment splits, or at best, the spiral crack leading upwards becomes visible so that there is only a precarious hold of the proximal fragment and it is not safe to walk the patient. Therefore choosing this method must be resisted and the fracture treated as though it was a trochanteric fracture but using a longer plate with 7–12 holes as necessary.

Fractures of the lower third of the femur are often T-shaped with the stem of the T passing down between the condyles into the knee. A special pin and plate (Howmedica, London, England) which is inserted laterally, but which has a medial threaded aperture in the nail to take a bolt with a washer, allows compression of the two condyles and their firm fixation to the femoral shaft. This allows walking and the usual further rehabilitation (BROWN and D'ARCY 1971).

2. Fractures of the Patella

There are two types: one has separated fragments which means the lateral part of the quadriceps expansion has been torn; the fragments are removed at operation and the quadriceps expansion repaired. A routine pressure dressing is applied at the end of the operation and one or two plaster bandages put over the whole. This gives an eggshell thickness plaster cast which is very light, but with the pressure dressing it is quite sufficient to prevent flexion while allowing early walking with full weight-bearing. The other type of patella fracture is linear or stellate, but with no separation. Provided the patient can lift the straight leg operation is not indicated and a similar eggshell plaster to that described is applied and the patient allowed to walk and to remain at home.

3. Fractures of the Tibia

Fractures of the tibia are treated as at any other age, but sometimes those of a very osteoporotic shaft do best with an intramedullary rod. This can be a Küntscher nail, the entry point being the anterior extracapsular part of the tibial plateau. Because the upper part of the tibial shaft is directed more posteriorly than the rest, this part of the plateau is directly over the medulla of the tibial shaft and the straight nail goes down easily to obtain a good fixation.

4. Fractures of the Ankle and Foot

A heavy walking cast often incapacitates the elderly and everything possible should be done to curtail its use. Therefore even the simple Pott's fracture is best screwed securely so that the patient may be independent quickly and with only a firm supportive bandage. For other fractures of the foot that do not lend themselves to internal fixation, it is often possible to use elastic adhesive bandaging instead of plaster; the patient will readily put up with a slight extra discomfort when the position is explained and the alternative described.

II. The Pelvis and Trunk

1. Pelvis

Most of these injures are not severe, but often masquerade as a fracture of the hip. Examination, if not meticulous, may miss the tenderness in one or more of the rami and, because no fracture is seen in the vicinity of the hip, the injury to the pelvis is overlooked. Fractures of one or both of the pubic rami can be treated by an explanation to the patient there is only a slight crack and that although it will be uncomfortable no harm will come of walking; a frame is used and shortly the patient is independent. Severe fractures of the pelvis which are unstable should if possible be treated by external fixation as at other ages.

2. Spine

The osteoporotic crush fracture is extremely common and it is worth noting the natural history. At first the osteoporotic vertebra is of normal shape but as the osteoporosis continues the bone mass is diminished and the bone is weaker. Eventually the weakened bone can no longer fully withstand the stresses upon it and it is at this stage that pain may occur although radiologically there will still be a normal shape. Once the bone crushes into the characteristic wedge, the pain from the stressing of the bone is no longer present.

Sometimes, before the vertebra has actually crushed with normal everyday activity, some simple ill-judged step or slight jolt is sufficient to cause the vertebral collapse with moderate pain. Such patients are admitted but they should be given as many pillows as possible for comfort and encouraged to sit. Once the latter is achieved the patient may sit out of bed and then stand and walk with a frame. Again a full explanation is needed (refraining from the expression "a broken back") to reassure the patient that the pain is no reason to stay in bed. This form of fracture has, of course, medico-legal implications and the proper knowledge of the aetiology is important.

III. The Arm

1. Neck of Humerus

The fractured neck of humerus can be so painful that it necessitates admission to hospital in which case the simple procedure of inserting a Rush pin through the head of the humerus and down its shaft is sufficient to control the pain, if not completely fix the fracture. A triangular sling allows the patient to be up and independent. The shoulder is mobilised early.

2. Dislocation of the Shoulder

After the usual reduction, excercises should be started as soon as the pain is improved, usually in 1 to 2 days. Early mobilisation is always indicated in the elderly.

3. The Elbow

Bad fractures at the elbow are best left to early mobilisation on the "bag of bones" principle, but the fracture of the olecranon can be fixed with a Rush pin supplemented by an Attenborough spring (Howmedica, London, England). This allows early movement.

4. The Colles' Fracture

This is treated in the usual way, but exemplifies the proper organisation and management of elderly outpatients with fractures described in Sect. D.

D. Outpatient Management of Fractures in Elderly Patients

A properly organised fracture clinic and follow-up system is both cost-effective in staff and patient time and produces better results. The best example is one of the commonest injuries in the elderly, the Colles' fracture. After diagnosis and manipulation when necessary a padded backslab is applied. The patient then attends physiotherapy for individual treatment as often as necessary to disperse the swelling of, and restore movement to, the fingers and thumb. The patient then attends the fracture clinic and has the plaster completed and is referred to the occupational therapy workshop, and is given tasks to do in the company of all the other patients with various fractures. Once the patient has achieved sufficient expertise and function of hand, elbow, and shoulder to be left to continue unaided workshop attendance ceases.

Once the plaster has been removed it is usual to find that there is full movement of the whole arm with only some slight restriction of wrist movement; normal use will soon restore the movement and the patient need attend no more. If this form of organisation is applied to all fractures, then the results improve and the time taken to achieve them is shortened.

E. Pathological Fractures and Metastatic Paraplegia

A pathological fracture should be treated by fixation like any other fracture, however grave the condition; such a fracture is painful and fixation is the only satisfactory method of relieving the pain. There need be no fear of fungation of the carcinoma through the wound. Radiotherapy or other treatment is much easier with internal fixation than with plaster casts.

Paraplegia or paraparesis from metastatic deposits is a grave emergency. No time must be lost before doing a radiculograph. It should be done not the next day, but as soon as the clinical examination has established the diagnosis of paraplegia. First, ordinary radiographs may or may not show the site of the deposit, but the clinical examination will have established the approximate level. The radiculograph follows. It will either show a block to the dye, or the dye will flow freely up the intradural space. The latter indicates the arterial supply to the cord has been interrupted and that decompression will be of no avail. When the level of the block has been found the patient is taken to theatre for immediate decompression. The reason for the great urgency is the bladder. If it is affected by the lesion and remains so for more than a few hours it has little chance of recovery. The patient may or may not recover from the paraplegia after operation, but if the bladder remains functioning what life is left to the patient has a far better quality than otherwise.

F. Radiculography

A water-soluble radiopaque fluid, metrizamide (Amipaque), is used, it gives an excellent outline of the structures including nerve roots and can be used when a computerised axial tomographic scan is not available or as an adjunct to it. It is useful in almost all spinal conditions associated with space-occupying lesions, especially to show up blocks from metastatic deposits or fractures and for assessing the cause of nerve root irritation such as from a prolapsed intervertebral disc or a spinal tumour. There are some slight complications to the use of metrizamide; it can occasionally give painful spasms in the lower limb and even more rarely higher up, even when injected into the lumbar area, but the spasms are transient and soon pass. Sedation and strong analgesia is indicated.

Myelography can be used in the elderly, but its use in the younger patient, or one with a considerable expectancy of life, is contraindicated because of the occasional interstitial neuritis the follows if the iodophendylate (Myodil) is left within the dura; it is often difficult to ensure that all of it is removed without proper neuroradiological techniques. Nevertheless, if a geriatric patient presents with a paraparesis or similar urgent condition it may be used if there is no other method available.

G. Scintigraphy

In geriatric patients with orthopaedics problems usually the $^{99}Tc^{m}$ scan is used which shows a "hot" spot where there is osseous activity. It is valuable in assessing bone metastases, loosening of implants, including hip and knee replacements, and for stress fractures.

I. Metastatic Deposits

A skeletal survey by radiography may not show the early deposit, but usually the bone scan will. Because it includes the whole skeleton it gives a very comprehensive examination. However, in the geriatric patient it is often academic to know the answer in terms of total body involvement and it is more important to know if a long bone is involved and if so whether a pathological fracture is likely to occur; for this, plain radiography is satisfactory.

II. The Loose Prosthesis

This will show as an area of increased activity around that part that is loose. After a new joint has been inserted increased activity on scanning the joint remains for about 1 year and then fades. A further increase at this stage indicates failure of fixation, but not necessarily that the joint is infected.

III. Stress Fractures

Some elderly people have pain in the hip (or shin or ankle) caused by a stress fracture. Scintigraphy will show this lesion much earlier than it will show on a radiological plate. Sometimes the stress fracture is so high up in the neck of the femur that, like ony other ordinary fracture at this site, it will cause avascular necrosis (DEVAS 1974). Avascular bone should show no activity on scintigraphy.

H. Computer Assisted Tomography

This investigation is of very great value in the elderly in assessing the lumbar spine for stenosis because it gives a very accurate picture of not only the bony canal, but the soft tissues within it, including disc protrusions or other soft tissue space-occupying lesions that may affect the cord or cauda equina. The machine will scan segments at varying distances apart, but for assessing lumbar stenosis four "cuts" per centimetre is ample and often two is sufficient. This will allow an accurate assessment of the site and severity of the stenosis and will indicate those sites that need decompression.

A further benefit is that often in lumbar stenosis one or more lumbar nerve roots have become compressed by an overhang of bone forming posterior to the nerve root and just proximal to the foramen through which it passes and which may also be stenosed. No other investigation will demonstrate this so well although radiculography will show a cutoff in the filling of the nerve root sleeve. Cervical spinal tomography is also valuable for determining the site and size of posterior bar formation at the level of the discs, the extent of facet arthritic encroachment on the neighbouring structures and the state of the atlantoaxial complex. This may be a great benefit in the diagnosis and treatment of the elderly patient with rheumatoid arthritis. For the confirmation of spinal lesions, such as those already described, radiculography is usually sufficient to outline the extent of the problem, and in the old person it may save a long and arduous journey to a place where a scanner is available.

I. Spinal Stenosis

This very serious condition has had much attention paid to it over the last decade or so and the interest and research has been such that a great deal more is known about the aetiology than before. Nevertheless, treatment is not yet fully agreed, partly because there has been insufficient time for long series of cases to be reviewed with a satisfactory length of follow-up.

The symptoms of spinal stenosis are bizarre to such an extent that the patient may be thought to be neurotic or suffering from dementia or brain failure. Therefore it is important to remember that the condition not only exists, but is quite common. At first the patient may merely complain of weakness of one or other leg, perhaps with pain. The weakness itself may seem peculiar in that it is present with certain actions or positions, but not with others. Thus an old lady complained that on entering a car and having sat on the seat she was unable to lift her leg into the car; but she was quite able to walk to or from the car. The usual symptom of presentation is that patients say that after walking a certain distance the legs feel peculiar and will not continue to take the weight any longer and that they fear that the legs will give way or some other disaster will befall them. The description of what would happen if rest, sitting or even leaning cannot be done is always rather vague and there is rarely any account of the patient actually being deposited on the ground by the legs giving way. At the same time the sensory subjective changes may include all forms of odd feelings: hot[2] or cold water running down the leg, formication, a feeling of swelling, bursting, tightness and so on. After a further lapse of time with no dramatic episodes, the patient will be found to have become almost chair-ridden, rising only for the most important activities and unable to got any distance beyond the door.

Pain in the back, or down the legs may or may not be present; in general it is not relevent to the degree of stenosis, but to the preexisting condition. Thus, as part of the disease process, the discs may be prominent but insufficiently so to cause nerve root compression until the rest of the canal is made smaller by the progress of the stenosis.

There is a congenital variety of stenosis which, if not causing symptoms in its own right will predispose the individual to the occurrence of the condition later in life with the advent of osteoarthritis, osteoporosis and disc generation, perhaps with an element of spondylolisthesis. It is most usual for the stenosis to develop as a combination of degeneration of the joints in the region of the fourth lumbar vertebra and bulging discs. That this should be the place for the stenosis to occur is not surprising because in the normal anatomy this is the narrowest portion of the lumbar spine. Iatrogenic spinal stenosis may follow poor techniques of spinal fusion with the new bone mass, always posterior, bulging anteriorly to compress the cord beneath it.

K. The Practical Management of Arthroplasties in the Elderly

The elderly person will often demand a joint replacement because the joint or joints concerned are threatening independence or that the pain and disability is

[2] Hot water "running down the leg" (or up) is a most descriptive symptom and the author can vouch for its existence, having had it himself when a large lumbosacral disc caused compression of the nerve root

making life not worth living. Although joint replacement should not be considered as a life-threatening procedure, nevertheless the better the management the better the mortality rate, and, almost equally important, the better the morbidity rate.

The old person is quite prepared to take a chance on an operation, but no surgeon should offer arthroplasty without the confident expectation of a mortality below 1% and no sepsis. To continue to replace joints when the sepsis rate is higher than 2% shows a tragic disregard of both the patient's well-being and the essentials of geriatric orthopaedic organisation.

There are certain geriatric problems and others are purely orthopaedic, but both are easily overcome. For example, cardiac abnormalities are no contraindication to surgery after the condition has been assessed and stabilised. On the other hand, certain chronic respiratory problems such as chronic bronchitis and emphysema are best treated over a period of time to make sure that after the operation there will be no problem with the routine rehabilitation.

From the orthopaedic side the joints to be replaced must be considered. Thus, if a patient has a bad hip and a bad knee it is wise to do one at a time and always to do the knee first. This is because it is easier to rehabilitate the knee in the presence of a bad hip (for the latter is almost invariably stable) than vice versa. Sometimes considerable thought needs to be given to deformity or limited movement of the knee, whereas a "stiff" hip will respond after arthroplasty and will give a reasonable range of movement; the same is not true of the knee which rarely improves more than 30° above the range of movement before operation. This is true of the younger patient, but the very old with the loss of muscle power concomitant with their age find it difficult to achieve even this. Therefore there should be a period of muscle development and mobilisation before the operation. It must also be remembered that the bone will be osteoporotic and a patient who is otherwise very fit may walk too much after the hip or knee is no longer painful and produce a stress fracture: therefore careful activity control is needed.

Hospitals are among the worst places for old people and it is imperative that the stay should be carefully planned so that as soon as sufficient morbility and independence is regained, the patient may leave. This needs considerable preplanning and all arrangements should have been made before the patient is admitted. It should, perhaps, again be noted that this applies to the lower social groups in particular; it is the ordinary everyday person, whose daily income is matched by expenditure, who needs all possible help.

I. The Programme

The patient is seen at the first consultation by the surgeon. The clinical manager's department will have processed the referral letter before the patient arrives so that radiographs may be available; either taken beforehand or on arrival according to local practice, the distance from the patient's home and the patient's general condition. It is important to gain the total confidence of the patient at this first consultation; to be able to say to the patient exactly what is wrong and what will be done and to answer questions. Most elderly patients, on seeing a surgeon tend to become somewhat nervous or anxious and they may be unable to ask those questions that they need to ask, or worse, do not take in everything that has been said to them in the consultation. Thus, it is quite common for such a patient who has had the whole procedure explained, to ask the nurse afterwards "Are they going to operate?" This also applies the other way round and the surgeon may not have been given a lot of information with a direct bearing on the patient's progress or well-being. Should any medical complication be found or be suspected it is at this stage that the patient will be referred to the geriatrician for an opinion and, usually, treatment before admission.

At the close of the consultation the patient is given an appointment to attend an assessment clinic in the near future. According to whether or not the patient will have to wait any time for the operation, there will be a second assessment nearer the date of admission. If the delay is only a few weeks there is only need for one. It is important at this point to note that a short delay is not harmful, but beneficial, for several reasons which will become apparent as well as that already mentioned, that the patient may remember vital facts that were not produced at the first interview. The patient is then seen at the assessment clinic which should be 3 to 6 weeks before admission.

II. The Assessment Clinic

At this clinic are present members of the clinical manager's staff: physiotherapists, occupational therapists and nursing staff. The medical social worker may attend, but usually the necessary details will also be covered by the clinical manager. Each patient's assessment should take some 2 hours; this gives an unhurried approach. It does not mean that only one patient is seen every 2 hours; on the contrary, the numbers can continue steadily, but by keeping each patient moving slowly, confusion is reduced, memory sustained, faces remembered and awareness increased.

The patient will be seen by every member of the team first alone and then all together. The clinical manager will be checking all the patients details and recording them in a special folder which will accompany the patient round the assessment clinic, during the time in the ward, on transfer to the geriatric orthopaedic unit or the low dependency nursing unit (convalescent home). In this folder the whole team will record relevant information. The proposed admission and discharge dates will be checked and later, at every stage, the patient's progress will be assessed against that put down as a proposed an feasible course.

The manager will inquire into all previous medical problems to make sure that these coincide with those listed in the medical notes and will arrange for an up-to-date list of drugs being taken to be available from the family doctor and also of any other treatments from other sources. The manager will let the primary health care team know of the proposed dates of admission, discharge and method thereof, and will confirm the latter to make sure the health visitor or another member of the primary health care team calls on the patient at home on the afternoon of discharge; all discharges are arranged in the morning for this purpose. Next the clinical manager will check the domestic situation and find out about family, friends, neighbours, etc., who might come in and help. The manager will ensure that the time of admission does not clash with a holiday taken by the family or friends that live with the patient.

The manager will also look into the financial background of the patient both to ensure there is no hardship at present and to find out if the patient might be able to afford a short holiday as convalescence. Old people automatically become anxious about their financial affairs, feeling perhaps that they are much poorer than they are and continue to scrimp and save against the supposed rainy day to come, not realising that already there is a downpour upon them.

Finally the manager will explain what happens on admission, on preparation for the theatre, on being anaesthetised and on waking up with the myriad of coils of tubing passing to and from the patient. Many old people do not realise that all the tubes are normal and, if they are not told beforehand, believe that some awful complication or catastrophy has occurred and that all is lost. Having completed this thorough briefing, the manager will take the patient to the physiotherapist.

The physiotherapist will do a full muscle and joint assessment and will learn the home conditions so that capabilities required after operation can be achieved. If there is weakness or stiffness of the joint or joints concerned isometric excercises will be given for muscle strengthening and simple nonresistance exercises to improve the range of movement. These may be done at home or at the physiotherapy department according to needs and circumstances. The patient will also be shown the method of being helped out of bed the day after the operation, the technique of walking, helped for the first few days after operation, by walking frame which is so much more satisfactory than crutches, especially for the elderly. The physiotherapist then hands the patient on to the occupational therapist, who will be most interested in the capabilities of the patient in regard to the activities of daily living and the most important assessment of the mental state that ordains these activities. The occupational therapist will discuss the home and its problems, stairs, kitchen, steps to the front door, how far are the shops, who will do the shopping, the heating in the house, beds and bedding and all things relevant to the life of an old person, particularly one who lives alone. It is always to be remembered that an old person exists in great part by reflex action, each one stimulating the next as the day wears on and once the pattern is broken then it may take a considerable while for it to be regained, this depending on the degree of brain failure that may be present. The occupational therapist may check on the ability of the patient in dressing and undressing if circumstances warrant it, and in the general performance of the natural functions.

Finally, the nurse will interview the patient, noting the patient's likes and dislikes, how, when and what drugs are taken, and how easy it is to sleep. The nurse will enquire after the bowel habits and advise the patient on what to bring to hospital, what the patient should ask her friends to bring, what will be needed for going home and so on. The nurse will finally check again the list of allergies and other important nursing information. Further, the patient is told that a commode will be available beside the bed from the second day after the operation rather than the bedpan, but that this will be discontinued in favour of walking to the lavatory as soon as possible. The patient is told about the catheter that will be put in before the operation and that it will be removed within 48 hours, but that it is there for comfort rather than necessity and, of course, that it ensures a dry bed. Many old people are a little bit incontinent and make very great efforts to hide this from others because in their eyes it is shameful and thus to be reassured is a relief to them. The period of no eating and drinking is explained to the patient and it is done with great care so that the patient fully understands. Before the operation the patient need not necessarily be kept in bed until the premedication is given so it is possible to eat or drink. If the patient is considered untrustworthy in this respect the nurse will make a note of it and the patient's movements may be confined to bed or the chair beside it, before the operation. It is convenient at this time to go into any dietary peculiarities; to plan any weight reduction diets; to ensure that diabetic patients know about their particular problems and that for the first few days no extra food in the form of sweets or fruit is to be taken without permission.

The patient, who has been able to take a leisurely pace through the assessment is then seen by the whole group together and the highlights discussed with the patient and any final questions answered. The patient may then go home or be refered to the anaesthetic clinic. Before closing the patient's folder the members of the team present will have a discussion about any relevant problem or difficulty that may have appeared, or might appear, so that it can be prevented before it occurs. The assessment over, and all details recorded, the patient is admitted in due time to the ward.

III. Admission

Normally the patient will come in the afternoon before the operation. Longer that this is not necessary and is contraindicated. The longer the patient is "nursed", which includes even the inactivity of having all hotel services, the worse for the patient. Activity is the adjuvent of the old, both mentally and physically. The patient need not be put to bed at once but may remain dressed and should be encouraged to unpack personal belongings and to tidy them away in the bedside locker. The patient should be walked to the bathroom and lavatory to be shown where these essentials are.

Before the operation an antibiotic is given. This will conform to any allergies the patient may have and any locally resistant strains of bacteria that may be known to exist, but other than this should have a broad spectrum and should be nontoxic. In this respect the cephalosporins are favoured, having intramuscular and oral varieties; 500 mg should be given by intramuscular injection 4 hours before the premedication and another 500 mg with the premedication. After the operation the antibiotic will be continued by injection at the rate of 500 mg cephalosporin four times a day until the patient is taking fluids by mouth satisfactorily, when it may be changed to the oral route, continuing for 5 days.

Particular care must be given to this antibiotic cover if the surgeon is to preserve an infection-free record for arthroplasties. There is no one secret that ensures success, but rather attention must be given to a myriad of details, the omission of any one being a possible loophole through which the infection may pass.

Thus, the junior surgical staff will examine every part of the patient's body for any septic spots, sores or intertrigo, not forgetting the scalp and the webs of the toes. The state of the mouth will have been noted and if necessary attended to at the assessment, but this must again be checked. All systems are, of course examined carefully; fresh blood is taken for cross-matching against that reserved for the patient by the haematology department, but other than this there should be little in the way of "routine" tests, all of which will have been accomplished at assessment.

IV. Skin Preparation

This may seem to be another detail, but if sepsis after operation is to be eliminated then it must be considered as a most essential and important procedure, over which great thought and care should be taken and, if it is left to a junior nurse, than the nurse in charge should check that all steps have been properly taken. The patient will have an ordinary bath or shower the night before operation. The hair in particular will be examined and shampooed if there is the slightest indication for so doing, despite the hair care advice given at assessment. The following day the patient may have another bath, using a bactericidal soap, or a bed bath.

After this the part is carefully cleaned and painted with the desired skin preparation lotion. This must be chosen not for its smell or colour, but for its effectivenes; the fact that it does have an easily perceptible colouring is an added bonus for then any unprepared area is clearly seen. The organic iodine preparations are highly satisfactory in all respects. The whole hindquarter, from the navel to the toes must be prepared for a hip replacement and from the groin for a knee replacement. Nothing less will do. It is only by scrupulouse care that sepsis can be avoided and any shortcut is disastrous in the longer term. The part is swathed in sterile towels and the patient is taken to the theatre, which preferably should be a clean air theatre.

V. The Clean Air Theatre

The routine is well established, but laminar air flow theatres may not be satisfactory for all replacements, such as total knees, if the air flow has to come from the head of the table. For hips the air flow will come from the foot of the table, and over the towelled legs; from the head it carries dust from the anaesthetist and the patient. This is a point which must be considered. The Charnley–Howarth type of enclosure is most satisfactory.

After the patient has been anaesthetised on the operation table in the anaesthetic room the preparation for the operation is done by a theatre nurse with sterile equipment, outside the theatre. First a plastic apron, self-adhesive at the top, is placed around the upper part of the limb to seal off the perineum. The limb is repainted with the preparation required and carefully towelled making sure that, expecially for the hip, there is ample space for the surgical approach and that the towels are all fixed so that they will not slip during the second preparation or during the operation.

Properly prepared, the patient is taken on the operation table into the theatre and there given another skin preparation and is draped yet again, but over the existing sterile towelling which is not disturbed. The actual part to be operated upon has a self-adhesive clear plastic film placed over it, sealed round its edges by the towels so that no skin is open to the field of operation. If it is a knee replacement the cuff of the tourniquet will have been applied beforehand. This is connected after entry into the theatre to its pressure supply, the leg is elevated for 3 minutes and the pressure let into the cuff abruptly, and not slowly, so that the arterial supply is cut off at the same time as the venous drainage. An operation wound with no blood in it is less likely to infection than otherwise. The time of application of the tourniquet is noted and the operation begun. It is important here to note that the whole theatre team must be ready and waiting for the patient and not the other way round. Tight theatre discipline must be maintained throughout; staff may not come and go; those that start must finish; the special gowns must be worn correctly; two pairs of gloves are essential, hair must not be visible, and so on.

VI. The Operation

The actual surgical steps will vary according to the procedure and will not be gone into in detail here, but certain points particularly important in the elderly will be considered. First, the approach to the hip for its replacement must always be lateral or anterolateral. There is no indication for either the anterior or posterior approach, and both have strong contraindications. Again, sepsis is the important consideration for although the patient will have been catheterised, accidents in this respect can occur and the posterior wound can become bathed in urine, or worse, faeces, if, as occasionally happens, diarrhoea occurs after operation. This emphasises the importance of the nursing assessment enquiry into the bowel habits. Secondly, after the posterior approach the old and feebler patient is less likely to turn and alter weight distribution on the buttocks than is the case with younger patients; and finally, drainage tubes are a little more awkwardly placed. There are certain other more controversial orthopaedic reasons against the posterior approach, but certainly in less-experienced hands the dislocation rate after operation may be higher. The main contraindication to the anterior approach is again the slightly increased chance of wound sepsis caused by the sweating in the inguinal crease and the fact that here the wound may cause irritation and cause the patient to scratch. Orthopaedically it gives a much inferior access to the hip.

For the knee, the incision should be almost straight down from the centre point over the quadriceps tendon to the patella when a gentle slight lateral curve is made only to return to the midline at the lower patellar border. The skin is dissected with great care off the capsule and the patella, and skin towels then applied. The medial skin flap must not be folded back upon itself but must have a rolled-up swab wrapped under it so that it is rolled and not creased, for the latter, particularly with degenerate vessels will cause thrombosis in skin capillaries. The capsule is incised medially and reflected laterally with the patella; thus, on closure, it gives added layers of protection to the joint beneath it.

VII. Physiotherapy in the Recovery Room

The patient, once awake but still in the recovery ward will be seen by the physiotherapist and made to do the isometric exercises that have already been tought. Although some centres like to use calf stimulators during the operation in an attempt to prevent venous stasis, it is still very important to start active muscle contractions as soon as possible. The exercises are continued regularly when in bed even after walking has started.

VIII. Infection

There are two forms of infection after a total joint replacement, primary, within a few weeks of operation and late, perhaps 2–3 years later. The former is an ordinary wound infection, but the latter may be from a hidden infection at the cement–bone interface which takes a long time to develop. Antibiotic-containing cement may have an advantage here in preventing this, but the cement is slightly weakened by the antibiotic in it. The presence of a large foreign body is conducive to infection, especially in the debilitated patient such as those with rheumatoid arthritis or in general from other chronic illness, and many old people fall into the latter category. These patients should all be given antibiotics freely if they have had a total replacement whenever there is the suspicion of infection or even of a transient bacteraemia such as occurs with a tooth extraction. So particular emphasis must be paid to preventing infection in the elderly who may be more prone to it and with less resistance than the younger adult. Late infection is probably considerably less in those patients for whom very full precautions have been taken and it is most important to remember the possibility of this happening in the future and thereby ensuring that all steps to avoid it are taken.

IX. Care After Operation

The patient who has had a total hip or knee replacement should get up the following day. It should always be part of the definitive programme that, the day after operation the patient is assisted out of bed, stood with the help of a walking frame, walked a step or two to a chair and allowed to sit for a time depending on the overall condition. Tubes from drips and drains are no contraindication to this, and on the second day the drainage bottles and, if the catheter is still in, the urine bag, are tied to the walking frame; longer walks are taken, the patient gains confidence and is soon able to be in and out of bed without assistance. As soon as the last tube is removed the patient gets dressed; this is often the third day. If the catheter has to remain in the bladder, this is no bar to dressing but a urine bag strapped to the thigh must be used.

When the occupational therapist considers that the patient has regained sufficient of the activities of daily living to leave the ward the patient will be discharged from the acute unit to whatever place was arranged at the assessment, whether it be straight home or to an intermediate place such as convalescence or a low dependency nursing unit.

The patient, having left the acute ward at 8 days or so should be seen in about 3 weeks for a further haemoglobin estimation in case it falls; this, if it does, may slow up the progress of the patient. Further physiotherapy or occupational therapy is not given routinely; if the patient can do all the activities of daily living and continues to walk as much as possible then that is sufficient, and the patient may cease further visits to the clinic.

L. Conclusion

The care of the elderly patient with an orthopaedic complaint is most stimulating; sharing the responsibility for the total care of the patient gives intense satisfaction to the whole team, including the surgeon and the physician, and undoubtedly benefits the well-being and progress auf the patient. Never should the orthopaedic surgeon deny the elderly patient an operation when it will restore a satisfactory quality of life, however short that may be, to the patient who needs it. Properly managed such a philosophy will always benefit both patient and surgical team alike.

References

1. Barnes R, Brown JT, Garden RS, Nicoll EA (1976) Subcapital fractures of the femur. J Bone Joint Surg [Br] 53:2–24
2. Brown A, D'Arcy J (1971) Internal fixation for supracondylar fractures of the femur in the elderly. J Bone Joint Surg [B] 53:420
3. D'Arcy J, Devas M (1976) Treatment of fractures of the femoral neck by replacement with the Thompson Psothesis. J Bone Joint Surg [B] 58:279–286
4. Devas M (ed) (1977 a) Geriatric orthopaedics. Academic Press, London
5. Devas M (1977 b) Aetiology of acetabular erosion after Thompson replacement for fractured necks of femur. J Bone Joint Surg [B] 59:128
6. Fenton L (1981) Fractures of the femoral nec: Changing incidence. Br Med J 283:1217
7. Irvine RE, Baquall MK, Smith BJ (1977) The older patient, 3rd edn. University Press, London
8. Wild D, Nayak USL, Issacs B (1981) How dangerous are falls in old people at home? Br Med J 282:266–268

Anesthesiology

Anesthesia

E. RÜGHEIMER

A. Introductory Remarks

Over the last 20 years the number of geriatric patients subjected to elective or emergency surgical interventions has increased both absolutely and relatively. Some of the factors that have contributed to this state of affairs are (HAMER 1975):

1. The advances achieved in almost all areas of medicine. This applies in particular to the expanded possibilities of preoperative diagnostic procedures and to improved postoperative treatment.
2. The enormous expansion of surgical indications made possible by an improvement in our knowledge of pathophysiologic relationships, and the development of modern surgical techniques.
3. The present standard of the procedures and the overall potential of modern anesthesiology.

Only 50 years ago, the upper age limit for surgical intervention was considered to be 55 years; today, more than 10% of surgical patients are older than 70 years.

Table 1 shows how the age distribution of surgical patients has changed over the last 30 years. Compared with 1952, the number of patients older than 60 years had, by 1981, increased from 16.6% to 28.2%, that of patients over 70 years old from 5.2% to 12.5%. Older collective statistics from the period prior to 1960 reveal an overall mortality rate for elderly patients of between 11.1% and 21.6% (HERRION et al. 1960; STAHLGREN 1961). Data published in subsequent years show only slight changes in this situation (Table 2). All these data show that the mortality rate of geriatric patients is considerably greater than that of surgical patients as a whole, for whom, as shown in Table 1, it is about 2%, values in the literature ranging between 1.3% and 4.9% (KOHN et al. 1973; HAMER 1975). A detailed evaluation of the complication and mortality risk in the geriatric patient is, however, only possible on the basis of an analysis of the influence of previous diseases, surgery, and anesthesia on the nature and incidence of the complications. These points are dealt with in Sect. C.

Almost all the statistics show that with increasing age, the mortality rate tends to rise. This means that in the group of patients over 90 years old, it is greater than in 80- to 89-year-old patients, and in this group, in turn, it is higher than in 70- to 79-year-old patients (BERGMANN 1963; MAYRHOFER 1970; PULVER and OTTEN 1970; LUTZ et al. 1972; BÜNTE 1979; PALMBERG and HIRSJÄRVI 1979; HEBERER 1982; KALLINA 1982). An exception may be found in the data published by STAHLGREN (1961), who described a lower mortality rate in patients over 80 years

Table 1. Age distribution of patients of the Department of Surgery of the University of Erlangen-Nürnberg in 1952 compared with 1981

Age (years)	1952		1981	
	No.	(%)	No.	(%)
0– 10	189	8.0	1,023	10.9
11– 20	300	12.7	929	9.8
21– 30	340	14.4	819	8.7
31– 40	325	13.7	835	8.9
41– 50	440	18.6	1,307	14.0
51– 60	350	14.8	1,824	19.4
61– 70	247	10.9	1,489	15.8
71– 80	123	5.2	957	10.4
81– 90	12	0.5	190	2.0
91–100	0	0	10	0.1
Unknown	28	1.2		

Table 2. Mortality in the elderly following various surgical interventions. Review of the literature since 1961

Reference	Minimum age (years)	No.	Mortality (%)
STAHLGREN (1961)	70	105	15.3
WILDER and FISHBEIN (1961)	80	207	33.0
BERGMANN (1963)	80	427	14.8
MARSHALL and FAHEY (1964)	80	443	19.4
COGBILL (1967)	65	223	20.6
LORHAN (1967)	80	710	27.4
VON BRAMANN and HEROLD (1969)	80	699	18.6
MAYRHOFER (1970)	80	125	13.6
PULVER and OTTEN (1970)	80	450	33.0
DENNEY and DENSON (1972)	90	272	29.0
LUTZ et al. (1972)	70	30,126	8.8
KOHN et al. (1973)	80	599	17.5
MILLER et al. (1977)	90	147	12.2
RIFAT (1977)	65	869	20.8
DJOKOVIC and HEDLEY-WHYTE (1979)	80	500	6.2
KRAAS et al. (1979)	70	1,005	21.0
PALMBERG and HIRSJÄRVI (1979)	70	590	9.2
WEISS and LESMICK (1980)	65	100	11.0
STEPHEN (1981)	70	840	5.7
FARROW et al. (1982)	65	18,860	6.3
KALLINA (1982)	70	220	5.5

old than in those under 80 years old, and in the reports by SALEHI (1979) who, in urologic operations, found a constant mortality rate between the eighth and tenth decades of life. KOHN et al. (1973) made similar observations in patients over 90 years old. These publications do not indicate whether this flattening off of the mortality rate in very old age is due to a more stringent application of in-

Table 3. Frequency of preexisting disorders of various organ systems in geriatric surgical patients. All data given as percentages

Reference	STAHLGREN (1961)	VON BRAMANN and HEROLD (1969)	PULVER and OTTEN (1970)	KOHN et al. (1973)	MILLER et. al. (1977)	KRAAS et al. (1979)	STEPHEN (1981)	HALJAMÄE et al. (1982)	HEBERER (1982)	MICHEL and KÖRNER (1983)	OSSWALD et al. (1983)
Minimum age (years)	70	80	80	80	90	70	70	70	70	75	60
Cardiovascular	43	52.6[a] 17.3[b]	53	56.9	81.6	41	–	78	39.5	73.5	70.6
Hypertension	–	–	–	–	21.8	–	46.6	21	18.0	–	–
Respiratory	29	36.4	21	33.2	28.6	26	–	14	18.0	51.4	17.6
Central nervous system	–	–	29	16.2	35.4	–	–	39	–	12.5	–
Fluid/electrolytes	6	7.1	–	–	–	–	–	14	–	–	–
Hypovolemia	35	–	–	–	–	–	–	–	–	–	–
Anemia	–	26.2	–	–	17.7	33	–	24	–	–	–
Genitourinary	17	5.2	–	17.0	–	22	32.1	–	4.2	27.5	6.0
Liver	4	–	–	2.8	–	–	17.6	–	–	7.0	6.2
Diabetes	–	–	–	23.0	11.6	12	9.4	10	11.2	28.8	12.1

[a] Cardiac; [b] Vascular

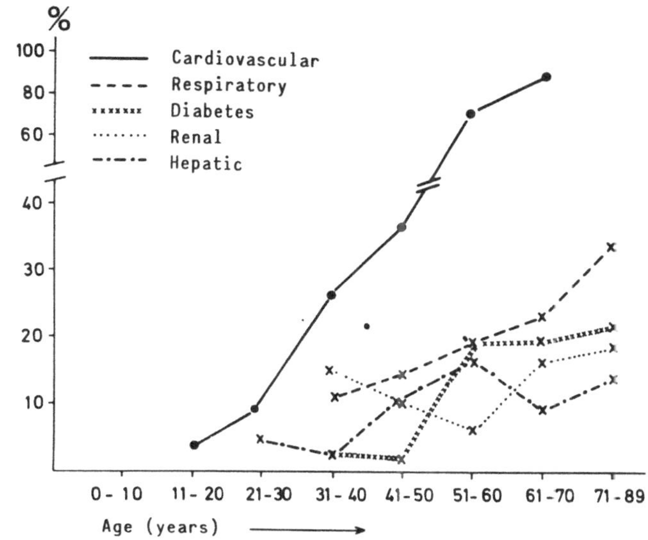

Fig. 1. Frequency of various preexisting diseases in surgical patients of different ages. (After STRIEBEL et al. 1981, with permission)

dication criteria, or to the good physiologic status of the patients who had survived beyond the age of 80 years.

Apart from the more nonspecific influence of age on the overall risk, that of the patient's preoperative general condition can be most readily evaluated and quantified. Of particular importance are the associated diseases of major organ systems that are commonly found in the elderly (Table 3). These include cardiovascular and respiratory diseases, metabolic, hepatic, and renal diseases, hypovolemia, and overweight.

Without a doubt, the most common diseases of the elderly involve the cardiovascular system. They include cardiac failure, coronary heart disease, arrhythmias, hypertension, and arteriosclerosis. Such diseases are observed in more than 50% of geriatric patients, while respiratory disorders are seen in 25%–35%. Among the remaining pathologic findings, hypovolemia, anemia, diabetes mellitus, and functional disorders of the central nervous system deserve particular attention. Figure 1 shows the age dependency of the occurrence of the major preexisting diseases in surgical patients. Cardiovascular, respiratory, renal, and electrolytic disorders double the incidence of anesthesia-related complications (STRIEBEL et al. 1981). In surgical patients older than 60 years, OSSWALD et al. (1983) found a two- to fourfold incidence of preexisting disorders of the major organ systems compared with a group of patients under 60 years old. The intra- and postoperative occurrence of cardiovascular complications was also higher in the older group (Table 4).

Table 4. Frequency (%) of intra- and postoperative cardiovascular complications. (After OSSWALD et al. 1983)

	During anesthesia		In recovery room	
	<60 years	>60 years	<60 years	>60 years
Hypotension	0.9	2,9[b]	0.8	2.8[a]
Hypertension	0.9	3.7[b]	2.6	9.3[a]
Arrhythmias	1.6	3.9[b]	3.1	2.7

[a] $P<0.01$
[b] $P<0.001$

B. Changes of Aging: Anesthesiologic Aspects

I. Cardiovascular System

To date, no general diminishment of the contractility of the heart muscle cell with increasing age has been demonstrated, although the cardiac reserves available for increased physical exercise have been shown to be reduced. The reasons for this must be assumed to be specific changes in the biochemistry and energy turnover of the myocardial cell (LAKATTA 1979; MILLER 1981). In addition to a reduction in resting cardiac output, a further expression of the deterioration in the mechanical performance of the heart is a diminishment in the maximum heart rate during exercise. The maximum oxygen consumption drops from more than 2,000 ml/min to 1,400–1,500 ml/min. This corresponds to a small increase in cardiac output (BRANDFONBREUER et al. 1955; GRANATH et al. 1964).

The following observations may be interpreted as signs of an age-related change in the autonomic system (LAKATTA 1979):

1. The heart rate response to dynamic exercise is reduced by about 20% at age 75 years, as compared with age 20 years.
2. The chronotropic effect of the β-receptor stimulant isoproterenol is diminished (Fig. 2). In contrast, the maximum heart rate achievable with pacing is age independent. The inotropic response to catecholamines and digitalis glycosides is also diminished in isolated heart muscle preparations, but not that to paired stimulation (LAKATTA and YIN 1982).
3. The sensitivity of the baroreceptor reflex system also decreases with age. Under controlled conditions, an elevation of blood pressure by a given amount results in a smaller increase in heart rate than in young adults.
4. Aging causes a significant attenuation of the increase in heart rate induced by hypoxia or hypercapnia.
5. The stress of sustained isometric handgrip results in an increase in blood pressure and heart rate, which is attenuated with increasing age. The parallel increase in plasma catecholamines is, however, not diminished, and may even be greater, than in young adults.

These observations indicate that a diminishment of the sensitivity to sympathicoadrenergic stimulation is involved in the reduced adaptability of the elderly

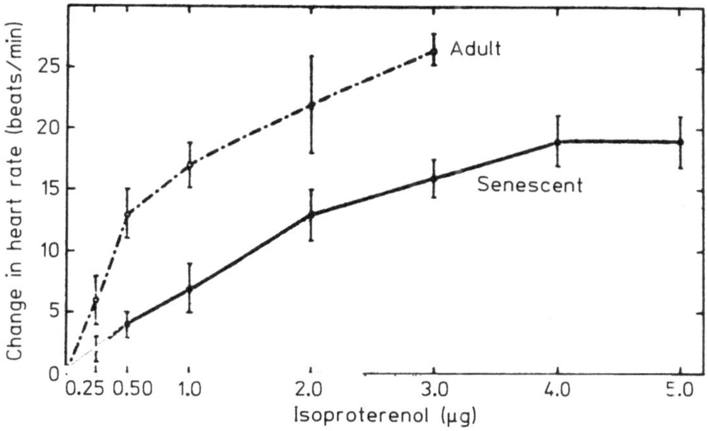

Fig. 2. The effect of age on the increase in heart rate in humans in response to varying concentrations of isoproterenol (mean ± standard error). At all concentrations above 0.25 µg, the effect of age on the response is significant at $P<0.005$. (LAKATTA 1979). From Fed Proc, with permission of Fed Am Soc Exp Biol

heart to changes in the demands made on it. The possible reason for this may be a decline in activity (FLEISCH 1981) or a reduction in the number of a β-adrenoceptors (WEISS et al. 1979). As yet unclear is the significance of the parasympathetic system and its interaction with the sympathetic system for the change in the regulatory capacity of the cardiovascular system. Clinical experience shows that the geriatric patient often presents with bradycardia, which responds only poorly to atropine (VIRTANEN et al. 1982). This has been confirmed by systematic electrocardiographic (ECG) investigations of the effects of a partial vagal block with atropine (DAUCHOT and GRAVENSTEIN 1971). Furthermore, aging brings an increase in the weight of the heart and left ventricular hypertrophy (LINZBACH and AKUAMOA-BOATENG 1973 a; GERSTENBLITH et al. 1977). Whether this is associated with any change in the distensibility of the myocardium is not clear (LAKATTA and YIN 1982).

Increasing age also results in changes in the vascular system. The peripheral vascular resistance increases by 25%–30% between the ages of 30 and 70 years (WEZLER 1958), and the elastic distensibility of the arterial system, in particular the aorta, is diminished (SIMON and MEYER 1958). This latter can readily be deduced from the increase in the arterial pulse wave velocity (WEZLER and BÖGER 1939; SCHIMMLER 1965). In parallel with this development, the arterial blood pressure also increases with age (WEZLER and BÖGER 1939; MASTER and LASSER 1961). This applies in greater measure to the systolic pressure than to the diastolic, so that in old age, disproportionate systolic hypertension is more frequently observed (KOCH-WESER 1978).

The importance of the changes in the cardiovascular system brought about by aging for practical anesthesiology may be described in the following points:

1. The incidence of cardiac disease increases with age (Table 5 and Fig. 1). The most important of these conditions are coronary heart disease, arrhythmias,

Table 5. Frequency of cardiovascular disturbances in the elderly. (After HAMER 1975)

	Frequency (%)	Minimum age (years)
Hypertension	75	70
General atherosclerosis	35	70
Compensated cardiac failure	80	70
Coronary heart disease	60	60
Coronary artery occlusion	40	55
Arrhythmias	90	80
Pathologic ECG	77	60
Pulmonary sclerosis	60	60

and congestive heart failure. Abnormal ECG findings must be expected in more than 50% of patients older than 70 years (MIHALICK and FISCH 1974), and coronary heart disease in almost 100% (WEDGWOOD 1973; BURCH 1975). Morphologically, more than one pathologic finding is usually detected in the heart, so that the term "polypathia of the heart" was coined (LINZBACH and AKUAMOA-BOATENG 1973b). These diseases restrict the compensation possibilities of the heart additionally to the greater or lesser physiologic diminishment in its performance (HAMER 1975).

2. The result of this is that in geriatric patients, pharmacotherapy of the cardiovascular system in the perioperative phase is the rule rather than the exception. On account of the changes in autonomic tone and pharmacodynamics, however, such therapy differs quantitatively compared with younger patients. This applies in particular to the commonly required use of glycosides and catecholamines.

3. The arterial hypertension frequently observed in old age increases the risk of cardiovascular complications, even when only the systolic pressure is appreciably elevated beyond normal (KOCH-WESER 1978; KANNEL et al. 1981). Milder forms of hypertension do not lead to an increase in the perioperative complication rate when, by means of complete intra- and postoperative monitoring, any and all circulatory instabilities are immediately detected and treated: in contrast, in severe, untreated hypertension (with diastolic values in excess of 110 mmHg), an increased incidence of perioperative myocardial infarction and cerebrovascular accidents must be expected (GOLDMAN and CALDERA 1979; PRYS-ROBERTS 1979; TOWNE and BERNHARD 1980; STEPHEN 1981).

II. Respiratory System

In common with the cardiovascular system, the respiratory system, too, is subject to age-related changes which become manifest as an increasing decline in the toleration of physical effort. This decrease in the respiratory reserve can be measured as a regression of a large number of ventilation and arterial oxygenation parameters (Fig. 3). It must, however, be remembered that the "normal" values usually applied to patients over 60 years old should not unreservedly be considered rep-

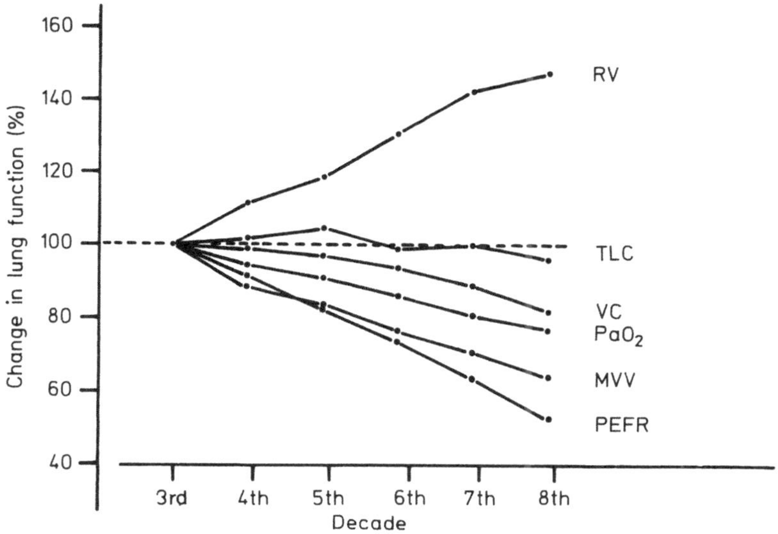

Fig. 3. The effect of age on lung function parameters presented as percentage changes of values in the third decade of life. *RV* residual volume; *TLC* total lung capacity; *VC* vital capacity; PaO_2 partial pressure of oxygen in arterial blood; *MVV* maximal voluntary ventilation; *PEFR* peak expiratory flow rate. (Modified after CHOWANETZ and SCHRAMM 1981)

resentative, since for these age groups adequately large, homogeneous groups of normal subjects with no pathologic disorder are hardly available (CHOWANETZ and SCHRAMM 1981).

The total lung capacity remains virtually constant, while the vital capacity declines by about 25 ml every year. As a result, the residual volume increases between the ages of 20 and 70 years by about 40%. The functional residual capacity (FRC) is believed to be considerably less dependent on age; according to ULMER et al. (1976), in subjects of normal weight, it increases between the ages of 20 and 70 years by only 13%–14%, although according to data quoted by HEDLEY-WHYTE et al. (1976), the increase is at least 20%.

During the course of aging, the elastic recoil pressure of the lungs decreases, so that static lung compliance becomes greater. In contrast, the compliance of the thoracic wall becomes smaller, so that the resulting overall compliance changes but slightly. Accordingly, the total lung capacity does not change, while the declining elasticity of the lung results in an increase in residual capacity and FRC at the expense of the vital capacity (PIERCE and EBERT 1958; TURNER et al. 1968; HEDLEY-WHITE et al. 1976; HARTUNG 1977).

The influence exercised by age alone on airway resistance is small. On relaxed breathing, this parameter is constant, while on deep expiration, airway resistance increases with age (ISLAM et al. 1978). In part, this difference is due to the dependence of the airway resistance on the intrathoracic gas volume (ULMER et al. 1976).

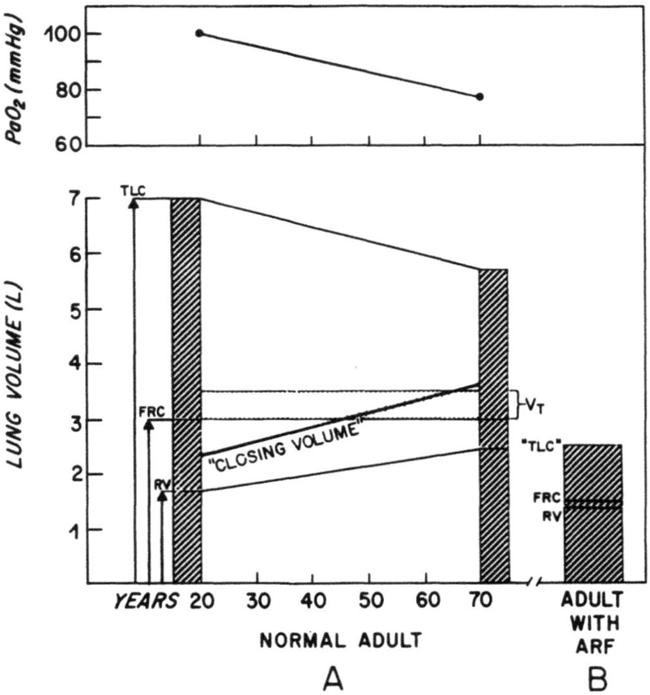

Fig. 4. Changes in PaO_2 and lung volumes with age in normal adults in the supine position (*A*), and typical values for lung volumes in an adult patient (*B*) with acute respiratory failure (*ARF*). PaO_2 partialpressure of oxygen in arterial blood; *RV* residual volume; *FRC* functional residual capacity; *TLC* total lung capacity; V_T tidal volume. (PONTOPPIDAN et al. 1972). Reprinted by permission of the New England Journal of Medicine 287:690–698, 1972

Numerous clinical studies have shown that the closing volume increases linearly with increasing age (HOLLAND et al. 1968; LEBLANC et al. 1970; DON et al. 1971; MANSELL et al. 1972; BEGIN et al. 1975). When the volume of the lungs decreases during expiration, small airways close, in particular in the dependent parts of the lungs, where the expiratory volume is greater and the distending transpulmonary pressures smaller. The lung volume at which noticeable airway closure just begins, is defined as the closing volume. In contrast to the FRC, which decreases by about 20% on changeover from an erect to a supine position, the closing volume is largely independent of the position of the body. For this reason, in the supine position, the closing volume equals the FRC as early as the age of 40–45 years, but in the seated or standing subject only at ages over 60 years (LEBLANC et al. 1970; DON et al. 1971; MANSELL et al. 1972, BEGIN et al. 1975), as shown in Fig. 4.

The underlying cause of an increase in closing volume with age is believed to be a reduction in the elastic recoil of the lungs (HOLLAND et al. 1968). Airway closure has consequences in particular for the regional distribution of the respiratory gases within the lungs, and impairs the adaptation of ventilation to perfu-

Table 6. Frequency of abnormal preoperative lung function in 311 unselected male patients undergoing general surgical procedures

Age (years)	Frequency of ventilatory abnormalities detected with spirometry (%)	
	Total	Moderate and severe
<30	40.7	13.0
30–40	43.7	18.1
40–50	50.0	20.4
50–60	46.6	25.0
60–70	69.6	41.2
>70	75.7	43.3

sion. This is considered the most important reason for the drop in arterial PO_2 values shown in Fig. 3 and 5 (Pontoppidan et al. 1972), but further causes for the diminishing arterial oxygenation seen in advanced age cannot be excluded (Hedley-Whyte et al. 1976).

Under resting conditions, the pressure in the pulmonary circulation does not change. With increasing age, however, the rise in pulmonary artery pressure under load increases, the corresponding changes in pulmonary vascular resistance being nonuniform (Emirgil et al. 1967; Gloger 1972). As in the case of the positive chronotropic response of the heart, the ventilatory response to hypoxemia and hypercapnia in the elderly is reduced by 40%–50% (Kronenberg and Drage 1973).

The significance of these changes for anesthesia in geriatric patients rests, in particular, on two points:

1. As in the case of the cardiovascular system, in the respiratory system, it must be expected that bronchopulmonary diseases will be superimposed on disturbances of pulmonary function owing to physiologic changes of aging. With increasing age, such diseases become more and more common, as the figures in Table 6 demonstrate in an exemplary manner.

2. Important though previous bronchopulmonary diseases are for the patient about to undergo surgery, they are by no means the sole risk factors associated with the respiratory system that can affect the intra- and in particular the postoperative course. Anesthesia and the operation can also impair the mechanics of respiration and the exchange of gases, and further aggravate the preexisting age- and disease-related impairment of pulmonary function (Pecora 1969; Falke 1976; Laver et al. 1976; Braun and Voigt 1978; Landauer 1979; Wolff 1979). These anesthesia- and surgery-related mechanisms will be described briefly here.

All surgical interventions lead to a postoperative decline in pulmonary function which manifests itself, globally, as a reduction in vital capacity and FRC (Fig. 5). Major underlying causes are postoperative pain and the immobilization of the patient by confinement to bed (often without change of position), which together with the intestinal atony that often presents, results in an elevation of the diaphragm. As a result, respiration becomes, shallower and more rapid, sigh-

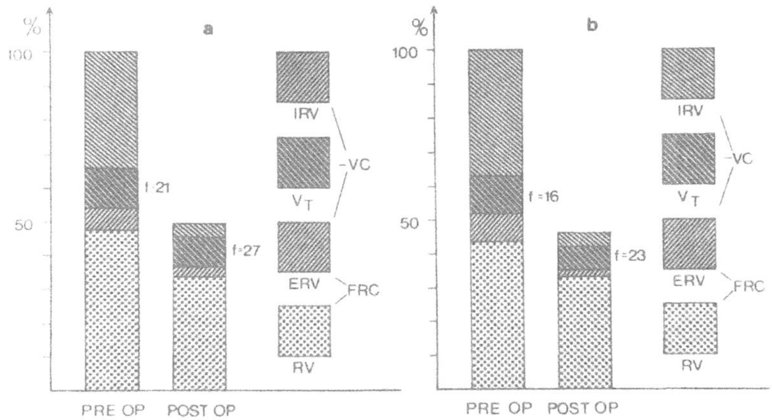

Fig. 5. Influence of **a** upper abdominal (Whipple's procedures) and **b** thoracoabdominal procedures (left thoracic gastrectomies) on lung volumes. Preoperative values = 100%; *N* 10 in both groups; *f* respiratory frequency; V_T tidal volume; *IRV* inspiratory reserve volume; *ERV* expiratory reserve volume; *RV* residual volume; *VC* vital capacity; *FRC* functional residual capacity

ing and the coughing mechanism are hindered, or completely suppressed. Considerable mismatching of ventilation and perfusion occurs, together with increased dead space ventilation. This leads to arterial hypoxemia (MARSHALL and WYCHIE 1972). Such disturbances are most marked after thoracic and upper abdominal surgery. Following laparotomy, the vital capacity is reduced on average by 50%, and the FRC by 20%. Complete compensation is achieved at the earliest after several days or, after thoracotomies, only after weeks.

Anesthesia, too, has a variety of effects on the intra- and postoperative pulmonary function (MARSHALL and WYCHIE 1972; REHDER et al. 1975; FALKE 1976; BRAUN and VOIGT 1978; WOLFF 1979; GELB et al. 1981). Compliance and the FRC decrease and the difference between closing volume and FRC becomes greater (KITAMURA et al. 1972; REHDER et al. 1977). As a result, regional perfusion–ventilation inhomogeneities increase and a right-to-left shunt develops. Under general anesthesia, such changes can occur even with spontaneous respiration, and are more marked under relaxation and controlled respiration. Both extrapulmonary and pulmonary causes can be specified.

Extrapulmonary factors that might be mentioned are the positioning of the patient (supine, prone, or lateral position maintained without change over a lengthy period), and changes in muscle tone resulting from both loss of consciousness and relaxation (FROESE and BRYAN 1974; REHDER et al. 1975; LAVER et al. 1976). Pulmonary factors acting in the same direction are the ventilation pattern in controlled respiration together with resulting changes in the pulmonary circulation (which, in turn, lead to regional perfusion–ventilation inhomogeneities), occasionally occurring interstitial pulmonary edema, particularly in dependent regions, retention and inspissation of secretions, and, finally, the direct pharmacologic effects of anesthetic agents on the bronchial system, alveoli, pulmonary

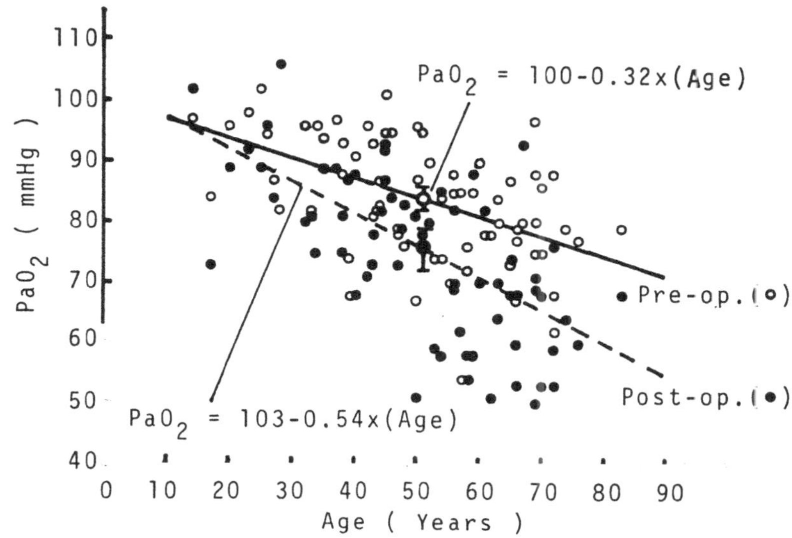

Fig. 6. Relationship between arterial oxygen tension (PaO_2) and age during breathing of room air. (KITAMURA et al. 1972). From Anesthesiology, with permission of J. B. Lippincott

circulation, and regulation of respiration. With respect to the anesthetic agents, four aspects are of particular importance:

1. They have an influence on lung compliance and airway resistance (GELB et al. 1981).
2. Fat-soluble inhalation anesthetics impair the function and synthesis of the surfactant lining the alveoli (LANDAUER 1979). An additional contribution to this effect is made by the ventilation pattern (REHDER et al. 1975).
3. Numerous anesthetics inhibit the hypoxic pulmonary vasoconstriction that serves to adapt perfusion to ventilation (BJERTNAES 1977; MATHERS et al. 1977).
4. Depending upon the composition of the inspired gas, absorption in alveolar zones distal to closed airways can result in the collapse of the alveoli and the development of atelectasis. The overall effect of the operation- and anesthesia-related changes is to lead to an increase in alveoloarterial O_2 partial pressure difference, and a lowering of arterial O_2 partial pressure (PaO_2). Together, these changes give rise to the age-associated PaO_2 decrease, as is impressively shown in Fig. 6 (KITAMURA et al. 1972).

III. Brain

In advanced age, there is an increase in degenerative and vascular diseases of the brain with typical morphological and pathophysiologic changes. They reveal characteristic clinical correlates (BLESSED 1980). Senile dementia due to degenerative causes, including presenile and senile dementia of the ALZHEIMER type, can be distinguished from lesions (multi-infarction type) with a vascular background.

The former account for 60%–70%, the latter for 20%–25%, and mixed forms for 15%–20% of diseases of this type (HACHINSKI et al. 1974; TOMLINSON 1980; HOYER 1981). The longer a state of dementia persists, and the more marked its clinical symptomatology, the greater do cerebral perfusion and metabolism deviate from normal. In parallel with this, the concentration and distribution of neurotransmitter vary in various parts of the brain (CARLSSON 1981).

Age-related, but not pathologic, changes involving the central (e.g., decline in neuronal metabolism), or the peripheral, nervous system (e.g., a decrease in nerve conduction velocity), have no direct effects on anesthesia and surgery, but, as an underlying cause of the increasing sensitivity to the effects of anesthetic drugs with increasing age, must be taken into account (MILLER 1981). Further, the clinical observation can often be made that certain cerebral function characteristics of the elderly are more marked in the postoperative phase, and delay or prevent recovery. These include cognitive performance, emotional state, and reduction of activity, coupled with diminished motivation. If during anesthesia and surgery, disturbances of cardiovascular, respiratory, and metabolic homeostasis occur, complete decompensation of the reduced cerebral reserves can occur.

IV. Other Organs

Other organs (liver, kidney) or functional systems (fluid and electrolyte balance, metabolism, endocrine system) also undergo changes with age. However, these are not so directly important for anesthesia as are pathologic states of these organs that more frequently occur in advanced age, although they are by no means specific to the geriatric patient. More detailed information may be obtained from the respective chapters in this book.

V. Pharmacology

With increasing age, changes occur both in pharmacokinetics and in pharmacodynamics. The reduction in renal and hepatic metabolization and excretion functions and a decrease in plasma binding, together with a decline in the lean body mass and muscle mass relative to the total body weight, result in increased plasma concentrations and a reduction in the elimination rate of drugs (GREENBLATT et al. 1982). In principle, however, drugs have the same effects in old patients as in young patients. So far, no unequivocal evidence has been found for a change in drug–receptor binding and response.

1. Pharmacokinetics

Changes in pharmacokinetics have been described for atropine, barbiturates (thiopental), benzodiazepines, opioids (narcotic analgesics), muscle relaxants, inhalation anesthetic agents, and other drugs. In the case of intravenously administered atropine, the elimination half-life $t_{1/2}$ increases markedly with age, while the clearance Cl drops to less than 50% (VIRTANEN et al. 1982). In the case of thiopental, too, $t_{1/2}$ increases (Fig. 7), while Cl remains virtually age independent (JUNG et al. 1982). Of the numerous benzodiazepines, diazepam has been thor-

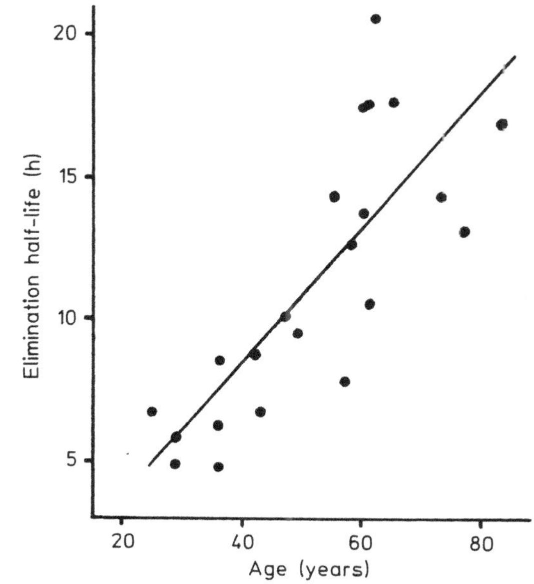

Fig. 7. Relationship between the elimination half-life of thiopental and age. The *full line* was determined by linear regression analysis ($r = 0.80$; $P < 0.001$). (JUNG et al. 1982). From Anesthesiology, with permission of J. B. Lippincott

oughly investigated. It behaves in a similar manner to thiopental, that is $t_{1/2}$ increases between the ages of 20 and 80 years, from 20 to 90 h, while Cl, although revealing considerable individual fluctuations, remains constant (KLOTZ et al. 1975). Also the opioids, exemplified by morphine (STANSKI et al. 1978) and fentanyl (BENTLEY et al. 1982), reveal an increase in $t_{1/2}$, and a decrease in Cl with age.

Furthermore, CHAN et al. (1975) reported that after identical doses, the serum concentration of pethidine is higher in patients over 70 years old than in those under 30 years old. The most thoroughly investigated relaxant agent is probably pancuronium, which is also characterized by an appreciable reduction of Cl and an increase in $t_{1/2}$ (MCLEOD et al. 1979; DUVALDESTIN et al. 1980).

Inhalation anesthetics of the halogenated hydrocarbon group differ principially from injected agents with respect to their pharmacokinetic behavior, since they are taken up via the lungs, from which they are also largely eliminated. It is possible that their rate of uptake is reduced in old age, for it has been shown that the alveolar equilibrium concentration of halothane and methoxyflurane is achieved more rapidly in children than in adults (EGER et al. 1971).

2. Pharmacodynamics

It is known, on the basis of clinical experience, that elderly patients have a reduced anesthetic requirement (MILLER 1981). This has been established scientifically in investigations of dose–effect relationship. All patients older than 65 years premedicated with morphine lost consciousness at a thiopental dose of 1.8 mg/kg while 20- to 40-year-old patients required a dose of 2.8 mg/kg (MURAVCHICK and MANDEL 1982). After administration of barbiturates, ODUAH (1970) found a cor-

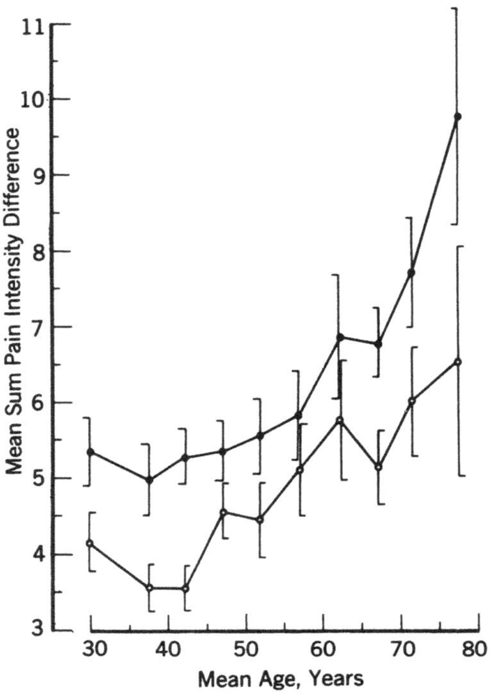

Fig. 8. Change of mean sum pain intensity difference with age. Patients received 20 mg pentazocine (*open circles*) or 10 mg morphine sulfate (*full circles*). (BELVILLE et al. 1971). Reprinted by permission from JAMA 217:1835–1841. Copyright 1971, Am Med Ass

relation between age and duration of sleep. Intravenous administration of 4.5 mg/kg thiopental caused 30-year-old subjects to sleep for an average of 4 min, while 70-year-old subject slept for an average of 15 min. After administration of hexobarbital, the sleep durations were about 1.5 and 4.5 min, respectively.

The dose-related efficacy of diazepam increases with age, as was shown by REIDENBERG et al. (1978) and the BOSTON COLLABORATIVE SURVEILLANCE PROGRAM (1973). BELLVILLE et al. (1971) investigated the postoperative analgesic effectiveness auf 10 mg morphine and 20 mg pentazocine in 712 patients aged between 30 and 80 years. The suppression of pain was more clearly marked in the group of elderly patients than in the younger patients (Fig. 8).

A change in the intensity of the effect of muscle relaxants with age is not so evident. Org NC 45 (norcuronium) reveals a moderate, but statistically significant, increase in effect in patients older than 60 years (D'HOLLANDER et al. 1982). In contrast, the effect of pancuronium does not change with age (DUVALDESTIN et al. 1980). The reduced alveolar requirement of the volatile anesthetic agents halothane, enflurane, and isoflurane, indicated by a decrease in minimum alveolar concentration (MAC), is well documented (GREGORY et al. 1969; GION and SAIDMAN 1971; STEVENS et al. 1975), as can be seen in Fig. 9.

In the use of local anesthetic agents for regional anesthesia there are also marked differences between young and old adults. BROMAGE (1969) was able to quantify the decline in dose requirement per spinal segment with increasing age, in epidural anaesthesia (Fig. 10), and this was later confirmed by, among other workers, SHARROCK (1978). In contrast to lidocaine or mepivacaine, for the long-

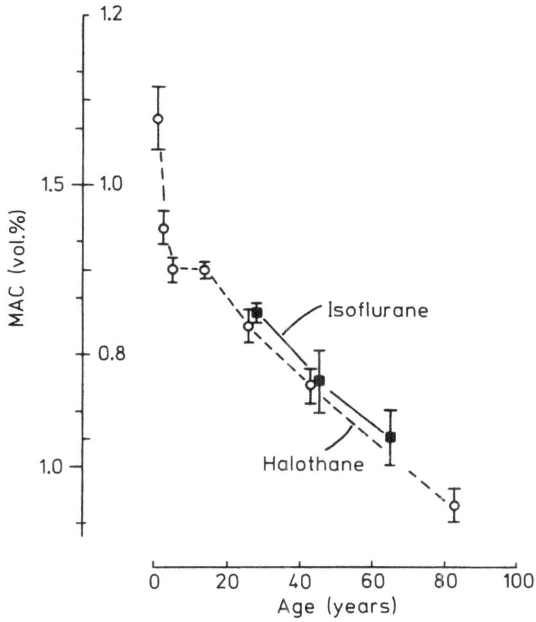

Fig. 9. Dependence on age of minimum alveolar concentrations (*MAC*) of halothane and isoflurane. (STEVENS et al. 1975). From Anesthesiology, with permission of J. B. Lippincott

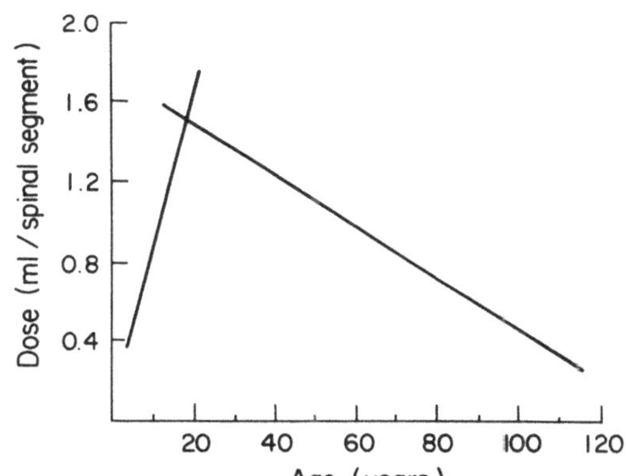

Fig. 10. Segmental epidural dose requirements of 2% lignocaine hydrochloride with 1:200,000 epinephrine, related to age between 4 and 102 years. From Br J Anaesth 41:1016–1022, 1969 (modified by MILLER 1981). Reprinted by permission of Macmillan Press and Churchill Livingstone

acting local anesthetic bupivacaine used for brachial plexus blockade, a positive correlation has been found between age and duration of effect (BROMAGE and GERTEL 1972).

C. Hazards of Anesthesia and Surgery

I. Preoperative Status

1. Quantification of the Anesthetic Risk

The anesthetic risk is difficult to define unequivocally, since intra- and postoperative complications are influenced not only by the anesthesia itself, but also by

Table 7. Classification of physical status by the American Society of Anesthesiologists (ASA)

1	A normal healthy patient
2	A patient with a mild systemic disease
3	A patient with a severe systemic disease
4	A patient with an incapacitating systemic disease that is a constant threat to life
5	A moribund patient not expected to survive 24 h with or without operation

preexisting diseases and the surgical intervention. A separation of the anesthesiologic from the overall surgical risk is hardly possible (PETER et al. 1980; KEATS 1983). These complex interactions make it difficult preoperatively to systematize all the relevant risk factors in such a manner that the significance of each individual factor, in accordance with its complication incidence, can be taken into account and a prediction as to the course of the procedure made.

The most commonly employed classification scheme is that published by the American Society of Anesthesiologists (ASA) involving five categories (Table 7). In numerous studies involving large groups of patients, it has been shown that the complication and mortality rates correlate with the ASA class. However, on account of the considerable variations in the manner of determining mortality rate (on the operating table, 48 h or 7 days postoperative, in-hospital mortality), quantitatively greatly differing data are presented (VACANTI et al. 1970; LUTZ et al. 1972; MARX et al. 1973; DJOKOVIC and HEDLEY-WHYTE 1979). On the basis of a comparison of the reported figures, it may be concluded that the ASA classification does not permit any useful prediction for the individual case. One of the reasons for this is that the scheme takes account neither of the surgical intervention itself, nor of the age of the patient.

In recent years, in particular in Germany, improved and more detailed classifications that give particular consideration to these two factors have been elaborated. In this connection, not only is a rough subjective assessment of the general state undertaken, as in the case of the ASA scheme, but the assessment also employs examination findings as a basis (LUTZ 1980; PETER et al. 1980).

2. Prediction of Cardiovascular and Pulmonary Risks

In both the intra- and the postoperative phases, the patient is at greatest risk from cardiovascular and pulmonary complications. Cardiac failure, shock, myocardial infarction, pulmonary embolism, cerebral vascular insults, and pneumonia, together with sepsis, are the major causes of death (WILDER and FISHBEIN 1961; LORHAN 1967; PULVER and OTTEN 1970; MILLER et al. 1977; STEPHEN 1981). A preoperative quantification of these risks makes good sense, since it permits the entire perioperative care to be tailored to the specific requirements of the individual case. As already mentioned, general classification schemes such as that of the ASA grouping are not suitable for the preoperative assessment of such specific risks.

GOLDMAN et al. (1977) have described a multifactorial index of the cardiac risk borne by surgical patients which, based exclusively on the results of noninvasive

Table 8. Clinical factors independently related to perioperative cardiac complications. (GOLDMAN et al. 1977)

Criteria[a]	Multivariate discriminant function coefficient	Points
1. History		
a. Age >70 years	0.191	5
b. MI in previous 6 months	0.384	10
2. Physical examination		
a. S_6 gallop or JVD	0.451	11
b. Important VAS	0.119	3
3. ECG		
a. Rhythm other than sinus or PAC on last preoperative ECG	0.283	7
b. >5 PVC/min documented at any time before operation	0.278	7
4. General status		
$PO_2 < 60$ or $PCO_2 > 50$ mmHg, $K < 3.0$ or $HCO_3 < 20$ mequiv./l BUN > 50 or Cr > 3.0 mg/dl, abnormal SGOT, signs of chronic liver disease or patient bedridden from noncardiac causes	0.132	3
5. Operation		
a. Intraperitoneal, intrathoracic, or aortic operation	0.123	3
b. Emergency operation	0.167	4
Total possible		53

[a] MI denotes myocardial infarction; JVD jugular vein distension; VAS valvular aortic stenosis; PAC premature atrial contractions; ECG electrocardiogram; PVC premature ventricular contractions; PO_2 partial pressure of oxygen; PCO_2 partial pressure of carbon dioxide; K potassium; HCO_3 bicarbonate; BUN blood urea nitrogen; Cr creatinine; SGOT serum glutamic oxaloacetic transaminase

examination procedures, permits quite an accurate prediction of expected intra- and postoperative cardiac complication (myocardial infarction, pulmonary edema, ventricular tachycardia, cardiac death) on the basis of a point scoring system (Table 8). In the practical clinical situation, of course, the GOLDMAN scheme cannot be used in detail for every geriatric patient; it has, however, considerably extended our knowledge about the factors which in high-risk patients need to be taken into particular account preoperatively, and it has provided the stimulus for employing noninvasive procedures to establish indications for accurate and invasive intra- and postoperative monitoring and treatment, such as can be effected by means of the Swan–Ganz catheter (DEL GUERICO and COHN 1980; VAN AKEN et al. 1982.

In patients presenting with cardiac failure, the use of the functional classification of the New York Heart Association (NYHA) offers a possibility for risk assessment (HEINRICH et al. 1982a). In particular after intrathoracic and intra-abdominal operations, the postoperative mortality rate is closely correlated with the

NYHA class (SIEGEL 1976). Since this classification is effected exclusively on the basis of the medical history, it demonstrates the importance of the preoperative history under exercise conditions.

If not treated, arterial hypertension also represents a risk factor (FOËX and PRYS-ROBERTS 1974; HARTUNG et al. 1983). A correlation between the degree of hypertension and its therapy on the one hand, and the incidence of intra- and postoperative complications on the other has, however, not been shown for mild and moderate hypertension (GOLDMAN and CALDERA 1979; STEPHEN 1981), with the exception of certain operations such as carotid endarterectomy, in which preoperative hypertension correlates with an elevated postoperative complication rate (BOVE et al. 1980; ASSIDAO et al. 1982).

A complication that is particularly feared is postoperative myocardial infarction (TOMPKINS and ARTUSIO 1964; PLUMLEE and BOETTNER 1972; TARHAN et al. 1972; STEEN et al. 1978). It is reported to occur in 0.13%–0.66% of patients with no prior myocardial infarction; as a postoperative reinfarction, however, it has a reported incidence of 6%–8%. The mortality rate in this latter case is between 60% and 70%. The danger of a postoperative reinfarction occurring is particularly great if surgery is carried out within 6 months after a prior myocardial infarction (up to 50%); after this time period, it has a constant incidence of about 5% (TARHAN et al. 1972; STEEN et al. 1978).

Point scoring systems similar to the GOLDMAN scheme already described, have also been developed to assess pulmonary risk (HAMER 1977; B. A. SHAPIRO 1980). Both schemes divide the pulmonary risk into three classes (slight, moderate, and high risk). The most important parameters evaluated are the preoperatively measured spirometric parameters (forced vital capacity FVC, and forced expired volume in 1 s FEV_1).

II. Surgical Procedure

General figures on the mortality rate of geriatric patients (see Table 2) are of only limited value, since they permit no prediction of the individual risk. In addition to the previous diseases, the operation per se also has a major influence on the outcome. The individual factors of the surgical intervention that are of importance here, are discussed in the following sections.

1. Nature of the Operation

The incidence of complications, together with mortality rate, are greater after intracranial, intrathoracic, and intra-abdominal operations than after more peripheral surgery. Among 2,391 deaths in patients of all age groups after an overall total of 108,878 anesthetic procedures, FARROW et al. (1982) found that most deaths occurred after intracranial (19.7%), intrathoracic (8.6%), and upper abdominal (6.6%) operations, while the lower abdomen revealed only 2.8%. In patients older than 70 years, laparatomies precede one-half of all cases of death, while thoracotomies, in contrast to peripheral interventions, more rarely contribute to the overall mortality rate (BÜNTE 1979). The reason for this is the small number of intrathoracic interventions performed in old patients, in whom surgery involving the abdomen and limbs greatly predominates.

Various statistics on geriatric surgical patients show that about 25%–40% undergo general surgical interventions and operations on the limbs, while about 20% are submitted to urologic surgery (WILDER and FISHBEIN 1961; LORHAN 1967; VON BRAMANN and HEROLD 1969; MILLER et al. 1977). Interventions considered to be especially typical of old age are, in particular, certain procedures of limb surgery, e.g., operative management of fractures close to the hip joint, including hip joint replacement (KALLINA 1982), numerous vascular surgical procedures (HERMAN 1980), and, among the urologic operations, transuretheral resection of the prostate (SALEHI 1979).

2. Repeat Operations

If, during on and the same hospitalization for treatment, or within a period of 1 month, several interventions have to be carried out in the same patient, the mortality rate increases only slightly. LORHAN (1967) found a mortality rate of 26.5% in octogenarians subjected to repeat interventions, in comparison with an overall 22.3% for 871 evaluated operations. In the same age group, PULVER and OTTEN (1970) found a mortality rate of 39% in patients undergoing a second operation, as compared with 33% for single operations.

3. Duration of Anesthesia and Surgery

It is generally assumed that there is a relationship between the duration of the anesthesia or intervention, and mortality. Such a relationship can, indeed, be shown for the overall surgical patients (LUTZ et al. 1972). For interventions lasting less than 120 min, the complication rate is 3% and the 4-week mortality rate 2.4%. For longer-lasting operations, both figures increase and, for a duration of operation of more than 5 h, the complication rate is 14% and the mortality rate 17.4%. Similar figures have been reported for patients older than 70 years (SHELBY and LORHAN 1968; MAYRHOFER 1970; LEWIN et al. 1971; PALMBERG and HIRSJÄRVI 1979).

In contrast, COGBILL (1967) found virtually no difference in mortality rates for operations lasting less than 2 h and those lasting more than 2 h. MILLER et al. (1977) also failed to establish any unequivocal relationship between anesthesia duration and mortality rate, but did find fewer postoperative complications after anesthesia lasting less than 1 h. Postoperative myocardial infarction, one of the most common causes of death in geriatric patients, occurs at a greater frequency after operations lasting more than 150 min (DJOKOVIC and HEDLEY-WHYTE 1979).

4. Elective vs Emergency Surgery

Numerous studies have shown that the mortality rate among elderly patients is appreciably higher after emergency interventions than after elective operations. However, since the groups of patients investigated vary widely, and the definitions of the terms "emergency" and "elective" were by no means identical in all studies, available quantitative data fluctuate considerably. According to COGBILL (1967), the mortality rate associated with emergency surgery is greater than that for elective surgery by a factor of only 1.3. On the other hand, for operations on the biliary system, an "increase factor" of 16.7 has been reported (SHELBY and LORHAN 1968). The majority of the investigations report an increase of two- to three-fold (HERRION et al. 1960; MAYRHOFER 1970; KRAAS et al. 1979; PALMBERG and HIRSJÄRVI 1979; SALEHI 1979; HEBERER 1982).

A clear correlation has also been demonstrated between the occurrence of intraoperative complications and surgical urgency (LUTZ et al. 1982). These include, in particular, such cardiovascular complications as hypotension, cardiac rhythm disorders, cardiac arrest, or death on the operating table. In addition, complications due to technical difficulties, and aspiration during emergency procedures, also occur more frequently.

III. Anesthesia

In common with all other age groups, various anesthetic procedures are available for geriatric patients. Basically, for numerous operations, a choice is possible between general and local or regional anesthesia. Of greater importance than a decision for one or the other procedure, is the experience of the anesthetist in the use of the procedure to be employed (HAMER 1975; MILLER et al. 1977; LAWIN 1982).

In a number of comparative studies, the alternative use of general anesthesia and regional anesthesia (preferentially spinal anesthesia) for operations on the lower half of the body was investigated. In patients over 60 years old, DRIPPS et al. (1961) found no difference in the mortality rate in a group of 18,737 Patients undergoing spinal anesthesia, as compared with another group of 14,487 patients with general anesthesia. After eliminating deaths due to the underlying disease or surgery, however, the percentage of anesthesia-related deaths was higher in the general anesthesia group than in the group receiving spinal anesthesia (10% and 6.7% of the overall mortality, respectively). Deaths due to anesthesia, however, occurred only when the physical status was impaired. BERGMANN (1963, 1970) found, in operations on the limbs, a lower overall mortality rate (14%) under spinal anesthesia than under general anesthesia (18%), although, on average, the general condition of patients receiving spinal anesthesia was poorer. In the regional anesthesia group, NOLTE et al. (1974) established appreciably fewer intraoperative complications, in particular hypotension and cardiac arrhythmias, but also a lower mortality rate up until the third postoperative week. Only after the third postoperative week was the mortality rate equal in both procedures. More recent studies reveal a similar tendency (MCLAREN et al. 1978; SALEHI 1979; TOLKSDORF et al. 1980).

In a long-term follow-up of women over 70 years old operated on for hip joint fractures (WICKSTRÖM et al. 1982), no effect of the anesthesia procedure on survival rate was determinable up to 12 months postoperatively (Fig. 11). A comparison was made between two inhalation anesthetic agents (halothane, enflurane),

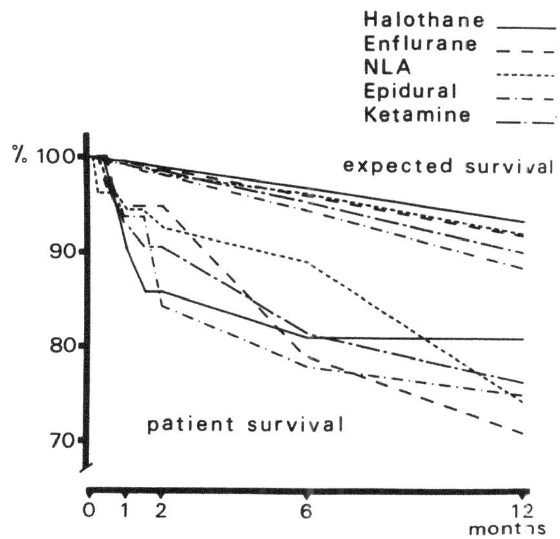

Fig. 11. Rates of survival of five groups of female geriatric patients, aged 70 years or more, anesthetized with five different anesthetic methods for hip fracture surgery. The expected rates of survival of five equally large groups of women of the same age distribution are shown for comparison. (WICKSTRÖM et al. 1982, with permission)

two intravenous anesthetic methods (neuroleptanalgesia, ketamine), and epidural anesthesia. Further follow-up for up to 4 years also revealed no differences that might have been traced back to the anesthetic procedure. In contrast, patient age and the type of hip fracture (neck of the femur, trochanter) did have an unequivocal influence on the subsequent outcome. The early postoperative course depended upon the preoperative state of the patient, but not on the anesthetic procedure.

In view of these results, some authors recommend using regional anesthesia in all cases in which it is technically possible (MAYRHOFER 1969; FOLDES 1974; CARMACK 1975; MILLER 1981), while for special clinical pictures (e.g., coronary heart disease, predicted high loss of blood) others favor general anesthesia on account of its greater ease of control (LAWIN 1965). However, a critical remark is in order here. None of these studies was carried out on a prospective randomized basis, so that, at present, it is not possible to make any well-founded statement as to whether regional anesthesia is fundamentally superior to general anesthesia.

D. Preoperative Management

I. Diagnosis and Treatment of Preexisting Disease

A thoroughgoing preoperative examination of the geriatric patient by the anesthetist is one of the most important prerequisites for an intra- and postoperative course that is as free as possible from complications. Such an examination includes history taking, physical examination, and evaluation of the laboratory results, and represents the basis for the preoperative therapeutic measures that in many cases have to be taken, as well as for premedication (MAYRHOFER 1969). The diagnostic program must, in particular, cover the following organs and functional systems (HAMER 1975).

1. Cardiovascular system
2. Respiratory system
3. Blood (hemoglobin, hematocrit, thrombocytes, clotting, plasma proteins)
4. Kidneys
5. Liver
6. Cerebrovascular system
7. Fluid and electrolyte balance
8. Metabolism (state of nutrition, diabetes)

Together with the clinical picture (in particular, the history of the patient's physical performance and cerebral status), the results of these examinations permit an assessment to be made of the major functional decrements and adaptation losses, and also reveal the deviations from the norm that have to be compensated, and possible diseases with associated risks that need to be treated (ROIZEN 1981). As far as possible, preoperative immobilization should be avoided.

1. Cardiovascular System

Since diseases of the heart and the vessels increase the morbidity and mortality of anesthesia and surgery, and are common in the elderly (cf. Fig. 1 and Tables 3 and 4), routine preoperative measures providing information as to disturbances of the cardiovascular system are essential. Detailed medical history, careful physical examination, ECG, and chest X-rays form the basis of evaluation. In the majority of patients with these techniques, the severity of cardiac or vascular disorders can be determined and their implications for the outcome can be assessed. Complementary diagnostic procedures must be tailored to the individual patient and selected for their relevant in formation yield. In this connection, exercise ECG, echocardiography, myocardial scintigraphy, cardiac catheterization, and angiography may be mentioned (FOËX 1981).

If cardiac failure presents, the first decision to be taken is whether a complete noninvasive, or possibly invasive, diagnostic work-up is necessary, or even possible. This will apply, in particular, to valvular diseases (mitral or aortic valvular stenosis), which represents a considerably increased risk. A further decision to be taken is whether the patient will need intra- and postoperative invasive monitoring. This includes a central venous catheter, wich is also often indicated for other reasons, an arterial catheter, and finally, if the preoperative diagnostic work-up shows it to be necessary, a Swan-Ganz pulmonary catheter (DEL GUERICO and COHN 1980; VAN AKEN et al. 1982).

2. Preoperative Cardiac Therapy

The preoperative treatment of chronic congestive heart failure is oriented to the usual recommendations, namely diuretics and digitalis (RÜGHEIMER 1974; MOFFITT 1978). Excessive diuresis in the geriatric patient can produce not only a deficit of sodium and, in particular, potassium, but also hypovolemia. The latter condition can be largely excluded clinically if neither postural hypotension nor hypotension associated with tachycardia presents (Goldman and Wolf 1980; Miller 1981).

The prophylactic use of digitalis in the elderly patient is a matter of controversy (Löllgen et al. 1983). In a sufficient myocardium, prophylactic digitalization does not lead to any improvement in cardiac output. Digitalization neither changes the resting stroke volumen or cardiac output, nor is a load-dependent increase in the two parameters observed, as can typically be achieved in cardiac failure. The indiscriminate use of digitalis must therefore be avoided. The therapeutic spectrum is small, and the adverse effects of digitalis toxicity are not negligible, in particular in the postoperative phase (Chung 1981 a). Digitalized patients frequently have cardiac arrhythmia problems (Vanik and Davis 1968; Juler et al. 1969; Janis 1978; Tyras et al. 1979).

In contrast to the indication list drawn up by Deutsch and Dalen (1969), which unequivocally recommends prophylactic digitalization of the surgical patient, today, most anesthetists go along with the recommendations of Laver and Lowenstein (1980). Preoperative digitalis is indicated only in manifest cardiac failure and in atrial flutter or fibrillation with rapid ventricular response (more than 80 beats/min; prior to abdominal or intrathoracic interventions, it may be given when a prior myocardial infarction as occurred, or when vetricular function is abnormal. The value of preoperative digitalization has been confirmed in patients with moderately diminished cardiac function, which presents in about 80% of patients with signs of ischemia in the ECG (Bille Brahe 1982).

In the majority of cases, patients with symptomatic coronary heart disease (angina pectoris) are usually managed with nitrates, β-blockers or calcium antagonist. These drugs must not be discontinued pre- or postoperatively; this applies in particular to the β-blockers, since otherwise the danger of a myocardial infarction is increased owing to a withdrawal rebound syndrome (Chung 1981 b; Goldman 1981; Pontén et al. 1982).

As for coronary heart disease, similar considerations also apply to arterial hypertension. Antihypertensive treatment must be continued up until surgery, and then postoperatively. This applies in particular to β-blockers and clonidine, since for both drugs, a withdrawal rebound syndrome has been described which can acutely endanger the patient (Bruce et al. 1979; Planz et al. 1982). Preexisting untreated hypertension should be controlled preoperatively if very marked (grade III or IV), or if signs of hypertensive complications are present. Whether mild forms of hypertension represent an indication for immediate treatment is not certain (Goldman and Caldera 1979; Marshall 1981).

Cardiac arrhythmias are common in elderly patients. They need to be evaluated in particular with respect to their potential progression to dangerous arrhythmic states, or their importance as markers of coronary heart disease. In the case of severe forms that appear threatening (e.g. suspected sick sinus syndrome, tachy-brady-arrhythmias, paroxysmal atrial tachycardia with block, numerous ated in particular with respect to their potential progression to dangerous arrhythmic states, or their importance as markers of coronary heart disease. In the case of severe forms that appear threatening (e.g. suspected sick sinus syndrome, tachy-brady-arrhythmias, paroxysmal atrial tachycardia with block, numerous premature ventricular contractions), treatment should be determined in cooperation with the cardiologist, and provisions made for the use of the temporary pacemaker (LAPPAS et al. 1977; ATLEE 1980; EWY 1980).

An integral component of the preoperative treatment of the cardiovascular system is the compensation of disturbances in blood volume and blood composition (anemia, hypovolemia) and in the fluid and electrolyte balance, hypokalemia and hyperkalemia both playing an important role (MAYRHOFER 1969; HEINRICH et al. 1982b). A drop in the total amount of potassium within the body is no rarity in elderly patients, but is difficult to diagnose (GOLDMAN and WOLF 1980).

3. Respiratory System

The first step is history taking, the task of which is to identify pulmonary diseases, smoking habits, sputum production, and exercise tolerance. The physical examination comprises observation, palpation, percussion, and auscultation. In the elderly patient, an X-ray of the chest is always indicated. For an evaluation of function, modern spirometers are available. The examination program comprises FVC, FEV_1, and the peak expiratory flow rate. With the aid of these parameters, and with consideration being given to the nature and localization of the surgical intervention, the pulmonary risk can be estimated and the preoperative treatment regimen decided (HAMER 1977; HENSLEY and FENCL 1980; B. A. SHAPIRO 1980; WIRÉN and JANZON 1983).

If the FVC amounts to only 80% of normal, and if the value $(FEV_1/FVC) \times 100$ is between 70% and 60%, no appreciable impairment of the surgical mortality is to be expected. If the FVC value is 60%–30%, and the quotient between 60% and 45%, surgical mortality will be increased, in particular when upper abdominal or thoracic surgery is planned. In such a case, intensive preoperative therapy should be instituted. At an FVC below 30% and $(FEV_1/FVC) \times 100$ below 45%, the pulmonary risk is high. The surgical indication must be reviewed and, as far as possible, surgery postponed until later. Intensive physiotherapeutic treatment prior to surgery is mandatory. For further diagnostic clarification, a thorough pulmonologic function investigation is required (HONIG 1983), including determination of the intrathoracic air volume, residual volume and FRC, resistance measurements, blood gas analyses in the resting state and after exercise, and measurement of the diffusion capacity. In the presence of pathologic findings in the chest X-ray, further differentiated radiologic diagnostic procedures, including computerized tomography should be employed. After weighing up the pros and cons of surgical intervention, the following invasive procedures may be employed: bronchoscopy, thoracoscopy, mediastinoscopy, with the aim of obtaining in accurate categorization of the pulmonary risk involved.

Pulmonary diseases that lead to respiratory failure in the preoperative phase include, in particular, such diseases of the airways as bronchial asthma and chronic obstructive pulmonary disease (COPD), infections such as tracheobronchitis or pneumonia, noninfectious parenchymal diseases, affections of the chest wall, neuromuscular diseases, disturbances of respiratory control, cor pulmonale and (especially in the case of emergency interventions) numerous acute disorders of the respiratory function (RÜGHEIMER 1970; HENSLEY and FENCL 1980). All these problems should, as far as possible, be given causal treatment.

The main aim of respiratory therapy is the treatment of obstructive ventilation disorders. It comprises the following measures (HAMER 1977):

1. Breathing exercises
2. Intermittent positive pressure breathing (IPPB)
3. Local and systemic drug therapy

In the preoperative phase, breathing exercises are certainly of value, provided enough time is vailable (FITZAL 1982). The greatest value of such exercises is the fact that they represent active instruction and psychologic preparation of the patient for what to expect and the demands to be met, postoperatively. The patient is familiarized with the postoperative course, and with the procedures and techniques of respiratory therapy employed (B. A. SHAPIRO 1980). In the case of old patients, the importance of this point should not be underestimated.

IPPB therapy is aimed at training inspiration and the coughing mechanism, and thus removal of secretion, improving the distribution of ventilation and the application of drugs in the bronchial tree (SHAPIRO et al. 1977; RÜGHEIMER 1982). Although the usefulness of IPPB is variously assessed, and has repeatedly been completely called into question by some authors (HEDLEY-WHYTE et al. 1976), new investigations on the basis of exact experimental planning and measuring methods unequivocally show that this technique improves pulmonary function both preoperatively and postoperatively (POWERS and MORRISON 1978; O'DONOHUE 1979; RICHARD and GEORGE 1981).

In recent years, methods aimed at actively training the voluntary inspiration of the patient using so-called incentive spirometers, have come into widespread use (BARTLETT et al. 1973). Their effectiveness is, however, clearly lower than that of IPPB (WELCH et al. 1980; BRANDL 1983; DOWNS 1983), as can be seen in Fig. 12 which compares the effects of IPPB and sustained maximal inspiration (SMI) on various lung function parameters.

The most important drugs for local use in the form of aerosols, or via IPPB, are bronchodilators, mucolytics, corticosteroids, and antibiotics. The former are used preferentially to treat obstructive ventilation disorders (RÜGHEIMER 1982). In principle, the same groups of drugs can be used systemically when the indication is appropriate (SHAPIRO et al. 1977; RAU 1978; ZIMENT 1978; BONNER 1983).

4. Fluid and Electrolyte Balance

Of particular quantitative and qualitative importance in the geriatric patient is the fluid and electrolyte balance. The overall water content and its distribution within the extracellular space and the intracellular space, blood volume, and electrolytes, are all closely coupled with cardiovascular and respiratory function. In the elderly patient, dehydration is the rule rather than the exception (MAYRHOFER 1969). It contributes to the fact that cardiac and renal reserves are reduced as compared with younger patients, and should therefore be carefully treated in the preoperative phase. This is unavoidable when, on account of the underlying disease, the water, electrolyte, and protein losses exceed the usual amount of 1,500–2,000 ml/day (LORHAN 1955). On the other hand, too vigorous a substitution must be

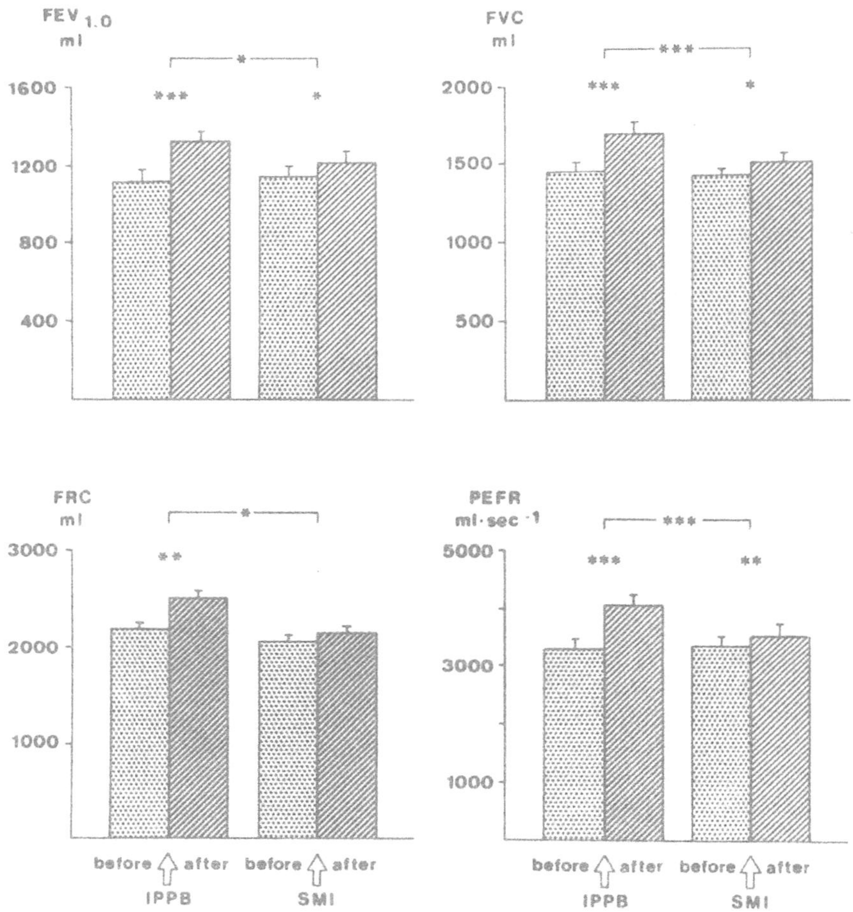

Fig. 12. Influence on lung function parameters of two preoperative respiratory therapy maneuvers (mean $\pm$ standard error). *IPPB* intermittent positive pressure breathing; *SMI* sustained maximal inspiration; *FVC* forced vital capacity; *FEV_1* forced expiratory volume in 1 s; *PEFR* peak expiratory flow rate; *FRC* functional residual capacity; $*P<0.005$; $**P<0.01$; $***P<0.001$

avoided, since otherwise there is a danger of oversubstitution with injurious effects on the heart, lungs, kidneys, and brain. If the urgency of the operation permits, compensatory measures should therefore be effected slowly. The most important monitoring parameters are urine excretion, central venous pressure, serum electrolytes, and serum osmolality (GIESECKE 1981; HEINRICH et al. 1982b).

II. Premedication

The aim of premedication is, by the administration of drugs, to prepare the patient for anesthesia. Thus, premedication will be determined by the nature of the anesthesia. Orginally, it served mainly to compensate for adverse effects (e.g., hypersecretion when using diethyl ether) or for shortcomings of a procedure (e.g., imperfect analgesia in anesthesia with barbiturates alone). The introduction of methods free from such adverse reactions or shortcomings and whose main effects are well balanced with respect to the major components of anesthesia, namely analgesia, unconsciousness, muscle relaxation, and vegetative damping has resulted in a change in the task of premedication more toward the psychologic preparation of the patient, so that the erstwhile schematic, anesthesia-oriented medication has now given way to individual, patient-oriented management.

Accordingly, preparation of the patient for anesthesia is usually limited to elimination of anxiety. The main means of achieving this is to talk to the patient. Benzodiazepines, which, as far as their pharmacologic effect is concerned, largely fulfill the requirements to be met by a good premedication agent, nevertheless often lead to adverse reactions, articularly in geriatric patients. Because of this, their use must be thoroughly weighed up beforehand.

For sedation and tranquilization, barbiturates and "major tranquilizers" (neuroleptic agents such as promethazine and droperidol) are available (STOELTING 1981). The indication for these drugs is not fundamentally different than in young patients, but the dosage should be lower than in the latter (BEATTIE and SELLERS 1979). Here, too, adverse reactions must be expected in the old patient. In doubtful cases, the rule "when in doubt, leave it out" should be applied (CARMACK 1975).

Analgesia is only rarely required. If analgesic agents are thought to be desirable for premedication, low-dose opioids are injected. Morphine, pethidine and fentanyl have all proved particularly useful, the latter in combination with droperidol as Thalamonal or Innovar. On account of their depressive effect on respiration, which is more marked in combination with sedatives, these substances must, of course, be prescribed only in the lowest dosages and only when constant observation of the patient is guaranteed.

When diethyl ether was used as the sole anesthetic, the use of anticholinergic agents was indispensable to suppress the excessive secretion in the airways. In modern anesthesia, this indication is now only of secondary importance, so that these substances should only be prescribed when really required (MILLER 1981). They are then most expediently administered intravenously, immediately prior to the induction of anesthesia. Scopolamine should not be given since, in contrast to young patients, it can cause restlessness and confusion in elderly patients (CARMACK 1975). Atropine, on the other hand, has a more cardial vagolytic than central nervous effect, although in geriatric patients the former is often not at all marked (compare Sect. B. I).

E. Anesthetic Management

The selection and technical implementation of the anesthetic procedure, and monitoring during anesthesia, must take account of the anatomic and physiologic peculiarities, and the numerous associated diseases, of the geriatric patient. Toothlessness, loose teeth, trophic jaws, and flabby facial skin and cheeks make the use of the face mask difficult. Arthritic changes in the temporomandibular joints and the cervical vertebral column represent an obstacle to intubation (MILLER and COULTHARD 1981). The stiffening up of old joints requires great care with extreme positioning maneuvers, in particular when the patient has been given muscle relaxants. Care must also be taken to avoid pressure damage to the skin and the subcutaneous tissues, which in the elderly patient can easily lead to decubitus ulcerations. Since old skin is atrophic, adhesive tape should be used only sparingly (MILLER 1981).

I. Regional Anesthesia

In conjunction with the surgical trauma, every form of regional anesthesia must be considered just as individually as every form of general anesthesia. However, a number of basic aspects can be mentioned. It is generally believed that local anesthesia impairs homeostasis to a smaller degreee than does general anesthesia (DUDZIAK and KLEIN 1982). A major advantage is considered to be the preservation of consciousness:

1. Any signs of acute cardiac or cerebral insufficiency that might occur during surgery can more readily be detected in the conscious patient.
2. Since the patient remains conscious, the transition phase from anesthesia to wakefulness is obviated. In elderly people, this transition phase is often prolonged, so that, following general anesthesia, early mobilization and return to as normal a daily routine as possible, can prove difficult.

However, this advantage of regional anesthesia can also prove a disadvantage in very old patients with cerebral insufficiency. Such patients are not infrequently excessively anxious, uncooperative, show psychomotor agitation, and thus tolerate the intervention poorly. Attacks of angina pectoris, or hypertensive crises may be provoked. Sedation is often something of a problem, since to "break through" the agitated state, high doses of sedatives, hypnotics, or neuroleptic agents are necessary. The danger of respiratory and circulatory depression that then threatens may be more acute than that associated with general anesthesia, although, in principle, epidural anesthesia is more bland than neuroleptanalgesia with respect to its depressive effect on respiration and metabolism in old patients (STEFÁNSSON et al. 1982c).

The same remarks also apply to the circulation, provided that adequate volume replacement is ensured, and too great an extension of the block (nervi accelerantes) is avoided. The differences are, however, often only slight. MARSHALL and WYCHIE (1972) observed a continuous drop in arterial O_2 partial pressure in the postoperative period after abdominal surgery under epidural anesthesia. This drop in pressure was not observed under general anesthesia, although the initial immediate postoperative values were lower than after epidural anesthesia. If sedation is necessary, the recommended drugs of choice are benzodiazepines administered in small doses (MILLER 1981), which, where necessary, can be combined with small amounts of the anesthetic agent ketamine (about 0.5 mg/kg). Although ketamine in very old patients can produce mild respiratory depression (STEFÁNSSON et al. 1982a), in comparison with the narcotic analgesics in clinical use, this is only of secondary importance.

The most important regional anesthetic procedures are epidural and spinal anesthesia used for the lower half of the body, and the various types of brachial plexus blocks for operations on the upper limbs. Of the various regional anesthesias produced close to the spinal cord, in geriatric patients, spinal anesthesia is usually preferred over epidural anesthesia, because it is quicker and technically easier to implement, and the incidence of postspinal headache diminishes with age (KORTUM et al. 1979; DRIESSEN et al. 1980). Epidural or spinal anesthesia is suitable for use in transurethral resection of the prostate and other genitourinary procedures, gynecologic operations, inguinal hernias, fractures of the hip joints and hip joint replacement, and all peripheral operations on the locomotor system or vascular system. After operations on the hip joint, it is believed that the incidence of thromboembolic complications is significantly reduced under spinal anesthesia (MCLAREN et al. 1978).

Particular attention should be paid to the following points. The doses required to achieve epidural anesthesia decrease with increasing age (see Fig. 10), and this probably also applies to spinal anesthesia (MILLER 1981). In addition, an increased toxic effect of local anesthetic agents must be expected. The sympatholytic effect associated with sensory and motor blockade, can, owing to vasomotor inhibition, lead to relative hypovolemia with considerable hypotension (COVINO 1978). Since elderly patients often have only moderately compensated hypovolemia, and a reduced cardiovascular regulation margin, the greatest attention should be paid to prophylaxis and early treatment of such conditions. In the selection of the local anesthetic agents and of the technique of implementation, there are no differences in the rules that otherwise apply to these forms of blockade (MURPHY 1981).

Brachial plexus blocks are indicated for all operations on the upper limbs, including the shoulder, and are thus employed in particular for repositioning and osteosynthesis. As a rule, no circulatory effects of plexus blocks need be feared. As an alternative procedure, intravenous regional anesthesia is available (WALLACE et al. 1982).

II. General Anesthesia

Irrespective of the nature of the anesthetic procedure, special attention must be given to a number of points with respect to induction. As already mentioned, elderly patients often present with a more or less compensated hypovolemia, and a prolonged circulation time. For this reason, adequate volume replacement prior to induction is extremely important (HALDEMANN et al. 1976). Anesthetic agents are to be administered in small incremental doses (LAWIN 1982) until an adequate depth of anesthesia has been achieved. Anatomic circumstances and the diminished respiratory reserves usually make it necessary to use intubation when employing general anesthesia. If the anesthesia is too light, laryngoscopy and intubation may be associated with a danger of detrimental circulatory stimulation, which manifests as an increase in heart rate, arterial and intracranial pressure. Additionally, ventricular arrhythmias may develop.

Increases in blood pressure induced by intubation are not, per se, dangerous, but they must be avoided when prior damage to heart and brain is present (FOX

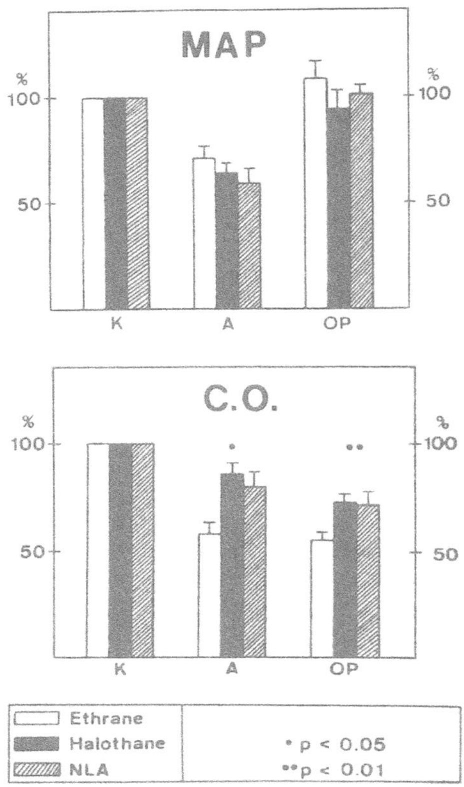

Fig. 13. Effects of various anesthetics on mean arterial pressure (*MAP*) and cardiac output (*C.O.*) of patients older than 70 years. *K* awake (control); *A* after induction of anesthesia; *OP* during operation. (After HALDEMANN et al. 1975, with permission)

et al. 1977). Such predamage is more frequently to be expected in elderly patients than in young adults. On account of the time factor, however, the routine use of topical anesthesia of the mucosa of the pharynx, larynx, and trachea prior to laryngoscopy, is adequately effective only if a waiting period of 1 min is observed. Thus, a twofold laryngoscopy must, in effect, be carried out prior to intubation (HAMILL et al. 1981). For this reason, an adequate depth of anesthesia as a prophylaxis against such reactions is of greater advantage in routine work.

Selection of the anesthetic agents often depends not only on their pharmacodynamic adverse reactions, but also on the experience the anesthesiologist concerned has acquired in the course of routine work with the respective techniques (LAWIN 1965; HAMER 1975). Among the undesired adverse effects of anesthetic agents, the greatest importance attaches to effects on the cardiovascular system, while effects on respiration, at least during surgery, can largely be neglected, since elderly patients generally have to be ventilated during anesthesia and, where required, can also be ventilated in the postoperative phase.

The inhalation narcotic agents halothane and enflurane, have a negative inotropic effect, and can lead to peripheral vasodilation. As a result, the cardiac output diminishes with increasing dose (HALDEMANN et al. 1975; MORR-STRATHMANN et al. 1975a, b), without any severe changes in metabolism occurring (STE-

Table 9. Simplified representation of cardiac and vascular effects of commonly used anesthetics. (After PASCH 1982)

	Myocardial performance[a]	Peripheral resistance[a]
Barbiturates	↓↓	↓↓
Althesin	↓↓	↓↓
Etomidate	(↓)	↓
Ketamine	(↓)	(↑) or (↓)
Droperidol	(↓)	↓↓
Benzodiazepines	(↓)	↓↓
Opioids	(↓)	(↓) or (↑)
Nitrous oxide	↓	(↑)
Halothane	↓↓	↓
Enflurane	↓↓	↓↓
Isoflurane	↓	↓↓

[a] ↑ Increase; ↓ decrease

FÁNSSON et al. 1982b). The circulatory effects of neuroleptanalgesia depend on the agents selected, and their dosage. If, following premedication with 2.5 mg droperidol, only fentanyl is employed, the cardiac output and other hemodynamic parameters remain unchanged during anesthesia (STEFÁNSSON et al. 1982c). If fentanyl is combined with droperidol, the cardiac output drops (HALDEMANN et al. 1975). Figure 13 shows a comparison of circulatory changes under halothane, enflurane, and neuroleptanalgesia. The combination benzodiazepine–fentanyl, appreciably lowers the mean arterial pressure. This effect is due not so much to a reduction of cardiac output, but rather to a drop in peripheral resistance (HALDEMANN et al. 1977). Ketamine employed as the sole anesthetic agent after premedication with 2.5 mg droperidol, has a different effect. In such a case, stimulation of the myocardium with an increase in cardiac output and left ventricular stroke index occurs (STEFÁNSSON et al. 1982a).

Overall, as already emphasized, these differences often have little significance for the clinical indication, since the personal experience of the anesthetist, and the influence of the surgical trauma, preponderate. As a basic rule, it is accepted that for all anesthetic agents, the dose must be decreased with increasing age, as was pointed out in Sect. B. V. This also applies to muscle relaxants, although less information is available on these drugs (MILLER 1981).

Primarily, anesthetic agents and anesthesia methods that neither reduce contractility nor increase the oxygen consumption of the myocardium, should be given preference. For this reason, the volatile inhalation anesthetics, the barbiturates, and ketamine are not the agents of first choice for anesthesia in the geriatric patient (Table 9).

Among the available general anesthetic procedures, intravenous anesthesia with emphasis being given to receptor-specific, opioid-mediated analgesia, in the form of neuroleptanalgesia, impair the cardiac performance least and, as a rule, without increasing the oxygen consumption of the myocardium (LOWENSTEIN and PHILBIN 1983). Moreover, modern variants avoid apparent disadvantages of standard neuroleptanesthesia. Owing to its virtual lack of adverse effects on the cardiovascular system – at least at the dose required for induction of anesthesia in combination with an opioid – etomidate suggests itself for use as a hypnotik agent which helps make the induction phase safe, reliable, and brief while, in addition, preventing any postoperative memories of intubation or surgery. The droperidol-specific side effect of hypotension during induction, due to the α-blocking effect, can be compensated for by volume replacement. The replacement of droperidol by a benzodiazepine reduces the circulatory reaction. In addition, this replacement also avoids psychopathologic reactions to the neuroleptic agents (RÜGHEIMER 1981). Unexplained is the mechanism which in some patients, particularly hypertensive subjects, leads to a hypertonic reaction during neuroleptanesthesia (EHEHALT and RUPP 1982). The addition of a small dose of a volatile inhalation anesthetic agent (0.2–0.4 vol.% enflurane) almost always leads to a drop in blood pressure to an ecceptable level, the small dose ensuring that the negative inotropic adverse reactions of the inhalation anesthetic agent remain negligible (RÜGHEIMER 1981).

Maintenance and withdrawal of anesthesia in the geriatric patient effected in the same manner as in younger adults. For reversing the effects of nondepolarizing relaxants, pyridostigmine has advantages compared with neostigmine, since it is associated with a reduced tendency to produce bradycardia and arrhythmias. This difference is particularly noticeable after halothane administration (OWENS et al. 1978). For the reversal of opiate-induced respiratory depression with naloxone, the same considerations apply as in the case of laryngoscopy and intubation. Naloxone leads indirectly, via a painful reaction, to a stimulation of the circulatory system that is of potential danger to the patient. Hypertension and arrhythmias, even left heart failure with pulmonary edema have been described (FLACKE et al. 1977; AZAR and TURNDORF 1979). For this reason, in patients with preexisting cardiac or cerebral "damage", the dose must be kept as small as possible, and postoperative ventilation be given preference over the risk attendant on naloxone administration.

III. Monitoring

The intensity of monitoring of the vital functions during the anesthesia depends not so much on the age of the patient, as on any preexisting diseases, and the nature and extent of the operation. In addition to the measurement of the arterial blood pressure and the heart rate, and the monitoring of ventilation parameters, the continuous recording of the ECG is a matter of course. This latter serves for the detection of arrhythmias and ischemic reactions. In suspected coronary heart disease, the lead V_5, in modified form, delivers the most reliable information on acute ischemia in the region of the left coronary artery (KAPLAN and KING 1976).

In the elderly patient, arrhythmias readily occur when, to preoperative hypokalemia and metabolic alkalosis, respiratory alkalosis due to hyperventilation during anesthetic ventilation is added, and, possibly, alkalizing solutions (lactated Ringer's solution) are additionally infused. Under such circumstances, digitalized patients are most likely to develop arrhythmias (JANIS 1978). For this reason, the continuous measurement of the end-expiratory CO_2 concentration is useful since with its aid, too marked a hypocapnia due to hyperventilation, can be avoided (LAWIN 1982).

In lengthy operations, measurement of the body temperature is to be recommended via nasopharyngeal, esophageal, or rectal sensors. Generous use should be made of central venous catheterization in order to be able to monitor the central venous pressure and, postoperatively, for longer-term infusion therapy. An arterial cannula is indicated whenever close monitoring of the arterial blood pressure and the arterial blood gases offers advantages, for example, in operations during which considerable loss of blood must be expected, or in the presence of congestive heart failure. In addition, the arteriovenous O_2 content difference can be determined by the additional measurement of the mixed venous O_2 saturation, as an indicator for the peripheral O_2 delivery. Routinely, measurement of the central venous oxygen saturation suffices, so that for this indication, a pulmonary catheter is not absolutely necessary (BRANDL et al. 1981).

Accurate monitoring of the myocardial performance is possible only with a Swan–Ganz catheter, which permits the measurement of the left ventricular filling pressure in the form of the pulmonary capillary wedge pressure (PCWP), and the cardiac output. This provides the basis for control of fluid therapy, the correction of too high or too low a filling pressure, and too low a contractility of the myocardium. For the indication, the criteria already mentioned in the discussion of preoperative preparation (Sect. D. I. 1) apply. The risks and expected advantage of these invasive methods must be weighed up in the individual case; in particular the question as to whether fewer invasive procedures would suffice must be carefully considered (MANGANO 1980; TARNOW 1982; SHAVER 1983). There is no reason for routine use of the Swan–Ganz catheter beyond a certain age limit.

F. Postoperative Care

On completion of surgery, the patient is transferred either to the recovery room or to the intensive care unit. This decision depends on the preexisting diseases and their treatment, the nature and extent of the operation, the management of anesthesia and possible complications that have occurred. In the majority of cases, the care normally afforded in the recovery room, where the patient is taken when spontaneously breathing, is completely adequate in the elderly, too. Here, care must be provided to ensure proper recovery from the residual effects of the anesthetic, adequate treatment of pain, provision of free airways, stabilization of the vital functions, and early diagnosis and treatment of any complications (A. G. SHAPIRO 1982). The task is, therefore, not reduced merely to keeping patients in recovery until they have "more or less regained consciousness", that is, until specific residual effects of the anesthetic have abated. Nor does it make good sense to subject all patients without exception to as comprehensive a monitoring program as possible. Of decisive importance is the principle of selection, that is, by employing the amount of diagnostic effort appropriate to the individual case, all those patients should be identified in good time for whom, owing to threatening or manifest complications, the whole spectrum of intensive diagnostic and therapeutic possibilities are required (GABEL and TONNESEN 1980).

Of particular importance is the transfer of information from the anesthetist and surgeon to the recovery area staff. An accurate description of the operation, the present state of the circulation, the ability of the patient to breathe spontaneously, the blood and fluid balance, the drugs employed, possible complications, and suggestions for the further procedure are all indispensable data (FEELEY 1981). Of extreme importance in the immediately postoperative phase are the detection and prevention of complications of the cardiovascular system and respiration. Owing to their importance, they will be discussed in detail in the following sections.

I. Circulatory Complications

Postoperative disorders of the cardiovascular homeostasis can have a wide range of causes. Heading the list are loss of blood and hypovolemia, hypothermia, hypoxia, hypercapnia, disturbance of the acid–base and electrolyte balance, pain, residual effects of anesthetic agents and their antagonists, and the indication for other drugs such as digitalis, antiarrhythmic agents, antihypertensives, anticholinergics, etc. These disorders add to cardiovascular diseases and diseases of other important function systems present preoperatively (PASCH 1982).

Routine monitoring (GABEL and TONNESEN 1980) also includes careful physical examination (skin color and temperature, state of consciousness, motoricity, auscultation, palpation of pulse, and evaluation of the state of filling of the veins of the neck). The cardiac rhythm is monitored via the ECG, the blood pressure measured at regular intervals. Loss of fluid from wounds, drains, via aspiration and tubes, together with urine excretion must be recorded. Such laboratory parameters as concentration of hemoglobin, hematocrit, electrolyte status, and blood gas analysis are obtained as required. Further measures such as measurement of the central venous pressure, a central venous blood gas analysis, and direct recording of the arterial pressure are only exceptionally indicated. When severe complications present, an invasive and comprehensive diagnostic work-up is, of course, necessary, of which the most important procedure is the placement of a Swan–Ganz catheter in the pulmonary artery. Such invasive diagnostic measures, including the resulting therapy, however, belong to the instrumentarium of the intensive care unit (QUINN and QUEBBEMAN 1981).

The most important clinical symptoms that justify further diagnostic and/or therapeutic measures, are hypotension, hyertension, and arrhythmias. Postoperatively, the most probable course of hypotension is hypovolemia or the failure of the pumping action of the heart. Rapid and reliable differential diagnosis is not always easy, since hypovolemic and cardiogenic shock have common cardinal symptoms (centralization, tachycardia). If the clinical signs of acute left ventricular failure (dyspnea, pulmonary congestion, pulmonary edema) are not unequivocal, the first step is to look for signs of a myocardial infarction and rhythm disorders using a complete ECG lead program. If it is not possible to exclude either condition, the patient is transferred to the intensive care unit and treated as though suffering from a fresh myocardial infarction. If the suspected myocardial insufficiency is not confirmed, a postoperative drop in blood pressure is first considered to be due to hypovolemia, and treated accordingly (PASCH 1982).

Any marked cardiac failure (with or without infarction) requires intensive medical care, including measurement of the cardiac output and the PCWP. The aim of treatment is, by optimizing preload, afterload, and contractility, to achieve statisfactory perfusion of the organism (COHN and FRANCIOSA 1977; LAPPAS et al. 1977).

An arterial blood pressure above the initial preoperative level is frequently observed in the postoperative phase (STEPHEN 1981). In patients with a healthy circulatory system, such reactions are, as a rule, not dangerous, but in patients with previous cardiac or cerebral injury, frequently give rise to complications. The increased afterload can lead an elevated myocardial oxygen requirement, and trigger left ventricular failure with pulmonary edema. Finally, in rare cases, hypertensive encephalopathy can develop. In more than 8% of the cases, postoperative hypertension develops as early as 30 min after withdrawal of the anesthetic (GAL and COOPERMAN 1975). The same also applies to postoperative pulmonary edema which, in most cases arises out of a hypertensive episode, and is thus also most commonly seen within the first 30 min (COOPERMAN and PRICE 1970).

Possible causes of increases in blood pressure are, apart from the presence of hypertensive disease, a withdrawal syndrome (see Sect. D. I. 2), usually a markedly sympathetic activation by pain, hypothermia, hypercapnia, or hypoxemia. These factors can readily be treated causally. If such simple measures are not adequately successful, rapidly acting antihypertensive drugs must be employed. In the presence of threatening, or already manifest, left heart failure with pulmonary edema, as an initial measure, two bursts of a nitroglycerin spray (corresponding to 0.8 mg) are given sublingually, which results in prompt relief via venous pooling. Sublingual nifedepine (10–20 mg) may also lower blood pressure promptly (BEER et al. 1981). Apart from these drugs, other longer-acting substances such as clonidine, diazoxide, and hydralazine or dihydralazine, can be given parenterally in severe hypertensive episodes (PASCH 1982)

As in the case of hypotension and hypertension, arrhythmias in the postoperative phase are frequently an expression of hypoxia, acidosis, hypokalemia, digitalis overdose, or sympatheticotonia. These conditions are all responsive to causal treatment. Not all postoperative arrhythmias are in need of treatment. This is particularly true when they do not lead to mechanical circulatory depression and had long been known in the preoperative phase without giving rise to hemodynamic disorders. For the immediate diagnosis and treatment of arrhythmias, it is expedient to proceed in accordance with the scheme described by FINLAYSON (1979), which covers the most frequent situations (Figs. 14 and 15). If arrhythmias are the cause of a circulatory depression, and cannot be brought under control by simple measures, a thoroughgoing diagnostic work-up must be initiated, myocardial infarction excluded, and treatment continued in the intensive care unit (ATLEE 1980).

II. Respiratory Disorders

The development of postoperative respiratory failure is usually a multifactorial event. Often, it is difficult to establish the main cause in the individual case. Even though the course of the immediately postanesthesia phase is largely determined

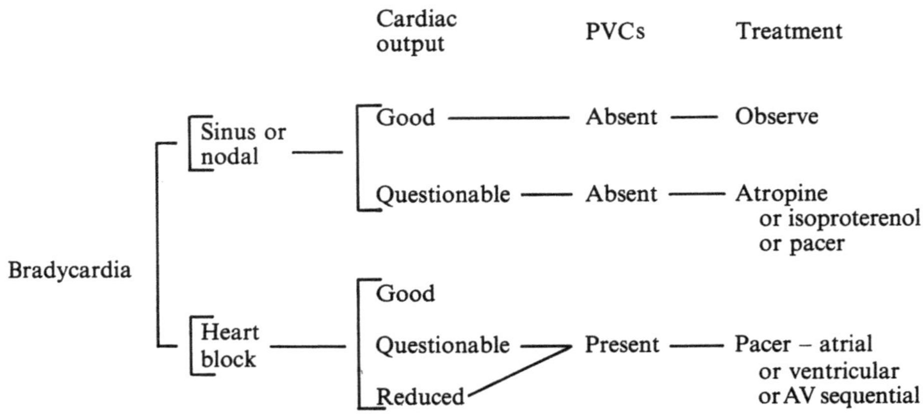

Fig. 14. Algorithm for the diagnosis and treatment of bradycardia. *PVCs* premature ventricular contraction. (FINLAYSON 1979). From FINLAYSON (1979) Postoperative intensive care. In: Kaplan JA (ed) Cardiac anesthesia. By permission of Grune & Stratton

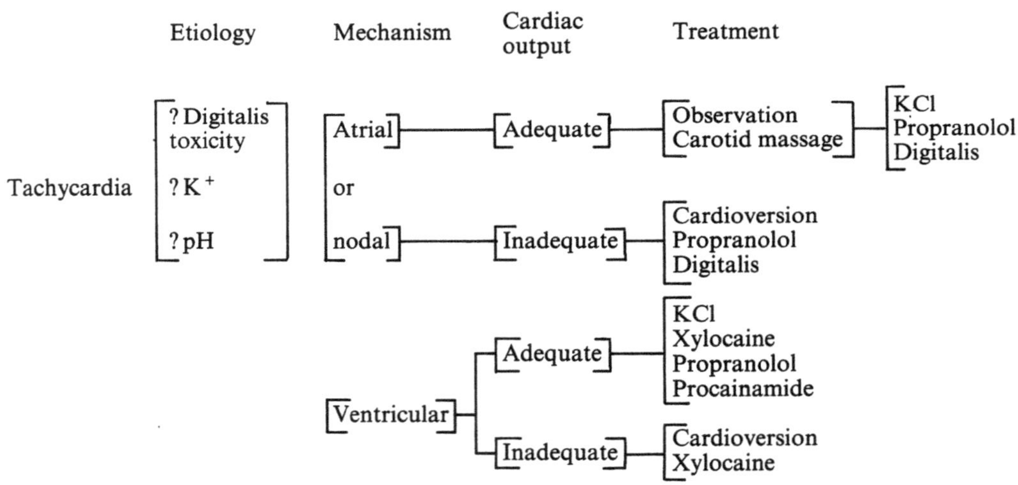

Fig. 15. Algorithm for the diagnosis and treatment of tachycardia. (FINLAYSON 1979). From FINLAYSON (1979) Postoperative intensive care. In: Kaplan JA (ed) Cardiac Anesthesia. By permission of Grune & Stratton

by the pharmacology of the anesthetic procedure employed, subsequently, the effects of the surgical intervention itself acquire increasing importance for the impairment of the pulmonary performance (BRANDL 1982). The most important forms of postoperative respiratory complications are hypoventilation, hypoxemia, and mechanical obstruction of the airways. They are further differentiated in Table 10.

In the pathogenesis of hypoventilation, central respiratory depression by narcotic analgesics, and peripheral muscular paralysis due to relaxants play a major

Table 10. Factors contributing to postoperative respiratory failure. (After BRANDL 1982)

Hypoventilation	
Central respiratory depression	Narcotic analgesics Benzodiazepines Hypnotics Inhalational anesthetics
Peripheral respiratory depression	Muscle relaxants Inhalational anesthetics Other drugs (e.g., antibiotics) Neuromuscular diseases
Hypoxemia	
Hypoventilation	See above
Diffusion hypoxia	Nitrous oxide
Increased right-to-left shunt	Aspiration Atelectasis Pneumothorax Pulmonary edema
Ventilation–perfusion mismatch	Positioning Artificial ventilation
Pain-induced reflexes	Thoracic and upper abdominal procedures
Increased O_2 consumption	Shivering Increased cardiac output
Obstruction	
Postoperative bleeding	Struma resections Carotid endarterectomies
Airway obstruction	Tongue Secretions
Laryngospasm	Reflex-induced
Bronchospasm	Allergic COPD

role. This can be observed in particular in elderly patients, who manifest an increased sensitivity to narcotic analgesics (BELLVILLE et al. 1971). Attention has already been drawn to this in Sect. B. V. These relationships make it clear that in the geriatric patient, particularly careful monitoring of the respiration in the postoperative phase is necessary. Apart from the clinical observation and recording of the most important circulatory parameters (ECG, arterial blood pressure), the respiratory rate should also be recorded, which can be done most expediently with the aid of a thorax impedance measurement with the ECG electrodes. In high-risk patients, monitoring of ventilation parameters (tidal volume, FVC) must also be done at intervals of about 15 min. Finally, in doubtful cases, an arterial blood gas analysis is necessary.

Arterial hypoxemia in the postoperative phase can have a number of causes. In addition to the hypoventilation just discussed, a number of anesthesia- and operation-related factors can be considered, mention of which has already been made in Sect. B. II. In this connection, pain is undoubtedly of major importance. It leads to shallow breathing, a reluctance of the patient to change position, ab-

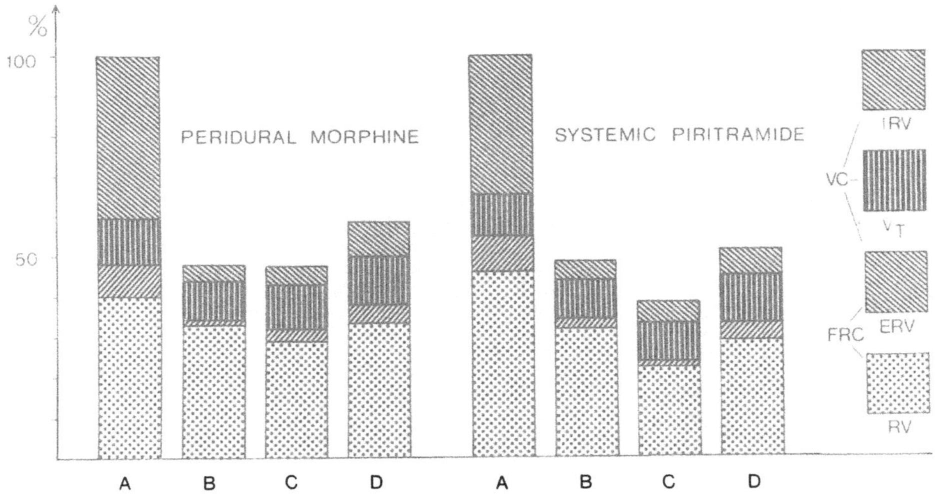

Fig. 16. Comparison of the effects of epidural and systemic postoperative analgesia on lung volumes in patients with partial resections of the pancreas (Whipple's procedure). $N=6$ in both groups; *A* preoperative (control); *B* 1 h postoperatively; *C* 2 h postoperatively with analgesic therapy; *D* 1 day postoperatively with analgesic therapy. Same symbols as in Fig. 5

sence of a cough effort, and a reflex increase in tone of the muscles effecting expiration. As a result, there is a drop in the functional residual capacity, retention of secretion, impairment of surfactant, and development of microatelectasia as early as the first 24 h postoperatively.

For this reason, great importance attaches to the postoperative amelioration of pain (DOWNS 1983). This applies in particular in the case of thoracic and upper abdominal procedures. As a rule, analgesics having a peripheral effect are inadequate; rather, narcotic analgesic agents must be employed. These are, however, themselvess associated with the risk of central respiratory depression. A point that has to be considered in old patients is that considerably lower doses, as compared with young adults, suffice to produce adequate analgesia (see Fig. 8). For this reason, an attractive alternative is postoperative epidural anesthesia. Although this had been recognized by SIMPSON et al. as early as 1961, this form of treatment has only recently achieved widespread acceptance (SEELING et al. 1982), with the development of new catheter materials and techniques for continuous epidural anesthesia.

The injection of opioids, predominantly morphine, into the epidural space, has further expanded the spectrum of postoperative regional analgesia. In contrast to the injection of local anesthetic agents, no motor blockade occurs, analgesia is adequate, the patients are not sedated as in the case of systemic administration of opioids, and the danger of central respiratory depression is considerably reduced. However, the question as to whether the epidural application of morphine in the geriatric patient has advantages over conventional analgesia, has not yet been resolved clinically (KLINCK and LINDOP 1982). In Fig. 16, the postoperative changes of lung volumes, and the effects on them of systemic or epidural opioid administration are shown.

Airway obstruction is a rare cause of postoperative respiratory failure, but always has a very acute course. Immediate intervention is necessary to eliminate the cause (e.g., an afterbleed in the neck region or in the airways themselves, paralysis of the recurrent laryngeal nerve), but also gradually developing obstructions due to the tongue falling back into the pharynx, accumulation and inspissation of secretion within the airways, acute exacerbation of a chronic obstructive pulmonary disease, or bronchial asthma also require aggressive therapy. Not infrequently, laryngoscopy and reintubation become necessary.

References

Assidao, CB, Donegan JH, Whitesell RC, Kalbfleisch JH (1982) Factors associated with perioperative complications during carotid endarterectomy. Anesth Analg 61:631–637

Atlee JL (1980) Diagnosis and therapy of perioperative arrhythmias. In: Brown BB (ed) Anesthesia and the patient with heart disease. Davis, Philadelphia, pp 137–172

Azar I, Turndorf H (1979) Severe hypertension and multiple arterial premature contractions following naloxone administration. Anesth Analg 58:524–525

Bartlett RH, Gazzaniga AB, Geraghty TR (1973) Respiratory maneuvers to prevent postoperative pulmonary complications. A critical review. JAMA 224:1017–1021

Beattie BL, Sellers EM (1979) Psychoactive drug use in the elderly: the pharmacokinetics. Psychosomatics 20:474–479

Beer N, Gallegos I, Cohen A, Klein N, Sonnenblick E, Frishman W (1981) Efficacy of sublingual nifedipine in the acute tratment of systemic hypertension. Chest 79:571–574

Begin R, Renzetti AD, Bigler AH, Watanabe S (1975) Flow and age dependence of airway closure and dynamic compliance. J Appl Physiol 38:199–207

Bellville JW, Forrest WH, Miller E, Brown BW (1971) Influence of age on pain relief from analgesics. A study of postoperative patients. JAMA 217:1835–1841

Bentley JB, Borel JD, Nenad RE, Gillespie TJ (1982) Age and fentanyl pharmacokinetics. Anesth Analog 61:968–971

Bergmann H (1963) Zur Indikation der Spinalanästhesie in der Alterschirurgie. Anaesthesist 12:233–236

Bergmann H (1970) Die derzeitige Stellung der Lokalanaesthesie. In: Hutschenreuther K, Bihler K, Fritsche P (eds) Anaesthesie in extremen Altersklassen. Springer, Berlin Heidelberg New York, pp 219–232 (Anaesthesiologie und Wiederbelebung, vol 47)

Bille Brahe NE (1982) Digitalization of surgical patients with impaired left ventricular function. Dan Med Bull 29:45–58

Bjertnaes LJ (1977) Hypoxia-induced vasoconstriction in isolated perfused lungs exposed to injectable or inhalation anesthetics. Acta Anaesthesiol Scand 21:133–147

Blessed G (1980) Clinical aspects of senile dementias. In: Roberts PJ (ed) Biochemistry of dementia. Wiley, Chichester, pp 1–14

Bonner JT (1983) Preoperative preparation. In: Kaplan JA (ed) Thoracic anesthesia. Livingstone, New York, pp 171–196

Boston collaborative surveillance program (1973) N Engl J Med 288:277–280

Bove EL, Fry WJ, Gross WS, Stanley JC (1980) Hypotension and hypertension as consequences of baroreceptor dysfunction following carotid endarterectomy. Surgery 85:633–637

Bramann H von, Herold G (1969) Anaesthesie bei über 80jährigen. Anaesthesist 18:321–325

Brandfonbreuer M, Landowne M, Shock NW (1955) Changes in cardiac output with age. Circulation 12:557–566

Brandl M (1982) Ursachen, Diagnostik und Therapie der postoperativen Ateminsuffizienz. In: Ahnefeld FW, Bergmann H, Burri C, Dick W, Halmágyi M, Hossli G, Rügheimer E (eds) Aufwachraum – Aufwachphase. Eine anästhesiologische Aufgabe. Springer, Berlin Heidelberg New York, pp 150–166 (Klinische Anästhesiologie und Intensivtherapie, vol 24)

Brandl M (1983) Präoperative Atemtherapie. Perimed-Verlag, Erlangen Anästhesiologie und Intensivmedizin, 24, pp 206–213

Brandl M, Pasch T, Kamp HD, Haertl L (1981) Comparative study on the calculation of intrapulmonary right-to-left shunt using central venous and mixed venous blood. Crit Care Med 9:272

Braun V, Voigt E (1978) Die Rolle von ventilatorischen Verteilungsstörungen bei der späten postoperativen Hypoxämie nach Oberbauchlaparotomien. Ein Beitrag zum Risiko von Oberbauchlaparotomien bei respiratorischer Vorschädigung. Anaesthesist 27:163–171

Bromage PR (1969) Ageing and epidural dose requirements. Br J Anaesth 41:1016–1022

Bromage PR, Gertel M (1972) Improved plexus blockade with bupivacaine hydrochloride and carbonated lidocaine. Anesthesiology 36:479–487

Bruce DL, Croley TF, Lee JS (1979) Preoperative clonidine withdrawal syndrome. Anesthesiology 51:90–92

Bünte H (1979) Allgemeine Faktoren, die das Operationsrisiko im Alter erhöhen. In: Rehm J (ed) Der alte Mensch in der Chirurgie. Springer, Berlin Heidelberg New York, pp 36–41

Burch GE (1975) Interesting aspects of geriatric cardiology. Am Heart J 89:99–114

Carlsson A (1981) Aging and brain neurotransmitters. In: Platt D (ed) Funktionsstörungen des Gehirns im Alter. Schattauer, Stuttgart, pp 67–81

Carmack CA (1975) Anesthesia and preoperative evaluation. In: Greenfield LJ (ed) Surgery in the aged. Saunders, Philadelphia, pp 14–23

Chan K, Kendall MJ, Mitchard M, Well WDE (1975) The effect of aging on plasma pethidine concentration. Br J Clin Pharmacol 2:297–302

Chowanetz W, Schramm A (1981) Lungenfunktion und Alter. Münch Med Wochenschr 123:1621–1623

Chung DC (1981 a) Anaesthetic problems associated with the treatment of cardiovascular disease. I. Digitalis toxicity. Can Anaesth Soc J 28:6–16

Chung DC (1981 b) Anaesthetic problems associated with the treatment of cardiovascular disease. II. Beta-adrenergic antagonists. Can Anaesth Soc J 28:105–113

Cogbill CL (1967) Operations in the aged. Mortality related to concurrent disease, duration of anesthesia, and elective or emergency operations. Arch Surg 94:202–205

Cohn JN, Franciosa JA (1977) Vasodilator therapy of cardiac failure. N Engl J Med 297:27–31 and 254–258

Cooperman LH, Price HL (1970) Pulmonary edema in the operative and postoperative period. Ann Surg 172:883–891

Covino BG (1978) Cardiovascular effects of spinal and epidural anesthesia. Regional-Anaesthesie 1:23–26

Dauchot P, Gravenstein JS (1971) Effects of atropine on electrocardiogram in different age groups. Clin Pharmacol Ther 12:274–280

Del Guerico LRM, Cohn JD (1980) Monitoring operative risk in the elderly. JAMA 243:1350–1355

Denney JL, Denson JS (1972) Risk of surgery in patients over 90. Geriatrics 27:115–118

Deutsch S, Dalen JE (1969) Indications for prophylactic digitalization. Anesthesiology 30:648–656

D'Hollander A, Massanx F, Nevelsteen M, Agoston S (1982) Age-dependent dose – response relationsship of Org NC 45 in anaesthetized patients. Br J Anaesth 54:653–657

Djokovic JL, Hedley-Whyte J (1979) Prediction of outcome of surgery and anesthesia in patients over 80. JAMA 242:2301–2306

Don HF, Craig DB, Wahba WM, Couture JG (1971) The measurement of gas trapped in the lungs at functional residual capacity and the effects of posture. Anesthesiology 35:582–590

Downs JB (1983) Postoperative respiratory care. In: Kaplan JA (ed) Thoracic anesthesia. Livingstone, New York, pp 635–663

Driessen A, Mauer W, Fricke M, Kossmann B, Schleinzer W (1980) Prospektive Untersuchungen zum Pathomechanismus des postspinalen Kopfschmerzes an einem ausgewählten Krankengut. Regional-Anaesthesie 3:38–41

Dripps RD, Lamont A, Eckenhoff JE (1961) The role of anesthesia in surgical mortality. JAMA 178:261–266

Dudziak R, Klein G (1982) Vor- und Nachteile von Regionalanaesthesie im Vergleich zur Allgemeinnarkose. Langenbecks Arch Chir 358:331–334

Duvaldestin P, Berger JL, Saada J, Desmonds JM (1980) Pancuronium: pharmacokinetics and pharmacodynamics in the elderly. Anesthesiology 53:S 284

Eger EI, Bahlman SH, Munson ES (1971) The effect of age on the rate of increase of alveolar anesthetic concentration. Anesthesiology 35:365–372

Ehehalt V, Rupp D (1982) Adrenerge Kreislaufreaktionen bei Neuroleptanalgesien. Anaesthesist 31:77–81

Emirgil C, Sobol BJ, Campodonico S, Herbert WH, Mechkati R (1967) Pulmonary circulation in the aged. J Appl Physiol 23:631–640:

Ewy GA (1980) Preoperative evaluation of patients with electrocardiographic conduction defects. In: Brown BB (ed) Anesthesia and the patient with heart disease. Davis, Philadelphia, pp 121–136

Falke K (1976) Anästhesiemethoden und -beatmung bei Patienten mit eingeschränkter Lungenfunktion. In: Ahnefeld FW, Bergmann H, Burri C, Dick W, Halmagyi M, Rügheimer E (eds) Der Risikopatient in der Anästhesie. 2. Respiratorische Störungen. Springer, Berlin Heidelberg New York, pp 100–113 (Klinische Anästhesiologie und Intensivtherapie, vol 12)

Farrow SC, Fowkes FGR, Lunn JN, Robertson IB, Samuel P (1982) Epidemiology in anaesthesia. II. Factors affecting mortality in hospital. Br J Anaesth 54:811–817

Feeley TW (1981) The recovery room. In: Miller RD (ed) Anesthesia, vol 2. Livingstone, New York, pp 1335–1360

Finlayson DC (1979) Postoperative intensive care. In: Kaplan JA (ed) Cardiac anesthesia. Grune and Stratton, New York, pp 473–490

Fitzal S (1982) Methodik der Atemtherapie. In: Benzer H, Frey R, Hügin W, Mayrhofer O (eds) Anaesthesiologie, Intensivmedizin und Reanimatologie, 5th edn. Springer, Berlin Heidelberg New York, pp 798–805

Flacke JE, Flacke WE, Williams GD (1977) Acute pulmonary edema following naloxone reversal of high-dose morphine anesthesia. Anesthesiology 47:376–378

Fleisch JH (1981) Age-related decrease in beta adrenoceptor activity of the cardiovascular system. Trends Pharmacol Sci 2:337–340

Foëx P (1981) Preöperative assessment of the patient with cardiovascular disease. Br J Anaesth 53:731–744

Foëx P, Prys-Roberts C (1974) Anesthesia and the hypertensive patient. Br J Anaesth 46:575–588

Foldes FF (1974) Wahl des Anästhesieverfahrens bei geriatrischen Patienten; Lokal- oder Allgemeinanästhesie? In: Ahnefeld FW, Halmágyi M (eds) Anaesthesie im Alter. Springer, Berlin Heidelberg New York, pp 57–58 (Anaesthesiologie und Wiederbelebung, vol 83)

Fox EJ, Sklar GS, Hill CH, Villanueva R, King BD (1977) Complications related to the pressor response to endotracheal intubation. Anesthesiology 47:524–525

Froese AB, Bryan AC (1974) Effects of anesthesia and paralysis on diaphragmatic mechanics in man. Anesthesiology 41:242–255

Gabel JC, Tonnesen AS (1980) Postoperative care of the patient with heart disease. In: Brown BB (ed) Anesthesia and the patient with heart disease. Davis, Philadelphia, pp 173–188

Gal J, Cooperman LH (1975) Hypertension in the immediate postoperative period. Br J Anaesth 47:70–74

Gelb AW, Southorn P, Rehder K (1981) Effect of general anaesthesia on respiratory function. Lung 159:187–198

Gerstenblith G, Frederiksen J, Yin FCP, Fortuin NJ, Lakatta EG, Weisfeldt ML (1977) Echocardiographic assessment of a normal adult aging population. Circulation 56:273–278

Giesecke AH (1981) Perioperative fluid therapy – crystalloids. In: Miller RD (ed) Anesthesia, vol 2. Livingstone, New York, pp 865–883

Gion H, Saidman LJ (1971) The minimum alveolar concentration of enflurane in man. Anesthesiology 35:361–364

Gloger K (1972) Die Altersabhängigkeit des Pulmonalarteriendruckes während stufenweise gesteigerter Ergometerarbeit. Z Kreislaufforsch 61:728–737

Goldman L (1981) Noncardiac surgery in patients receiving propranolol. Case reports and a recommended approach. Arch Intern Med 141:193–196

Goldman L, Caldera DL (1979) Risks of general anesthesia and elective operation in the hypertensive patient. Anesthesiology 50:285–292

Goldman L, Wolf MA (1980) The heart and circulation. In: Vandam LD (ed) To make the patient ready for anesthesia: Medical care of the surgical patient. Addison-Wesley, Menlo Park, pp 1–17

Goldman L, Caldera DL, Nussbaum SR, Southwick FS, Krogstad D, Murray B, Burke DS, O'Malley TA, Goroll AH, Caplan CH, Nolan J, Carabello B, Slater EE (1977) Multifactorial index of cardiac risk in noncardiac surgical procedures. New Engl J Med 297:845–850

Granath A, Jonsson B, Strandell T (1964) Circulation in healthy old men. Studied by right heart catheterization at rest and during exercise in supine and sitting position. Acta Med Scand 176:425–446

Greenblatt DJ, Sellers EM, Shader RI (1982) Drug disposition in old age. New Engl J Med 306:1081–1088

Gregory GA, Eger EI, Munson ES (1969) The relationship between age and halothane requirement in man. Anesthesiology 30:488–491

Hachinski VC, Lassen NA, Marshall J (1974) Multi-infarct dementia: a cause of mental detoriation in the elderly. Lancet II:207–210

Haldemann G, Schmid E, Frey P, Hossli G, Schaer H (1975) Wirkung von Ethrane auf die Kreislaufgrößen geriatrischer Patienten. Anaesthesist 24:343–346

Haldemann G, Wüst HP, Hossli G, Schaer H (1976) Die Auswirkungen einer Volumenrestitution mit Dextran-Ringlerlaktat auf den kreislaufdepressorischen Effekt von Ethrane bei geriatrischen Patienten. Anaesthesist 25:522–525

Haldemann G, Hossli G, Schaer H (1977) Die Anaesthesie mit Rohypnol (Flunitrazepam) und Fentanyl beim geriatrischen Patienten. Anaesthesist 26:168–171

Haljamäe H, Stefánsson T, Wickström I (1982) Preanesthetic evaluation of the female geriatric patient with hip fracture. Acta Anaesthesiol Scand 26:393–402

Hamer P (1975) Die Narkose in der Geriatrie. Prakt Anasth 10:59–69

Hamer P (1977) Pulmonales Risiko sowie prä- und postoperative Atemtherapie des alten Menschen in der operativen Medizin. Z Gerontol 10:445–456

Hamill JF, Bedford RF, Weaver DC, Colohan AR (1981) Lidocaine before endotracheal intubation: Intravenous or laryngotracheal? Anesthesiology 55:578–581

Hartung HJ, Osswald PM, Roller G, Lutz H (1983) Kreislaufkomplikationen bei Hypertonikern während der perioperativen Phase. Anasth Intensivther Notfallmed 18:196–198

Hartung W (1977) Pathologie der Alterslunge. Z Gerontol 10:385–392

Heberer G (1982) Einführung: Perioperative Aspekte zur Chirugie des alten Menschen. In: Heberer G, Witte J (eds) Chirurgie im hohen Alter. Perioperative Aspekte. Perimed, Erlangen, pp 9–13

Hedley-Whyte J, Burgess GE, Feeley TW, Miller MG (1976) Applied physiology of respiratory care. Little, Brown, Boston

Heinrich H, Ahnefeld FW, Kilian J, Seeling W, Sigel H, Spilker ED (1982a) Der kardiozirkulatorische Risikopatient in der Anästhesie. I. Präoperative Diagnostik und Risikobeurteilung. Herz Kreisl 14:429–437

Heinrich H, Ahnefeld FW, Kilian J, Nechwatal W, Seeling W, Sigel H, Stauch M (1982b) Der kardiozirkulatorische Risikopatient in der Anästhesie. II. Präoperative Vorbereitung. Herz Kreisl 14:598–610
Hensley MJ, Fencl V (1980) Lungs and respiration. In: Vandam LD (ed) To make the patient ready for anesthesia: medical care of the surgical patient. Addison-Wesley, Menlo Park, pp 18–43
Herman BE (1980) Vascular surgery in the aged. Mt Sinai J Med 47:215–217
Herrion PW, Jesseph JE, Harkins HN (1960) Analysis of 600 major operations in patients over 70 years of age. Ann Surg 152:686–695
Holland J, Milic-Emili J, Macklem PT, Bates DV (1968) Regional distribution of pulmonary ventilation and perfusion in eldery subjects. J Clin Invest 47:81–92
Honig EG (1983) Preoperative evaluation. In: Kaplan JA (ed) Thoracic anesthesia. Livingstone, New York, pp 121–170
Hoyer S (1981) Pathopysiologische Muster der zerebralen Insuffizienz im Alter. In: Platt D (ed) Funktionsstörungen des Gehirns im Alter. Schattauer, Stuttgart, pp 53–60
Islam MS, Buckup K, Ulmer WT (1978) Altersabhängigkeit der mechanischen Eigenschaften der Lunge. Dtsch Med Wochenschr 103:1482–1485
Janis KM (1978) Anesthesia for the geriatric patient. 29th Annual refresher course lectures, no 115. American Society of Anesthesiologists, Park Ridge pp 1–11
Juler GL, Stemmer EA, Connolly JE (1969) Complications of prophylactic digitalization in thoracic surgical patients. J Thorac Cardiovasc Surg 58:352–360
Jung D, Mayersohn M, Perrier D, Calkins J, Saunders R (1982) Thiopental disposition as a function of age in female patients undergoing surgery. Anesthesiology 56:263–268
Kallina C (1982) Morbidity and mortality in elderly orthopedic patients. Surg Clin North Am 62:297–300
Kannel WB, Wolf PA, McGee DL, Dawber TR, McNamara P, Castelli WP (1981) Systolic blood pressure, arterial rigidity, and risk of stroke: the Framingham study. JAMA 245:1225–1229
Kaplan JA, King SB (1976) The precordial electrocardiographic lead (V_5) in patients who have coronary artery disease. Anesthesiology 45:570–574
Keats AS (1983) Role of anesthesia in surgical mortality. In: Orkin FK, Cooperman LH (eds) Complications in anesthesiology. Lippincott, Philadelphia, pp 3–13
Kitamura H, Sawa T, Ikezono E (1972) Postoperative hypoxemia: the contribution of age to the maldistribution of ventilation. Anesthesiology 36:244–252
Klinck JR, Lindop MJ (1982) Epidural morphine in the elderly. A controlled trial after upper abdominal surgery. Anaesthesia 37:907–912
Klotz U, Avant GR, Hoyumpa A, Schenker S, Wilkinson GR (1975) The effects of age and liver disease on the disposition and elimination of diazepam in adult man. J Clin Invest 55:347–359
Koch-Weser J (1978) Arterial hypertension in old age. Herz 3:235–244
Kohn P, Zekert F, Vormittag E, Grabner H (1973) Risks of operation in patients over 80. Geriatrics 28:100–105
Kortum K, Rössler B, Nolte H (1979) Morbidität nach Spinalanästhesie. Regional-Anaesthesie 2:5–11
Kraas E, Beyer HG, Schwermann R, Athanasiadis S (1979) Das Operationsrisiko bei Abdominaleingriffen im Alter in Abhängigkeit von der Operationsvorbereitung. In: Rehm J (ed) Der alte Mensch in der Chirurgie. Springer, Berlin Heidelberg New York, pp 8–14
Kronenberg RS, Drage CW (1973) Attenuation of the ventilatory and heart rate responses to hypoxia and hypercapnia with aging in normal men. J Clin Invest 52:1812–1819
Lakatta EG (1979) Alterations in the cardiovascular system that occur in advanced age. Fed Proc 38:163–167
Lakatta EG, Yin FCP (1982) Myocardial aging: Functional alterations and related cellular mechanisms. Am J Physiol 242 (Heart Circ Physiol 11):H927–H941
Landauer B (1979) Zur funktionellen Beeinflussung der Lunge durch Anaesthetica. Springer, Berlin Heidelberg New York (Anaesthesiology and intensive care medicine, vol 114)

Lappas DG, Powell WMJ, Daggett WM (1977) Cardiac dysfunction in the perioperative period: pathophysiology, diagnosis, and treatment. Anesthesiology 47:117–137
Laver MB, Lowenstein E (1980) Anesthesia and the patient with heart disease. In: Johnson RA, Haber E, Austen WG (eds) The practice of cardiology. Little-Brown, Boston, pp 1090–1109
Laver MB, Austen WG, Wilson RS (1976) Blood-gas exchange and hemodynamic performance. In: Sabiston DC, Spencer FC (eds) Gibbon's surgery of the chest, 3rd edn Saunders, Philadelphia, pp 1–51
Lawin P (1965) Alter Patient und Anästhesie. Anaesthesist 14:103–107
Lawin P (1982) Anästhesie und Alterspolypathie. Z Allg Med 58:262–270
Leblanc P, Ruff P, Milic-Emili J (1970) Effects of age and body position on "airway closure" in man. J Appl Physiol 28:448–451
Lewin I, Lerner AG, Green SH, Del Guerico LRM, Siegel JH (1971) Physical class and physiological status in the prediction of operative mortality in the aged sick. Ann Surg 174:217–231
Linzbach AJ, Akuamoa-Boateng E (1973a) Die Altersveränderungen des menschlichen Herzens. I. Das Herzgewicht im Alter. Klin Wochenschr 51:156–163
Linzbach AJ, Akuamoa-Boateng E (1973b) Die Altersveränderungen des menschlichen Herzens. II. Die Polypathie des Herzens im Alter. Klin Wochenschr 51:164–175
Löllgen H, Meuret G, Wiemers K, Just H (1983) Zur prophylaktischen perioperativen Digitalistherapie. Med Welt 34:1340–1343
Lorhan PH (1955) Geriatric anesthesia. Thomas, Springfield
Lorhan PH (1967) Anesthesia experiences with the octogenarian. Anesth Analg 46:601–606
Lowenstein E, Philbin DM (1983) Narcotic anaesthesia. In: Bullingham RES (ed) Opiate analgesia. Saunders, London, pp 5–15 (Clinics in anaesthesiology, vol 1, no 1)
Lutz H (1980) Präoperative Risikoeinschätzung nach objektiven Kriterien. Anasth Intensivther Notfallmed 15:287–292
Lutz H, Klose R, Peter K (1972) Die Problematik der präoperativen Risikoeinstufung. Anästhesiol Inform 17:342–351
Lutz H, Osswald PM, Bender HJ (1982) Risiken der Anaesthesie. Untersuchungen bei 153,660 Anaesthesieverläufen. Anaesthesist 31:1–5
Mangano DT (1980) Monitoring pulmonary arterial pressure in coronary-artery disease. Anesthesiology 53:364–370
Mansell A, Bryan C, Levison H (1972) Airway closure in children. J Appl Physiol 33:711–714
Marshall AJ (1981) Drug therapy of hypertension and ischaemic heart disease. Br J Anaesth 53:697–709
Marshall BE, Wychie MQ (1972) Hypoxemia during and after anesthesia. Anesthesiology 37:178–209
Marshall WH, Fahey PJ (1964) Operative complications and mortality in patients over 80 years of age. Arch Surg 88:896–904
Marx GF, Maeto CV, Orkin LR (1973) Computer analysis of postanesthetic deaths. Anesthesiology 39:54–58
Master AM, Lasser RP (1961) Blood pressure elevation in the elderly. In: Brest AN, Moyer JH (eds) Hypertension: recent advances. Lea and Febiger, Philadelphia, pp 24–34
Mathers J, Benumof JL, Wahrenbrock EA (1977) General anesthetics and regional hypoxic pulmonary vasoconstriction. Anesthesiology 46:111–114
Mayrhofer O (1969) Anästhesiologie. In: Doberauer W, Hittmair A, Nissen R, Schulz FH, Tuba J (eds) Handbuch der Praktischen Geriatrie, vol 3. Enke, Stuttgart, pp 22–105
Mayrhofer O (1970) Operationsrisiken alter Menschen unter besonderer Berücksichtigung der Arteriosklerose. MMW 112:2071–2077
McLaren AD, Stockwell MC, Reid VT (1978) Anaesthetic techniques for surgical correction of fractured neck of femur. Anaesthesia 33:10–14
McLeod K, Hull CJ, Watson MJ (1979) Effects of ageing on the pharmacokinetics of pancuronium. Br J Anaesth 51:435–438
Michel D, Körner HJ (1983) Operationsvorbereitung und Operationsrisiko bei unabweisbaren Notfalleingriffen am alten Menschen. Krankenhausarzt 56:30–32

Mihalick MJ, Fisch C (1974) Electrocardiographic findings in the aged. Am Heart J 87:117–128

Miller R, Marlar K, Silvay G (1977) Anesthesia for patients aged over ninety years. NY State J Med 77:1421–1425

Miller RD (1981) Anesthesia for the elderly. In: Miller RD (ed) Anesthesia, vol 2. Livingstone, New York, pp 1231–1246

Miller RW, Coulthard SW (1981) Anesthesia for the elderly and debelitated patient. Otolaryngol Clin North Am 14:715–722

Mofitt EA (1978) Preoperative evaluation of the patient with myocardial disease: Clinical review. Can Anaesth Soc J 25:457–461

Morr-Strathmann U, Huppertz K, Lawin P (1975a) Hämodynamische Untersuchungen während der Narkoseeinleitung mit Etomidate und Ethrane bei geriatrischen Patienten. Prakt Anasth 10:239–242

Morr-Strathmann U, Boeger OD, Foitzik H, Lawin P (1975b) Kreislaufuntersuchungen während Enflurane-Narkosen bei einem geriatrischen Krankengut. Prakt Anasth 10:69–72

Muravchick S, Mandel J (1982) Thiopental sleep dosages in geriatric patients. Anesthesiology 57:A327

Murphy TM (1981) Spinal, epidural, and caudal anesthesia. In: Miller RD (ed) Anesthesia, vol 1. Livingstone, New York, pp 635–678

Nolte H, Meyer J, Wurster J (1974) Morbidität und Mortalität geriatrischer Patienten unter Berücksichtigung verschiedener Anaesthesietechniken. In: Ahnefeld FW, Halmágyi M (ds) Anaesthesie im Alter. Springer, Berlin Heidelberg New York, pp 65–72 (Anaesthesiologie und Wiederbelebung, vol 83)

O'Donohue WJ (1979) Respiratory therapy. Chest 76:683–687

Oduah M (1970) Verhalten des Serumspiegels von Hexobarbital und Thiopental beim alten Patienten. In: Hutschenreuther K, Bihler K, Fritsche P (eds) Anaesthesie in extremen Altersklassen. Springer, Berlin Heidelberg New York, pp 165–171 (Anaesthesiologie und Wiederbelebung, vol 47)

Osswald PM, Hartung HJ, Bender HJ, Becker P, Lutz H (1983) Zeitpunkt und Häufigkeit perioperativer Herzkreislaufkomplikationen bei geriatrischen Patienten. Anasth Intensivther Notfallmed 18:193–195

Owens WD, Waldbaum LS, Stephan CR (1978) Cardiac dysrhythmia following reversal of neuromuscular blocking agents in geriatric patients. Anesth Analg 57:186–190

Palmberg S, Hirsjärvi E (1979) Mortality in geriatric surgery. With special reference to the type of surgery, anaesthesia, complicating diseases, and prophylaxis of thrombosis. Gerontology 25:103–112

Pasch T (1982) Ursachen, Erkennung und Behandlung von Störungen nach Anästhesie und Operation: Herz-Kreislauf. In: Ahnefeld FW, Bergmann H, Burri C, Dick W, Halmágyi M, Hossli G, Rügheimer E (eds) Aufwachraum – Aufwachphase. Eine anästhesiologische Aufgabe. Springer, Berlin Heidelberg New York, pp 167–180 (Klinische Anästhesiologie und Intensivtherapie, vol 24)

Pecora DV (1969) Predictability of effects of abdominal thoracic surgery upon pulmonary function. Ann Surg 170:101–108

Peter K, Unertl K, Henrich G, Mai N, Brunner F (1980) Das Anästhesierisiko. Anästhesiol Intensivmed 21:240–248

Pierce JA, Ebert RV (1958) The elastic properties of the lungs in the aged. J Lab Clin Med 51:63–71

Planz G, Beckenbauer U, Bundschu HD (1982) Response of plasma catecholamines and blood pressure to clonidine and to sudden withdrawal of the drug in subjects with essential hypertension. Int J Clin Pharmacol Ther Toxicol 20:474–478

Plumlee JE, Boettner RB (1972) Myocardial infarction during and following anesthesia and operation. South Med J 65:886–889

Pontén J, Biber B, Bjurö T, Henriksson BA, Hjalmarsen A (1982) β-receptor blocker withdrawal. A preoperative problem in general surgery? Acta Anaesthesiol Scand [Suppl] 76:32–37

Pontoppidan H, Geffin B, Lowenstein E (1972) Acute respiratory failure in the adult. N Engl J Med 287:690–698, 743–752, 799–806
Powers WE, Morrison DR (1978) Evaluation of inspired volumes in postoperative patients receiving volume-oriented IPPB. Respir Care 23:39–43
Prys-Roberts C (1979) Hypertension and anesthesia – fifty years on. Anesthesiology 50:281–284
Pulver KG, Otten M (1970) Die Allgemeinnarkose im Greisenalter. In: Hutschenreuther K, Bihler K, Fritsche P (eds) Anaesthesie in extremen Altersklassen. Springer, Berlin Heidelberg New York, pp 114–122 (Anaesthesiologie und Wiederbelebung, vol 47)
Quinn K, Quebbeman EJ (1981) Pulmonary artery pressure monitoring in the surgical intensive care unit. Benefits vs difficulties. Arch Surg 116:872–876
Rau JL (1978) Respiratory therapy pharmacology. Year Book Medical, Chicago
Rehder K, Sessler AD, Marsh HM (1975) General anesthesia and the lung. Am Rev Respir Dis 112:541–563
Rehder K, Marsh HM, Rodarte JR, Hyatt RE (1977) Airway closure. Anesthesiology 47:40–52
Reidenberg MM, Levy M, Warner H (1978) Relationship between diazepam dose, plasma level, age, and central nervous system depression. Clin Pharmacol Ther 3:371–374
Richard RR, George RB (1981) Improving postoperative tidal volumes. Respir Care 26:985–986
Rifat K (1977) Anesthésie-réanimation chez le sujet agé en traumatologie. Ann Anesthesiol Fr 18:493–498
Roizen MF (1981) Routine preoperative evaluation. In: Miller RD (ed) Anesthesia, vol 1. Livingstone, New York, pp 3–19
Rügheimer E (1970) Die akute Ateminsuffizienz in der prä- und postoperativen Phase von Noteingriffen. Langenbecks Arch Chir 327:896–905
Rügheimer E (1974) Die cardiale Vorbereitung zum operativen Eingriff in Narkose. In: Lawin P, Morr-Strathmann U (eds) Deutsche Gesellschaft für Anaesthesie und Wiederbelebung. Jahrestagung vom 23. bis 26. November 1972 in Hamburg. Springer, Berlin Heidelberg New York, pp 18–30
Rügheimer E (1981) Neuroleptanästhesie. In: Ahnefeld FW, Bergmann H, Burri C, Dick W, Doenicke A, Halmágyi M, Hossli G, Rügheimer E (eds) Die intravenöse Narkose. Springer, Berlin Heidelberg New York, pp 175–191 (Klinische Anästhesiologie und Intensivtherapie, vol 23)
Rügheimer E (1982) Inhalationstherapie. In: Benzer H, Frey R, Hügin W, Mayrhofer O (eds) Anaesthesiologie, Intensivmedizin und Reanimatologie, 5th edn. Springer, Berlin Heidelberg New York, pp 788–798
Salehi E (1979) Narkoserisiko in der geriatrischen Urologie. Aktuel Gerontol 9:75–81
Schimmler W (1965) Untersuchungen zu Elastizitätsproblemen der Aorta. Statistische Korrelation der Pulswellengeschwindigkeit zu Alter, Geschlecht und Blutdruck. Arch Kreislaufforsch 47:189–233
Seeling W, Altemeyer KH, Berg S, Feist H, Schmitz JE, Schröder JM, Ahnefeld FW (1982) Die kontinuierliche thorakale Periduralanaesthesie zur intra- und postoperativen Analgesie. Anaesthesist 31:439–448
Shapiro AG (1982) Introduction and overview. In: Israel JS, De Kornfeld TJ (eds) Recovery room care. Thomas, Springfield, pp 3–7
Shapiro BA (1980) Evaluation of respiratory function in the perioperative period. 31st annual refresher course lectures, no 107. Am Soc Anesthesiol, St. Louis, pp 1–8
Shapiro BA, Harrison RA, Trout CA (1977) Clinical application of respiratory care. Year Book Medical, Chicago
Sharrock NE (1978) Epidural anesthetic dose responses in patients 20 to 80 years old. Anesthesiology 49:425–428
Shaver JA (1983) Hemodynamic monitoring in the critically ill patient. N Engl J Med 308:277–279
Shelby EA, Lorhan PM (1968) Age as a factor in mortality after cholecystectomy. Anesth Analg 47:733–736

Siegel JH (1976) General considerations in the surgical management of the aged and high-risk patient. In: Siegel JH, Chodoff P (eds) The aged and high risk surgical patient: medical, surgical and anesthetic management. Grune and Stratton, New York, pp 1–22

Simon E, Meyer WW (1958) Das Volumen, die Volumendehnbarkeit und die Druck-Längen-Beziehungen des gesamten aortalen Windkessels in Abhängigkeit von Alter, Hochdruck und Arteriosklerose. Klin Wochenschr 36:424–432

Simpson BR, Parkhouse J, Marshall R, Lambrechts W (1961) Extradural analgesia and the prevention of postoperative respiratory complications. Br J Anaesth 33:628–641

Stahlgren LH (1961) An analysis of factors which influence mortality following extensive abdominal operations upon geriatric patients. Surg Gynecol Obstet 113:283–292

Stanski DR, Greenblatt DJ, Lowenstein E (1978) Kinetics of intravenous and intramuscular morphine. Clin Pharmacol Ther 24:52–59

Steen PA, Tinker JH, Tarhan S (1978) Myocardial reinfarction after anesthesia and surgery. JAMA 239:2566–2570

Stefánsson T, Wickström I, Haljamäe H (1982a) Hemodynamic and metabolic effects of ketamine anesthesia in the geriatric patient. Acta Anaesthesiol Scand 26:371–377

Stefánsson T, Wickström I, Haljamäe H (1982b) Cardiovascular and metabolic effects of halothane and enflurane anesthesia in the geriatric patient. Acta Anaesthesiol Scand 26:378–385

Stefánsson T, Wickström I, Haljamäe H (1982c) Effects of neurolept and epidural analgesia on cardiovascular function and tissue metabolism in the geriatric patient. Acta Anaesthesiol Scand 26:386–392

Stephen CR (1981) Influence of hypertension on cardiovascular accidents associated with anesthesia in the elderly. In: Rügheimer E, Zindler M (eds) Anaesthesiology. Proceedings of the 7th World Congress of Anaesthesiologists, Hamburg, september 14–21, 1980. Excerpta Medica, Amsterdam, pp 470–475

Stevens WC, Dolan WM, Gibbons RT, White A, Eger EI, Miller RD, de Jong R, Elashoff RM (1975) Minimum alveolar concentrations (MAC) of isoflurane with and without nitrous oxide in patients of various ages. Anesthesiology 42:197–200

Stoelting RK (1981) Psychological preparation and preoperative medication. In: Miller RD (ed) Anesthesia, vol 1. Livingstone, New York, pp 95–105

Striebel JP, Scherrer R, Stähler-Hambrecht I, Lutz H (1981) Wertigkeiten verschiedener Parameter bei der präoperativen Beurteilung des Anästhesie-Risikos. In: Haid B, Mitterschiffthaler G (eds) Zentraleuropäischer Anaesthesiekongreß, vol 1. Springer, Berlin Heidelberg New York, pp 50–60 (Anaesthesiologie und Intensivmedizin, vol 139)

Tarhan S, Moffitt EA, Taylor WF, Ginliani ER (1972) Myocardial infarction after general anesthesia. JAMA 220:1451–1454

Tarnow J (1982) Swan-Ganz catheterization. Application, interpretation and complications. Thorac Cardiovasc Surg 30:130–136

Tolksdorf W, Raiss, G, Striebel JP, Lutz H (1980) Intra- und postoperative pulmonale Komplikationen bei transurethralen Prostataresektionen in Intubationsnarkose und rückenmarksnaher Leitungsanästhesie. In: Wüst HJ, Zindler M (eds) Neue Aspekte der Regionalanaesthesie 1. Springer, Berlin Heidelberg New York, pp 146–160 (Anaesthesiologie und Intensivmedizin, vol 124)

Tomlinson BE (1980) The structural and quantitative aspects of the dementias. In: Roberts PJ (ed) Biochemistry of dementia. Wiley, Chichester, pp 15–52

Tompkins MJ, Artusio JF (1964) Myocardial infarction and surgery: a five year study. Anesth Analg 43:716–720

Towne JB, Bernhard VM (1980) The relationship of postoperative hypertension to complications following carotid endarterectomy. Surgery 88:575–580

Turner JM, Mead J, Wohl ME (1968) Elasticity of human lungs in relation to age. J Appl Physiol 25:664–671

Tyras DH, Stothert JC, Kaiser GC, Barner HB, Codd JE, Willman VL (1979) Supraventricular tachyarrhythmias after myocardial revascularization: A randomised trial of prophylactic digitalization. J Thorac Cardiovasc Surg 77:310–314

Ulmer WT, Reichel G, Nolte D (1976) Die Lungenfunktion. Physiologie und Pathophysiologie, Methodik, 2nd edn. Thieme, Stuttgart

Vacanti CJ, Van Houten RJ, Hill RC (1970) A statistical analysis of the relationship of physical status to postoperative mortality in 68,388 cases. Anesth Analg 49:564–566
Van Aken H, Baum J, Lawin P (1982) Präoperative Bestimmung der Starling-Kurve bei kritisch Kranken. Dtsch Med Wochenschr 107:735–740
Vanik PE, Davis HS (1968) Cardiac arrhythmias during halothane anesthesia. Anesth. Analg 47: 299–307
Virtanen R, Kanto J, Iisalo E, Iisalo EUM, Salo M, Sjövall S (1982) Pharmacokinetic studies on atropine with special reference to age. Acta Anaesthesiol Scand 26:297–300
Wallace WA, Guardini R, Ellis SJ (1982) Standard intravenous regional anaesthesia. Br Med J 285:554–556
Wedgwood J (1973) Cardiovascular disease in the old. Br Med J 3:622–626
Weiss B, Greenberg L, Cantor E (1979) Age-related alterations in the development of adrenergic denervation supersensitivity. Fed Proc 38:1915–1921
Weiss MF, Lesmick GJ (1980) Surgery in the elderly: attitudes and facts. Mt Sinai J Med 47:208–214
Welch MA, Shapiro BJ, Marcurio P, Wagner W, Hirayama G (1980) Methods of intermittent positive pressure breathing. Chest 78:463–467
Wezler K (1958) Die physiologische Altersinsuffizienz des Herzens. Verh Dtsch Ges Herz Kreislaufforsch 24:74–104
Wezler K, Böger A (1939) Die Dynamik des arteriellen Systems. Ergeb Physiol 41:291–606
Wickström I, Holmberg I, Stefánsson T (1982) Survival of female geriatric patients after hip fracture surgery. A comparison of 5 anesthetic methods. Acta Anaesthesiol Scand 26:607–614
Wilder RJ, Fishbein RH (1961) Operative experiences with patients over 80 years of age. Surg Gynecol Obstet 113:205–212
Wirén JE, Janzon L (1983) Respiratory complications following surgery. Improved prediction with preoperative spirometry. Acta Anaesthesiol Scand 27: 476–479
Wolff G (1979) Die respiratorische Insuffizienz in der Chirurgie. Schweiz Med Wochenschr 109:1552–1561
Ziment I (1978) Respiratory pharmacology and therapeutics. Saunders, Philadelphia

Surgery

Gastrointestinal Surgery in the Elderly

D. E. F. TWEEDLE and P. F. SCHOFIELD

A. Introduction

In writing about gastroenterological surgery in the elderly, we have chosen to emphasise those problems which are either especially common in the elderly or difficult to manage in the older patient. For these reasons, this chapter is not intended to be comprehensive, but stresses those conditions which are of outstanding importance in the geriatric age group, namely hiatus hernia and oesophageal reflux, oesophageal and gastric cancer, peptic ulcer, gallstones, pancreatic tumours, diverticular disease of the colon, colorectal tumours, inflammatory bowel disease and the problems of faecal incontinence and prolapse of the rectum.

B. Hiatus Hernia and Reflux Oesophagitis

The typical symptom of reflux oesophagitis, postural heartburn, is often associated with hiatus hernia, but the demonstration of a hiatus hernia is not the crucial factor affecting the decision to operate in elderly patients with reflux. It is well recognised that a sliding hiatus hernia can be demonstrated in 30% of an asymptomatic population and that symptomatic oesophageal reflux can be demonstrated in large numbers of patients who do not have hiatus hernias, so that the coexistence of symptomatic oesophageal reflux with a hiatus hernia may well be fortuitous (PRICE and CASTELL 1978). If the clinician is uncertain of the validity of the history, objective confirmation of the frequency and severity of the reflux may be obtained by monitoring oesophageal pH over 24 h (DEMEESTER et al. 1976).

Although the incidence of acute, gross haemorrhage from hiatus hernia is very low, anaemia due to chronic blood loss is common. Some surgeons are of the opinion that the incidence of chronic haemorrhage from hiatus hernia is increased if the hernia is irreducible and this is more likely to occur in a paraoesophageal hernia when the blood supply has become embarrassed. At least 60% of patients become symptom free or their symptoms are greatly reduced by adequate medical treatment, including elevation of the head of the bed, avoidance of stooping, avoidance of activity that increases intraabdominal pressure, losing weight and stopping cigarette smoking (ATKINSON 1967). Metoclopramide improves oesophageal motility, reduces dysphagia and increases lower oesophageal sphincter tone. Antacid–alginate compounds are more effective in relieving heartburn than simple antacids (STANCIU and BENNETT 1974). Although the formation of a stricture may influence the decision concerning surgery, repeated dilatations using the

Table 1. Deaths from cancer in England and Wales 1966–1970 (per million) (Office of population census and surveys 1975)

	Men						
	55–	60–	65–	70–	75–	80–	85+
Colon and Rectum	433	740	1186	1835	2666	3491	4628
Stomach	540	923	1412	1957	2538	2708	2838
Pancreas	204	318	473	648	833	932	1038
Oesophagus	114	181	287	389	580	707	812
Gallbladder	31	50	75	108	149	142	200

	Women						
	55–	60–	65–	70–	75–	80–	85+
Colon and Rectum	402	586	875	1319	1937	2603	3609
Stomach	213	357	580	939	1395	1813	2299
Pancreas	112	182	267	389	512	625	752
Oesophagus	55	92	130	199	299	397	500
Gallbladder	29	52	92	141	171	201	190

Eder–Puestow dilators can be performed without a general anaesthetic as an out-patient procedure in elderly patients (ROYSTON et al. 1976).

Surgery should be reserved for those patients with complications and those in whom medical treatment gives inadequate control of symptoms. Although it has been emphasised that thoracotomy can be performed in the elderly with an over-all mortality of 6% (WELLINGTON and LYNN 1966), most surgeons would wish to avoid thoracotomy in patients over the age of 65 years and would choose to perform the antireflux procedure from within the abdomen. Consequently, many surgeons choose to perform a Nissen fundoplication (NISSEN 1956). This simple operation can be performed comparatively easily within the abdomen with very little postoperative upset. A great majority of patients become symptom free or their symptoms are considerably reduced, but some complain of gastric distension which they cannot relieve by eructation.

C. Carcinoma of the Oesophagus

It is apparent from Table 1 that carcinoma of the oesophagus is a disease of old age, its incidence and resulting mortality increasing particularly above the age of 70 years. The majority of tumours are squamous carcinomas, but about 10% of tumours occurring in the lower third are adenocarcinomas. It has been suggested that squamous carcinoma of the oesophagus can be treated more effectively by radiotherapy than by surgery (PEARSON 1971), but most authorities believe that surgical excision is the best method of treatment, and have used radiotherapy as an adjunct to surgical excision or for palliation. The majority of patients are mal-

Table 2. Carcinoma of the oesophagus: Operative mortality and survival

Reference	Country	Cases	Mortality (%)	5-year survival[a]
NAKAYAMA (1968)	Japan	310	10	30 (9)
COLLIS (1971)	England	314	14	36 (12)
MILLER (1961)	Scotland	175	31	22 (13)
VAN ANDEL et al. (1979)	Holland	81	21	18 (21)
DARK et al. (1981)	England	449	8	48 (17)

[a] Figures in parentheses are percentages

nourished and there are those who believe that nutritional repletion before surgery should be an important component of their treatment (MULLER et al. 1981). If a patient undergoes thoracotomy, macroscopic resection of the growth is usually feasible, but it is well recognised that microscopic extension in the submucosa of the oesophagus and into the surrounding mediastinal tissues renders resection incomplete in the majority of cases. The ability to demonstrate extraluminal extension of the tumor would be a major advance and would reduce the incidence of inappropriate thoracotomy. Mediastinoscopy and computer assisted tomography are being assessed for this purpose in a number of centres throughout the world. Many surgeons now perform a total oesophagectomy regardless of the site of the tumour, mobilising the stomach for anastomosis in the neck (MCKEOWN 1976). Anastomotic leakage is now an uncommon event and postoperative deaths are usually due to respiratory or cardiovascular complications. The operative mortality of oesophagectomy is high, even in experienced hands, and the 5-year survival is poor (Table 2). COLLIS (1971) has emphasised that operative mortality is related to experience, half of his first 50 cases died in the postoperative period, but only 12% of his patients died after operation when he had performed more than 300 oesophagectomies, a feature recently confirmed by DARK et al. (1981). The survival figures in Table 2 may appear to be poor, but in the northwest of England, any male reaching the age of 65 years has only an 80% chance of surviving to the age of 70 years and a 60% chance of reaching 75 years. Actuarial survival after resection for carcinoma of the oesophagus may be higher than was formerly imagined. A patient who survives for 2 years after oesophagectomy for carcinoma is unlikely to die from residual or recurrent malignancy.

Thoracotomy is not indicated in at least 20% of patients presenting with carcinoma of the oesophagus, because the patients' general condition makes the chance of recovery extremely remote. The recent development of endoscopic intubation of oesophageal strictures is a major advance in the palliation of unresected tumours (ATKINSON and FERGUSON 1977). The mortality of endoscopic intubation is much less than intubation at laparotomy under general anaesthesia (JOHNSON et al. 1976). If the neoplastic stricture is too tight to admit the semirigid tube, it can be dilated with Eder–Puestow dilators. Intubation is effective palliation, but does not appear to influence long-term survival. Following intubation, patients take an ordinary diet, but must mince all their food and use soda water to prevent tube blockage. Despite this, about 8% of tubes become blocked and endoscopic means have to be employed in an attempt to overcome the blockage. A further problem is that 10% of tubes become displaced and new tubes have to be inserted. In future it may be possible to perform a partial, intraluminal resection of a tumour using laser beams directed endoscopically.

D. Carcinoma of the Stomach

It can be seen from Table 1 that the mortality rate for carcinoma of the stomach increases considerably in people over the age of 60 years. The incidence of gastric cancer designated as "early" has risen to over 30% in Japan (TAKAGI 1981). Elsewhere in the world it varies from less than 1% to 11% (JOHANSEN 1976). As might be expected, the results of treatment of "early gastric cancer" differ dramatically from those obtained in patients with lymphatic dissemination or serosal invasion (IMANAGA and NAKAZATO 1977). The dramatic difference between the incidence of early gastric cancer in Japan and that in the rest of the world may lie in the endoscopic screening programmes for asymptomatic patients conducted by the Japanese or may reflect a true geographical variation in disease. Such screening can be justified in Japan where gastric cancer is three times as common as in Europe. In Europe screening could be undertaken in patients particularly at risk including those suffering from pernicious anaemia, chronic atrophic gastritis, gastric polyps, Ménétrier's disease and in those who have had a gastrectomy or gastroenterostomy.

Surgical technique may be more important than has previously been recognised in attempting curative resections. Most surgeons recognise the need for en bloc dissection of adequate lengths of healthy intestine, mesentery, and lymph nodes when operating for colonic carcinoma, but may neglect a similar approach for carcinoma of the stomach. The Japanese surgeons resect the lymphatic drainage of the stomach in a similar manner to the colon. Many patients who have undergone attempted curative resections for gastric cancer have been found to have evidence of presumed recurrence in the gastric remnant. Evidence has been available for many years that invasion of the duodenal mucosa frequently occurs in gastric carcinomas arising in the pyloric antrum (CASTLEMAN 1936). As elsewhere in the gastrointestinal tract, the line of resection should be adequately clear from malignant tissue evident to the naked eye and the specimen should include the omenta and lymphatics. The results of some European and Japanese surveys are compared in Table 3.

As the majority of patients in Europe present with serosal and lymphatic involvement and attempted curative resection would be inappropriate for elderly patients, the majority will be receiving palliative treatment. For these patients, resection of the tumour rather than proximal bypass increases the length of survival and the quality of life. If the patient has a distal tumour, the surgeon should perform a distal gastrectomy rather than a gastrojejunostomy.

Proximal tumours present a difficult problem. Proximal or total gastrectomy is often technically very difficult to perform through the abdomen alone and the mortality and morbidity of thoracoabdominal gastrectomy is high in this aged

Table 3. Survival following laparotomy for gastric cancer

Reference	Country	Total patients	5-year survival	
			Overall (%)	Curative resection (%)
BROOKES et al. (1965)	Britain	5,441	4.5	15.6
INBERG et al. (1975)	Finland	1,614	6.5	27
MUTO et al. (1968)	Japan	2,014	18	26
IMANAGA and NAKAZOTO (1977)	Japan	1,628	45	64

population. If the tumour is comparatively hard and encircles the cardia, it may be possible to intubate it using an endoscope. Sometimes the commercially available tubes are rather short for this purpose and although impacted correctly, the distal end of the tube may become blocked by spread of the tumour. Gastric carcinomas are often soft and do not encircle the entire lumen of the stomach so that intubation is impossible. Perhaps in the future it may be possible to destroy the major portion of the intraluminal tumour by laser photocoagulation.

E. Peptic Ulceration

In the older patient gastric ulceration is nearly as common (45%) as duodenal ulceration (55%) (LEUZ and HAECK 1972), which contrasts with the younger patient in whom duodenal ulceration is much more common. The commonest age of onset of gastric ulceration is between 50 and 59 years in women, and between 60 and 69 years in men, 60% of these patients being male. In duodenal ulceration the first symptoms occur most frequently between the ages of 30 and 39 years in men and between 40 and 49 years in women, but 10%–15% of patients present after 60 years of age (KAPLAN et al. 1972a; LEUZ and HAECK 1972). As in younger age groups, duodenal ulceration is four times more common in males than in females. In patients over the age of 60 years, haemorrhage is a more frequent complication than perforation in duodenal ulceration whilst perforation is a more common complication than haemorrhage in gastric ulceration.

In many of these patients, peptic ulceration may be provoked by medical treatment for arthritis. The effect of aspirin and steroids is well known. Unfortunately, the newer nonsteroidal anti-inflammatory agents such as indomethacin may produce ulceration as severe as that produced by steroids (THOMPSON 1980). The natural history of these ulcers appears to differ from those arising in patients not receiving anti-inflammatory agents. They are more resistant to medical treatment and more prone to complications such as bleeding and perforation.

It is well recognised that elderly patients tolerate acute gastrointestinal haemorrhage very badly and mortality rises dramatically according to the quantitiy of blood lost. Mortality is usually below 10% in patients who have lost less than 3 l blood before operation, but increases to 35%–50% in patients who have lost more than 4.5 l (KAPLAN et al. 1972b; LEUZ and HAECK 1972). Consequently, surgery should be undertaken early in the elderly patient with bleeding peptic ulceration. Although these features have been confirmed in many subsequent reviews, there is still a tendency for many physicians to fatally delay a surgical opinion in the elderly patient. Preliminary endoscopic determination of the site of bleeding does not appear to have influenced the mortality (HOARE 1980). However, this should not be advanced as an argument for abandoning this investigation because the presence of a definite chronic ulcer is one of several factors which influence the decision to proceed to surgery. If the results of treatment are to improve, accurate diagnosis is essential and it can sometimes be extremely difficult to locate the source of bleeding at laparotomy. Furthermore, the surgeon may by protected from the uncommon but acutely embarrasing predicament of finding himself operating in the abdomen when the pathology can only be effectively dealt with through the chest.

The most recent therapeutic measure suggested in the management of upper gastrointestinal tract bleeding is laser photocoagulation via an endoscope. The results of nonrandomised studies suggest that immediate haemostasis can be obtained in approximately 80% of patients (LAURENCE et al. 1980). The incidence of rebleeding immediately after laser photocoagulation is much lower than that in control patients (MACLEOD et al. 1983; SWAIN et al. 1983). However, there has been no suggestion that laser photocoagulation can induce healing of ulcers. The place of this method is not established, but a number of randomised trials comparing laser photocoagulation with surgery are being undertaken throughout the world.

I. Gastric Ulceration

It is the authors' experience that chronic gastric ulceration occurring at any age is less amenable to medical treatment than duodenal ulceration. Nevertheless, a trial of medical treatment for uncomplicated ulceration should precede surgical treatment. Patients may be treated with H_2 receptor antagonists such as cimetidine and ranitidine, but the colloidal bismuth preparation De-Nol, appears to be as effective (MARTIN et al. 1981).

Gastroscopy is essential before treatment of any gastric ulcer because it is necessary to exclude malignancy. Pathological material should be obtained by brushing for cytology and forceps biopsy for histological examination. The authors have seen patients in whom mucosal healing occurred across malignant gastric ulcers under treatment with cimetidine.

Surgery may be indicated for failure of medical treatment, unremitting pain or complications such as anaemia, haemorrhage or perforation. Although vagotomy, with or without local excision of the ulcer has been advocated for the treatment of gastric ulceration (CADE et al. 1979), most surgeons believe that gastrectomy including the ulcer in the resected portion of the stomach is the optimal treatment. Even in patients with ulcers high on the lesser curve of the stomach, it is usually possible to excise the ulcer within a tongue of tissue and then reconstitute the lesser curvature using Pauchet's manoeuvre. Most surgeons reestablish intestinal continuity with a Billroth I anastomosis rather than a Billroth II or Polya anastomosis. Any of these anastomoses can be performed in the traditional manner using sutures or by using stapling instruments. It is suggested that after adequate training, surgeons can perform gastrectomy more rapidly using stapling instruments which may be an important consideration in elderly patients.

Most patients with anaemia due to gastric ulceration respond to treatment with oral iron. Unfortunately, those patients with gastric ulceration as a consequence of medical treatment for arthritis frequently fail to respond to such treatment and in many patients it is necessary to treat the ulcer surgically in order that the patients may continue with their anti-inflammatory treatment. When first presented with such a problem, the less experienced surgeon might baulk at the idea of performing a gastrectomy to allow continuing anti-inflammatory treatment for arthritis. There is no doubt that many elderly patients with severe arthritis are better advised to accept the potential morbidity and mortality after partial gastrectomy than to be subject to constant pain and to be confined to a wheelchair. When surgery is undertaken for acute bleeding from a gastric ulcer, the choice lies between excision of the ulcer with vagotomy or gastrectomy.

Perforation occurs in approximately 15% of patients requiring surgery for gastric ulceration. Although operative mortality increases from 7% in patients less than 60 years old to 37.5% in patients over the age of 75 years, there is no evidence that performing lesser procedures than gastrectomy reduces operative mortality. Indeed, in one study, the converse was true when 20% of patients over the age of 60 years died after simple suture closure of the ulcer compared with 9% after partial gastrectomy (KAPLAN et al. 1972b). Although biopsies may be taken from the ulcer before simple suture closure, the biopsy may not be representative and malignant change cannot be excluded by this technique.

II. Duodenal Ulceration

The majority of patients over the age of 60 years presenting to the hospital for the first time with symptoms of duodenal ulceration have had symptoms for many years. However, by way of contrast, some elderly patients with duodenal ulceration present with massive gastrointestinal haemorrhage and deny any previous dyspeptic history. It is unusual for the surgeon to be requested to operate on an elderly patient with a duodenal ulcer for dyspepsia alone and surgery should never be contemplated unless there has been an adequate trial of medical treatment with H_2 receptor antagonists or the colloidal bismuth preparation De-nol (MARTIN et al. 1981).

As with haemorrhage from gastric ulceration, surgery should be considered early in the treatment of elderly patients (ALLAN and DYKES 1976). At the present time, truncal vagotomy and pyloroplasty with suture of the bleeding vessels in the base of the ulcer is the most commonly performed operation (HEGGATY et al. 1973). In patients with perforation, the mortality and morbidity following truncal vagotomy and pyloroplasty is no greater than after suture closure alone and thus the curative operation is to be preferred. Elderly patients presenting with pyloric stenosis due to duodenal ulceration are often malnourished with compromised renal function. It is well worth delaying the surgical treatment for a few days so that the patient can be rehydrated and renal function improved. During this time the stomach should be cleansed by repeated gastric lavage.

Table 4. Age distribution of patients undergoing surgery for cholelithiasis and choledocholithiasis May 1976–Aug 1981

Age	Cholecystectomy alone	Cholecystectomy and choledocholithotomy	Choledocholithotomy alone	Endoscopic choledocholithotomy
10+	2			
20+	29	4		4
30+	48	7		2
40+	49	7		8
50+	59	11	1	6
60+	62	23	2	14
70+	27	26	6	26
80+	5	5	4	12
90+		1	1	
Total	281	84	14	72

F. Gallstones

Cholelithiasis and choledocholithiasis are the most common gastroenterological conditions requiring abdominal operation in an elderly population. From Table 4 it is apparent that the most frequent age of presentation for cholelithiasis is the seventh decade of life and for choledocholithiasis the eight decade.

I. Cholelithiasis

Patients may present with flatulent dyspepsia, biliary colic, acute cholecystitis or empyema. Surgeons believe that the natural history of cholelithiasis with recurrent attacks of dyspepsia, colic, and infection indicates the need for operation in most patients. Occasionally, elderly patients may be unfit for surgery, but it must be remembered that elderly patients withstand infection badly and patients presenting with acute cholecystitis or empyema may suffer septicaemia. Recently, there has been considerable interest in the nonoperative treatment of gallstones but the long-term results of gallstone dissolution therapy appear to be disappointing (Ruppin and Dowling 1982). As most patients with stones in the gallbladder not only have lithogenic bile, but also have diseased gallbladders, cholecystectomy is usually indicated. As can be seen from Table 5 elective cholecystectomy carries a low morbidity and mortality, even in elderly patients.

It is rarely necessary to carry out the operation as a matter of urgency and emergency cholecystectomy should be reserved for patients with evidence of spreading peritonitis due to free perforation. In patients with acute cholecystitis with no evidence of spread of infection, early surgery within a few days does not seem to be particularly hazardous and often is not technically difficult. No obvious benefit has been demonstrated for either early or delayed cholecystectomy in this situation (Essenhigh 1968; Glenn 1977).

Cholecystostomy has been advanced as being particularly applicable to the treatment of acute cholecystitis and empyema of the gallbladder in elderly

Table 5. Mortality and morbidity following operations for cholelithiasis and choledocholithiasis May 1976–Aug 1981

	Cholecystectomy alone	Cholecystectomy and choledochotomy	Choledochotomy alone	Endoscopic choledochotomy
Total patients	281	84	14	72
Deaths	1	5	1	1
Pancreatitis	0	5	1	6
Septicaemia	2	11	2	4
Subphrenic abscess	1	4	1	0
Wound infection	21	19	3	0
Chest infection	24	15	3	0

patients (GLENN 1977), but most surgeons consider cholecystostomy inferior to cholecystectomy. Theoretical advantages of the former are not reflected in the reported mortality rate because, in common with other biliary operations in aged patients, the major cause of death is septicaemia. The only indication for cholecystostomy, rather than cholecystectomy, is gross inflammatory change wich renders anatomical dissection extremely hazardous with considerable danger of damaging the common duct. In the authors' experience, provided a surgeon of experience carries out the operation, this situation almost never pertains and in a long surgical experience, the authors have only been forced to this expedient on two occasions. There is no excuse for cholecystostomy being performed by a junior surgeon when cholecystectomy could be performed by a more experienced surgeon.

II. Choledocholithiasis

The morbidity and mortality due to choledocholithiasis is considerably greater than that associated with cholelithiasis at all ages. As with cholelithiasis, patients may present with flatulent dyspepsia or biliary colic, but a large number present with obstructive jaundice, cholangitis or pancreatitis. Patients with stones in the common bile duct are particularly prone to complications due to infection. Organisms can be cultured from bile in the ducts in approximately 90% of these patients (GALLAGHER et al. 1982). Although some patients with cholangitis respond to conservative management, many patients require urgent surgery before the infection can be controlled.

Stones can be removed from the common bile duct by either surgical choledocholithotomy or after endoscopic sphincterotomy. The results shown in Table 5 confirm previous reports that the mortality of exploration of the common bile duct is much greater than that following cholecystectomy alone and increases with age (MCSHERRY and GLENN 1980). However, mortality is only a part of the picture and it is evident from Table 5 that the incidence of septic complications following surgical choledocholithotomy is considerable. The mortality and morbidity associated with endoscopic sphincterotomy is much lower in our hands. We found that all stones were removed or passed spontaneously from the duct in 90%

of patients undergoing endoscopic sphincterotomy and in 94% of patients undergoing surgical choledocholithotomy (TWEEDLE and MARTIN 1981). The great majority of patients undergoing endoscopic sphincterotomy had already undergone cholecystectomy.

III. Cholelithiasis and Choledocholithiasis

What of patients who have cholelithiasis and choledocholithiasis? Many surgeons would argue that they should undergo cholecystectomy and choledocholithotomy at the same time. However, as the morbidity and mortality following surgery is largely due to stones in the duct, such patients might be treated better by preliminary endoscopic choledocholithotomy and subsequent surgical cholecystectomy (TWEEDLE and MARTIN 1981). More recently it has been the authors' practice in the very elderly patient to remove the stones from the duct by endoscopic means, but to leave the stones in the gallbladder. So far, only one patient has required subsequent cholecystectomy, but this study has been in progress for only 3 years and involves less than 50 patients.

When operating on an elderly patient with recurrent choledocholithiasis, it is important to ensure adequate duct drainage so that any further stones will pass. There is controversy as to whether choledochoduodenostomy or transduodenal sphincteroplasty is the best method to achieve this (BERLATSKY and FREUND 1981; JONES and SMITH 1952). It is difficult to compare these two procedures, but if choledochoduodenostomy is performed it should be located at the lowest possible point in the common duct so as to reduce the size of the "sump" and the incision should measure 2–3 cm so as to ensure adequate drainage and reduce the chance of stenosis. At operation for recurrent stones, some surgeons prefer to explore the common bile duct via the duodenum. A sphincteroplasty is performed and the stones removed from below. This procedure has the advantage that the sometimes difficult dissection needed to visualise the common bile duct is unnecessary. In patients with papillary stenosis and recurrent pancreatitis, sphincteroplasty is the operation of choice as the opening of the pancreatic duct may be in the stenosed ampulla and choledochoduodenostomy will not relieve the obstruction. The sphincteroplasty should be adequate in size, extending through the muscle coat of the duodenum so that the sphincter is divided and the opening at the lower end of the common bile duct is adequate. There is very little evidence to support the concept that cholangitis is an ascending phenomenon and much to suggest that it is a consequence of inadequate drainage of the duct. Both methods of draining the common bile duct may be performed without increasing the mortality or the morbidity of choledocholithotomy and the surgeon operating on an elderly patient should not be deterred from these procedures if they are indicated.

IV. Complications of Gallstones

1. Acute Pancreatitis

The commonest cause of acute pancreatitis in our practice is choledocholithiasis and consequently as might be expected from Table 4 the incidence of acute pancreatitis increases with age. A high intake of alcohol is the second most common aetiological factor, whilst postoperative or posttraumatic pancreatitis is uncommon, with a high mortality (TRAPNELL 1966). The mortality of acute pancreatitis also increases with age and the majority of patients die from pulmonary or renal failure. Surgical intervention is rarely indicated in the acute stage unless it is thought that unresolving pancreatitis is due to a stone impacted in the ampulla of Vater (KELLY 1980). However, we now remove such stones by endoscopic sphincterotomy (SAFRANY and COTTON 1981). At a later stage the surgeon may be required to drain a pancreatic abscess or pseudocyst.

2. Carcinoma of the Gallbladder

Carcinoma of the gallbladder is a rare tumour whose incidence increases greatly with age (Table 1). During the last years the mortality (which reflects the incidence as the condition is almost invariably and rapidly fatal) has decreased considerably in Britain, the United States and Canada, but has increased considerably in Sweden (DIEHL and BERAL 1981). Although it is often stated that gallstones are an important factor in the aetiology of this tumour, the evidence is inconclusive. The changing incidence in the countries discussed was inversely related to the changes in cholecystectomy rates, providing support for an aetiological role. However, the incidence of neoplasia is less than 2% in all the patients with cholelithiasis and long-term follow-up of patients with asympatomatic calculi has shown an incidence of less that 1% (LUND 1960; MCFARLANE and GLENN 1967). Attempted curative resection is possible in less than 10% of patients and the majority die within 6 months of diagnosis. If gallstones are an important aetiological factor in the development of carcinoma of the gallbladder it has been estimated that there would be one less death for every 100 cholecystectomies performed during the previous year (DIEHL and BERAL 1981). As the mortality of elective cholecystectomy in an aged population may exceed 1%, surgeons may ignore the possible potential for neoplasia when considering cholecystectomy in elderly patients.

G. Carcinoma of the Pancreas

Carcinoma of the pancreas occurs in 8 per 100,000 of the population in western Europe and its incidence is increasing. In 1971 it was the fifth most common cause of death from malignancy in Great Britain. The incidence increases with age (Table 1) and the majority of patients are now over the age of 60 years. When the carcinoma is in the head of the pancreas the patient usually presents with obstructive jaundice and weight loss. Some may be free of pain, but there is usually a history of persistent backache. A distended gallbladder is frequently palpable in the abdomen and the liver may also be palpable owing to cholestasis rather than metastatic disease. Diagnosis tends to be delayed if the tumour is in the body or tail of the pancreas because ill-defined back and abdominal pain may defy diagnosis until the disease is very advanced. These tumours are rare and clinical suspicion is necessary to initiate the appropriate investigations.

The development of ultrasonography, endoscopic retrograde pancreatography, computerised axial tomography and percutaneous transhepatic cholangiography has allowed the diagnosis to be made with far greater certainty before operation. Recently, preoperative tissue confirmation of the diagnosis has been achieved in many institutions by ultrasonically guided percutaneous needle biopsy (HANCKE et al. 1975). Histological confirmation of carcinoma of the head can be made with safety at operation by transduodenal biopsy (TWEEDLE 1979).

The majority of patients undergo some form of surgical procedure, but even with small tumours confined to the head of the pancreas, an attempted curative resection is a formidable procedure and the operative mortality of published series from experts in the field varies from 10% to 30%. A recent review of 61 publications involving 15,000 patients showed that, on average, 78% of patients underwent laparotomy, but in some hospitals less than 50% reached this stage. Only 11% underwent resection and 0.4% survived for 5 years (GUDJONSSON et al. 1978). The majority of elderly patients undergoing laparotomy for carcinoma of the pancreas have bypass operations rather than resection. Obstruction to the lower end of the common bile duct can be relieved by cholecystojejunostomy or choledochoduodenostomy. There is some disagreement as to whether gastrojejunostomy should always be performed at the same time to obviate future obstruction in the second part of the duodenum. We have found that 25% of patients palliated by simple bypass ultimately developed duodenal obstruction and so we recommend a gastrojejunostomy with a cholecystojejunostomy as a Roux loop. Patients with severe pain who are undergoing bypass operations may experience considerable relief following coeliac ganglionectomy although this may be a temporary phenomenon. The role of biliary decompression by prostheses inserted either percutaneously (HOEVELS 1978) or endoscopically (HUIBREGTSE and TYTGAT 1982) remains to be assessed.

H. Carcinoma of the Periampullary Region

This term is used by many to encompass malignant tumours arising in the second part of the duodenum, the ampulla of Vater or the intrapancreatic portion of the common bile duct. Periampullary tumours account for at least 25% of tumours in this region. The mortality from pancreaticoduodenectomy is the same whether it is carried out for a periampullary tumour or carcinoma of the head of the pancreas, but the long-term survival for the former is much better. The reported 5-year survival of 25% may justify radical resection in this group of patients (WARREN et al. 1975; FORREST and LONGMIRE 1979) and for this reason, histological diagnosis should always be obtained in patients with tumours in this region. Tumours of the ampulla of Vater often grow slowly and local resection with reanastomosis of the pancreatic and bile ducts to the duodenom may be possible.

J. Carcinoma of the Large Intestine

This is one of the commonest malignant processes and although it is a disease which may occasionally affect the younger patient, the main bulk of patients present in the older age groups (see Table 1). GOLIGHER (1941) showed that the maximum incidence was in the seventh decade whilst DE JODE (1982) showed that in his practice the maximum incidence was in the eighth decade.

The clinical presentation of patients with large bowel tumour depends on the site of the tumour. Typical presentation in the case of rectal carcinoma involves obvious passage of blood with a feeling of incomplete emptying which may amount to tenesmus. Left colonic tumours tend to present with an alteration in bowel habit which is frequently associated with manifest bleeding; abdominal pain of a colicky type is quite frequent due to partial obstruction and complete intestinal obstruction is most commonly seen in large bowel tumours of this situation. The patients with carcinoma of the right colon present with less specific symptoms, particularly anaemia and weight loss, without manifest alteration in bowel habit. Pain may occur in this group, but if so it gives the appearance of intermittent low small bowel colic. All elderly patients with unexplained anaemia, colicky abdominal pain, abdominal pain of less clearly specified nature of recent origin, alteration in the bowel habit or the passage of blood per rectum should be fully assessed.

Clinical examination may reveal a mass on abdominal palpation or may reveal a tumour palpable on rectal examination. Part of the clinical assessment of these patients is sigmoidoscopy with either a rigid instrument or a short flexible sigmoidoscope. Further assessment should be by double-contrast barium enema, supplemented in cases of doubt by bimanual examination under anaesthesia and/or colonoscopy.

One of the more common errors made by medical practitioners is to accept that the patient does not have large bowel disease because there is apparently normal radiology of the large bowel. It cannot be stressed too often that the majority of large bowel tumours are within the reach of either digital examination or the rigid sigmoidoscope so that digital and endoscopic assessments are essential. The development of the newer fibre optic instruments has allowed more refined endoscopic techniques to be used for assessing the colon. Nevertheless, it remains true that clinical awareness and persistence with investigation when there is a strong suspicion of a colonic lesion is much more important in terms of diagnostic accuracy than the sophistication of the equipment.

It is as well to be aware of the disease processes that may well be associated with a higher incidence of large bowel carcinoma. There is a slightly increased chance of large bowel malignancy in patients who have had gallbladder disease (LOWENFELS 1980), carcinoma of the breast or carcinoma of the endometrium (SCHOENBERG et al. 1969). Of more significance are the known premalignant conditions of long-standing ulcerative colitis and polyposis coli. Patients with ulcerative colitis require a surveillance programme after the disease has been present for 10 years and this is best effected by annual colonoscopy with biopsy so that if there is any suggestion of malignant transformation the appropriate surgery can be carried out. In polyposis coli the condition is invariably premalignant so that excisional surgery is indicated and it has usually been carried out before old age. Consideration of this disease raises the topic of the relationship of colonic malignancy to benign colonic tumours. Many pathologists believe that most carcinomas of the colon arise owing to malignant change in a preexisting adenoma

(MORSON 1974). There is no doubt that villous adenomas have a highly malignant potential, but simple tubular adenomas seem to be much less likely to undergo malignant transformation if they are small.

I. Colonic Adenomas

Simple tubular adenomas often produce no symptoms though they may present with colonic bleeding or descend through the anal canal and the patient complains of material prolapsing. Rarely they may initiate a colonic intussusception. Villous adenomas are frequently situated in the rectum or sigmoid colon where they produce a typical history of the frequent passage of mucoid diarrhoea owing to the excessive mucous production by such tumours. The story is quite typical and may, on rare occasions, be associated with hypokalaemia because of excessive potassium loss in the mucus. On rare occasions, the patient may present because of profound weakness from the hypokalaemia. Many villous tumours can be palpated per rectum, but they are often quite soft and very easily missed. The findings are much more abnormal on sigmoidoscopy than on palpation. Villous tumours may be localised but can spread, becoming circumferential and involving large areas of the rectum. Since malignant transformation in these tumours is so common, it is important to make this assessment before planning treatment. If the tumour is palpable, we have always found that an area of hardness within the tumour is a reflection of malignant change and such an area should be identified and investigated by multiple biopsies. If there is no hard area in the tumour then in all probability the tumour is benign, but it is still desirable that multiple biopsies are taken to confirm this.

1. Treatment

If a tubular adenoma has undergone malignant change, but it can be adequately excised through a normal stalk, then this type of treatment is satisfactory. If there is malignant change in a villous tumour then it should be treated as for as carcinoma. Benign adenomas can usually be readily removed either by transanal operation or by colonoscopic removal with a diathermy snare. Rarely, if an adenoma is at a flexure, it can be difficult to snare it and under these circumstances we advise removal at laparotomy via a colotomy in a fit patient, if the tumour is more than 1.5 cm in diameter. If the tumour is smaller and is producing little in the way of symptoms, or the patient is unfit, it seems a sensible policy to place the patient on endoscopic follow-up, though this situation is rare.

Benign villous tumours, if small, can be dealt with in the same fashion as tubular adenomas, but when the villous tumour is large, particularly if it occupies more than half the circumference of the bowel, formal surgical excision is necessary. If the tumour involves the rectum down to the upper anal canal, then a transanal submucous dissection, as described by PARKS (1968) can be used in many cases, but on some occasions it is necessary to carry out a posterior approach to the rectum as described by MASON (1972). If the lower rectum is not involved, then a circumferential tumour can be dealt with by an appropriate resection with anastomosis from the abdominal route.

II. Large Bowel Carcinoma

1. Prophylaxis

In patients who are at high risk, namely those with either established long-standing ulcerative colitis, or a strong family history of carcinoma of the colon, an annual colonoscopy surveillance programme is required. At this colonoscopy biopsies should be taken and any adenoma found should be removed. It is more difficult to know whether a surveillance programme is justified in the general population. There has been strong advocacy for the use of Hemoccult to detect occult blood in the faeces to give a subgroup on whom colonoscopy would be valuable and groups in Germany (FRUHMORGEN 1978) and the United States (WINAWER 1980) have produced results to support this. However, using Hemoccult to screen populations in England has produced very poor yields in the three studies which have presently been reported (MILLION et al 1980; HARDCASTLE et al. 1980; FARRANDS et al. 1981). It is our impression that screening the general population by Hemoccult is not cost-effective.

2. Treatment of Carcinoma of the Colon

The majority of patients which colonic carcinoma are treated by conventional excision, which in the left colon is either sigmoid colectomy or left hemicolectomy with a high tie of the appropriate artery of supply, and in the right-sided lesions a right hemicolectomy. We tend to use a high tie because it makes mobilisation of the colon easier, rather than because of any advantage that it might confer in terms of long-term survival. Primary end-to-end anastomosis is satisfactory and with modern techniques anastomotic leakage should be very rare other than in very low anterior resection. Since the low anterior resections seem to be particularly at risk, it has been our policy to cover this type of operation by means of a defunctioning dependent loop colostomy (SCHOFIELD et al. 1980).

It should be borne in mind that some patients have multiple carcinomas of the colon. The usually quoted incidence of multiple tumours, that is 3% synchronous and 3% metachronous (BUSSEY et al. 1967) is lower than that which we have observed. Indeed, in our practice we have found that 12% of patients with large bowel carcinoma have synchronous tumours. It seems likely that this is due to patients with carcinoma of the colon having multiple polyps, more than one of which undergoes malignant change. It is certainly important to recognise these patients during investigation, for we feel that there is a definite place for total colectomy and ileorectal anastomosis in patients who have either multiple carcinomas or carcinoma with many adenomas. In fact, this operation does not appear to throw any greater strain on the patient than the ordinary segmental resection. The problems of colorectal surgery chiefly arise from sepsis and this can be minimised by operating on an empty colon produced by total gut irrigation and the routine use of peroperative antibiotics.

3. Treatment of Rectal Carcinoma

The standard methods of surgical treatment of carcinoma of the rectum are still abdominoperineal excision of the rectum with terminal colostomy, and anterior resection of the rectum. It is clear that carcinomas in the rectal ampulla have to be treated by abdominoperineal resection. Equally clearly, patients with tumours in the upper third of the rectum should be treated by anterior resection. The difficulty lies in the patients with tumours in the middle third of the rectum, that is between 6 and 10 cm from the anal verge. Provided an adequate excision of such a tumour can be carried out, removing the malignant tissue with a reasonable clearance of normal tissue, anterior resection is desirable, but may be technically difficult. In the past, the technical difficulties have been overcome by various types of pull-through procedure but the development of mechanical circular stapling devices has made very low anastomosis between the rectum and colon much easier and since the advent of this instrument, it has largely replaced pull-through procedures. Undoubtedly stapling has increased the numbers of reconstructive resections which the surgeon is now willing to attempt (HEALD 1980). In the last few years in our practice, the number of abdominoperineal resections has fallen from a little under 50% to a little over 30% of the rectal carcinomas treated, owing to the improved facility for doing very low anterior resections.

4. Other Methods

Occasionally it may be justified to use local treatment for carcinoma of the rectum. The local methods available are local excision (MORSON et al. 1977) local diathemy destruction (CRILE and TURNBULL 1972) and endorectal contact radiotherapy (PAPILLON 1975). Local excision is suitable for malignant change in a polyp and may be useful in some small sessile lesions which are apparently confined to the mucosa. Diathermy destruction should only be used if the tumour occupies less than one-third of the circumference of the rectum and is less than 3 cm in its greatest diameter. If larger tumours than these are treated, the results are poor even in terms of palliation, but in the very poor risk patient with the small lesion, the method can produce good palliation with a moderate prospect of longer-term survival. Provided the cases are satisfactorily selected, endocavity contact radiotherapy, as suggested by PAPILLON (1975) of Lyon, has been shown to produce good long-term results. It should be emphasised however, that only a very small subgroup of patients with carcinoma of the rectum are suitable for local treatment.

5. Supplementary Treatment

As an adjuvant to surgery, radiotherapy has been used both before and after operation for carcinoma of the rectum. The present available evidence suggests that low dosage preoperative radiotherapy offers little benefit (MEDICAL RESEARCH COUNCIL 1982) but the early results from a number of studies suggest that rather higher dosage radiotherapy to the locally advanced rectal tumour may be combined with surgery to advantage (MITTELMAN 1980). Low dosage radiotherapy has not been associated with any increased morbidity or mortality, but the higher dosage schedules may make anterior resection more hazardous, though there is, as yet, insufficient data on this point (ROMSDAHL and WITHERS 1978).

Chemotherapy, either with single agents or by combination, does not seem to offer significant advantage to the patient with colorectal cancer and is of little value in the treatment of recurrent disease (MANSOUR et al. 1980).

K. Anal Tumours

Malignant tumours of the anal canal and perianal region are much less common than carcinoma of the rectum. Most of these tumours are squamous cell carcinomas though occasionally a true basal cell carcinoma is seen in the perianal skin. The anal canal may be involved by a downgrowth of an adenocarcinoma or be involved by the rare cloacogenic carcinoma or malignant melanoma. Pretreatment biopsy is essential. Small squamous cell carcinomas of the perianal skin or of the anal canal (less than 3 cm) can be treated locally by either excision or implantation of appropriate radio isotopes. Larger anal canal tumours, adenocarcinomas, cloacogenic carcinomas and malignant melanomas should be treated by abdominoperineal excision. Although some have reported good results by adding mitomycin C treatment to radiotherapy we have not found any additional benefit from chemotherapy.

L. Diverticular Disease

Diverticular disease of the colon shows great variation in incidence in different countries, which is believed to be due to dietary rather than genetic factors. In the United Kingdom and the rest of western Europe, where the diet tends to produce little residue, diverticular disease is common. Indeed, at the age of 60 years, one-third of the population have diverticular disease and at the age of 80 years, more than half of the population have diverticular disease (PARKS 1968). Fortunately, this disease is usually asymptomatic, but symptoms may occur in the absence of inflammation, owing to associated colonic spasm with the production of high intraluminal pressure. The diverticula are produced because of this increased intraluminal pressure which causes the formation of so-called false diverticula at points of weakness in the colonic muscle wall. Thus, the diverticula are outpouchings of the colonic mucosa through the muscular wall of the colon. Associated with the outpouchings it is usual to see moderate muscle hypertrophy in the colon.

Most commonly the diverticula are concentrated in the sigmoid loop with perhaps scattered diverticula elsewhere in the colon, but less commonly the diverticula are more evenly distributed throughout the whole of the colon. Since diverticular disease is so common in the older patient, it presents a considerable problem to know whether symptoms should be ascribed to diverticular disease. Indeed, in the absence of complications of the diverticular disease, it should be understood that any symptoms arising in diverticular disease are due to the increased intraluminal tension and colonic spasm rather than to the diverticula themselves. Uncomplicated diverticular disease may be associated with ill-defined abdominal pain with perhaps some alteration in the bowel habit, but is not associated with bleeding. These patients should be fully screened to exclude any other colonic pathology, but once this has been done they should be managed conservatively with advice about high residue diet and bran supplements. If these measures are pursued enthusiastically it is unusual for there to be indication for operative treatment for uncomplicated diverticular disease. The few cases that do come to surgery are best dealt with by complete resection of the sigmoid colon with the anastomosis being made between the mobilised descending colon and the upper rectum. Some years ago, REILLY (1965) suggested longitudinal division of the hypertrophied colonic muscle as an operative treatment. Although myotomy does appear to produce short-term reductions of intraluminal pressure, these improvements do not persist. The procedure is not without the hazard of perforation and since the morbidity and mortality is little different from the more certain sigmoid colectomy, the procedure has fallen out of favour with most surgeons. Attempts to modify the procedure have not received any general acceptance.

The usual reasons for surgery in diverticular disease are the development of complications and although these complications are relatively rare, they are important causes of serious problems in the elderly. The particular complications that we see are those due to infection and massive bleeding.

I. Infective Complications

The area of diverticular disease which becomes infected is almost invariably the sigmoid colon and when this occurs, the patient will get more severe pain localised to the left iliac fossa, often associated with an attack of diarrhoea, possibly followed by constipation. The patient may be pyrexial and abdominal examination usually shows tenderness in the left lower quadrant. This type of problem will often settle down with a short course of antibiotics and is not an indication for surgery. However, if the inflammation worsens, surgery may be indicated. Situations which may require surgical treatment are the development of a localised abscess, evidence of spreading peritonitis and fistula formation. If there is evidence of a spreading peritonitis then the patient should have an emergency laparotomy at which it may be found that there is a purulent or a faeculent peritonitis. The operative strategies for dealing with this problem have ranged through simple drainage of the pelvis with repair of any perforation, drainage of the pelvis with a transverse colostomy, excision of the diverticular mass with end colostomy and closure of the rectal stump, to excision with primary anastomosis. In the very ill patient with faecal peritonitis or with a large fixed abscess we are inclined to drain the pelvis and carry out a proximal dependent loop colostomy, but in most instances we feel that excision of the inflamed sigmoid colon is the best policy. In our view, when there is gross sepsis it is unreasonable to carry out a primary anastomosis so we close the rectum and bring out the proximal colon as a colostomy. The second stage procedure after this operation is to reestablish intestinal continuity. This may be technically difficult, but frequently it is surprisingly easy, provided adequate time has been left for the sepsis to resolve, say 6 months. The reconnection procedure has been made much easier since the introduction of the circular stapling devices which can be passed through the rectum and which make anastomosis to the mobilised left colon relatively easy. The main point which should be emphasised in all anastomoses for diverticular disease is that the suture line should definitely be in the upper rectum with no area of lower sigmoid unresected because this tends to produce recurrent problems.

II. Fistulas

Infection in diverticular disease may produce an enterocutaneous fistula to the skin of the abdominal wall or to the buttocks through the ischiorectal fossa. It may produce a colovaginal or colovesical fistula. Fistulas to the vagina may produce relatively minor leakage and can sometimes be managed conservatively, but most external fistulas and virtually all colovesical fistulas require surgical treatment. In our experience, about 80% of colovesical fistulas are due to diverticular disease, 15% are due to carcinoma, usually colonic, and only a few are due to other inflammatory bowel disease. If colovesical fistulas are not treated surgically, the patient gets recurring urinary tract infections, which in many instances become life-threatening as well as unpleasant. Treatment is by excision of the sigmoid colon together with its diverticular disease with the adherent bladder wall, which usually is a relatively small amount of the bladder near its dome. The bladder can be closed easily with two layers of catgut and drained postoperatively by a urinary catheter. The usual anastomosis between the mobilised left colon and the upper rectum is easily carried out. If possible, the omentum should be positioned between the suture line in the bladder and the suture line in the upper rectum. If there has to be extensive dissection in the pelvis then the operation is covered by a dependent loop colostomy which is closed at 8 weeks. Usually it is not necessary to fashion a colostomy and the operation is carried out in one stage.

III. Massive Bleeding

Massive colonic bleeding in the elderly is an unusual problem, but for many years the principal cause has been felt to be bleeding associated with generalised diverticular disease and most often bleeding has occurred from the right colon. The recognition of angiodysplasia (WHITEHOUSE 1973) which appears to affect the right colon in the elderly patient and produce massive bleeding, has introduced another dimension to this problem. However, the recognition of this pathology has not in any significant way changed the clinical management. Our policy when an elderly patient comes in with apparent colonic bleeding of a massive nature is first to resuscitate the patient by adequate blood transfusion and then to establish that there is no upper gastrointestinal cause for the bleeding by an emergency gastroduodenoscopy. We fell this is a very important early step in the diagnosis for when gastrointestinal bleeding is massive, the nature of the blood passing per rectum can be quite misleading as to the site of the bleed and on several occasions we have felt, on clinical grounds, quite confident that we were dealing with a colonic bleed, only to find that on endoscopy the patient had a chronic duodenal ulcer, which was the source of the problem. Once we have established that the bleeding is colonic, the next step in management depends on whether the patient continues to bleed. If, after transfusion of 4–5 U blood, the patient is still not stable, then we go straight to emergency angiography to locate the source of bleeding preparatory to surgery. This group represents less than 10% of the patients who come in with a massive colonic bleed, for in our practice most patients stop bleeding shortly after admission. In the majority of patients who stop bleeding, angiography is not useful unless they have a further bleed. Indeed, we only submit patients to angiography when we have decided that they require surgery. This group of patients is taken from the angiographic suite to theatre and the appropriate operation is carried out. Usually the bleeding point is demonstrated in the right colon, when a right hemicolectomy is performed. If angiography does not localise the bleeding, then a total colectomy with ileostomy and mucous fistula is the procedure of choice.

In the major group of patients bleeding stops; then they are left under observation and investigation is by barium enema on day 1 and colonoscopy after 4 or 5 days. We have found that attempting to carry out colonoscopy at an early stage does not produce useful information because of the residual blood in the colon. The only difficulty of this form of management is the few patients who rebleed shortly after the barium study, for this can complicate angiography.

If the colonoscopy reveals stigmata indicating angiodysplasia, then this can be dealt with by diathermy or laser photocoagulation, though there is no real evidence that this is useful in preventing subsequent bleeds. In our experience, most patients recover from their bleed and go for long periods before they have a subsequent problem and it has not been our policy to suggest interventional surgery in these patients after a first bleed. If, however, the bleeding is recurrent and massive, it may be that the lesser risk is to carry out a total colectomy, though this is never a very satisfactory solution, for these patients are often aged and barely fit for such major surgery.

M. Colitis in the Elderly

Inflammatory bowel disease, either Crohn's disease or ulcerative colitis, is most often a disease of the young. However, a small proportion of patients who appear to have inflammatory bowel disease present with their first symptoms over the age of 60 years (Carr and Schofield 1982). There can be little doubt that some of these patients do have true inflammatory bowel disease. It is usually confined to the colon and in our practice localised Crohn's disease, particularly Crohn's proctitis, is the commonest variety. Although it is usual for the older patient to have a relatively localised colitis or proctitis, when there is a total or subtotal colitis the disease is often severe. Our own experience accords with that of Watts et al. (1966) when he reports a mortality of more than 20% associated with an acute attack of total colitis over the age of 60 years. These patients are much more prone to complications, e.g. massive bleeding, perforation and toxic dilation. Unfortunately, because of the patient's age, surgery tends to be withheld and it seems to us that the only way to improve the high mortality in this group of patients would be to be more aggressive with regard to surgical treatment.

On the other hand, ischaemic colitis is a disease which usually affects the older patient with hypertension (Marston et al. 1966). Clinically the patient has a sudden attack of abdominal pain with diarrhoea and bleeding. The most usual site for colonic ischaemia is near the splenic flexure, but other areas in the colon may be involved and, indeed, the colon can be widely affected by an ischaemic process which is difficult to distinguish from inflammatory bowel disease. The blood supply of the colon is derived from the branches of the superior and inferior mesenteric arteries which anastomose and send straight vessels to supply the colon. In the usual type of ischaemic colitis it is felt that it is these vasa recta which become blocked and produce ischaemia. There are three potential outcomes to the reduced flow produced by vessel blockage: one is complete necrosis of the colonic wall; the second is colonic ischaemia with resolution, producing a fibrous colonic stricture; and the third is ulceration of the colonic mucosa with subsequent complete recovery. If necrosis occurs, the patient will present with signs of peritonitis and would require an appropriate resection of the bowel, but the usual ischaemic colitis patient resolves without surgery and the diagnosis is only confirmed if adequate barium contrast radiology is carried out within the first couple of weeks. If subsequent symptoms develop, then consideration has to be given to either removal or bypassing of a stricture, if present.

N. Rectal Prolapse and Incontinence

Rectal prolapse may be partial or total. Partial prolapse occurs when rectal mucosa prolapses through the anal sphincter, which is associated with excessive straining. This is to be distinguished from prolapsing haemorrhoids and from total rectal prolapse. Provided the practitioner insists on seeing the prolapse, there really is no difficulty in distinguishing between mucosal and total prolapse. Total rectal prolapse occurs predominantly in childhood and old age and there are very few cases in younger adults. Indeed, in adults in our practice, the problem is seen almost entirely in elderly women and the average age in the 80 patients that we have operated on is in the late 70s.

Partial anal prolapse can be dealt with adequately by local anal operations; in minor degrees of prolapse by injection, but in more major degrees of prolapse by excision as for haemorrhoids. The patient needs to be instructed about straining if the condition is not to recur. As far as total prolapse is concerned, local anal operations are valueless. Some 25 years ago, one of us had the opportunity to review the figures from 50 Tiersch operations of encirclement of the anus with silver wire, carried out for total rectal prolapse by an expert anal surgeon. The patients suffered problems from faecal impaction owing to the wire being too tight, persisting prolapse, ulceration of the wire knot and many other problems, so that in fact within 1 year of operation, 46 of the patients had had the wire removed. We cannot believe that the operation will be much more satisfactory if other materials are used for it seems illogical to attempt to prevent a total prolapse which is, in effect, an intussusception, by any operation at the outlet. The rectum must be pulled up by some abdominal operation.

It is significant that abdominal operations for rectal prolapse are well tolerated by the elderly and we have not had a single death in the 80 elderly patients in whom we have carried out an abdominal repair. The abdominal operations for total rectal prolapse must involve the removal of the deep pouch of pelvic peritoneum and the fixing of the rectum to the sacrum, either by an Ivalon (polyvinyl alcohol) sponge (WELLS 1959) or by Mersilene (braided polyester) mesh. We prefer the latter, the so-called RIPSTEIN (1965) method, in which a 2–3 cm band of Mersilene is passed loosely round the mid to low rectum and fastened as a sling to the midsacrum immediately above the levatores ani. The results from this procedure are eminently satisfactory. Of the 80 operations, 79 have been satisfactory in controlling the prolapse and the single recurrence is easily managed by the patient.

Most of the patients that we see with this problem are worried by the prolapse rather than by any associated incontinence. Indeed, when the prolapse is repaired, continence which is satisfactory to the individual is usual in most instances, either immediately or within a few weeks, but a few patients do have persisting troublesome incontinence.

Incontinence in the elderly is a subject which requires considered attention. It may be due to overflow from faecal impaction, it may be due to neurological disease, colonic disease or it may be idiopathic. A patient who is less active and on a more restricted diet with aging, may develop constipation, rectal inertia and a tendency to overflow diarrhoea because the anal spincter is reflexly relaxed owing to the full rectum. If this is the problem, then adequate emptying of the rectum of the hard stool and clearing of the colon, together with dietary advice and possibly the use of suppositories will relieve the problem. When the problem is due to neurological, colonic, rectal or anal disease, then the treatment should be directed towards the cause. However, there is a small subgroup of elderly patients where no cause can be demonstrated which properly can be called idiopathic. The sphincter muscles are lax and there is no anal reflex. If pressure measurements are made of the sphincters, there is little demonstrable tone and the few patients with persisting incontinence after rectal prolapse repair seem to have the same physiological disturbance. This group of patients respond well to the operation of postanal repair, that is dissection behind the anus between the internal and external sphincters and plication of the muscles of the pelvic floor behind the rectum. There are very few patients whose rectal incontinence is truly idiopathic, but in this small number the results of postanal repair have been satisfactory. PARKS (1977), who described the repair and who has reported a large series, finds the operation satisfactory in 80%–90% of cases.

References

Allan R, Dykes P (1976) A study of the factors influencing mortality rates from gastrointestinal haemorrhage. Q J Med 45:533–559

Atkinson M (1967) Hiatus hernia. Br Med J 4:218–221

Atkinson M, Ferguson R (1977) Fibreoptic endoscopic palliative intubation of inoperable oesophagogastric neoplasms. Br Med J 1:266–267

Berlatsky U, Freund H (1981) Choledochoduodenostomy in the treatment of benign biliary tract disease. Am J Surg 141:90–93

Brookes VS, Waterhouse JAH, Powells DJ (1965) Carcinoma of the stomach: A 10 year survey of the results and of the factors affecting prognosis. Br Med J 1:1577–1583

Bussey HJR, Wallace MH, Morson BC (1967) Metachronous carcinoma of the large intestinal and intestinal polyps. Proc R Soc Med 60:208–210

Cade D, Allan D (1979) Longterm follow-up of patients with gastric ulcer treated by vagotomy, pyloroplasty and ulcerectomy. Br J Surg 66:46–47
Carr N, Schofield PF (1982) Inflammatory bowel disease in the older patient. Br J Surg 69:223–225
Castleman B (1936) Extension of gastric carcinoma into the duodenum. Ann Surg 103:348–352
Collis JL (1971) Surgical treatment of carcinoma of the oesophagus and cardia. Br J Surg 58:801–804
Crile G, Turnbull RB (1972) The role of electrocoagulation in the treatment of carcinoma of the rectum. Surg Gynaecol Obstet 135:391–396
Dark JF, Mousalli H, Vaughan R (1981) Surgical treatment of carcinoma of the oesophagus. Thorax 36:891–895
DeMeester TR, Johnson LF, Joseph GJ, Toscano MS, Hall AW, Skinner DB (1976) Patterns of gastroesophageal reflux in health and disease. Ann Surg 184:459–470
Diehl AK, Beral V (1981) Cholecystectomy and changing mortality from gallbladder cancer. Lancet II:187–189
Essenhigh DM (1968) Perforation of the gallbladder. Br J Surg 55:175–178
Farrands PA, Griffiths RL, Britton DC (1981) The Frome experiment – value of screening for colo-rectal cancer. Lancet I:1231–1232
Forrest JF, Longmire WP (1979) Carcinoma of the pancreas and periampullary region. Ann Surg 189:129–138
Fruhmorgen P (1978) In: Grundmann E (ed) Colon cancer. Fischer, Stuttgart, p 127
Gallagher P, Ostick G, Jones D, Schofield PF, Tweedle DEF (1982) Intraoperative microscopy of bile – is it useful? Br J Surg 69:473–474
Glenn F (1977) Cholecystectomy in the high risk patients with biliary tract disease. Ann Surg 185:185–191
Goligher JC (1941) The operability of carcinoma rectum. Br Med J 2:393–397
Gudjonsson B, Livston EM, Spiro HM (1978) Cancer of the pancreas. Cancer 42:2494–2506
Hancke S, Holm HH, Koch F (1975) Ultrasonically guided percutaneous fine needle biopsy of the pancreas. Surg Gynaecol Obstet 140:361–364
Hardcastle JD, Balfour TW, Amar SS (1980) Screening for symptomless colorectal cancers by testing for occult blood in general practice. Lancet I:791–793
Heald RJ (1980) Towards fewer colostomies – the impact of circular stapling devices in a district hospital. Br J Surg 67:201–202
Heggaty MM, Schofield PF, Grime R (1973) The management of upper gastrointestinal tract haemorrhage. Br J Surg 60:275–279
Hoare AM (1980) Endoscopic diagnosis. Br J Hosp Med 23:347–356
Hoevels J, Lunderguist A, Ihse J (1978) Percutaneous transhepatic intubation of bile duct for combined internal-external drainage in preoperative and palliative treatment of obstructive jaundice. Gastrointest Radiol 3:23–31
Huibregtse K, Tytgat GN (1982) Palliative treatment of obstructive jaundice by transpapillary introduction of large bore bile duct endoprosthesis. Gut 23:371–375
Imanaga H, Nakazato H (1977) Results of surgery for gastric cancer and effect of adjuvant Mitomycin "C" on cancer recurrence. World J Surg 1:213–221
Inberg MV, Heinonen R, Rantakokko V, Viikari SJ (1975) Surgical treatment of gastric carcinoma: A regional study of 2,590 patients after a 27 year period. Arch Surg 110:703–707
Jode LR de (1982) Prospects in large bowel cancer. J R Soc Med 75:301–302
Johansen AA (1976) Early gastric cancer in current topics in pathology. In: Morson BC (ed) Pathology of the gastrointestinal tract. Springer, Berlin Heidelberg New York, p 1
Johnson IR, Balfour RQ, Bourke JB (1976) Intubation of malignant gastroesophageal strictures. J R Coll Surg Edinb 21:225–228
Jones SA, Smith LL (1952) Transduodenal sphincteroplasty for recurrent pancreatitis. Ann Surg 136:937–947
Kaplan MS, List JW, Stemmer EA, Connolly JE (1972a) Surgical management of peptic ulcer disease in the aged patient. Arch Surg 104:667–671

Kaplan MS, List JW, Stemmer EA, Connolly JE (1972 b) Surgical management of upper gastrointestinal bleeding in the aged patient. Am J Gastroenterol 58:109–123
Kelly TR (1980) Gallstone pancreatitis: the timing of surgery. Surgery 88:345–350
Laurence BH, Vallon AG, Cotton PB, Armengol Miro JR, Salord Oses JC, Le Bodiac L, Sudry P, Fruhmorgen P, Bodem F (1980) Endoscopic laser photocoagulation for bleeding peptic ulcers. Lancet I:124–125
Leuz CA, Haeck W (1972) Peptic ulcer surgery in the elderly in a community hospital. Mich Med 71:613–614
Lowenfels AB (1980) Gallstones and the risk of cancer. Gut 21:1090–1092
Lund J (1960) Surgical indications in cholelithiasis; prophylactic cholelithiasis; prophylactic cholecystectomy elucidated on the basis of long-term follow-up on 526 non-operated cases. Ann Surg 151:153–162
MacLeod IA, Mills PR, MacKenzie JF, Joffe SN, Russell RI, Carter DC (1983) Neodymium yttrium aluminium garnet laser photocoagulation for major haemorrhage from peptic ulcers and single vessels: a single blind controlled study. Br Med J 286:345–348
Mansour EG, MacIntyre JM, Johnson R, Lerner HJ, Muggia FM (1980) Adjuvant studies in colorectal carcinoma: Experience of the Eastern Co-operative Oncology Group (ECOG). Preliminary report. In: Gerard A (ed) Progress and perspectives in the treatment of gastrointestinal tumour. Pergamon, Oxford, p 68
Marston A, Pheils MT, Thomas ML, Morson BC (1966) Ischaemic colitis. Gut 7:1–10
Martin DF, Hollanders D, May SJ, Ravenscroft MM, Tweedle DEF, Miller JP (1981) Differences in relapse rates of duodenal ulcer after healing with Cimetidine or Tripotassium Dicitrato Bismuthate. Lancet I:7–10
Mason AY (1972) Trans-sphincteric exposure of the rectum. Ann R Coll Surg Engl 51:320–331
McFarlane JR, Glenn F (1967) Carcinoma in choledochal cyst. J A M A 202:1003–1006
McKeown KC (1976) Total three stage oesophagectomy for carcinoma of the oesophagus. Br J Surg 63:259–268
McSherry CK, Glenn F (1980) The incidence and causes of death following surgery for non-malignant biliary tract disease. Ann Surg 191:271–275
Medical Research Council (1982) A trial of pre-operative radiotherapy in the management of operable rectal cancer. Br J Surg 67:775–780
Miller C (1961) Carcinoma of thoracic oesophagus and cardia. Br J Surg 49:507–522
Million R, Howarth J, Turnberg E, Turnberg LA (1980) Faecal occult blood screening in general practice. Gut 21:921
Mittelman A (1980) Adjuvant chemotherapy and radiotherapy following rectal surgery. An interim report from the Gastrointestinal Tumour Study Group (GITSG). In: Gerard A (ed) Progress and perspectives in the treatment of gastrointestinal tumours. Pergamon, Oxford, p 61
Morson BC (1974) Evolution of cancer of the colon and rectum. Cancer 34:845–849
Morson BC, Bussey HRJ, Samourian S (1977) Policy of local excision for early cancer of the rectum. Gut 18:1045–1050
Muller JJ, Brenner U, Dienst C, Pichlmaier H (1981) Preoperative parenteral feeding in patients with gastrointestinal carcinoma. Lancet I:68–70
Muto M, Maki T, Majuna S, Yamaguchi I (1968) Improvement in the end results of surgical treatment of gastric cancer. Surgery 63:229–235
Nakayama K (1968) Atlas of Gastrointestinal Surgery. Lippincott, Philadelphia, p 167
Nissen R (1956) Eine einfache Operation zur Beeinflussung der Refluxoesophagitis. Schweiz Med Wochenschr 86:590
Office of population census and surveys (1975) Cancer mortality in England and Wales, 1911–1970. Studies on medical and population subjects No 29. Her Majesty's Stationery Office, London, pp 20–35
Papillon J (1975) Intracavity irradiation of early rectal cancer for cure: a review of 186 cases. Cancer 36:696–701
Parks AG (1968) A technique for excising extensive villous papillomatous change in the lower rectum. Proc R Soc Med 61:441–442

Parks AG (1977) Postanal pelvic floor repair. In: Todd IP (ed) Colon, rectum and anus, 3rd edn: Operative Surgery. Butterworths, London, p 249
Parks TG (1968) Post-mortem studies on the colon with special reference to diverticular disease. Proc R Soc Med 61:932–934
Pearson JG (1971) The value of radiotherapy in the management of squamous oesophageal cancer. Br J Surg 58:794–798
Price S, Castell DO (1978) Esophageal mythology J A M A 240:44–46
Reilly M (1965) Sigmoid myotomy. Clin Gastroenterol 4:121–145
Ripstein CB (1965) Surgical cure of massive rectal prolapse. Dis Colon Rectum 8:34–38
Romsdahl MW, Withers HR (1978) Radiotherapy combined with curative surgery. Its use as therapy for carcinoma of the sigmoid colon and rectum. Ann Surg 113:446–453
Royston CMS, Dowling BL, Gear MWL (1976) Oesophageal dilatation using the Eder Puestow dilators. Am J Surg 131:697–700
Ruppin D, Dowling H (1982) Is recurrence inevitable after gallstone dissolution by bile-acid treatment? Lancet I:181–185
Safrany L, Cotton P (1981) A preliminary report: Urgent duodenoscopic sphincterotomy for acute gallstone pancreatitis. Surgery 89:424–428
Schoenberg BS, Greenberg RA, Eisenberg H (1969) Occurrence of certain multiple cancers in females. J Natl Cancer Inst 43:15–32
Schofield PF, Cade D, Lambert ME (1980) Dependent loop colostomy: Does it defunction the distal colon? Br J Surg 67:201–202
Stanciu C, Bennett JR (1974) Alginate/Antacid in the reduction of gastro-oesophageal reflux. Lancet I:109–111
Swain CP, Brown SG, Salmon PR, Kirkham JS, Northfield TC (1983) Controlled trial of Nd YAG laser photocoagulation in bleeding peptic ulcers. Gut 24:967
Takagi K (1981) The incidence of early gastric cancer since the advant of endoscopy. In: Fielding JWL, Newman CE, Ford CHJ, Jones BG (eds) Gastric Cancer. Pergamon, Oxford, p 159 (Advances in the biosciences, vol 32)
Thompson MR (1980) Indomethacin and perforated duodenal ulcer. Br Med J 1:448
Trapnell JE (1966) The natural history and prognosis of acute pancreatitis. Ann R Coll Surg Engl 38:265–287
Tweedle DEF (1979) Peroperative transduodenal biopsy of the pancreas. Gut 20:992
Tweedle DEF, Martin DF (1981) Choledocholithiasis – surgical or endoscopic lithotomy? Gut 22:888
Van Andel JG, Dees J, Dijkhuis CM, Fokkens W, Van Houten H, De Jong PC, Van Woerkom-Eykenboom WMH (1979) Carcinoma of the oesophagus – results of treatment. Ann Surg 190:684–689
Warren KW, Choe DS, Plaza J, Relihan M (1975) Results in radical resection for periampullary cancer. Ann Surg 181:534–540
Watts JM, Watkinson G, Goligher JC (1966) Early course of ulcerative colitis. Gut 7:16–31
Wellington JL, Lynn RB (1966) Thoracic surgery in the elderly. Canad Med Assoc J 95:252–256
Wells C (1959) New operation for rectal prolapse. Proc R Soc Med 52:602–603
Whitehouse GH (1973) Solitary angiodysplastic lesions in the ileo-caecal region diagnosed by angiography. Gut 14:977–982
Winawer SJ (1980) Screening for colo-rectal cancer: an overview. Cancer 45:1093–1098

Surgery in Old Age-Fractures

J.K. WEBB

A. Introduction

The ever-increasing geriatric population has led to greater concern for the management of fractures and in particular the development of ideas and solutions to these problems. In Great Britain the population over 65 has increased by 800,000 in the past decade, causing a major financial crisis in surgical centres. The North American continent faces similar problems in that 1 person in 9 is over 65; by the year 2000 this figure is expected to be 1 in 8.

The elderly person is less mobile and often, despite successful treatment of the fracture is a failure in terms of returning to the community. The fracture is just one more insult to the aged patient and the associated complications may lead to the demise of the patient, in spite of the most sophisticated medical care.

The principle of care remains the same in the elderly as the young: union of the fracture and return to normal function. The goal may be difficult to achieve, but one for which we must strive!

The ability to predict the outcome of the patient following fractures is difficult. The primary mortality within one month of surgery is approximately 15% –20% (RISKA 1970). Routine medical and mental assessment in the elderly should allow the surgeon to judge what treatment would benefit the patient and whether an operation is indicated: the patient's age is the most significant factor, but operative technique and duration of operation affect the mortality: arguably the more skilled surgeon should operate on the most elderly.

The elderly patient must be fully assessed before surgery and in an ideal world, should be seen by a geriatric team and associated medical conditions treated (SYLVESTER et al. 1977). Little evidence exists to suggest a few days delay before surgery increases the morbidity or mortality, especially if cardio-vascular problems can be controlled during this time. The Nottingham Ortho-Geriatric Unit reported that the period in hospital was reduced by 27% when a combined approach was applied (BOYD et al. 1982). The assessment of the fracture is of paramount importance, and in the elderly we must exclude underlying causes, particularly those metabolic factors which predispose to fractures. These insufficiency fractures include

Osteoporosis
Osteomalacia
Paget's Disease
Rheumatoid Arthritis
Fibrous Dysplasia
Osteopetrosis
Scurvy
Post-radiation
Hyper-parathyroidism.

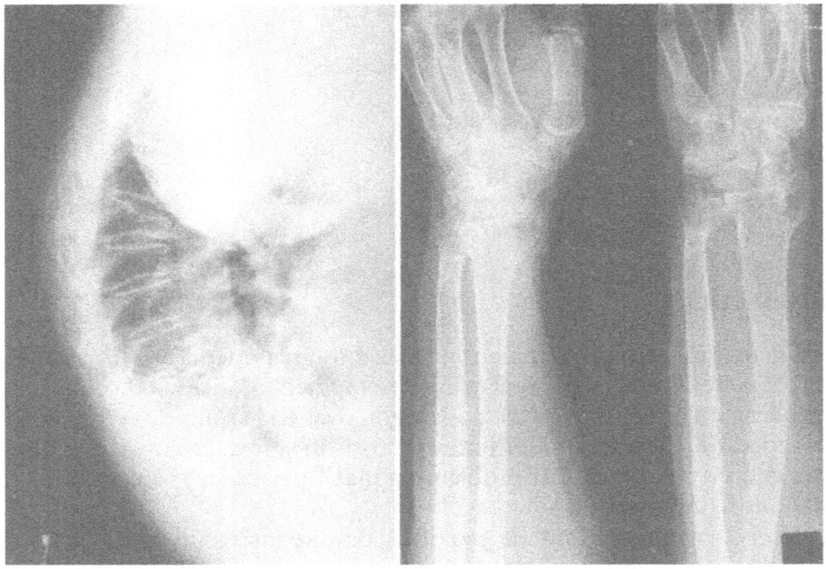

a b

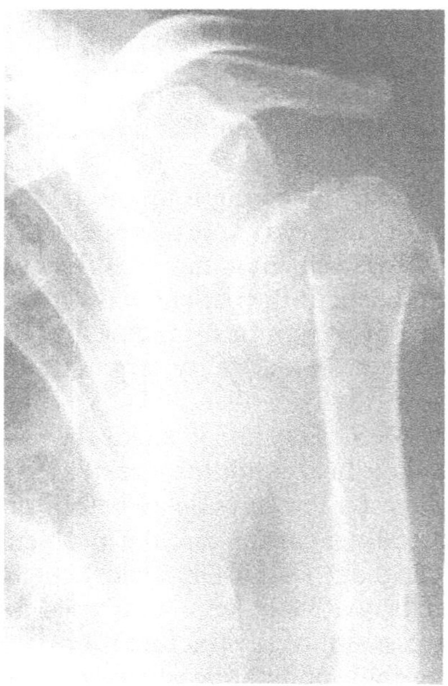

c

Fig. 1 a–c. A 76-year-old woman with osteoporosis. **a** Vertebral fractures, **b** Colles' fracture, and **c** upper humerus fracture

B. Osteoporosis

Some degree of osteoporosis accompanies normal aging and the most prevalent expression of the condition is the increased liability to fracture.

The most common fractures are of the vertebral body (Fig. 1), the wrist and femoral fractures; the latter reaching almost epidemic proportions in the aging population of affluent countries.

Osteoporosis can be defined as that condition in which there is a deficiency of the tissue within the anatomical bone; the bones which remain being normal by present day criteria. This deficiency involves trabecular and compact bone, and all the bones are affected to some extent (CHALMER 1973). The commonest form of osteoporosis is that which affects post-menopausal women and the elderly. There is considerable disagreement as to the mechanisms operating to produce a common end result (ADAMS 1981) but everyone agrees that patients have too little bone to maintain the structural integrity of the skeleton. The patterns of loss are age-related; loss of trabecular and cortical bone may differ (RIGGS et al. 1981) and the patterns of fracture may represent variable losses from these different compartments. Vertebral crush fractures are probably due to a loss of trabecular bone while femoral fractures are due to a combined loss of cortical and trabecular bone (HORSMAN et al. 1980).

The osteoporotic patient is characterised by easy fractures of the vertebral bodies, femur, proximal humerus and distal radius (Colle's). SAVILLE (1970) found that about 32% of his patients had a preceeding history of fractures affecting the distal forearm, neck of femur or humerus. NORDIN et al. (1979) reported about 27% of their patients with spinal osteoporosis had a previous history of a Colles' fracture.

The disabling deformity of osteoporosis is a progressively increasing kyphoscoliosis: in the early stages of the disease there appears a lower dorsal kyphosis – "Dowager's Hump". The patient presents with pain in the back. Classically we recognise two forms of presentation; the local pain associated with the fracture and the concommitant radicular pain, and secondly the associated severe pain of muscle spasm. The latter settles with a short period of bed rest and analgesics. There is no evidence that a few days in bed will cause any significant loss of bone. The diagnosis of osteoporosis is made on clinical, radiological and histological grounds, other causes of insufficiency fractures must be excluded.

The possibility of tumours must be considered, especially myelomatosis in spinal fractures. The radiological signs of vertebral body fractures are increased radio-translucency of the bones, prominence of the vertical trabeculae and endplate, irregular or assymetrical biconcavity of the vertebral bodies and wedge-compression fractures. The finding of a single wedge-fracture in an elderly woman is of doubtful significance in terms of osteoporosis, although this may point to a more serious disease such as metastatic spread. Measurement of the metacarpal cortical thickness is of little value in the diagnosis among individual patients. The assessment of trabecular pattern of the proximal femur (Fig. 2), (SINGH et al. 1970) is thought to provide a good means of identifying a patient with osteoporosis; but does suffer from observer error. Bone biopsy is the most reliable indicator of osteoporosis.

In the therapy of osteoporosis, prevention of bone loss as a prophylactic measure should be considered separately from treatment of the disease after the fracture has occurred. Evidence suggests that oestrogen deficiency is associated with an early accelerated bone loss and replacement is effective in reducing cortical bone loss when compared with untreated groups. Its use is still controversial, the weight of evidence suggests that there is an increased incidence of carcinoma of the uterus in women on oestrogen replacement (RYAN 1982); D & C is recom-

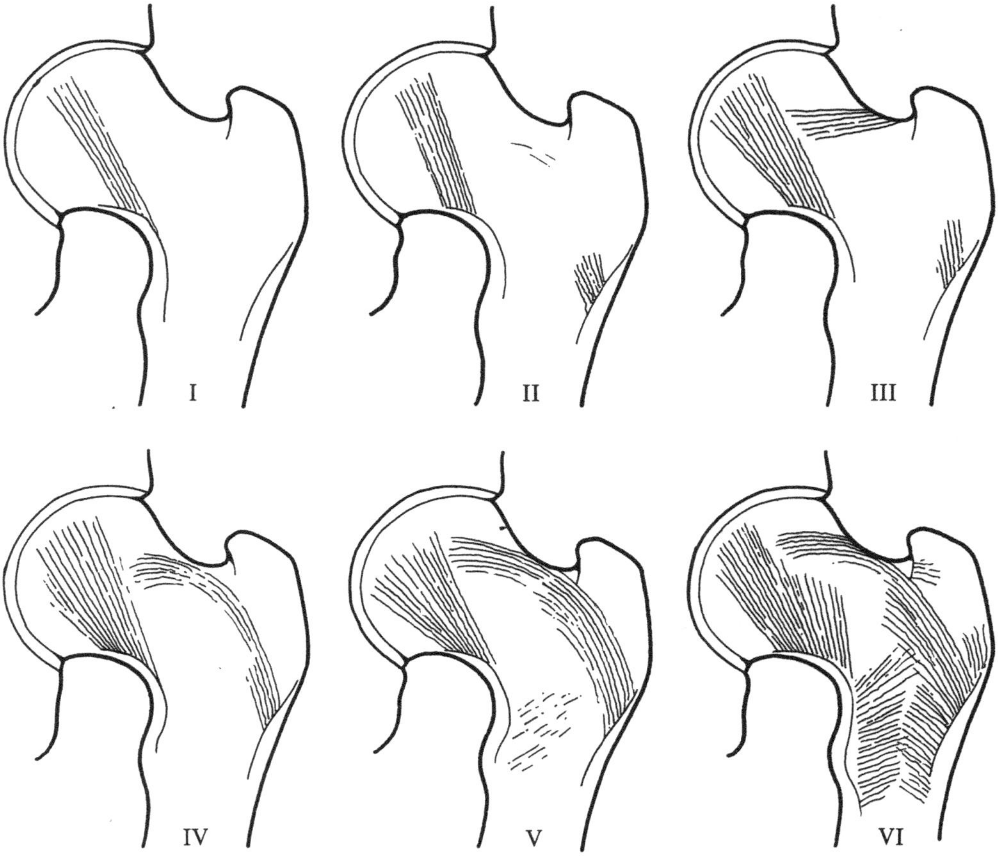

Fig. 2. Grades I to VI. Trabecular pattern used to judge 6 grades of osteoporosis. (After SINGH et al. 1970)

mended every 18 months. An additional factor is that oestrogen therapy has been shown in one study to be effective in preventing cortical bone loss for about 8 years, then there is a gradual loss (LINDSAY et al. 1980).

The primary criterion for effectiveness in the treatment of patients with osteoporotic fractures is a reduction in fracture rate. Preliminary data suggests that treatment with calcium and oestrogens slows subsequent bone loss in patients with osteoporosis and there may be a significant reduction in fracture rate (RIGGS et al. 1981; HUTCHINSON et al. 1979).

The role of fluoride treatment for post-menopausal women is ill-defined; there is usually an increase in bone formation and in particular an increase in the axial skeleton. RIGGS (1983) demonstrates a decrease in the bone-mineral density of the radius. This report suggests that fluoride therapy may protect against vertebral fractures but does not protect and may even increase the incidence of long-bone fractures. This condition is the curse of the orthopaedic surgeon, and the enemy of the patient: all the literature warns the surgeon of the disappointing results and the need for caution in the use of implants, and these patients are precisely the ones that require internal fixation and early mobilisation.

This chapter is in essence the problems of osteoporosis and possible ways to overcome these problems.

C. Osteomalacia

In osteomalacia there is probably an increased mass of bone but much of this is incompletely mineralized. Bone of normal mineral content is removed by the usual process of bone resorption and replaced by bone in which there is less mineral than normal. In the elderly this can present as the classical condition; with associated muscle weakness, pain and the presence of pseudo-fractures. However, it usually presents in a sub-clinical form. The high incidence of this condition in the elderly has many causes, in particular reduced exposure to sunlight, poor dietary intake, and often to drugs, in particularly anti-convulsant therapy. This defective mineralisation may contribute to a decrease in the tensile strength of the skeleton and the prevelance of osteomalacia among fracture patients is five times higher than in unselected hospital admissions of the elderly (ANDERSON 1966; CHALMER et al. 1968). O'DRISCOLL (1973) suggested that a sub-capital fracture which lacks a spike of calcar femorale attached to the inferior aspect of the head is mainly associated with osteomalacia. The practical message is always to exclude the condition if in doubt. The radiological hallmark of this condition is a Looser's zone which is a ribbon-like area of demineralisation (DENT and STAMP 1977), but only occurs in the most severely affected cases. In the elderly biochemical investigations can often be misleading: the alkaline phosphatase is often raised in the elderly in any case, because of coincidental liver disease or Paget's disease. The reduction of the plasma phosphatase is the most useful indicator of osteomalacia, but may be impaired by poor glomerular function. In uncomplicated femoral neck fractures the alkaline phosphate does not begin to rise until the second week (HOSKING 1978) and measurements in the first week have the same diagnostic significance as those in non-fracture patients. Bone biopsy and the measurement of undecalcified cancellous bone will show both that the osteod is increased in thickness and that it covers more of the mineralized surface than normal. Management of these patients should include treatment of the underlying nutritional, intestinal, hepatic, and renal problems. Vitamin D should be given in conventional doses (25–75 μg daily; 1,000–3,000 IU). Some elderly patients will require greater doses, but newer hydroxylated derivatives should not be used unless closely biochemically monitored; the risk of hypercalcaemic intoxication must be appreciated. They should only be prescribed if healing does not occur despite the use of regular medication.

D. Paget's Disease

Paget's disease is also common in the elderly, although why it should show a predilection to the elderly is not clear. It is characterised by a greatly increased turnover of bone.

Pain is the common presenting symptom, although deformity can be the cause for patient's concern. Pain, particularly if unresponsive to simple analgesics is the most common indication for treatment. Calcitonin 100 MRC units, twice weekly can be effective although there is a great variation in response. Pain relief generally occurs within the first few months, if no response occurs then treatment should be discontinued. There is no close correlation between relief of pain and a fall in bone turnover. The use of the first generation compounds, disodium etidronate (EHDP) can be shown to be more effective than calcitonin in reducing pain. There appears to be an increased risk of long bone fractures particularly with doses > 5 mg/kg, which appear to begin at sites of fissure fractures (KHAIRI et al. 1977; CANFIELD et al. 1977). Lower doses (400 mg) may reduce but not eliminate this risk but the biochemical changes are also less complete. EHDP 400 mg daily will reduce the alkaline phosphotase levels by approximately 50%.

Bone pain or fracture is the usual cause for presentation to the orthopaedic surgeon. Fissure fractures are often seen on radiographs and their treatment can be a dilemma. If they become acutely painful this is a sign of impending fracture and internal fixation is required. There is little evidence that they are healed by calcitonin (REDDEN et al. 1981). The risk of the fissure fracture extending is small, operative treatment should be considered in whom the development of acute pain suggests that a fracture is extending.

Operative intervention is indicated in fissure fractures of the femoral neck because complete fractures carry a high risk of non-union. Deformity is relatively slight in the trochanteric region so a fracture can be treated with a short nail. Femoral-shaft fractures must have their deformity corrected at the same time and then an intramedullary-nail introduced. Non-operative treatment can occasionally be recommended if the initial deformity is corrected. Surgery is to be recommended in the majority of fractures (Fig. 3).

E. Fractures

I. Femoral Neck

Femoral neck fractures are almost reaching epidemic proportions in the elderly.

Fractures of the femoral neck are of two types: either sub-capital or transcervical. Femoral neck fractures suffer from all the problems associated with the healing of intra-capsular fractures elsewhere in the body, but the most relevant fact is that the femoral head is rendered largely avascular by displacement and even with optimum treatment, signs of subsequent avascular necrosis and collapse usually occurs.

Management of the sub-capital fracture remains controversial and there are strong advocates of either internal fixation or hemi-arthroplasty (BARNES et al. 1970). The causes of failure are innumerable, such as cutting out of the nail or penetration into the acetabulum. Inadequate reduction is the commonest cause that leads to many failures (GARDEN 1971). The common problem of penetration of the cutting-edge of the nail through the femoral head into the hip-joint is more likely to occur in the osteoporotic patient; to prevent this problem

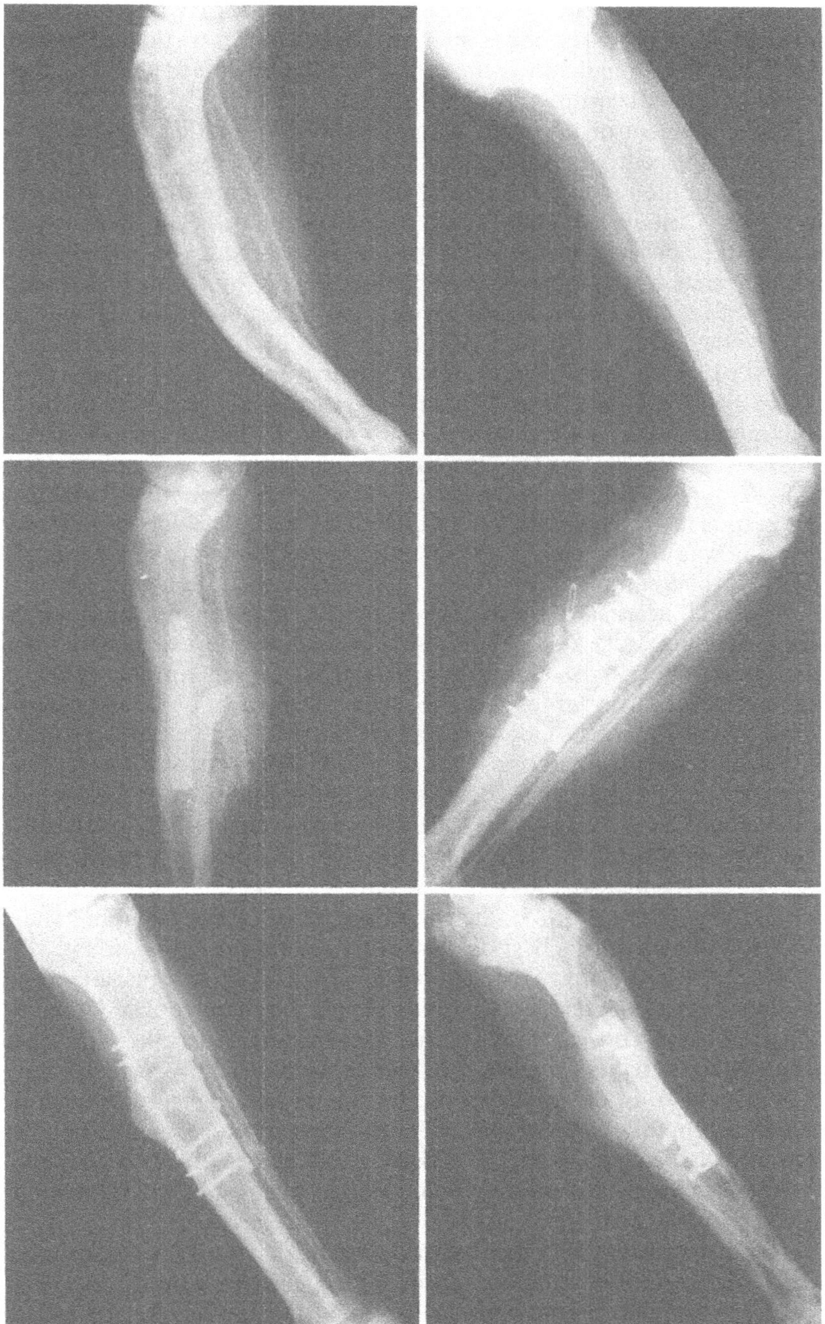

a

b

c

Fig. 3 a–c. Paget's disease of the tibia. **a** Fracture in deformed bone, **b** postoperative, and **c** united fracture the sliding nail-plate has been devised. Biochemical testing has shown that a large threaded screw provides, better internal fixation than a tri-flanged nail (BRODETTI 1960). The sliding nail allows the screw to collapse with the head and lessens the chance of the nail cutting through the head.

The placement of the screw is most important and ideally should be placed just below the centre of the head. It has been shown by GARDEN (1971) that the alignment of the reduction is important in determining the outcome of the fracture. This is known as "The Garden Alignment Index". This is an attempt to determine the accuracy of reduction and a perfect reduction is 160/180; the first number refers to the angle of an inclination made by the medial trabeculations of the head to that of the medial cortex, and the second figure indicates the angle made by the head as it aligns itself with the neck of the lateral radiograph. In 1935 PAUWELS divided the obliquity of the fracture line in three types; type one 30°, type two 50°, and type three 70°, and suggested that sheer forces in the more vertical fractures led to a higher rate of non-union; this has never been substantiated. CASSELBAUM and NUSENT (1963) found no significant difference in the end results, whatever type of fracture had occurred. BOYD and SALVATORE (1964) found 17% non-unions in type two and 8% in type three, and concluded that Pauwels classification was of little value and that it did not take into account the posterior obliquity of the fracture.

Avascular necrosis of the femoral head is the major complication of these fractures, in the literature at least 30%–40% of cases develop segmental avascular necrosis in the superior and anterior region of the head. GARDEN (1971) states that this complication is more likely to occur if there is obvious posterior angulation. If the alignment index shows that the head is in a varus position as well as severe posterior angulation, then there is 100% chance of developing necrosis of the femoral head. Review of cases in our hospital showed a 14% head collapse at three months; although only half of these patients required further surgery for pain. The treatment of this necrosis will depend upon symptoms; the literature suggests that as many as 50% of cases remain asymptomatic, which concurs with our findings (PRINCE 1983). If symptoms occur, then providing the patient's condition allows, this is best dealt with by a total hip replacement.

Whether hemi-arthroplasty should be undertaken as a primary procedure is still debated and the results of various papers are often contradictory. The morbidity appears to be less if an anterior approach is undertaken for replacement, although some papers suggest a higher morbidity with prosthetic replacement (HUNTER 1969). In certain cases the prosthetic replacement has been proved to have unacceptably high complications and, in certain series, the failure rate has been recorded as high as 41.5% (GREER and NIEMANN 1971) if possible. The use of cement in hemi-arthroplasty would suggest the results are significantly better (SONNE-HOLME et al. 1982).

Another problem with hemi-arthroplasty is that with osteoporotic bone there is a risk of acetabular erosion and migration (Fig. 4). This can occur in as high as 10% of patients (D'ARCY and DEVAS 1976). Acetabular erosion has lead to the development of the two bearing prosthesis; between the acetabulum and the prothesis, and within the prosthesis. The Monk "soft-top" endoprothesis showed an incidence of pain in 70% of patients at two years (WEBB et al. 1980) and also

a

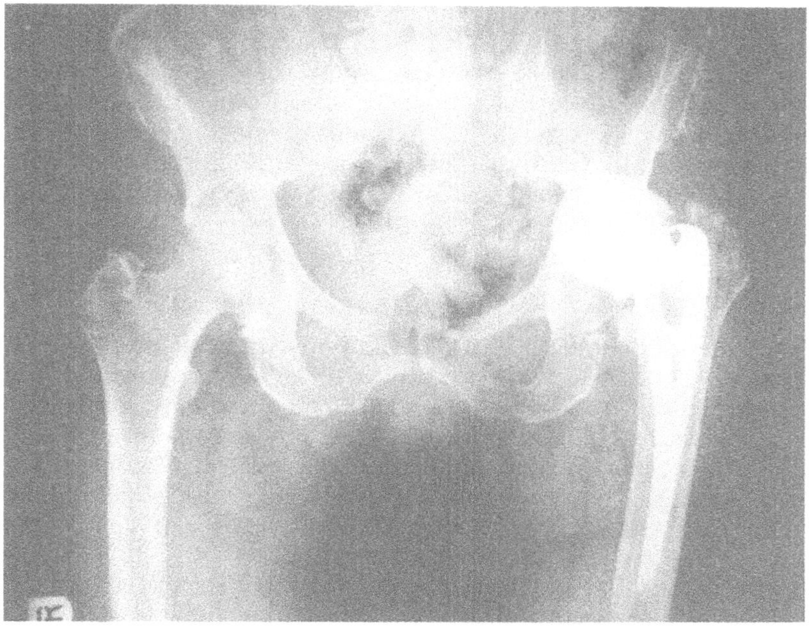

b

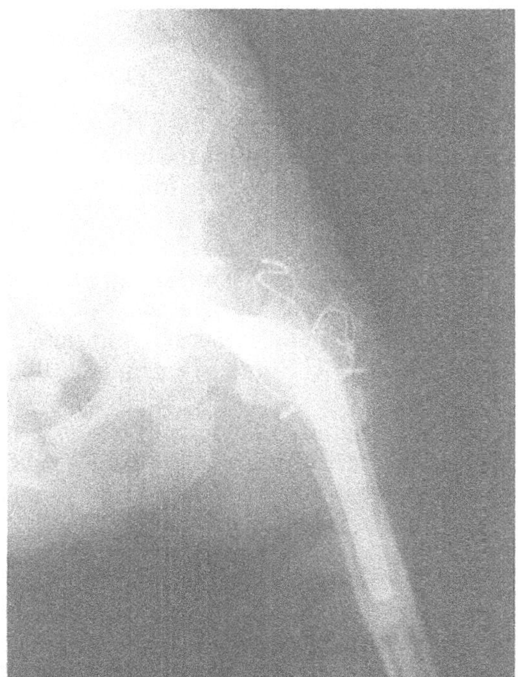

Fig. 4 a, b. a Acetabular protrusion of an Austin-Moore prothesis. b Conversion to a total hip replacement showed inherent design faults resulting in excessive wear of the polyethylene component. DEVAS and HINVES (1983) developed a concentic double-articulated prothesis; the polyethylene cup is covered by a steel outer shell. 72% of patients were satisfactory at one year; although results of standard hemi-arthroplasty are similarly quoted (KENNEDY 1982). Acetabular erosin did not occur but follow-up is far too short. In conclusion: there appears to be little to choose at the present time for either technique! Standard replacement is, however, easier and in most hands quicker.

II. Trochanteric Fractures

Trochanteric fractures can be divided into two types; the stable and unstable type (EVANS 1949; STEEN-JENSEN 1980) (Fig. 5). The stable trochanteric fractures are best treated with a sliding nail-plate; the failure rate using this technique is less than 5%, whereas in the unstable fractures, the sliding nail-plate has been shown to be a suitable implant with a failure rate of less than 6%, in comparison with a McLaughlin nail-plate and Jewitt nail of which nearly half fail on technical grounds, despite resonable reduction (STEEN-JENSEN et al. 1980). Technical failure in itself does not spell disaster for the patient, but 12%–17% of patients with McLaughlin and Jewitt nail-plates needed revision. The success of the sliding-nail plate suggests the demise of the displacement osteotomy in most unstable fracture.

III. Diaphyseal Fractures

The attitude towards treatment of these fractures veers towards non-operative intervention. It is strange how the upper femoral fractures are aggressively treated, but caution occurs with these fractures. The failure of internal fixation accounts for this attitude.

The active geriatric patient can be managed on traction, followed by a functional-brace; however, the upper third fracture and the necessity of an abduction device makes it unwieldy. The most suitable method of fixation is either, if it is a spiral or short oblique fracture, intra-medullary nailing supplemented by either cerclage wire or cerclage nylon bands (PARTRIDGE and EVANS 1982); methylmethacrylate may also be necessary. If, however, there is considerable comminution the most suitable method of fixation is a Zickel nail. This is technically quite demanding, with a significant morbidity, but is probably the only method which will enable a patient to mobilise within the first 5–7 days.

Most diaphyseal fractures of the middle and distal third of the femur can be managed by traction for a period of 4–6 weeks, followed by the application of a lightweight functional-brace (MOONEY et al. 1970). As far as stabilisation of osteoporotic bones with internal fixation is concerned, the results can be dissapointing. If internal fixation is to be undertaken (Fig. 6) it is important to take measures to prevent failure. Fully threaded cancellous screws may be needed to obtain a good hold of the soft bone; if a poor screw-bone purchase is obtained then bone cement is necessary. The plate and screws are applied and then removed. Slow setting cement is then injected into the already prepared holes, and the plate and

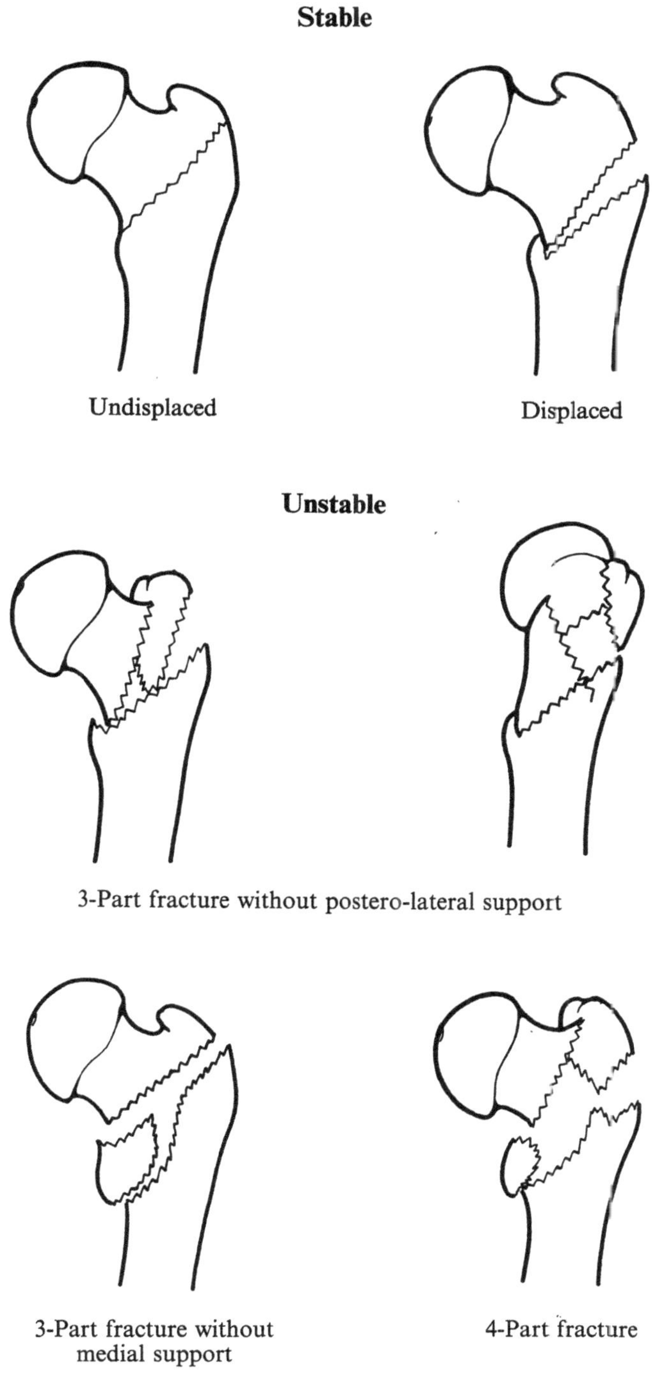

Fig. 5. Classification of trochanteric fractures. (After STEEN-JENSEN et al. 1980)

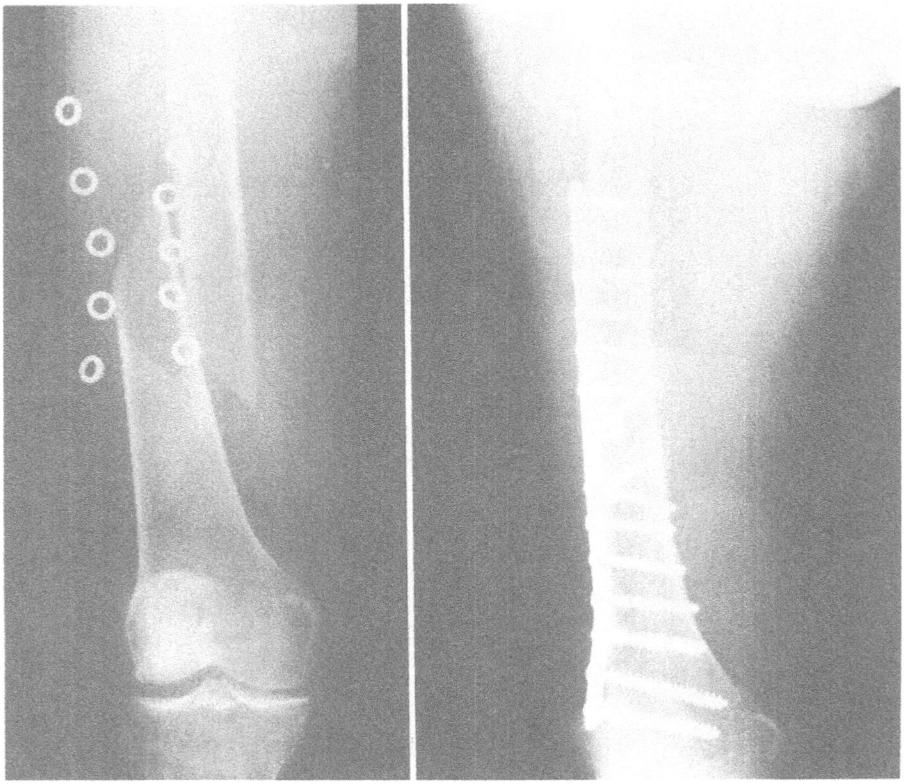

a b

Fig. 6. a Lower third fracture of the femur. **b** Internal fixation using A0 femoral plate, cancellous screws and bone cement

srews reapplied; a cancellous bone-graft is then used. Instead of using cement it is possible to use a plate and Parnam Bands; or a plate and a second polypropylene plate on the opposite cortex to allow the screws to penetrate for purchase (GALLANNAUGH 1975). These latter two techniques lead to considerable soft tissue stripping and the inevitable blood supply damage and should not be recommended in most cases. Post-operative care should include a functional-brace. It should be stressed that this sugery is difficult and the surgeon must be well acquainted with methods of internal fixation. Better to treat on traction if in doubt!

IV. Supracondylar Fractures

In the past there has been considerable reluctance to treat supracondylar fractures with internal fixation, the reasons being inadequate fixation and it has been stressed that there is a significant risk of infection and non-union, and for this reason most surgeons have advocated closed treatment (RIGGINS et al. 1972). Articles in the past have found more favourable results with closed methods of treatment (NEER et al. 1967; STEWART et al. 1966).

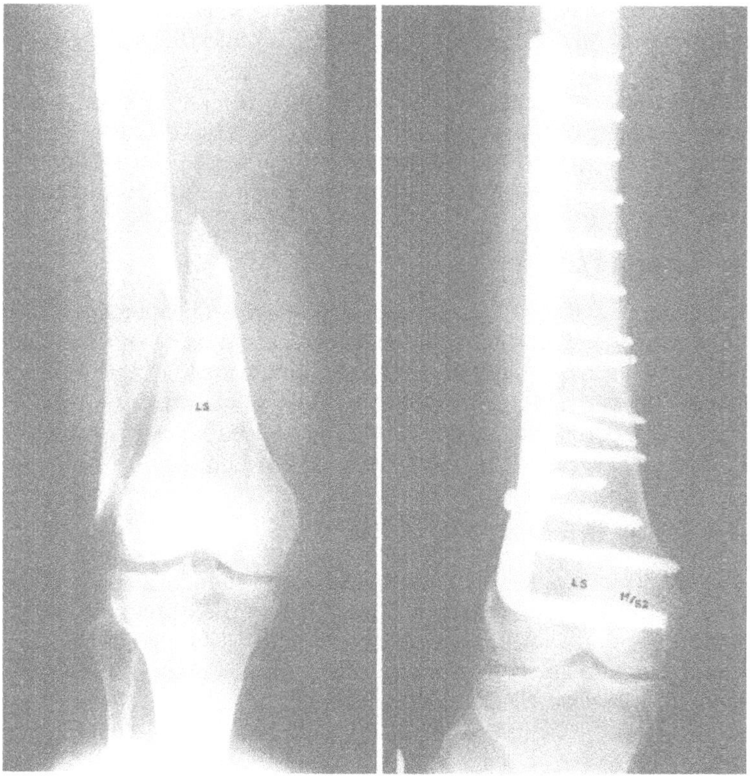

a b

Fig. 7. **a** Supracondylar fracture of the femur. **b** Eleven weeks later

SCHATZKER et al. (1974) found substantially better results in supracondylar fractures if anatomical reduction and rigid fixation were achieved, and they stressed the importance of using the guidelines laid down by the A0 group. The undisplaced or easily reduced fractures are probably best treated with traction or a long-leg cast, later being changed to a functional-brace. In the severely osteoporotic patient, internal fixation will fail catastrophically unless the fixation is supplemented by cement or nylon circlage. If severe comminution is encountered then the femur should be shortened to enhance stability. Good results have been reported in the elderly (MIZE et al. 1982). The supracondylar plate and lag screw (Fig. 7) has its advocates; if used correctly (which is technically difficult), then reported results are good with a very low failure rate in the elderly patient (GILES and KEEVER 1982).

V. Tibial Plateau Fractures

Plateau fractures are commonly seen in the elderly and in the majority of cases should not be treated surgically. The results of non-operative treatment are only satisfactory in a third of patients and in the surgical group less than half the patients had a successful outcome (SCHATZKER et al. 1979). SCHATZKER has grouped these fractures into 6 types but it would appear that the osteoporotic bone tends to compress and become comminuted which makes internal fixation difficult. Surgery should not be advocated unless the knee is unstable in either varus or valgus or there is considerable compression of the condyle of at least 1–1.5 cm; then the depressed articular cartilage can be elevated and held by packing the under-surface with bone cement and using a buttress plate.

VI. Tibial Fracture

Most fractures of the tibia should be treated by non-operative methods. The poor nutrition of the overlying skin leads to breakdown of wounds and the inevitable infection. The use of light-weight braces below the knee leads to early walking and union with excellent results. There are few indications for internal fixation of this common fracture and, indeed, it should be treated with a functional brace. The results in the elderly are satisfactory (DIGBY et al. 1983).

VII. Ankle Fracture

The ankle fractures are best treated by closed reduction and immobilisation in either a long-leg or short-leg cast, depending on the stability. The results of internal fixation are disappointing (BEAUCHAMP et al. 1982); the incidence of complications was significantly higher in women, due to osteoporosis and wound breakdown. There was little difference in function.

VIII. Upper Limb Fractures

The essential aspect in these fractures is function. There is little to be achieved by difficult surgery; early function must be encouraged by an enthusiastic team of physiotherapists and occupational therapists. In the majority of fractures the arm is splinted for comfort then early movement is encouraged. The common fracture of the lower end of the radius can be reduced and held in a splint for 3 weeks; however, it should be realised that the reduction usually slips in the elderly. Treatment must be directed towards function. Reconstructive procedures commonly advocated in the young cannot be applied to the elderly.

F. Conclusion

The management of fractures in the elderly is a subject ignored in most textbooks. Chapters are devoted to the minutia of insignificant fractures but little is written to guide us through the perils of treating the old person.

The purpose of this article is to draw attention to this ever-increasing problem. Nothing new is suggested, indeed one may conclude that little has changed over the years. The hope is the surgeon will be stimulated to be more positive and not let the old person languish in bed. The goal of treatment remains the same; bony union with good function.

References

Anderson G (1966) Bone grafts for delayed union and non-union of the tibia. J Bone Joint Surg [Br] 48:591
Adams PH (1981) Osteoporosis. Clin Rheum Dis 7:557–593
Barnes R, Boyd HB, Salvatore JE (1970) Problems in the treatment of femoral neck fractures. Proc R Soc Med 63:1119–1120
Beauchamp CG, Clay NR, Thexton PW (1982) Displaced ankle fractures in patients over fifty years of age. J Bone Joint Surg [Br] 65:329–332
Boyd HB, Salvatore JE (1964) Acute fracture of the femoral neck: internal fixation or prosthesis? J Bone Joint Surg [Br] 46:1066–1068
Boyd RV, Compton E, Hawthorne J, Kemm JR (1982) Orthogeriatric rehabilitation ward in Nottingham. Br Med J 284:1856–1857
Brodetti A (1960) The blood supply of the femoral neck and head in relation to the damaging effects of nails and screws. J Bone Joint Surg [Br] 42:749–801
Canfield R, Rosner W, Skinner J, McWhorter J, Resnick L, Feldman F, Kammerman S, Ryan K, Kanigonus B, Bohne W (1977) Diphosphate therapy of Paget's disease of bone. J Clin Endocrinol Metab 44:96–106
Casselbaum WH, Nugent G (1963) Predictability of bony union in displaced intracapsular fractures of the hip. J Trauma 3:421–424
Chalmer J (1973) Distribution of osteoporotic changes in the ageing skeleton. Clin Endocrinol Metab 2:203–220
Chalmer J, Conacher WDS, Gardner DL, Scott PJ (1968) Osteomalacia – a common disease in elderly women. J Bone Joint Surg [Br] 49:403–423
D'Arcy J, Devas M (1976) Treatment of fractures of the femoral neck by replacement with the Thompson prosthesis. J Bone Joint Surg [Br] 58:279–286
Dent & Stamp (1977) Vitamin D, ricketts and osteomalacia. In: Arioli LV, Krane SM (eds) Metabolic bone disease. Academic, New York, p 237–306
Devas M, Hinves B (1983) Prevention of acetabular erosion after hemiarthroplasty for fractured neck of femur. J Bone Joint Surg [Br] 65:548–551
Digby JM, Holloway GMN, Webb JK (1983) A study of function after tibial cast bracing. Injury 14:432–439
Evans EM (1949) Treatment of trochanteric fractures of the femur. J Bone Joint Surg [Br] 31:190–203
Gallannaugh SC (1975) High density polyethylene plate for fracture fixation in the elderly. Br Med J 4:560
Garden RS (1971) Malreduction and avascular necrosis of sub-capital fractures of the femur. J Bone Joint Surg [Br] 53:183–197
Gartland JJ (1982) A challenge for Orthopaedic Surgeons. J Bone Joint Surg [Br] 64:159–160
Giles J, Keever JE (1982) Supracondylar plate and lag-screw. J Bone Joint Surg [Br] 64:864–870
Greer RB, Niemann KNW (1971) Fractures of the hip. Geriatrics 126:86–92
Horsman A, Nordin BED, Aaron J, Marshall DH (1980) Osteoporosis. Recent advances in pathogenesis and treatment. University Park Press, Baltimore, pp 175–184.
Hosking DJ (1978) Changes in serum alkaline phosphatase after femoral fractures. JBJS 60B:61–65
Hunter GA (1969) A comparison of the use of internal fixation and prosthetic replacement for fractures of the neck of the femur. Br J Surg 56:229–232
Hutchinson TA, Polansky SM, Feenstein AR (1979) Post-menopausal oestrogen protection against fractures of the hip and distal radius. Lancet 2:705–709
Kennedy WR (1982) Treating femoral neck fractures with the Cathecal prosthesis: a preliminary report. Contemp Orthop 4:97–105
Khairi MRA, Altman RD, De Rose GP, Zimmerman J, Shenk RK, Johnston CC (1977) Sodium etidronate in the treatment of Paget's disease of bone – a study of long-term results. Ann Intern Med 78:656–663

Lindsay R, Fogelman I, Hart DM (1980) In: De Luca HF, Frost HM, Lee WSS, Johnston CC Jr, Parfitt AM (eds) Osteoporosis recent advances in pathogenesis and treatment. University Park Press, Baltimore, pp 399–406

Mize RD, Bucholz RW, Grogan DP (1982) Surgical treatment of displaced, comminuted fractures of the distal end of the femur. J Bone Joint Surg [Br] 64:864–870

Mooney V, Nickel VL, Harvey JP, Snelson R (1970) Cast brace treatment for fractures of the distal part of the femur. J Bone Joint Surg [Br] 52:1563–1578

Neer CS, Grantham SA, Shelton ML (1967) Supracondylar fractures of the adult femur. J Bone Joint Surg [Br] 49:591–613

Nordin BED, Horsman A, Marshall DH, Harries F, Jakerman W (1979) In: Barzel US (ed) Osteoporosis II. Grane and Stratton, New York, pp 183–203

O'Driscoll M (1973) Sub-capital fracture types and osteomalacia and Vitamin D deficiency. J Bone Joint Surg [Br] 55:882

Partridge AG, Evans PEL (1982) The treatment of fractures of the shaft of the femur using nylon cerclage. J Bone Joint Surg [Br] 64:210–214

Pauwels (1935) Der Schenkelhalsbruch: ein mechanisches Problem. Ferdinand Enke

Prince HGP (1983) Personal communication

Redden JF, Dixon J, Vennart W, Hoskings DJ (1981) Management of fissure fractures in Paget's disease. Int Orthop 5:103–106

Riggins RS, Garrick JG, Lipscum PR (1972) Supracondylar fractures of the femur: a survey of treatment. Clin Orthop 82:32–36

Riggs BL, Wahner HW, Dunn WL, Mazess RB, Offord KP, Melton JL (1981) Differential changes in bone mineral density of the appendicular and axial skeleton with ageing and relationship to spinal osteoporosis. J Clin Invest 67 (II):328–335

Riggs BL (1983) Treatment of osteoporosis with fluoride. In: Dixon A St J, Russell RGG, Stamp TBC (eds) Osteoporosis – a multi-disciplinary problem. Royal Society of Medicine, London, pp 231–236

Riska EB (1970) Factors influencing the primary mortality in the treatment of hip fractures. Injury 2:107–115

Ryan KJ (1982) Post-menopausal oestrogen use. Ann Rev Med 33:171–181

Saville PD (1970) In: Barzel US (ed) Osteoporosis. Grane and Stratton, New York, pp 38–46

Schatzker J, Horne G, Waddell J (1974) The Toronto experience with the supracondylar fracture of the femur – 1966–1972. Injury 6:113–128

Schatzker J, McBroom R, Bruce D (1979) The tibial plateau fracture – the Toronto experience 1968–1975. Clin Orthop 138:94–104

Singh M, Nagrath AR, Maimi PS (1970) Changes in trabecular pattern of the upper end of the femur as an index of osteoporosis. J Bone Joint Surg [Br] 52:457–467

Sonne-Holm S, Walter S, Steen-Jensen J (1982) Moore Hemi-Arthroplasty with and without bone cement in femoral neck fractures: a clinical controlled trial. Acta Orthop Scand 53:953–956

Steen-Jensen J (1980) Classification of trochanteric fractures. Acta Orthop Scand 51:803–810

Steen-Jensen J, Tondevold E, Sonne-Holm S (1980) Unstable trochanteric fractures: a comparative analysis of the methods of internal fixation. Acta Orthop Scand 51:949–962

Stewart MJ, Sisk TD, Wallace SL (1966) Fractures of the distal third of the femur: a comparison of methods of treatment. J Bone Joint Surg [Br] 48:784–807

Sylvester BS, Boston D, Grant C, Galasko CSB (1977) Peak flow measurements as a guide to prognosis in patients undergoing hip surgery. J Bone Joint Surg [Br] 59:500–501

Webb PJ, Wright KWJ, Winter GD (1980) The Monk 'soft-top' endoprosthesis. J Bone Joint Surg [Br] 62:174–179

The Prostate in the Elderly

A. Basso

A. Introduction

Prostatic pathology, especially benign prostatic hyperplasia and adenocarcinoma, represents the most common cause of urologic problems in the aging male. Benign or malignant enlargement of the prostate can cause obstruction of the bladder outlet which typically gives the picture of prostatism. This is characterized by decreased force of the urinary stream, hesitancy, postvoid dribbling, sensation of not emptying the bladder, and nocturia. Frequency, urgency and urge incontinence may be associated and sometimes hematuria can occur.

These symptoms vary in intensity in the same individual, but generally they are slowly progressive and may culminate in acute urinary retention. The latter, not infrequently, is precipitated by alcohol ingestion, infections, or by drugs that increase the bladder neck tone (such as sinus decongestants) or those producing hypotonicity of the detrusor (such as tranquilizers and anticholinergic drugs).

Incomplete emptying of the bladder can progress and be responsible for obstructive uropathy with hydronephrosis and renal failure; it also creates a predisposition to urinary tract infections. Additional complications can result from bacteremia and septic shock, usually secondary to gram-negative bacteria.

When the obstruction is slowly progressive over a very long period of time, the patient may not notice any difficulty with urination. The condition is insidious, giving symptoms only after severe obstructive uropathy and chronic bladder distension and renal failure are present. This picture characterizes the silent prostatism which not infrequently is discovered during a workup for anorexia and anemia or for an abdominal mass.

B. Hormonal Control of Prostatic Growth

The growth of the prostate is mostly influenced by hormones of testes and hypophysis. Among them, testosterone is the most important, as demonstrated by the marked decrease in size of the prostate in castrated animals. A correlation between the testes and the prostate has been suspected at least since the nineteenth century, when bilateral orchiectomy was done for the purpose of controlling prostatic enlargement (White 1895; Cabot 1896). The procedure is no longer used for this indication, but these early reports have stimulated a long series of studies in order to elucidate the hormonal control of prostatic growth.

Testosterone is utilized by the prostatic epithelial cells after its conversion to dihydrotestosterone by enzymatic action of 5α-reductase (BRUCHOVSKY and WILSON 1968). Once dihydrotestosterone is formed, it is bound to a cytoplasmic receptor and transported into the nucleus where cellular protein synthesis and cell replication are initiated.

Testosterone is produced by the Leydig cells, which are stimulated by the luteinizing hormone (LH) originated from the pituitary. In turn, testosterone can suppress the secretion of LH, through the inhibition of the secretion of LH releasing hormone (LRH) from the hypothalamus. As described by EWING (1976), with advancing age the secretion of testosterone is reduced and the number and lipidic content of Leydig cells decrease.

The effect of the pituitary on the prostate is not only indirect, through the secretion of gonadotropins, but also direct, probably through the production of prolactin which, together with androgens, is essential for restoring full prostatic growth in hypophysectomized rats (GRAYHACK et al. 1955).

In contrast to androgens and prolactin, estrogens are known to curb prostatic growth when administered exogenously. This effect takes place primarily through the hypothalamic–pituitary-gonadal axis by inhibiting the secretion of LH, thus decreasing the level of serum testosterone (SCOTT et al. 1980). A small amount of estrogens is normally present in the serum of healthy males; after 50 years of age there is an increase of serum estradiol, although most of it is protein bound (VERMEULEN 1976).

Considering that dihydrotestosterone is the active androgen at the prostatic level, several researchers have investigated its possible involvement in abnormal prostatic growth. It is of interest that the level of dihydrotestosterone is increased in benign prostatic hyperplasia (SIITERI and WILSON 1970); there is also evidence that dihydrotestosterone and some of its metabolites can induce benign prostatic hyperplasia in castrated dogs, especially in the presence of estrogens (WALSH and WILSON 1976; DE KLERK et al. 1979). Also, it has been noted that there is an increase in nuclear androgen receptor content in spontaneous and experimental canine prostatic hyperplasia (TRACHTENBERG et al. 1982).

Although these experimental observations and the hormonal changes of the elderly male seem to substantiate the theory of a purely hormonal origin of benign prostatic hyperplasia, the etiology of this condition is still uncertain and, as stated by WALSH (1979), "at present an unifying thesis correlating the onset of benign prostatic hyperplasia with endocrinological factors is lacking". The knowledge of the influence of hormonal factors on prostatic growth has been extensively utilized in the treatment of prostatic adenocarcinoma, but this will be discussed later in this chapter.

C. Benign Prostatic Hyperplasia

Benign prostatic hyperplasia originates from the periurethral glands (Fig. 1) and displaces peripherally the true prostate which in this process is also compressed. Usually there is a well-defined cleavage plaen between the two structures, which makes the surgical enucleation of the hyperplastic tissue relatively easy. In con-

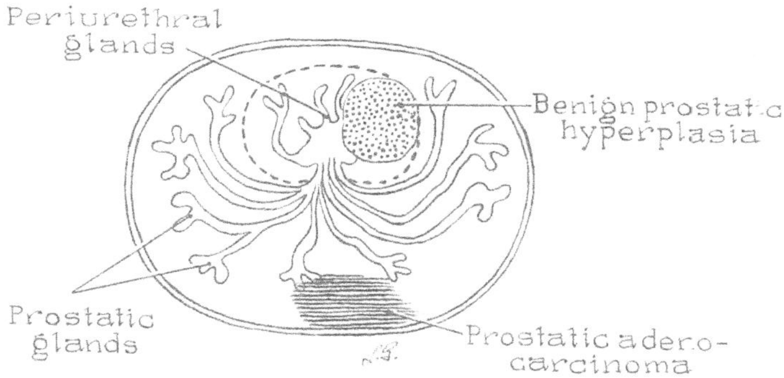

Fig. 1. Benign prostatic hyperplasia originates from the periurethral glands, while adenocarcinoma arises from the true prostate at the periphery. (After WEYRAUCH 1976)

trast, adenocarcinoma originates from the true prostate (Fig. 1); of course, the two conditions can coexist.

The symptoms caused by benign prostatic hyperplasia have already been described. It is important to know that they are not necessarily related to the size of the prostate, in that a hypertrophic medial lobe or a median bar may be very obstructive, but rectally the prostate may feel essentially normal. With the exception of these conditions, the prostate will be uniformly enlarged, smooth, and elastic.

The indications for treatment are based on the severity of symptoms and results of the urologic evaluation, which includes the intravenous pyelogram, the measurement of the postvoid residual, cystourethroscopy, and, in selected cases, urodynamic evaluation. When the elderly patient presents with voiding symptoms, it is important to keep in mind that these are necessarily not secondary to bladder outlet obstruction, even if the prostate may be enlarged at rectal examination.

Frequency, nocturia, urgency, and urge incontinence are irritative symptoms which could be secondary to bladder dysfunction with detrusor hyperreflexia encountered in some patients with cerebrovascular disease. With this condition, the postvoid residual is usually small. Furthermore, the endoscopic and radiologic evaluation of the urinary tract will fail to reveal obstructive changes; the cystometric study will show characteristic uninhibited contractions of the bladder. The use of anticholinergic medications such as propantheline bromide, or anticholinergic and musculotropic drugs such as oxybutynin may prove to be helpful in these patients.

Irritative urinary symptoms can also be secondary to prostatitis, which is more common in men less than 50 years of age, but this condition will be discussed later in this chapter.

Partial or complete urinary retention may also be related to functional conditions such as bladder dysfunction with detrusor areflexia secondary to diabetic neuropathy or abdominoperineal resection of the rectum. With these patients, the urologic evaluation will fail to demonstrate outlet obstruction; cystometric study together with clinical findings will be diagnostic.

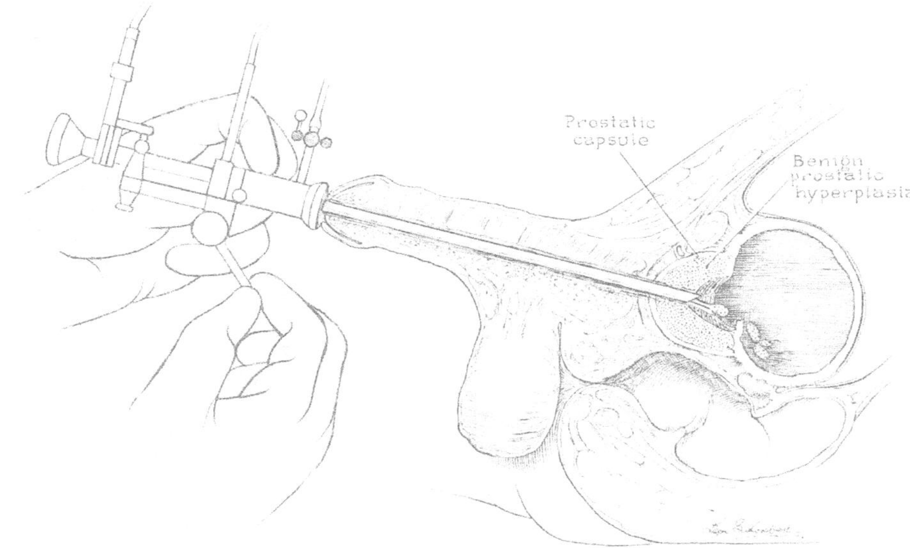

Fig. 2. Transurethral resection of the prostate. The capsule represents the compressed true prostate

In benign prostatic hyperplasia the treatment of choice is surgical and consists of the removal of the hyperplastic periurethral tissue, leaving the true prostate intact. This is a very important fact that should be explained to the patient, who, later on, could still be affected by cancer of the prostate, and consequently should be checked at least yearly for early detection of this condition. The excision of hyperplastic prostatic tissue may be done endoscopically, by transurethral resection, or by open procedures such as suprapubic, retropubic, or perineal prostatectomies (Figs. 2–5).

As pointed out by GRAYHACK and SADLOWSKI (1976), the results of these procedures are very good, with relief from the obstruction obtained rapidly and permanently in the majority of cases. Mortality rate is less than 1%, even though many relatively poor risk individuals are included in this group of patients.

Patients not infrequently express concern about impotence and incontinence after surgery, when these procedures are recommended. It is an important duty of the physician to disperse such fears, because potency is retained in most of the cases (87% in suprapubic prostatectomy and 95% in transurethral resection of the prostate according to FINKLE and PRIAN 1966) and incontinence is approximately 1% or less (GRAYHACK and SADLOWSKI 1976). All these procedures have the potential of producing incompetence of bladder neck with consequent retrograde ejaculation. This will cause sterility, but should not interfere with potency and/or sexual pleasure.

Because of the quick recovery and limited blood loss, transurethral resection of the prostate is the procedure preferably used in many institutions, especially in the United States. However, situations exist where open prostatectomy is pre-

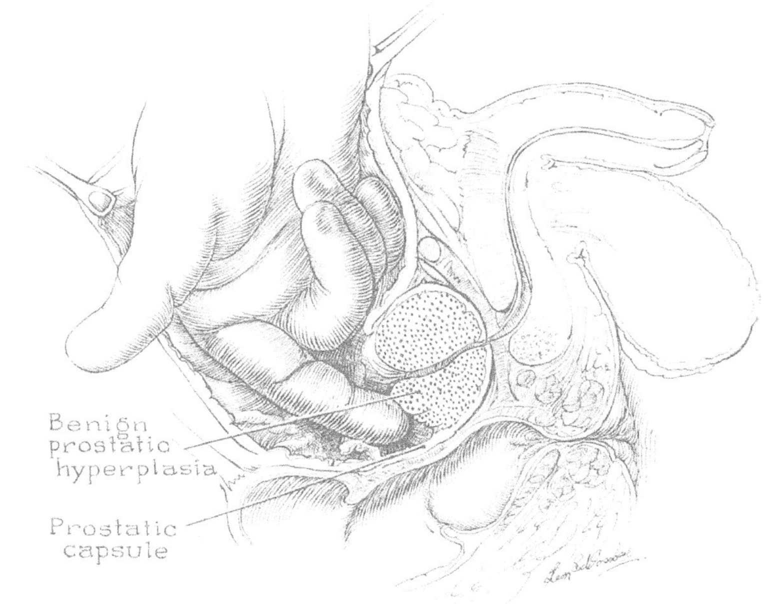

Fig. 3. Suprapubic prostatectomy. As in retropubic and perineal prostatectomies, only the hyperplastic prostatic tissue is enucleated while the compressed true prostate (capsule) is left in place

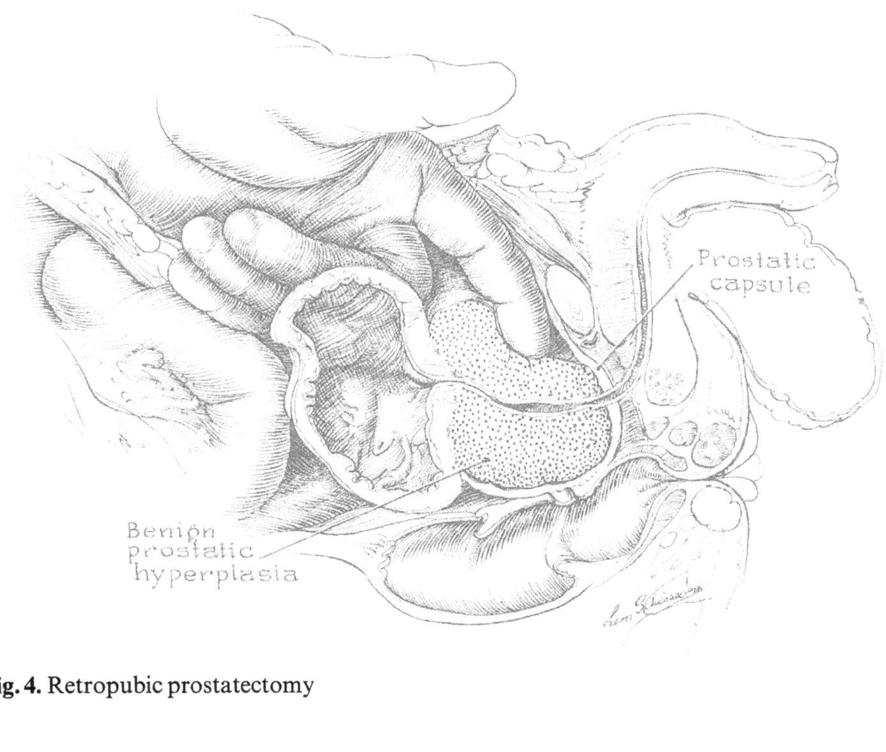

Fig. 4. Retropubic prostatectomy

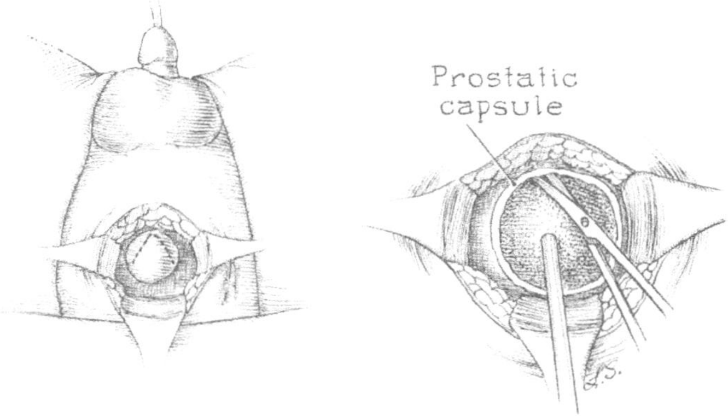

Fig. 5. Perineal prostatectomy

ferred. This depends on the amount and configuration of the hypertrophic tissue and on the presence of bladder lesions such as large calculi and diverticula. The training and the skill of the urologist are important factors in this decision. It is, in fact, essential to limit the resection time to 60–90 min because, if the resection is longer, the chances of complications such as hemodilution from absorption of irrigating fluid and urethral strictures are increased. Perineal prostatectomy, although very safe (YOUNG and DAVIS reported in 1926 a mortality rate of 3.2% in 1,000 cases), is used less at the present time, because more frequently than other procedures, it produces impotence by disturbing the innervation of the erectile system.

What are the alternatives to the surgical treatment of benign prostatic hyperplasia? Medical management has been directed towards the reduction of the hyperplastic tissue by hormonal manipulation or the relaxation of the bladder neck by the use of α-adrenergic blocking agents. While hormonal manipulation, although promising, does not seem to have practical value as yet, the α-adrenergic blocking agents could probably be used in selected conditions. However, in considering medical treatment for benign prostatic hyperplasia, one should keep in mind that at the present time there is no pharmacologic substitute for surgical therapy, when this is necessary because of irreversible urinary retention or chronic obstruction with renal damage.

The use of castration for control of prostatic enlargement has already been mentioned in the Sect. B. Although probably helpful, at the present time it has only historical value. In 1959, KAUFMANN and GOODWIN reported some favorable response to an estrogen–androgen combination, but the results were inconsistent. More recently, the so-called antiandrogens (i.e., cyproterone acetate, medrogestone, and flutamide) have been used. Although encouraging results have been reported (SCOTT and WADE 1969; RANGNO et al. 1971), they have been questioned because of a lack of appropriate controls. Of great interest, however, is the observation that there are distinct changes of the epithelial component of the benign hyperplastic nodular prostate, while the fibromuscular portion does not seem particularly affected (SCOTT and WADE 1969; SCOTT and DE KLERK 1976). This certainly leaves the field open for further investigation.

CAINE et al. (1981) have reported the use of an α-andrenergic blocking agent (phenoxybenzamine) to relieve symptoms in patients not having positive indications for surgery or in whom the operation was postponed; 200 patients were treated and 70%–80% of them were relieved of obstructive and irritative symptoms. Of the patients in whom the urine flow was measured, 46% showed an increase of 100% or more during treatment and about 25% had an increase of 50%-100%. In the control group, 12% had an improvement of 50%–100% and none had more than 100% amelioration. Only 10% of the patients had to stop the treatment because of side effects, mostly orthostatic hypotension.

For the patient with significant urinary retention, catheterization seems to be, at the present time, the only logical alternative to surgical treatment. When technically feasible, intermittent catheterization is preferable to indwelling catheters. This method is in fact associated with significantly fewer complications and leaves the patient reasonably unencumbered in his activities.

When an indwelling catheter must be used, the choice should fall on one made of inert materials such as silicone rubber, in order to decrease the chances of catheter incrustation and of vesicourethral irritation. The caliber should be 16 or 18 Fr. which is enough to provide good urinary flow, but at the same time allows free drainage of urethral secretions, minimizing the chances of infection and bacteremia. It is important also to provide a closed drainage system and to encourage fluid intake to ensure good urinary flow.

All these measures are helpful in controlling bacteriuria and decreasing chances of systemic urinary tract infection. However, in spite of all the care, a good number of patients will have positive urine cultures. This should not be an indication for antibiotic treatment unless there are systemic symptoms. Any attempt to sterilize the urine under other circumstances is futile and potentially dangerous, because of the development of more resistant bacterial strains which would make the control of infection more difficult, if mandatory.

In selected cases, a suprapubic indwelling catheter may be advisable. Although this will initially require a surgical procedure, it has the great advantage of bypassing urethral strictures and of risking fewer chances of infection of urethral origin. The decision to maintain urinary drainage with an indwelling catheter should be taken only if there are very serious reasons and no valid alternatives. On should never forget that the surgical risk is much less than the potentially grave consequences of gram-negative sepsis, which represents the major threat for patients with indwelling catheters.

D. Prostatitis

Prostatitis is more common prior to the age of 50 years; older men are characteristically affected by urinary tract infections complicating benign prostatic hyperplasia or urethral strictures. The possibility of prostatitis however, should be considered in the evaluation of the older man with voiding symptoms, because the therapeutic approach is very different from the one used in conditions causing obstruction of the bladder outlet. Typically, patients with prostatitis have very little if any postvoid residual. The intravenous pyelogram will not show abnormalities of the urinary tract, and their examination will not disclose the presence of a urethral stricture nor of significant prostatic enlargement.

The classification of prostatitis recommended by DRACH et al. (1978) represents a significant contribution in understanding this condition and outlining its treatment. Four clinical entities are considered: (1) acute bacterial prostatitis; (2) chronic bacterial prostatitis; (3) non bacterial prostatitis; and (4) prostatodynia.

I. Acute Bacterial Prostatitis

This does not present a problem of diagnosis and treatment. Usually the affected patients are acutely ill, febrile, and have severe frequency, dysuria, pollakiuria, or nocturia. Their urinary stream is decreased in force, mostly because they void in such small amounts. The prostate is very tender on palpation and the urine culture is positive. As a rule these patients will respond well to appropriate antibiotic treatment which, depending on the clinical picture, can be given parenterally or by mouth. Once the acute process is resolved, it is advisable to give oral medications for approximately 30 days in the effort to prevent the evolution to chronic prostatitis.

II. Chronic Bacterial Prostatitis

This condition is of more insidious onset. Discomfort in the genital or perineal area seems to be predominant and sometimes can be located in the groin or thighs. Frequency and dysuria may not be severe. Sometimes patients experience painful ejaculation and hematospermia. It is not unusual to elicit a history of recurrent epididymitis or of acute exacerbations. In these patients the examination of expressed prostatic secretions is very important, because the urine itself might not show abnormalities. The prostatic secretions will have more than 10–20 white cells per high power field. Lipid-laden macrophages (oval fat bodies) and decreased number of so-calles lecithin granules will be noted. The culture of these secretions, by definition, should be positive; most commonly the bacteria involved are gram-negative (*Escherichia coli, Klebsiella, Proteus,* and *Pseudomonas*), but gram-positive such as enterococci may be found.

The treatment of this condition may not be easy, not so much because of the tendency to develop resistant bacterial strains, but mostly because of the poor diffusion of antibiotics in the lumen of the prostatic glands. The diffusion of antibiotics in the prostate is directly proportional to their lipid solubility and ionization in the plasma and inversely proportional to their tendency to bind with proteins (STAMEY 1972). Most of the studies of drug diffusion have been done in dogs and for this reason in some instances may not necessarily reflect what happens in human pathology. For example, the pH of human prostatic secretions is higher than in dogs, especially if the prostate is infected (FAIR et al. 1979).

The drugs that appear to be more effective in the treatment of chronic bacterial prostatitis are trimethoprim–sulfamethoxazole (MEARES 1973, 1975), minocycline (FAIR 1974), erythromycin alone or associated with bicarbonate (MOBLEY

1974), carbenicillin indanyl sodium (OLIVERI et al. 1979), and kanamycin (STAMEY 1980). The efficacy of these treatments is variable, but a good clinical result can be expected in approximately 70% of patients.

III. Nonbacterial Prostatitis

Nonbacterial prostatitis causes symptoms similar to the chronic bacterial form with the exception of episodes of genitourinary infection such as epididymitis. The examination of expressed prostatic secretions will reveal a significant number of leukocytes and oval fat bodies and also decreased lecithin granules, but cultures will fail to demonstrate bacteria.

This is a very frustrating condition for the patient and the physician alike, because there is no specific treatment. More needs to be known of the etiology of this condition. In some cases the origin may be bacterial (*Chlamydia, Ureaplasma*), but generally the evidence of infectious origin is lacking (MEARES 1978; STAMEY 1980). At least initially, it seems reasonable to try treatment with erythromycin or tetracycline, but if the patient does not respond there is no reason to continue it. Prostatic massage, sitz baths, and anti-inflammatory drugs may be helpful in relieving the symptoms.

IV. Prostatodynia

Prostatodynia is characterized by symptoms similiar to nonbacterial prostatitis, but the expressed prostatic secretions will not show significant abnormalities. The etiology of this condition is unknown. From examination of the literature, it appears that probably the so-called prostatodynia is a manifestation of different clinical entities, among which at least three can be recognized: functional voiding disorders, tension of the pelvic floor, and emotional disturbances.

Functional voiding disorders can be demonstrated with urodynamic evaluation. They include detrusor–sphincter dyssynergia responding to the administration of phenoxybenzamine (MEARES 1978; STAMEY 1980), bladder hyperreflexia and bladder areflexia with nonrelaxing pelvic floor, which can be treated respectively with propantheline bromide and with diazepam (SIROKI et al. 1981). Pelvic floor tension myalgia has been described by SEGURA et al. (1979) and responds to exercise, warm baths and physiotherapy. Some patients may show evidence of psychiatric disorders and for them appropriate specialized evaluation is necessary. A good patient–physician relationship ist essential for all these patients, regardless of the origin of the symptoms, in order to uncover and alleviate emotional problems frequently associated with this condition.

E. Prostatic Adenocarcinoma

Prostatic adenocarcinoma is the second most common malignancy in American males and represents the third leading cause of cancer death in men beyond the age of 55 years (SILVERBERG and HOLLEB 1975). The pattern of diffusion of this

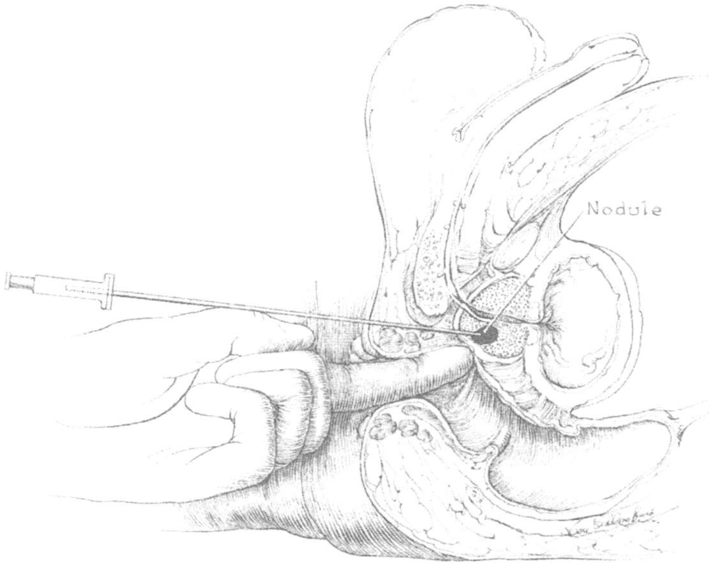

Fig. 6. Transperineal needle biopsy of prostatic nodule

cancer can be by local extension, which can progress to the point of causing ureteral obstruction, hematogenous dissemination to bones and internal organs (especially lungs), and lymphatic metastases.

It is important to remember that, although this malignancy can cause symptoms of urinary obstruction or pain due to metastases, the potentially curable early lesions are generally asymptomatic. They are most commonly discovered at routine rectal examination, which should be done yearly in every man above the age of 45 years. Characteristically, the rectal examination will reveal that the prostate has a circumscribed or diffuse induration with irregular surface, but it should not be forgotten that prostatic changes may be more subtle and that sometimes a prostate that feels benign on examination can contain cancer.

The clinical suspicion must be confirmed by tissue diagnosis. Specimens for this purpose may be obtained from the abnormal areas with a punch biopsy needle (Fig. 6) which may be used transperineally or, less frequently, transrectally. Samples for cytology may be secured by transrectal aspiration. This technique (Fig. 7) is used extensively in Europe and is relatively simple and atraumatic (STAEHLER et al. 1976). The accuracy of these methods is approximately 85%–90%. In selected cases where the biopsy has been negative and the patient would be a candidate for definitive therapy, open perineal biopsy can be considered to make sure that the sampling is taken from the affected area.

Once the diagnosis has been made, the tumor should be staged in order to decide the modality of treatment. The staging most commonly used in the United States is derived from the system introduced by WHITMORE in 1956. It is based on

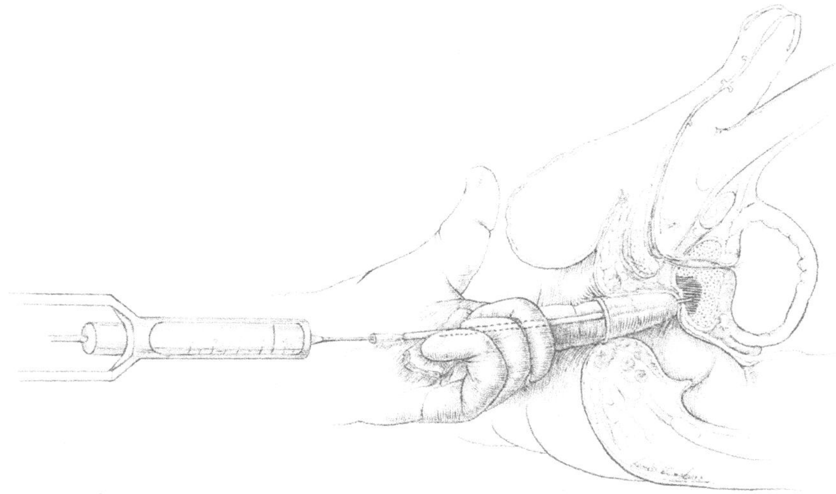

Fig. 7. Transrectal fine needle aspiration of prostatic nodule for cytodiagnosis

the appearance of the prostate at rectal examination and on the presence or absence of clinically demonstrable metastatic lesions. The detection of metastases and the evaluation of the extent of local spread is done by several modalities, the most common of which, at the present time, include determination of serum acid phosphatases, intravenous pyelogram, chest radiography, bone survey, and radionucleotide bone scan.

Stage I (now called A) is the clinically unsuspected cancer which is discovered by microscopic examination of prostatic tissue removed for seemingly benign prostatic enlargement causing obstruction. This represents approximately 10% of all cases. In stage II (B) the carcinoma is localized with the prostate and in stage III (C) it appears to be locally invasive. None of these stages has clinically demonstrable metastases. By contrast, stage IV (D) is characterized by the presence of metastases, regardless of the appearance of the prostate at rectal examination (Fig. 8). Approximately 80% of the patients have stage C or D lesions when first seen.

During the last decade, further subdivision of this classification has been made, based on anatomic and clinical considerations (JEWETT 1975) and also taking into account the presence or absence of lymph node metastases. Stage A tumors have been subdivided in to A_1 and A_2. The former are characterized by few foci of generally well-differentiated carcinoma; by contrast, the latter has diffuse microscopic invasion of mostly poorly differentiated neoplastic cells. These two types of tumors have a different natural history in that A_1 tumors do not tend to progress, whereas A_2 tumors have invasive potential.

Similarly, stage B tumors have been divided into B_1, or cancers clinically involving less than one lobe, and B_2, or cancers involving one lobe or more, but still confined within the prostate. These subdivisions have different prognosis. In fact

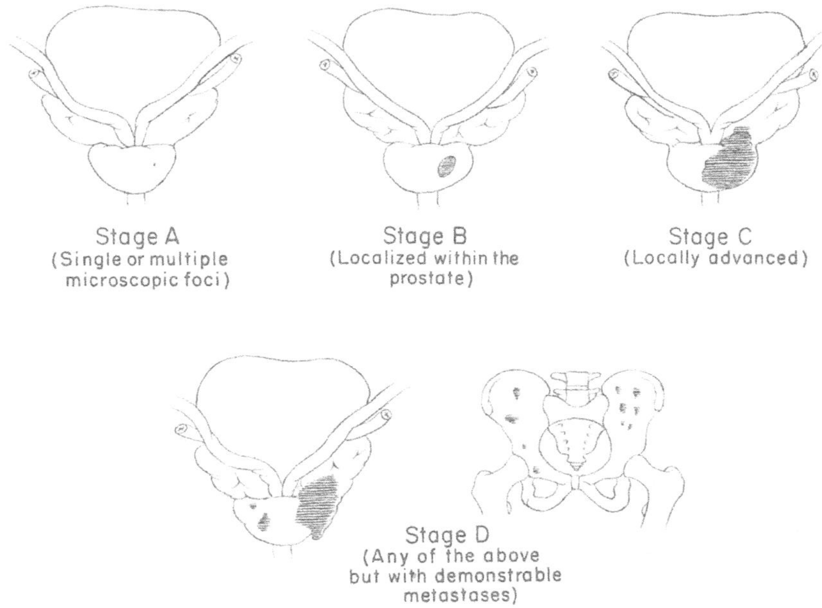

Fig. 8. Clinical staging of prostatic adenocarcinoma. (After BASSO, 1978; Original illustrator N. O. Hardy)

the majority of patients with stage B_1 carcinoma can be cured by radical prostatectomy, which is not nearly as successful in stage B_2 cancers.

Concerning the lymph node involvement in patients with carcinoma of the prostate, the average figures are approximately as follows: no nodal metastases in stage A_1, 25% in stage A_2, 15% in stage B_1, 30% in stage B_2, and 50% in stage C tumors (MCCULLOUGH 1980). The primary involvement is in the obturator, hypogastric, external iliac, presacral, and presciatic nodes. Although nodal metastases may indicate local tumor spreading, they may also be a sign of a systemic immunologic event (WAJSMAN 1981). The interpretation of this phenomenon notwithstanding, lymph node involvement is a sign of poor prognosis. In fact a high percentage of these patients will show rapid progression towards systemic disease, many of them within 2 years from the time of diagnosis, even if treatment has been instituted (PROUT et al. 1981; KRAMER et al. 1981).

As pointed out by PROUT et al. (1981), the early appearance of osseous metastases might indicate that these were already present at the time of diagnosis, but not detected with our methods. Since the presence of lymph node metastases so clearly influences the prognosis, irrespective of clinical staging, these patients have been assigned to a different stage (D_1). The detection of positive nodes is done preferably by pelvic lymph node dissection since the lymphangiogram alone does not seem to be accurate. There are indications, however, that a combination of lymphangiogram, fine needle biopsy, and tumor grading may be an acceptably accurate method of clinical evaluation of this possibility (WAJSMAN 1981).

Patients with clinically demonstrated metastases are considered now as stage D_2 (formerly stage IV or D).

The most widely accepted measures for treatment of prostatic adenocarcinoma are represented by surgery, radiation therapy, hormonal manipulation, and chemotherapy.

I. Surgical Treatment

Prostatovesiculectomy (radical prostatectomy) can be done by perineal or by retropubic approach. Radical perineal prostatectomy was perfected and standardized by YOUNG (1905) and is still widely used, although the retropubic procedure has gained popularity in our time. The only advantage of the retropubic approach is the possibility of doing a lymph node dissection through the same incision. In the hands of a skilled surgeon these procedures have a minimal mortality (2 deaths in 447 cases of perineal prostatectomy or less than 0.5% in the Johns Hopkins Hospital series), and very limited morbidity with moderate incontinence (not requiring protection) in not more than 2.5% (WALSH and JEWETT 1980). The major drawback of this procedure is impotence which occurs in at least 60% of patients (FINKLE and TAYLOR 1981; WALSH and DONKER 1982), but which can be corrected with the appropriate use of penile prostheses.

It is to be noted, however, that recently WALSH et al. (1983) have shown that the surgical technique can be modified to preserve the branches of the pelvic plexus that provide autonomic innervation to the corpora cavernosa. All of the patients who underwent this procedure experienced erections, indicating that it is possible to maintain sexual function after radical prostatectomy.

The largest series with follow-up of at least 15 years comes from Johns Hopkins Hospital (Baltimore, Maryland) and has been recently reviewed by WALSH and JEWETT (1980). A total of 57 patients with clinical stage B_1 tumors were treated between 1951 und 1963. Of them, 29 (51%) were alive and free of tumor after 15 years and 18 (32%) died without tumor. Only 10 (17%) had progression of the disease. The 51% survival is the same as the expected survival rate for this age group. These excellent results are even more significant if one considers that none of these patients was screened with bone scan or staged with node dissection.

During the same period, a group of 53 patients with clinical stage B_2 prostatic cancer underwent radical perineal prostatectomy. The 15-year survival rate free of tumor was 25%. In this group, 66% of patients had extraprostatic extension upon histologic examination. Their 15-year survival rate free of tumor was 13%. The remaining 34% had a tumor histologically confined to the prostate and had a 15-year survival rate of 50%, equal to an age-matched control population (ELDER et al. 1982).

At the present time, the role of pelvic lymph node dissection seems to be only for staging purposes. In fact, as pointed out by WALSH and JEWETT (1980), it is unlikely that all nodes, including the presacral and presciatic, can be removed without removing the rectum; furthermore, patients with positive lymph nodes seem to have poor prognosis, regardless of treatment, unless the involvement is very minimal.

II. Radiation Therapy

Radiation therapy is being used for definitive treatment of localized lesions and for palliation of bone pain in patients with metastatic tumors. The use of linear accelerator supervoltage radiotherapy has been popularized by BAGSHAW and colleagues who, in 1973, reported their results in 310 patients (RAY et al. 1973). The early 1970s have seen also the large-scale use of interstitial treatment with ^{125}I (WHITMORE et al. 1972) and ^{198}Au (CARLTON et al. 1975), the latter associated with external beam radiation.

The results of BAGSHAW et al. (1975) are very encouraging. Of 31 patients, 13 (42%) with stage B cancer and 8 of 28 (29%) with stage C lesions were reported alive without cancer 10 years or more after treatment. It is to be noted, however, that the number of patients followed for more than 10 years is very small and that other authors such as SEWELL et al. (1975) have reported rather poor results with a mortality from cancer of about 30% (5 of 17) in a group of patients with stage A or B lesions followed for 5–7 years.

A very disturbing observation in patients treated with radiation therapy is that approximately 60% of them continue to show cancer after the treatment has been completed (e.g., SEWELL at al. 1975; KIESLING et al. 1980; FREIHA 1982). Although it has been argued that the malignant cells noted in the biopsies are not biologically active, it is now known that these patients do not fare well. Indeed, from 30% (KIESLING et al. 1980) to approximately 50% (FREIHA 1982) of them show progession of the disease. Furthermore, about 50% of these biopsies show evidence of more undifferentiated tumors, and neoplastic cells present after 1 year of treatment will not disappear later (KIESLING et al. 1980). Of great interest in this regard is a study by PAULSON et al. (1982), indicating that in stage A_2 and B radical prostatectomy is more effective than megavoltage radiation in establishing disease control.

Complications of the treatment consist of irritative urinary symptoms and rectal tenesmus which usually are not lasting; impotence is present in about 40%–50% patients and absence of ejaculation is very common. Severe rectal lesions requiring colostomy are rare (1 of 430 patients in BAGSHAW's series reported in 1975). In patients who undergo extensive radiation because of node involvement, lymphedema can be noted. Because of these limitations, this form of treatment is not recommended in young patients with clearly resectable lesions, unless there are contraindications to surgery.

The use of interstitial therapy alone or in combination with external beam radiation has the advantage of giving a very high dose directly into the prostate. Although the results are very encouraging, its use is relatively too recent to allow an objective evaluation of the benefits of this treatment, especially in patients with stage B lesions.

Of great interest are the results reported by FLOCKS et al. (1975), in the treatment of stage C tumors with combined prostatectomy and interstitial irradiation with ^{198}Au. These authors have found that 147 of 244 patients (60.7%) with unknown lymph node status were alive at 5 years without evidence of tumor. In another group of 69 patients without lymph node metastases, the survival at 5 years was 74%, at 10 years 66.7%, and at 15 years 27.5%; if lymph nodes were involved

28 of 32 patients (87.5%) survived 5 years, but only 12.5% were alive at 15 years. These results are particularly significant if one considers that, according to these authors, the survival of these patients without treatment would be only 2–3 years.

III. Hormonal Therapy

Knowledge of the hormonal factors influencing prostate growth has been widely utilized in the treatment of prostatic adenocarcinoma. The modalities which have been used for this purpose are bilateral orchiectomy, administration of estrogens or antiandrogens, hypophysectomy, and adrenalectomy.

HUGGINS and HODGES (1941) introduced castration and estrogens in the treatment of advanced carcinoma of the prostate; in fact, estrogens can reduce the plasma testosterone to castration levels. In order to produce this effect, diethylstilbestrol should be used at the dose of 3 mg/day (SCOTT et al. 1980).

Before the publication of the VACURG (Veterans Administration Cooperative Urological Research Group) studies, hormonal manipulation was widely used in patients with prostatic carcinoma, regardless of its stage. VACURG was organized in 1960 for the purpose of evaluating the treatment of prostatic carcinoma in large-scale, randomized prospective trials. The results of this investigation can be summarized as follows: (1) administration of estrogens does not improve the survival of patients with stage A or B disease treated with prostatectomy; (2) delayed hormonal therapy is as beneficial as early hormonal therapy in affecting survival of patients with metastatic carcinoma; (3) the group treated with estrogens has a higher mortality rate because of cardiovascular complications; and (4) castration is as effective as estrogens or combination of the two (e.g. BYAR 1972, 1973; BLACKARD et al. 1973; BLACKARD 1975).

As a result of these findings, the use of hormonal manipulation, at least in the United States, is now mostly limited to cases with symptomatic stage D_2 carcinoma or with locally advanced tumors causing ureteral obstruction. The length of survival of untreated patients with stage D_2 cancer is variable, but averages between 1 and 2 years (WHITMORE 1956). According to the VACURG study, 10% of the patients treated with hormones will die within 6 months, 10% will live more than 10 years, and 80% will have an intermediate survival with 50% of the total living less than 3 years (JORDAN et al. 1977). Certainly, it would be very helpful to know in advance which patients would have a sustained remission under hormonal treatment. In this regard a recent study by BRENDLER and WALSH (1983) has shown that an index based on multiple enzymatic activities (such as androgen receptor content, tissue testosterone, dihydrotestosterone levels, and concentration of different enzymes of the androgen metabolism) may predict the response to endocrine therapy in prostatic carcinoma.

Relatively recently, antiandrogens, especially cyproterone acetate and flutamide, have been investigated. Although effective in the treatment of metastatic carcinoma of the prostate (e.g. SCOTT and SHIRMER 1966; SOGANI and WHITMORE 1979), they do not seem to be more effective than conventional hormonal treatment. Hypophysectomy and adrenalectomy can produce symptomatic relief in selected patients, but at the present time are very seldom used.

IV. Chemotherapy

Only recently, attention has been given to the use of chemotherapeutic agents in the treatment of prostatic adenocarcinoma. In the United States, the National Prostatic Cancer Project has been responsible for the organization of a nationally randomized study of these agents. At the present time, the only results available are from a study conducted in patients with stage D_2 disease not responding to hormonal treatment (SCHMIDT et al. 1980). Estramustine sulfate and cyclophosphamide are the most active of the drugs evaluated so far.

Estramustine sulfate couples the estrogenic action with a cytostatic or cytotoxic effect. It has been available in Europe for several years, being mostly utilized in the treatment of metastatic carcinoma (e.g. ALFTHAN and RUSK 1969; JÖNSSON and HÖGBERG 1971; NAGEL and KÖLLN 1972). Absence of myelosuppression is an important property of this drug and for this reason SCHMIDT et al. (1980) have used it in patients who had previously received radiation therapy. In 30% of them, an improved performance was noted and 30% had an objective response (regression of lesions in 6% and stabilization in 24%). The main limitation of this agent is that it causes gastrointestinal disturbances in a relatively high proportion of patients.

SCHMIDT et al. (1980) have also reported the results of treatment with cyclophosphamide in 41 patients. About 50% of them experienced relief of pain and 30% were able to improve their performance; an objective response was noted in 46% (regression of lesions in 7% and stabilization in 39%). Nausea or vomiting and decline of white cell count were frequently noted. From these observations it is clear that a good chemotherapeutic regime is not yet available, but it is possible that a combination of known agents or a newly discovered drug might in the future provide an answer to this problem.

V. Conclusions

What is the best therapeutic approach for prostatic adenocarcinoma? This is a subject of great controversy, which is sustained by the wide range of biologic malignancy of this cancer. This chapter will only give a guideline based on the available information. Important deciding factors are tumor grading and the patient's age. Both of them influence the prognosis because the invasive potential is indirectly proportional to the degree of tumor differentiation and to the age. Untreated patients in their eighties have a life expectancy similar to their comparison population whereas young patients, especially with undifferentiated cancers, have a poor prognosis if not treated aggressively (HANASH et. al. 1972).

It is probably best merely to keep stage A_1 tumors under observation, since they tend to remain dormant. By contrast, patients with stage A_2 tumors need additional treatment, especially if otherwise they have a long life expectancy. Although radical prostatectomy is feasible, it is more difficult because of previous prostatic surgery and has a higher incidence of urinary incontinence. For these reasons, radiation therapy seems to be a more appropriate form of treatment.

Stage B_1 tumors appear to be treated best with surgery when the patient has a life expectancy of at least 10 years; if surgery is contraindicated, external radiation treatment seem to be a valid alternative. Stage B_2 tumors are probably amenable to surgery if staging lymphadenectomy is negative or could be considered for definitive radiation therapy; if the pelvic lymph nodes are positive these tumors should be regarded as stage D_1 and in that case treatment is uncertain. External radiation therapy seems to be the best choice for stage C tumors, but a combination of surgery and interstitial radiation could be used.

Patients with stage D_1 tumors obviously have a systemic disease. They would be ideal candidates for chemotherapy and some of them might be selected for hormonal treatment, if the response to it could be anticipated; unfortunately, at the present time good chemotherapeutic regimes and universally accepted screening tests for hormonal dependence of tumors are not available. As a result the treatment of these patients is uncertain; however, a recent prospective study suggests that radiation therapy has some advantages over delayed hormonal therapy (PAULSON et al. 1982).

In stage D_2, hormonal manipulation, preferably in the form of castration, is indicated and at the present time is generally instituted when the tumor causes ureteral obstruction or the patient becomes symptomatic since there is no evidence that an early treatment produces better long-term results. If patients are refractory to hormonal manipulation, chemotherapy or radiation therapy to painful metastatic lesions could be used.

It is obvious that, in spite of the progress made in the knowledge of this disease, much needs to be learned. As pointed out by ELDER et al. (1980), it is possible that the discovery of new chemotherapeutic agents and methods of selecting patients for different modalities of treatment will improve our results in the battle against this common and possibly devastating disease.

Acknowledgments. The contribution of Leon Schlossberg (Assistant Professor of Art as Applied to Medicine, Johns Hopkins Hospital, Baltimore, Maryland), who drew the illustrations, is gratefully acknowledged.

References

Alfthan OS, Rusk J (1969) Estracyt in advanced prostatic carcinoma. Ann Chir Gynaecol 58:234–240

Bagshaw MA, Ray GR, Pistenna DA, Castellino RA, Meares EM Jr (1975) External beam radiation therapy of primary carcinoma of prostate. Cancer 36:723–728

Basso A (1978) The prostate in the elderly male. In: Reichel W, Schechter M (eds) The geriatric patient. HP Publishing Co, New York, p 123

Blackard CE (1975) The Veteran Administration Cooperative Urological Research group's studies of carcinoma of the prostate: a review. Cancer Chemother Rep 59:225–227

Blackard CE, Byar DP, Jordan WP Jr and the Veterans Administration Cooperative Research Group (1973) Orchiectomy for advanced carcinoma: a re-evaluation. Urology 1:553–560

Brendler CB, Walsh PC (1983) Predictors of response to endocrine therapy in carcinoma of prostate – Need for multiple discriminatory patients – Presentation at 78th Annual Meeting of AUA, Las Vegas (USA) April 17–21

Bruchovsky N, Wilson JD (1968) The conversion of testosterone to 5α-Androstan-17β-01-3-one by rat prostate in vivo and in vitro. J Biol Chem 243:2012–2021

Byar DP (1972) Treatment of prostatic cancer: studies by the Veterans Administration Cooperative Urological Research Group. Bull NY Acad Med 48:751–766

Byar DP (1973) The Veterans Administration Cooperative Urological Research Group's Studies of cancer of the prostate. Cancer 32:1126–1230
Cabot AT (1896) The question of castration for enlarged prostate. Ann Surg 24:265–309
Caine M, Perlberg S, Shapiro A (1981) Phenoxybenzamine for benign prostatic obstruction. Review of 200 cases. Urology 17:542–546
Carlton CE Jr, Hudgins PT, Guerriero WG, Scott R Jr (1975) Radiotherapy in the management of stage C carcinoma of the prostate. Trans Am Assoc Genitourin Surgeons 67:70–74
De Klerk DP, Coffey DS, Ewing LL, McDermott IR, Reiner WG, Robinson CH, Scott WW, Stranber JD, Talalay P, Walsh PC, Wheaton LG, Zirkin BR (1979) Comparison of spontaneous and experimentally induced canine prostatic hyperplasia. J Clin Invest 64:842–849
Drach GW, Meares EM, Fair WR, Stamey TA (1978) Classification of benign diseases associated with prostatic pain: prostatitis or prostatodynia? J Urol 120:266
Elder JS, Scott WW, Nyberg LM (1980) Overview of past and current philosophy of prostatic cancer. Prostate 1:287–301
Elder JS, Jewett JH, Walsh PC (1982) Radical perineal prostatectomy for clinical stage B_2 carcinoma of the prostate. J Urol 127:704–706
Ewing LL (1976) Testis: changes with age. In: Grayhack JT, Wilson JD, Scherbenske MJ (eds) Benign prostatic hyperplasia. US Government Printing Office, Washington DC, pp 195–204
Fair WR (1974) Diffusion of minocycline into prostatic secretions in dogs. Urology 3:339–344
Fair WR, Crane DB, Schiller N, Heston WDW (1979) A re-appraisal of treatment in chronic bacterial prostatitis. J Urol 121:437–441
Finkle AL, Prian DV (1966) Sexual potency in elderly men before and after prostatectomy. JAMA 196:139–143
Finkle AL, Taylor SP (1981) Sexual potency after radical prostatectomy. J Urol 125:350–352
Flocks RH, O'Donoghue EPN, Milleman LA, Culp DA (1975) Management of stage C prostatic carcinoma. Urol Clin North Am 2:163–179
Freiha FS (1982) quoted by: Stamey TA (1982) Cancer of the prostate. Monogr Urol 3:67–94
Grayhack JT, Sadlowski RW (1976) Current results of surgical therapy. In: Grayhack JT, Wilson JD, Scherbenske MJ (eds) Benign prostatic hyperplasia. US Government Printing Office, Washington DC pp 125–134
Grayhack JT, Bunde PL, Kearns JW, Scott WW (1955) Influence of the pituitary on prostatic response to androgens in the rat. Johns Hopkins Med J 96:154–163
Hanash KA, Utz DC, Cook EN, Taylor WF, Titus JL (1972) Carcinoma of the prostate: a 15 year followup. J Urol 197:450–453
Huggins C, Hodges CV (1941) Studies on prostatic cancer-I. The effect of castration, of estrogen and of androgen injection on serum phosphatases in metastatic carcinoma of the prostate. Cancer Res 1:293–297
Jewett HJ (1975) The present status of radical prostatectomy for stages A and B prostatic cancer. Urol Clin North Am 2:105–126
Jonsson G, Hogberg B (1971) Treatment of advanced prostatic carcinoma with Estracyt. Scand J Urol Nephrol 5:103–107
Jordan WP, Blackard CE, Byar DP (1977) Reconsideration of orchiectomy in the treatment of advanced prostatic carcinoma. South Med J 70:141–143
Kaufman JJ, Goodwin WE (1959) Hormonal management of benign obstructing prostate: use of combined androgen-estrogen therapy. J Urol 81:165–171
Kiesling VJ, McAninch JW, Goebel JL, Agee RE (1980) External beam radiotherapy for adenocarcinoma of the prostate: a clinical follow up. J Urol 124:851–854
Kramer SA, Cline WA Jr, Farnham R, Carson CC, Cox EB, Hinshaw W, Paulson DF (1981) Prognosis of patients with stage D prostatic adenocarcinoma. J Urol 125:817–891
McCullough DL (1980) Surgical staging of carcinoma of prostate. Cancer 45:1902–1905

Meares EM Jr (1973) Observations an activity of Trimethoprim-sulfamethoxazole in the prostate. J Inf Dis 128:S679–S685
Meares EM Jr (1975) Long-term therapy of chronic bacterial prostatitis with Trimethoprim-sulfamethoxazole. Can Med Assoc J 122:22S–25S
Meares EM Jr (1979) Urinary tract infections in men. In: Harrison JH, Gittes RF, Perlmutter AD, Stamey TA, Walsh PC (eds) Campbells' Urology, 4th edn. Saunders, Philadelphia, pp 509–537
Meares EM Jr (1980) Prostatitis Syndromes: new perspectives about old woes. J Urol 123:141–147
Mobley DF (1974) Erythromycin plus sodium bicarbonate in chronic bacterial prostatitis. Urology 3:60–62
Nagel R, Kolln CP (1972) Erfahrungen mit estracyt bei metastasierendem Prostatakarzinom. Acta Urol 3:241–246
Oliveri RA, Sachs RM, Caste PG (1979) Clinical experience with geocillin in the treatment of bacterial prostatitis. Curr Ther Res Clin Exp 25:415–421
Paulson DF, Cline WA Jr, Koefoot RB Jr, Hinshaw W, Stephani S, and Uro-Oncology Research Group (1982) Extended field radiation therapy versus delayed hormonal therapy in node positive prostatic adenocarcinoma. J Urol 127:935–937
Paulson DF, Lin GH, Hinshaw W, Stephani S and the Uro-Oncology Research Group (1982) Radical surgery versus radiotherapy for adenocarcinoma of the prostate. J Urol 128:502–504
Prout GR, Griffin DP, Daly JJ, Shipley WU (1981) Nodal involvement as prognostic indicator in prostatic carcinoma. Urology [Suppl] 17:72–79
Rangno RE, McLeod PJ, Ruedy J, Ogilvie RI (1971) Treatment of benign prostatic hypertrophy with medrogestone. Clin Pharmacol Ther 12:658–665
Ray GR, Cassidy JR, Bagshaw MA (1973) Definitive radiation therapy of carcinoma of the prostate: a report of 15 years experience. Radiology 106:407–418
Schmidt JD, Scott WW, Gibbons R, Johnson DE, Prout GR, Loening S, Soloway M, DeKernion J, Pontes YE, Slack NH, Murphy GP (1980) Chemotherapy programs of the National Prostatic Cancer Project (NPCP). Cancer 45:1937–1946
Scott WW, DeKlerk DP (1976) Benign prostatic hyperplasia: current status of medical treatment. In: Grayhack JT, Wilson JD, Scherbenske MJ (eds) Benign prostatic hyperplasia. US Government Printing Office, Washington DC, pp 135–151
Scott WW, Schirmer HKA (1966) A new oral progestational steriod effective in treating prostatic cancer. Trans Am Assoc Genitourin Surg 58:54–60
Scott WW, Wade JC (1969) Medical treatment of benign nodular prostatic hyperplasia with cyproterone acetate. J Urol 101:81–85
Scott, WW, Menon M, Walsh PC (1980) Hormonal therapy of prostatic cancer. Cancer 45:1929–1936
Segura JW, Opitz JL, Greene LF (1979) Prostatosis, prostatitis or pelvic floor tension myalgia? J Urol 122:168–169
Sewell RA, Braren V, Wilson SK, Rhamy RK (1976) Extended biopsy follow-up after full course radiation for resectable prostatic carcinoma. J Urol 113:371–373
Siiteri PK, Wilson JD (1970) Dihydrotestosterone in prostatic hypertrophy I. The formation and content of dihydrotestosterone in the hypertrophic prostate in man. J Clin Invest 49:1737–1745
Silverberg E, Holleb AI (1975) Major trends in cancer: 25 years survey. CA 25:2–8
Siroki MB, Goldstein I, Krane RJ (1981) Functional voiding disorders in men. J Urol 126:200–204
Sogani PC; Whitmore WF Jr (1979) Experience with flutamide in previously untreated patients with advanced prostatic cancer. J Urol 122:640–643
Staehler W, Ziegler H, Volter D, Schubert GE, Wartman WB (1976) Color atlas of cytodiagnosis of the prostate. Year Book Medical Publishers, Chicago, p 5
Stamey TA (1972) Urinary infections. Williams and Wilkins, Baltimore, p 191
Stamey TA (1980) Pathogenesis and treatment of urinary tract infections. Williams and Wilkins, Baltimore, pp 342–429

Stearns EL, MacDonnell JA, Kaufman BJ, Padua R, Luchman TS, Winter JSD, Faiman C (1974) Declining testicular function with age. Hormonal and clinical correlates. Am J Med 57:761–766

Trachtenberg J, Bujnovsky P, Walsh PC (1982) Androgen receptor content of normal and hyperplastic human prostate. J Clin Endocrinol Metab 54:17–21

Vermeulen A (1976) Testicular hormonal secretions and aging in males. In: Grayhack JT, Wilson JD, Scherbenske MJ (eds) Benign prostatic hyperplasia. US Government Printing Office, Washington DC, pp 177–182

Wajsman A (1981) Lymph node evaluation in prostatic cancer: is pelvic lymph node dissection necessary? Urology Suppl 17:80–82

Walsh PC (1979) Benign prostatic hyperplasia. In: Harrison JH, Gittes RF, Perlmutter AD, Stamey TA, Walsh PC (eds) Campbell's Urology, 4th edn. Saunders, Philadelphia, pp 949–964

Walsh PC, Donker PH (1982) Impotence following radical prostatectomy: insight into etiology and prevention. J Urol 128:492–497

Walsh, PC, Jewett JH (1980) Radical surgery for prostatic cancer. Cancer 45:1906–1911

Walsh PC, Wilson JD (1976) The induction of prostatic hypertrophy in the dog with androstenediol. J Clin Invest 57:1093–1097

Walsh PC, Lepor H, Eggleston JC (1983) Radical prostatectomy with preservation of sexual function: anatomical and pathological considerations. Prostate 4:473–485

Weyrauch HM (1967) Life after fifty: the prostatic age. The Ward Ritchie, Los Angeles, p 15

White JW (1895) The results of double castration in hypertrophy of the prostate. Ann Surg 22:1–80

Whitmore WF Jr (1956) Hormone therapy in prostatic cancer. Am J Med 21:697–718

Whitmore WF Jr (1973) The natural history of prostatic cancer. Cancer 32:1104–1112

Whitmore WF Jr, Hilaris B, Grabstald H (1972) Retropubic implantation of iodine-125 in the treatment of prostatic cancer. J Urol 108:918–920

Young HH (1905) The early diagnosis and radical care of carcinoma of the prostate: Being a study of 40 cases and presentation of a radical operation which was carried out in four cases. John Hopkins Med J 16:315–321

Young HH, Davis DM (1926) Young's practice of urology, Vol I. Saunders, Philadelphia, p 496

Thoracic Surgery in the Elderly: Heart and Vessels

M. PANETH

A. Definition

The elderly in this chapter are defined as patients over the age of 65 years. This is an arbitrary definition and in some units (and publications) 70 years is taken as the lower limit of this group of patients. It should be pointed out most emphatically that physiological rather than temporal age is significant and it is well known that a patient of 70 years but with well-preserved cardiorespiratory and renal reserves will have a better prognosis than a patient with the same correctable lesion in whom these reserves have been severely depleted. Since the more complex and severe congenital cardiac malformations often prove to be fatal in the first few months of life, it is obvious that they will not be encountered in this age group. On the other hand, the effects of ischaemia and degeneration will more frequently require surgical intervention.

B. Principles of Cardiac Surgery

The general principles which have made cardiac surgery safe apply with added emphasis of this group of patients. These principles are: support of the whole patient.

I. Support of the Whole Patient

Cardiopulmonary bypass is now an acceptably safe and well-established technique for the support of the vital organs during exclusion of the heart and lungs. This technique allows the surgeon to interrupt the function of the heart and lungs temporarily and thus to correct malformations and lesions which would otherwise be inaccessible. In the younger age group, and especially in infants, a considerable margin of safety is available since their powers of recovery are so good. The development of atheromatous lesions at the origins of the major branches of the aorta results in decreased perfusion to the corresponding territory. When coupled to a nonpulsatile and low pressure/low flow perfusion, ischaemic damage may result. Any bruit in a peripheral vessel (carotid, femoral) should be noted and may require further investigation. Thus carotid artery stenoses, if severe, will require correction before the patient is placed on cardiopulmonary bypass since it is this group of patients who are particularly at risk to develop an intraoperative hemiplegia. Equally, if there is a likelihood of intraaortic balloon counterpulsation

(Sect. E.I) being necessary after operation, knowledge of the arterial status of the limb is essential.

Patients with established benign essential hypertension also require a perfusion pressure higher than usual to maintain adequate tissue perfusion and to overcome undetected and untreatable stenoses in the smaller arteries supplying the central nervous system and kidneys. Renal function will require more thorough assessment and renal perfusion and urine production must be critically monitored and adequately maintained throughout the period of bypass. Periods of circulatory arrest, even at body temperatures considered safe in younger patients, should be kept shorter in this group since circulatory arrest and anoxia are not well tolerated.

In summary, the surgeon and supporting team must be aware of the fact that the function of a number of systems may be critically, although as yet subclinically, compromised and even slight reductions in the efficacy of perfusion and gas exchange may rapidly result in permanent and disastrous damage and thereby fatally affect what would otherwise have been a gratifying surgical result. The choice of oxygenator must also be taken into account. There should be a bias in favour of the use of membrane oxygenators as opposed to the bubble systems, since there is less blood damage and a much lower incidence of microbubble emboli reaching the patient's systemic arterial system. The theoretical advantages of pulsatile pumping systems, though considerable, have not been consistently observed in practice and although pulsatile perfusions are routinely employed in many centres, there is no clear-cut evidence to justify the increased cost and complexity of the perfusion technique which is involved.

II. Protection of the Heart

1. Coronary Perfusion

Theoretically the best protection of the myocardium should be obtained by maintaining coronary perfusion at normal levels and at normal temperatures, even in the completely unloaded heart. It could be argued that a normal coronary blood flow under these circumstances might in fact be too good and even harmful since the normal wall tension, in systole, is not generated by the empty heart and thus the intramyocardial coronary blood flow continues throughout the cardiac cycle. In practice it is certainly true that a normal electrocardiogram can be maintained by coronary perfusion, even though the flow pattern and volume are not normal. Such a state, indicative of a well-supported myocardium, is relatively easy to obtain in young adults, but in the elderly with some disease of the coronary arteries, and coupled with the technical difficulties of cannulating the coronary ostia satisfactorily while operating for aortic valve disease, the ideal situation is much more difficult to achieve and maintain.

2. Intermittent Ischaemia

This is achieved by intermittent occlusion of the ascending aorta. It is a fairly safe technique when coupled with moderate total body hypothermia (30 °C), but it is only possible when the ascending aorta remains intact, as in operations on the mitral valve, left ventricle or coronary arteries. It should be stressed that every time the pressure in the ascending aorta falls to zero with any part of the left heart open, the aortic valve leaflets will separate and the aortic root will empty of blood and fill with air. Every time the aortic clamp is released, the contained air in the aortic root will be forced into the coronary arteries as the aortic valve closes. Intermittent coronary ischaemia by this technique, for mitral valve replacement for instance, therefore has a cumulative deleterious effect, not only from the repeated ischaemic insult, but also from repeated coronary air embolism, particularly to the right coronary artery. Recurrent coronary air embolism does not occur when this technique of intermittent cardiac ischaemia is used for operations solely on the coronary arteries. On the other hand, intermittent coronary ischaemia is cumulative in itself and it has been shown that the aggregate ischaemic time should not exceed approximately 40 min at 30 °C.

3. Cold Cardioplegia

The technique of achieving profound myocardial hypothermia evolved from the technique of profound total body hypothermia which is still in use for the correction of complex congenital malformations in neonates and small infants. Hypothermia to 15 °C protects the myocardium and prevents damage from total myocardial ischaemia for up to 90 min. This technique offers the surgeon a still and bloodless heart and thus aids in the exposure and ease of operations on and inside the heart. Methods have been evolved to cool the heart uniformly and rapidly via its coronary bed by producing diastolic arrest with the use of solutions containing a high concentration of potassium ions and by bathing the heart both inside and out in cold physiological solutions. Care must be taken to prevent the heart from rewarming via the ambient temperature, from the radiant heat generated by the overhead theatre lights and from the surrounding tissues, lungs and descending aorta, which will still be maintained at moderate hypothermic levels.

In addition, and this applies particularly to patients with ischaemic heart disease, a significant volume of blood may enter the coronary bed by well-developed collateral channels and thus cause rewarming and also washout of the cold electrolyte solution. The effect of this collateral coronary flow can be reduced by reducing the perfusion pressure and temperature. In younger patients reduction in minute volume to reduce the pressure is quite safe, particularly when accompanied by a degree of moderate total body hypothermia, but, as pointed out before, pressure and temperature reduction may cause uneven perfusion and tissue temperatures in the presence of undetected stenoses in the primary and secondary branches of the aorta.

In summary, therefore, although coronary perfusion, either intermittent or continuous, depending on the local conditions, is still preferred by some surgeons, the majority of cardiac surgeons now prefer to protect the myocardium by instituting cold cardioplegia and maintaining the myocardial temperature between 5 ° and 15 °C until the cardiac part of the operation has been completed. At the same time it should be stressed that too low a temperature, as can be achieved with the use of ice slush in the pericardium, can and does cause permanent myocardial damage.

III. Correction of Lesion

This principle applies with rather more emphasis to this elderly group of patients since, with reduced reserves, they are less able to sustain the postoperative burden of a partially corrected lesion. For example, when the number of coronary arteries bypassed per patient is analysed, one finds that with increasing confidence and experience this number rises and this rise is accompanied by improved mortality and morbidity statistics. Elderly patients undergoing correction of mitral valve lesions do not tolerate a modest degree of aortic reflux since the regurgitant stream entering the left ventricle will tend to cause premature mitral valve closure and thus may result in a stormy postoperative course and an indifferent final result. On the other hand it is a matter of fine judgement to balance total correction of all lesions against the potential hazard of prolonged cardiac arrest and an extended total body perfusion time.

IV. Haemostasis

Haemorrhage is still the commonest complication of surgery and certainly postoperative blood loss after cardiac surgery is an important contributory factor to the patient's rate of recovery. Blood is a tissue and homologous blood, however carefully cross-matched, is a foreign tissue. Careful haemostasis with minimal dissection of tissue planes before heparinisation and prior to the insertion of the arterial and venous cannulae, will result in minimal blood loss into the pericardial cradle, less cardiotomy suction and therefore less damage to the blood components. Bleeding after the restoration of normal coagulation by administration of appropriate amounts of protamine will be reduced to reasonable levels. Blood replacement and demands on the blood transfusion services are then reduced to a minimum and homeostasis is easily achieved. The patient spends less time in the operating theatre with an open incision, the risk of sepsis is reduced and wound healing is improved with fewer postoperative hematomas and incidences of serosanguineous discharges. The upshot is that the patient spends less time in hospital during and after operation. This, of course, is an important consideration for all patients, but applies especially to the elderly who may develop severe symptoms of disorientation when they are suddenly translated from their stable environment to one which is totally strange and frightening to them. The cost of hospitalisation has to be borne either by the patient or by the State and in either event prolonged hospital stay is expensive, increases the average cost of treatment per patient, and denies another patient the use of that bed.

In some units, particularly in the United States, it has become a routine to reinfuse the blood recovered during the first 6 h via the pericardial drainage tubes. Since blood donors in some countries are not strictly supervised and are paid, the incidence of hepatitis is much higher than in other countries such as the United Kingdom where the blood transfusion service is free and is supported entirely by volunteer blood donors.

C. Technique

I. Exposure

For all intracardiac operations and those on the ascending aorta and origin of the great vessels, a vertical median sternotomy is universally accepted as the simplest and best. It affords easy access to the heart and great vessels. Cosmetic submammary skin incisions have no place at this age. If the pericardium is incised to the left of the sternum as a flap hinged laterally on the right and pulled out to be held by the right-hand blade of the sternal retractor, access to the right atrium, the right superior pulmonary vein and aorta is obtained and at the end of the operation the line of closure of the pericardium will be to the left of the sternum. This pericardial flap will protect the right ventricle at the time of resternotomy should this be necessary subsequently.

II. Cannulation

In this section, only the special precautions applicable to the elderly will be described since it is assumed that the reader is familiar with standard cardiopulmonary techniques using aortic and bicaval or right atrial cannulation.

1. Aorta

In these patients atheromatous changes may have occurred in the walls of the aorta and therefore special care must be taken during cannulation and clamping of the aorta that these atheromatous plaques, endothelial ulcers and calcifications are not loosened and displaced. In general the inner left lateral wall of the aorta is spared by these changes and this is therefore the preferred site for the insertion of the aortic perfusion cannula. For the same reason the application of side clamps prior to incising the cannulation site should be avoided, and the cannula should be inserted directly through the stab incision. Equally, when the aorta is occluded with a cross clamp, the arterial pressure should be allowed to fall to almost zero for a few seconds by stopping the arterial pump and allowing the venous blood to continue to drain into the oxygenator. A soft aorta is occluded gently by this manoeuvre and there is then less risk of injury to it. If there is the suspicion that calcified material or atheromatous plaques are likely to become dislodged either at the time of occlusion or when the occluding clamp is released, then precautions to prevent their embolisation, especially to the brain, must be taken by temporarily occluding the major branches of the aortic arch before the aortic occlusion clamp is either applied or released.

If it is thought that aortic cannulation is likely to be too hazardous then one should not hesitate to expose the common femoral artery in the groin and cannulate it for arterial return. This also applies if it is necessary to perform an extensive repair or resection of the ascending aorta up to the origin of the innominate (brachiocephalic) artery.

2. Right Atrium and Cavae

Bicaval cannulation is necessary for operations on the left and right atrioventricular valves, the atrial septum, the right ventricle and ventricular septum. Thus right atrial drainage via its appendage or through a pursestring suture in the wall of the right atrium, is sufficient for all operations on the left ventricle, coronary arteries, aortic valve and ascending aorta. Indeed, it is desirable to avoid the introduction of cannulae into the cavae and to snare them with tape whenever possible since these manoeuvres do result in an increased incidence of atrial dysrhythmias, probably by interfering with the sinoatrial node directly, or with its blood supply. Elderly patients react badly to postoperative dysrhythmias of any sort.

3. Left Ventricular Decompression

The purpose of a catheter inserted into the left ventricle usually via its apex is first to prevent the left ventricle from becoming overdistended with resulting stretch injury to the left ventricular muscle, and second to evacuate any residual air from the left side of the heart at the end of the intracardiac procedure and before the left ventricle is allowed to eject blood into the ascending aorta.

The left ventricular vent catheter can be inserted via a pursestring suture through a stab incision in the termination of the right superior pulmonary vein; it is advanced across the left atrium and then enters the left ventricle through the mitral valve. This route has the advantage that only the right side of the heart need be freed and this may be important in patients undergoing a reoperation in whom freeing the whole heart to gain access to the left ventricular apex is hazardous. The disadvantage of this route is that it is not so easy to be certain that all air has been evacuated from the left ventricle since the left ventricle cannot be satisfactorily manipulated. Also, if the vent catheter slips back into the left atrium unnoticed, then the left ventricle may not remain decompressed at all times. Since the effects of focal cerebral ischaemia are much more noticeable and permanent in elderly patients, the safest site for inserting the left ventricular vent catheter should be obtained.

Patients undergoing myocardial revascularisation only, in whom there is no aortic reflux, do not require left ventricular decompression since when the aortic cardioplegia catheter is placed on suction to remove the collateral coronary blood entering the heart, this decompresses the aortic root and the left ventricle. If on the other hand the technique of intermittent aortic occlusion is used, then it may be necessary to decompress the left ventricle if there is minimal, previously undetected, aortic reflux.

D. The Lesions

I. Congenital

As stated in Sect. A the more complex and immediately life-threatening malformations are not encountered at this age. On the other hand, congenital lesions which either remain undetected or were insignificant in early life may become more obvious and will then require correction.

1. Atrial Septal Defect

This relatively benign lesion resulting in a left-to-right shunt at atrial level is sometimes overlooked in childhood and adolescence. Since it does not usually result in a rise in pulmonary vascular resistance for many years, the continuing low pressure–high pulmonary flow situation produces enlargement of the right atrium, right ventricle and pulmonary arteries with plethoric lung fields. The commonest complication resulting from these changes is the onset of atrial fibrillation, and it is the development and investigation of this dysrhythmia which will eventually lead to the true diagnosis. It is arguable whether closing the atrial septal defect after atrial fibrillation is established is still indicated since even after a successful closure it is more than likely that the atrial dysrhythmia will rapidly reappear even if sinus rhythm has been obtained for a short period postoperatively.

The arguments in favour of closing the defect are first that atrial fibrillation will then not affect the systemic output so much, and second, an intact atrial septum will prevent the occurrence of a paradoxical embolus. This is a definite risk when the pulmonary vascular resistance rises. Closure of the defect is definitely contraindicated when investigations by cardiac catheterisation have proved that the pulmonary vascular resistance is now so high that the left-to-right shunt has been abolished or indeed reversed. Patients who have developed an Eisenmenger complex survive longer with the defect open than if an attempt is made to close it.

The defect in the atrial septum in this age group is usually large with poorly demarcated edges, and therefore patch closure using a woven polyester patch sutured in place with a continuous running suture of monofilament material is indicated to obtain secure abolition of the shunt without distortion of the remnants of the atrial septum. If on the other hand, as is more unusual, the defect is relatively small with well-developed edges all round, its direct closure in two layers with a continuous suture may be justified, provided traction on the atrial septum is avoided since this may lead to rhythm disturbances.

2. Persistent Ductus Arteriosus

The persistent ductus arteriosus which, like the atrial septal defect, is an obligatory intrauterine shunt, normally closes soon after birth. If it remains open, then it usually results in a left-to-right shunt, the blood being forced from the high pressure aorta into the low pressure pulmonary artery throughout the cardiac cycle. This imposes a volume load on the left side of the heart, ascending aorta and arch as far down as the origin of the ductus. In the elderly there will be a large left atrium, left ventricle, ascending aorta, and pulmonary plethora on the chest X-ray and quite often calcification may be seen in the region of the aortic end of the ductus.

The reason the ductus may have remained open is that usually it is broad and short and closure of such a ductus is by no means as simple and straightforward as would be the case in infancy and childhood. Both great arteries are now under increased tension and have become closely applied to each other, the long-standing elevation of the pulmonary artery pressure having taken up any length the ductus might have had in early life. These ductuses are unsuitable for closure by ligation in continuity and their division and suture may be hazardous first because of calcification at the aortic end of the ductus, and second because any remaining ductus tissue is friable and tears easily. Haemorrhage from a ductus under these conditions may rapidly prove fatal. It is therefore advisable to have the apparatus for the institution of left atrial–femoral bypass available if at the time of left thoracotomy it is judged that a direct attack on the ductus is too risky.

The left atrial–femoral bypass is set up by inserting an appropriate cannula into the left atrium via its appendage guarded by a pursestring, sucking an appropriate amount of blood from the left atrium by a roller pump and returning it via a cannula in the left femoral artery. Total heparinisation must be instituted prior to any cannulation and the left atrial–femoral bypass is then commenced. The left pulmonary artery is identified at its origin inside the pericardium and occluded. Next, the proximal aortic clamp is applied above the origin of the ductus and as the aorta is occluded the left atrial–femoral bypass is increased so as to maintain the upper limb blood pressure, monitored by radial artery cannula in the right wrist, at normal levels. This ensures that a normal and therefore adequate volume of blood is being supplied to the lower aortic segment via the left atrial–femoral bypass circuit; and thereby the blood supplied to the spinal cord is maintained and the risk of paraplegia from spinal cord ischaemia is averted. It is mandatory that the heart is kept beating since it has to supply the upper segment of the aorta which includes the head vessels and vessels to both upper limbs. When stability has been achieved the lower clamp distal to the ductus origin is applied and the excluded segment of the aorta is then opened by a longitudinal incision. The aortic ostium of the ductus is then seen and can be securely closed at leisure with a polyester patch sewn onto its margins with a continuous suture of monofilament material. After closing the aortotomy the aortic clamps are released in reverse order, the left atrial–femoral bypass is gradually discontinued, the left pulmonary artery is released, the cannulae are removed and protamine in appropriate quantities is administered to neutralise the circulating heparin. This technique is also applicable for the treatment of recurrent or recanalised or incompletely closed ductuses.

3. Coarctation

The only other congenital malformation likely to be found at this age is a coarctation of the aorta, but this is most unlikely to require correction since by this time a large number of collaterals will have developed in response to a haemodynamically significant obstruction. These collaterals are usually sufficient to prevent a rise in systemic blood pressure and the only reason for operating on a coarctation is to reduce the elevated upper limb pressure to normal.

II. Acquired

1. Ischaemia

a) Angina

Uncomplicated coronary ischaemia is the commonest form of acquired heart disease in the elderly and results form atheromatous plaques which cause narrowing and even complete obstruction of the major coronary arteries. Aortocoronary saphenous bypass grafts to circumvent the obstructed arteries is now a universally accepted operation and the only contraindications to it are the absence of angina coupled with an unacceptably poor left ventricular function which is judged to be irreversible.

The technique of operation does not differ from that employed generally in younger patients except that special attention should be paid to the state of the ascending aorta (see Sect. C.II.1). If there are extensive areas of calcification then it is advisable to attach the aortic ends of the grafts while the ascending aorta is still occluded and empty, performing open proximal anastomoses, rather than by the repeated application of a small partial occlusion clamp for each proximal end in turn. The risk of cerebral calcium embolism is thereby minimised. Although the elderly are less likely to indulge in strenuous exercise, nevertheless as complete a myocardial revascularisation as possible should be planned taking into account the state of the left ventricle and balancing the risks of prolonged cardiopulmonary bypass in this age group with the achievement of total relief from angina.

b) Left Ventricular Aneurysm

This is the result of a full thickness myocardial infarct, usually from total occlusion of the left anterior descending artery, if this vessel has been supplying a large part of the anterolateral wall of the left ventricle. The commonest site of the aneurysm is therefore the anteroapical aspect of the left ventricle and the aneurysm may cause angina, systemic emboli from contained thrombus, and ventricular tachycardia. Left ventricular failure may also be present, but the cause of this is more likely to be poor function of the remaining myocardium rather than the simple presence of an aneurysm. It has been shown that although subjective symptoms are improved after resection of an aneurysm, there has been no significant change for the better in any of the measurable parameters of left ventricular performance. The cause of the relief of angina after resection of an aneurysm without associated coronary artery bypass grafting is probably due to the fact that at least one of the diameters of the left ventricle has been reduced with consequent reduction in the wall tension generated during systole. In this respect alone the work of the left ventricle may have been reduced. Rarely is it necessary to graft the left anterior descending artery since even if a satisfactory graft is applied, it would only supply the scar tissue remaining and resulting from resection and repair of the aneurysm. On the other hand, it is becoming increasingly more evident that better postoperative results in this group are obtained if significant lesions in the other main branches of the coronary arteries are bypassed at the same time. The precautions taken in the presence of an unhealthy wall of the ascending aorta have been outlined in previous sections.

If there is a suspicion of thrombus in the left ventricle or its aneurysm, then the aorta should be occluded before the area of the aneurysm is manipulated, to open it or even to free it from adhesions to the pericardium. Myocardial protection should therefore be instituted at the time of aortic occlusion and the aneurysm only manipulated when it is safe to do so. Once exposed the aneurysm should be opened widely through the fibrotic left ventricular wall and all contained thrombus should be removed. At the same time the surgeon should inspect the inside of the ascending aorta through the aortic valve as far as the occlusion clamp, and also the left atrium via the mitral valve. Only when all visible thrombus has been removed is it safe to release the clamp on the ascending aorta should the technique of myocardial protection require this; but elective fibrillation of the heart must then be instituted and maintained until the incision in the left ventricle has been repaired and all air has been removed from the pulmonary veins, left atrium and left ventricle.

The left ventricular aneurysm is resected leaving a margin of about 0.5 cm fibrous tissue on each side of the incision and taking care to leave an adequate residual left ventricular cavity. The mitral valve mechanism should be inspected to ensure that it is intact. The fibrous edges of the incision in the left ventricle are then sutured together over two strips of polytetrafluoroethylene (PTFE) felt by a continuous horizontal mattress suture covered by a continuous over-and-over stitch. Any coronary anastomoses can then be performed either during the cardioplegic arrest (Sect. B.II.3), if this technique has been used, or by the intermittent aortic occlusion technique (Sect. B.II.2).

c) Ventricular Septal Defect

Ischaemic necrosis of the ventricular septum resulting in a ventricular septal defect occurs principally in two sites – anteroapical and inferobasal. Of these the former is the more common, but an associated left ventricular aneurysm of any size is unusual since the patient is unlikely to survive the double burden of a left ventricular aneurysm of any extent and the sudden development of a large left-to-right shunt resulting from perforation of the necrotic ventricular septum. In contrast, a small inferobasal aneurysm is often seen in posterior ventricular septal defects.

Ischaemic ventricular septal defects produce a sudden large left-to-right shunt, the size of which is limited by the development of pulmonary oedema and right ventricular failure. When measured by cardiac catheterisation and oximetry, it is rarely above 3 : 1 in the acute phase. Following a large infarct, the patient will suddenly develop acute dyspnoea, a raised central venous pressure, evidence of a low cardiac output, and a systolic thrill and murmur over the precordium. The diagnosis must be distinguished from acute massive mitral regurgitation due to papillary muscle rupture, and this can be done by cardiac catheterisation and angiography, or by the insertion of a Swan–Ganz catheter into the pulmonary artery for measurement of pulmonary arterial saturation and wedge pressure. Cardiac catheterisation involves transporting the patient to the cardiac laboratory and injecting contrast medium into the failing left ventricle with a risk of further, often catastrophic deterioration. However, the insertion of a Swan–Ganz catheter can be performed in the intensive care unit and the appropriate measurements can be obtained at the bedside with minimal upset to the patient. A rise in oxygen saturation at pulmonary artery level will pinpoint the diagnosis in favour of a ventricular septal defect.

Opinion is now veering towards early operation rather than supporting the patient for a few weeks to allow fibrous tissue to form around the edges of the ventricular septal defect and thereby to facilitate its later and theoretically more secure closure. Thus, if the clinical picture is one of deterioration, surgical intervention should be undertaken without delay. In both types of ventricular septal defects the best approach is through the ischaemic part of the left ventricle, but bicaval cannulation is advisable since the right ventricle will be opened during the intracardiac procedure. In the anteroapical type the exposure is relatively easy and is similar to the incision for a left ventricular aneurysm. The ventricular septal defect is readily seen as a ragged tear in the septum. No attempt at direct suture should be made as the necrotic myocardium does not hold sutures. A large patch of PTFE felt or woven polyester should be attached to cover the whole of the ventricular septum, placing the patch so as not to interfere with the chordae and papillary muscles of the mitral valve. The attachment should be carried out with mattress sutures backed with PTFE pledgets placed in healthy septal muscle. A continuous over-and-over stitch is also advisable for complete haemostasis at the edge of the patch. The free edge of the patch is brought out of the ventriculotomy and is incorporated in the repair of the ventricular incision. The same principle applies to the inferobasal type, but it should be borne in mind that these are anatomically closely related to the posteromedial papillary muscle of the mitral valve. The ventricular septal defect can always be clearly seen from its left side since this side of the ventricular septum is smooth. Attempts to close the defect via the tricuspid valve or through a ventriculotomy of the right ventricle are more likely to fail since the defect is difficult to identify among the trabeculations of this side of the septum and the patch application is likely to be less secure.

The immediate haemodynamic improvement in the patient's condition in these acute cases is most gratifying. If the patient can be maintained in a stable condition by pharmacological support, then it is worthwhile deferring the operation for about 2 weeks so as to allow the edges of the defect to become more clearly defined and fibrotic, and this together with the more stable cardiovascular state, makes the operation less hazardous.

d) Mitral Regurgitation

Following a myocardial infarct, mitral regurgitation will result if the ischaemic insult affects one or other of the papillary muscles. These muscles are supplied by end arteries. The posterior papillary muscle is more commonly involved in posteroinferior infarcts. Depending on the severity of the ischaemic attack, the muscle may fail to contract in a coordinated way with the rest of the left ventricle and thus allow the part of the mitral valve served by it to prolapse into the left atrium and regurgitation to occur. Alternatively one of the heads of the papillary muscle necroses and then ruptures causing torrential and sudden mitral regurgitation. If rupture of a papillary muscle accompanies extensive mural infarction of the left ventricle, then the double burden of regurgitation and grossly impaired left ventricular function proves to be rapidly fatal. Therefore, this combination of ischaemic lesions is not frequently found at surgery, but lesser degrees of myocardial ischaemia may still be tolerated and these patients demand urgent surgical correction. Preoperative investigations should be kept to a minimum, and cardiac catheterisation and angiography should be avoided since there is invariably severe pulmonary oedema and a low cardiac output.

At operation it is tempting to approach the lesion via a left ventriculotomy and this is technically quite possible if the extent and site of damage to the left ventricle permit a large enough incision to be made. Repair of the papillary muscle, either when stretched or ruptured, is not advisable since the result cannot be guaranteed immediately and the long-term competence of the valve is uncertain. Valve replacement, therefore, must be undertaken and the prosthesis of choice in this age group is a biological one; mounted xenografts are readily available (Sect. D.II.2.a). After completion of the valve replacement, the closure of the ventriculotomy can be used to eliminate the necrotic part of the left ventricle. In patients in whom left ventricular damage is not extensive enough to permit adequate exposure of the mitral valve, replacement should be performed via the conventional incision in the left atrium. The permanently damaged part of the left ventricle can also be dealt with by plication rather excision and repair. In general these patients are not only likely to require pharmacological support, but respond better to mechanical support of the circulation (Sect. E.I).

2. Degenerative

a) Valve Defects

Degenerative lesions affect the left-sided valves almost exclusively since these are under the greatest stress throughout life. In particular the mitral valve has to support the highest pressures during the cardiac cycle.

α) The Aortic Valve. The commonest degenerative lesion affecting this valve is calcification of its leaflets interfering with their proper movement. The calcification frequently affects the valve ring also and may even extend in "candle-grease" fashion to involve the ventricular aspect of the anterior leaflet of the mitral valve. Close inspection of the type of valve deformity will reveal that there is quite often a rudimentary (incomplete) commissure between the two coronary leaflets, and this results in a final valve opening in the shape of an anteroposterior slit extending between the other two commissures with a composite left-sided leaflet and a large normally sited right-sided leaflet. Strictly speaking this appearance, although now calcified, must originally have been congenital in origin, but the valve functioned satisfactorily until affected by degenerative changes. These bicuspid aortic valves rarely cause regurgitation.

In this group of patients the calcification is likely to be extreme and therefore special care should be taken not to injure the aortic ring, or the attachment of the anterior leaflet of the mitral valve. Calcification extending downwards onto this leaflet can be relatively safely and easily dissected off with a Watson-Cheyne dissector since it does not usually penetrate the full thickness of the leaflet. Calcification may also extend into the top of the ventricular septum involving both its membranous and muscular components and will be in close proximity to the conducting bundle of His, this bundle therefore being at risk. It should be noted that the patient exhibiting a bundle branch block in the electrocardiogram preoperatively is particularly liable to complete heart block after aortic valve replacement. An additional precaution taken during decalcification is the removal of all loose calcium fragments, clearing the left coronary ostium, the ascending aorta up to the level of the occlusion clamp, and also the left ventricular cavity; the latter is repeatedly washed out with large volumes of Ringer's lactate solution.

It is customary to start patients on anticoagulants, usually warfarin, following valve replacements so as to maintain the prothrombin time at 2–2.5 times the control value. After aortic valve replacement, provided the heart remains in sinus rhythm, as is usually the case, anticoagulants can then be tailed off on the assumption that the sewing ring of the prosthesis is now satisfactorily endothelialised. But if a mechanical prosthesis has been inserted, then it is mandatory that anticoagulants are maintained indefinitely. Elderly patients respond unfavourably to long-term anticoagulation and the incidence of anticoagulant-related complications is significantly higher in this age group. The preferred prosthesis is therefore the mounted xenograft (or free homograft, if the surgeon is familiar with its insertion).

β) The Mitral Valve. What has been said in the preceding section about the aortic valve also applies to this valve. It may not always be possible to decalcify the mitral ring and calcification affecting the posterior half of the ring should be cleared with great care. If it extends for more than a few millimetres in depth, it should not be removed since there is then a real danger of injury to the circumflex coronary vessels and left posterior atrioventricular junction. Injuries to these structures often prove fatal at the completion of the operation, from left ventricular failure and haemorrhage, respectively.

γ) Ruptured Chordae. Idiopathic rupture of the chordae controlling the posterior leaflet of the mitral valve is much more common than rupture of those controlling the anterior leaflet. These latter on the other hand are more commonly affected by the ravages of rheumatic fever or bacterial endocarditis. Nonrheumatic mitral regurgitation due to posterior chordal rupture is a condition eminently suitable for repair and accounts for about 10% of patients presenting with mitral regurgitation of recent onset. Indeed, valve replacement should be avoided if possible, since the normal mitral ring, unaffected by antecedent disease such as rheumatic fever, is flimsy, holds sutures poorly and there is an increased incidence of postoperative paraprosthetic mitral regurgitation.

The technique of repair of this lesion is standardised and consists of trapezoidal excision of the redundant and flail part of the posterior leaflet, the restoration of chordal continuity to the free margin of the leaflet by approximation of the edges of the resulting defect, and finally by the reduction of the size of the mitral ring to normal by plicating it with a double nonabsorbable suture of running horizontal interlocking mattress stitches. This plicating suture is based on the margins of the central fibrous body and therefore includes the posterior three-quarters of the mitral ring and is tied securely over small PTFE pledgets. The insertion of this suture is essential to maintain mitral competence and to prevent an intolerable disrupting strain on the leaflet suture line. This technique is also effective if the regurgitation is due to stretched rather than ruptured chordae.

Rupture of the chordae controlling the anterior leaflet does not lend itself so readily to conservative procedures because a similar technique involves excision of a part of the anterior leaflet with a consequent reduction in its area. It is the area of the anterior leaflet which determines the size of the mitral orifice and the restoration of competence after anterior mitral repairs quite often results in mitral stenosis; but for reasons already given, mitral valve replacement is safer in these cases.

b) Aorta

α) Annuloaortic Ectasia and Aneurysms. Annuloaortic ectasia due to cystic medial degeneration of the ascending aorta may occur at any age and its correction in the elderly differs in no way from the standard technique which involves excision of the whole affected segment of the aorta down to the aortic valve ring, preserving a button of the aortic wall around each coronary ostium, replacing the aortic valve with a composite graft, and reimplanting the coronary ostia in appropriately sited openings in this graft.

Aortic aneurysms should be repaired using the standard techniques, whatever their cause, since it is now well recognised that if they are enlarging over a period of observation then they will continue to do so because the wall tension increases with the increase in size, and the progressively thinned wall becomes progressively weaker. Delay, tempting in the elderly, until bone erosion or involvement of surrounding vital organs makes life intolerable, has nothing to recommend it.

β) Dissections of the Aorta. These lesions are seen more commonly in patients who are not only elderly, but also hypertensive. The origin of the dissection may be at an ulcerated atheromatous plaque, but frequently it is simply represented by a transverse tear in the otherwise healthy intima. Dissections involving the ascending aorta should be treated surgically without delay since the results of medical treatment are unsatisfactory. Often in these cases, any aortic regurgitation, if due to prolapse of a commissural pillar (usually the one between the right coronary and noncoronary leaflets), can be repaired by its secure reattachment using mattress sutures backed with PTFE pledgets both inside and outside the aorta. The dissected segment can then be excised and grafted, restoring a single true lumen distally by suture closure of the false channel. If the affected segment is still short, then an end-to-end repair of the ascending aorta can be achieved and this avoids the insertion of an artificial conduit. If the dissection has extended distally to involve the arch, then the restoration of a single true lumen as high as possible in the ascending aorta may be sufficient; but if there is interference with the origin of the head vessels and resulting cerebral dysfunction, then arch replacement may be necessary. For this, total body hypothermia to 15 °C is induced with cardiopulmonary bypass; the circulation is arrested and the arch is replaced by a graft.

The head vessels must be occluded during the period of repair to prevent cerebral air embolism and they are attached to the arch conduit by fashioning one large piece of the superior aspect of the aortic arch encompassing all their origins and inserting this into the conduit by a single anastomosis. This technique obviates the need for individual attachment of the arch vessels separately to the conduit and materially shortens the period of circulatory arrest.

Dissections involving the descending thoracic aorta are treated conservatively in the first instance by controlled hypertension using standard pharmacological agents. The aim is to maintain the systolic blood pressure at around 100–120 mmHg thereby diminishing the dissecting thrust of the left ventricle. Conservative management is continued for 6 weeks or so when the situation is reassessed, if necessary by repeat aortography. The indications for operation are continued pain, increase in size of the dissected segment, and rupture or impending rupture as shown by the development of bloody or blood-stained effusions. Interference with renal perfusion as shown by diminished urinary output, or the development of signs of ischaemia to the spinal cord, are rare complications, but demand urgent surgical intervention. On the other hand, once there is evidence of an upper motor neurone lesion involving the lower limbs, the incidence of postoperative paraplegia is high.

The technique of repair of descending thoracic aneurysms is essentially similar to the one indicated for closure of ductus with left atrial–femoral bypass (Sect. D.I.2). The upper extent of the dissection usually stops short of the origin of the left subclavian artery, but the lower limit may lie well below the level of the diaphragm. Provided a single true lumen is restored distally, it is not necessary to replace the entire dissected segment. Only the most severely dilated and diseased part needs replacement between proximal and distal occlusion clamps. The excluded part is opened longitudinally, the ostia of the intercostal arteries exposed thereby are oversewn, a tube graft of crimped woven polyester can then be inserted as an inlay and this graft may finally be wrapped by the remaining aortic wall, thus ensuring complete haemostasis easily.

E. Postoperative Support

I. Intraaortic Balloon Counterpulsation

This method of circulatory support is the only practical one of increasing the systemic output by an external source of energy. In principle it consists of a thin-walled balloon, attached to the end of a rigid catheter, which is placed in the descending aorta just below the origin of the left subclavian artery. Employing appropriate signals, either the R wave of the electrocardiogram or the upstroke of the arterial pulse trace, the balloon is actively and rapidly emptied by suction during left ventricular systole and is then fully and rapidly inflated after an appropriate period of delay. During left ventricular systole, therefore, the peripheral resistance facing the left venticle is reduced since the collapsing balloon offers additional space to the stroke volume. In early diastole rapid balloon inflation displaces its volume of blood retrograde to the head vessels and coronary arteries, and to a lesser extent prograde to the renal arteries. The systolic pulse wave generated by the heart is therefore augmented by a second pulse wave generated by balloon inflation. This starts ideally at the level of the dicrotic notch and ends well before the onset of the next systole. The area under this composite pulse wave is increased by the augmented wave, and is an index of increased systemic output. Clinically, properly used balloon counterpulsation results in improved myocardial and cerebral perfusion during diastole upstream from the balloon, and improved renal perfusion downstream from the balloon. Evidence of cardiac ischaemia and poor urine production is reversed.

Several precautions must be taken in practice. The femoral artery used for advancing the balloon in a retrograde direction must be of sufficient size to allow adequate perfusion of the ipsilateral limb. Atheromatous narrowing at the iliac or aortic bifurcation may prevent the further passage of the balloon catheter. Injudicious force will cause dissections with disastrous results. The balloon must be properly sited just below the left subclavian artery. Too high a position results in occlusion of the head vessels, whereas too low a position causes fatal splanchnic ischaemia and infarction. The timing of the balloon cycle is critical; too early inflation actually increases the resistance facing the left ventricle, and too late emptying may suck blood out of the coronary ostia.

In the elderly, atheroma of the lower limb vessels and iliac and aortic bifurcation frequently prevents satisfactory balloon insertion. In these patients, the balloon catheter can easily be introduced in the prograde direction through a small stab incision in the arch just below the origin of the left subclavian artery. If the balloon is inserted via the suprasternal notch through a separate skin incision, then the sternum can be approximated in the usual way. Removal of the balloon after successful weaning off then entails reopening the sternotomy and suture closure of the aortotomy. This is clearly a disadvantage of this technique since it involves the administration of a general anaesthetic and return to the operating theatre. But, if the standard femoral approach is not available, then this alternative is safe, easy and effective. The only other theoretical risk is that thrombus formed on the balloon will be wiped off at the aortotomy, and may then embolise the gut, liver, kidneys or lower limbs; but if the balloon has been kept moving during the weaning off period, and if heparin in standard dosage has been used to cover the period of balloon counterpulsation, then the risk of embolism is small and the effects of embolisation by recent and soft emboli could well be transient.

II. Left Ventricular Assist Devices

These have not yet achieved universal acceptance, are complex in their insertion and application and it is doubtful whether their use is justified in this age group. It is perhaps fair to say that these devices are still in the experimental stage and the indications for their use in this age group must therefore be exceptional.

Pulmonary and Oesophageal Surgery in the Elderly

H. C. NOHL-OSER

A. Pulmonary Surgery

I. Introduction

The place of pulmonary surgery in the elderly is obviously limited to those conditions especially afflicting old people, which cannot be treated by other means. Here the success of surgical intervention is even more dependent on the experience and skill of the surgeon than usual, because it is the correct assessment of the whole situation which plays the dominant role. The overriding principle generally is that surgical treatment should be the least that is necessary. Assessment of an elderly patient for possible lung surgery poses added difficulties, which are peculiar to aging. Apart from exploring alternative forms of treatment, the following aspects must be considered, so that a balanced judgement may be formed. These are: (a) the necessity for surgical treatment; (b) the general condition of the patient and therefore the risk involved; and (c) the quality of life to be expected after operation, taking into account the extent of lung resection necessary for cure and the patient's pulmonary reserves.

The first point is clear-cut in the case of bronchial carcinoma, where the outcome is invariably fatal, unless surgery, which alone holds out any hope, can be offered. Nor is there any doubt of the place of surgery in conditions, which could prove fatal, such as chest trauma, spontaneous pneumothorax or possibly giant emphysematous bullae. In other situations surgery is indicated because conservative measures have failed, as for instance in chronic empyema, where prolonged treatment by aspiration and antibiotics has been unsuccessful. On such occasions surgical treatment is advisable to eradicate chronic infection and restore health.

The second point is the problem of assessment and this is especially difficult in the elderly. Other factors, besides age, such as smoking habits and possible abuse of alcohol must be taken into account. This entails a searching enquiry into past history and a detailed medical examination, which will be outlined presently. Finally, the prediction of the possible quality of life after the operation is deduced from the results of special investigations, which are now available and which enable one to make a moderately accurate estimate of the effects of the operation on the cardiorespiratory reserves.

In elective surgery especially, accurate assessment and preoperative preparation are essential if acceptable results are to be obtained. On the other hand, it has been shown that prolonged preoperative hospitalization with bedrest exceeding 8 days, carries a complication rate of nearly 50% in geriatric patients, resulting in either postponement or even abandonment of planned surgical treatment (ECKERT et al. 1979). It is, therefore, of greatest importance, that the necessary investigations and treatment before the operation are carried out expeditiously. The extent of this preoperative preparation depends, of course, on the general condition of the patient and the nature of the underlying disease. In the case of bronchial carcinoma more extensive investigations are necessary than in other conditions needing surgical intervention and, as this disease is very common in the elderly, it will be discussed next, describing at the same time in detail the indispensable assessment that must precede any proposed major surgery.

II. Carcinoma of the Bronchus

The incidence of lung cancer has risen steeply since the Second World War, but even more significant is the increasing number of elderly patients referred to surgical units. This is well illustrated by Fig. 1. In spite of new developments in the treatment of malignancy by radiotherapy and chemotherapy, surgical treatment of lung cancer at present still offers the best prospect of cure.

1. Pathology

The pleomorphism of epithelial tumours of the bronchi and lung is well known (WILLIS 1960) and has been the main stumbling block in establishing a satisfactory classification.

However, the WHO classification (KREYBERG et al. 1967) is now generally accepted. It recognizes seven histological types, but the relative frequency of these varies from series to series, depending partly on the interpretation of the individual pathologist and partly on whether the statistics are based on surgical or necropsy studies. The histological types and their approximate incidence are shown in Table 1. There is a close relationship between the morphological type and the biological behaviour of the tumours. A very short description of each type is, therefore, not amiss.

The squamous cell carcinoma is a tumour of varying degrees of differentiation with much fibrous stroma between the sheets of carcinoma cells. Its growth takes the form of an endobronchial tumour, a peripheral round mass which may cavitate, or an infiltrating mural neoplasm. It metastasizes to the lymph nodes relatively late and is certainly the most favourable type from the surgical point of view.

The small cell carcinoma typically infiltrates the bronchial wall and spreads rapidly to the lymph nodes, so that it often presents itself radiologically as a "mediastinal tumour". Histologically it lacks stroma, the cytoplasm is so scanty that the dark staining nuclei appear to fill the cell entirely. The histological diagnosis of small biopsies of this tumour may be difficult to distinguish from similar appearance in malignant lymphomas, from the undifferentiated polygonal celled squamous carcinoma or even the benign carcinoid tumours, while crushed biopsies of chronic inflammatory tissue, on the other hand, may simulate a small cell carcinoma. Haematogenous spread occurs early with this tumour. All these features make this tumour highly malignant.

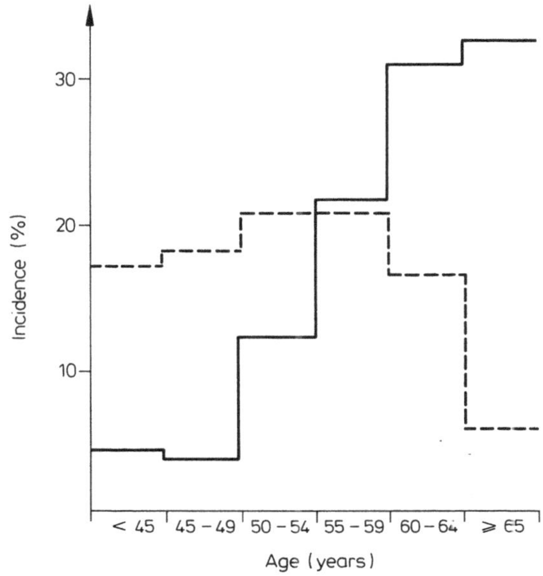

Fig. 1. A comparison of age distribution between two large series of patients treated surgically for lung cancer. It shows the increasing age at which patients are being accepted for surgery. *Full line* series of 663 patients (NOHL-OSER 1980); *broken line* series of 453 patients (BIGNALL and MOON 1955)

Table 1. Incidence of types of lung cancer

Histological type	Incidence (%)
Squamous cell carcinoma	45–50
Small cell carcinoma	35–40
Adenocarcinoma (including bronchioloalveolar carcinoma)	12
Large cell carcinoma	8–10
Mixed (e. g. carcinosarcoma)	Rare
Apudomas (carcinoid)	Relatively rare
Glandular (mucoepidermoid, adenocystic carcinoma)	Rare

The adenocarcinoma tends to be a peripheral lung carcinoma and over one-third of all cases arise in lung scars. More rarely polypoid endobronchial forms are seen. A third diffuse lymphangitic variety carries a bad prognosis and finally there is the disseminating pneumonic type, which in some cases produces much mucus. The scar variety, unless it invades the chest wall, is eminently suitable for resection and carries on the whole a good prognosis. The bronchioloalveolar carcinoma, where the carcinoma cells line the alveoli, is rare and hardly ever gives rise to extrapulmonary metastases and yet is not always amenable to surgery because of its frequent multicentric origin. The large cell carcinoma is an undifferentiated, relatively rare tumour, of which some may be unrecognized adenocarcinomas or even squamous cell tumours. Their malignancy equals that of the undifferentiated adenocarcinomas.

2. Staging

An internationally agreed staging system has been introduced (HARMER 1978), which records the size and situation of the tumour, the extent of lymph node involvement and the presence or absence of extrathoracic metastases. It is a complicated classification, which cannot be detailed here. Suffice to state that a growth in stage I is amenable to surgery and should carry a relatively good prognosis after surgical excision. Stage II is a more advanced condition, while stage III is usually no longer operable. Unfortunately the preoperative clinical staging cannot be as precise as postoperative staging with the pathological report on the surgical specimen available.

3. Presentation

Lung cancer occurs at any age, but becomes progressively more common in the older age groups. The death rate from lung cancer has been rising more steeply in women recently, so that it can no longer be said that this disease is rare in females. The early diagnosis of cancer of the lung is difficult, because of the variable ways it presents. The following are well recognized:

a) Symptomatically, with cough, bloodstained sputum, shortness of breath, loss of weight and pain in the chest.

b) By a febrile illness; a recent history of chest infection, which does not resolve or recurs after initial response to antibiotic treatment. The so-called virus pneumonia must be included in this group.

c) Unusual extrapulmonary manifestations (the so-called paraneoplastic syndromes).

d) As an asymptomatic lesion discovered on routine chest radiography.

a) Symptoms

Smoker's cough is all too common. A change in the nature of the cough, however, is important. Haemoptysis consists usually of bloodstained sputum rather than frank haemoptysis. It should never be ignored and must be investigated by bronchoscopy, even though the chest radiograph shows no abnormality. Chest pain, frequently described as mere discomfort, should never be dismissed as "rheumatism" or "fibrositis". It warrants radiological examination. Dyspnoea, a common symptom in bronchitis, emphysema and old age, should be heeded when of sudden and recent onset. Lassitude, although a vague symptom, may be encountered early in lung cancer and becomes significant if it persists after a febrile chest illness.

b) Febrile Chest Illness

The growth ultimately leads to bronchial obstruction, causing atelectasis of the lung segment involved; thus pneumonia, pleurisy, lung abscess and bronchiectasis may all be simulated. Temporary occlusion by secretions at the site of stenosis with distal infection causes transient pneumonia, which subsides as the bronchus becomes patent, only to recur when the bronchus becomes blocked again. This "recurrent 'flu" is a characteristic warning signal. Every patient recovering from a febrile chest illness should have a radiological examination and should not be considered as having recovered until the lung fields are absolutely clear. "Unresolved pneumonia" is a dangerous diagnosis; this should suggest the possibility of a neoplasm.

c) Unusual Manifestations

These modes of presentation often simulate disease affecting other parts of the body. The commonest is hypertrophic pulmonary osteoarthropathy, simulating rheumatism or arthritis and is usually associated with clubbing of the fingers and toes and subperiosteal bone deposition in radiographs of the long bones. It may sometimes be relieved by surgical means (see Sect. A.II.9). Carcinomatous neuromyopathy manifests itself bilaterally and typically involves the proximal muscles of the limbs. Lung cancer is said to be responsible for over 50% of all neuromyopathies (CROFT and WILKINSON 1965).

Endocrine disturbances are typically associated with the small cell type (oat cell) of tumour. Cushing's syndrome, dilutional hyponatraemia due to excessive secretion of the antidiuretic hormone, and hypercalcaemia are most frequently observed. Pain in the shoulder, often radiating down the arm, can frequently be caused by an apical tumour. Prolonged physiotherapy with no relief of pain is not an uncommon story. These apical tumours are easily missed on the routine posteroanterior chest films, as only the pleura is involved. An anteroposterior film of the apex or body-section radiography are indicated. Some tumours can be resected with relief of the severe pain.

d) Asymptomatic Lesions Discovered on Routine Chest Radiography

The majority of these lesions are solitary circumscribed pulmonary shadows, often described as "coin lesions". Over 50%–80% of these solitary shadows are malignant (GOOD and WILSON 1958; PRIDUN 1980). In some cases, body-section radiography may be of help. Malignancy can be suspected when the shadow shows lobulation or has an indefinite edge with radiating striae (so-called crab feet), extending into the surrounding lung parenchyma. Calcification in the lesion does not rule out malignancy (DAVIS et al. 1956; O'KEEFE et al. 1957). A cavity with a thick irregular wall due to necrosis of the tumour may be present. The presence of such a persistent shadow for a year or more without increase in size is no guarantee of its innocence. A needle biopsy usually establishes the diagnosis or may reveal a metastasis from a primary tumour elsewhere.

4. Diagnostic Investigations

Once the suspicion of lung cancer has been raised, a series of methodical investigations becomes necessary to establish or exclude the diagnosis. Although their purpose is principally diagnostic, they are also valuable in the assessment of operability.

a) Radiology

Most cases of bronchial carcinoma present with abnormal shadows, either the tumour mass itself or the changes following bronchial obstruction. Chest radiography should be carried out in at least two projections (straight posteroanterior and lateral projections). Centrally situated bronchial carcinoma causes simple atelectasis only when there is complete bronchial obstruction. More often sputum retention beyond the tumour stenosis causes segmental or lobar infective infiltration with possible abscess formation. Sometimes segmental collapse occurs, causing a sharply defined wedge-shaped shadow.

A carcinoma situated in the main bronchus will not show radiological changes until total obstruction occurs, but auscultation may reveal a persistent expiratory wheeze. It is in these patients that a radiograph taken during the expiratory phase may show obstructive emphysema. Body-section radiography, both posteroanterior and lateral views, will give further definition of the morbid anatomy (confirmation of cavitation, tumour edge, bronchial stenoses, tracheal narrowing, details of vascular and bronchial structure). Bronchography is rarely indicated. Other radiological investigations: pulmonary angiography, aortography, bronchial arteriography, intrathoracic venography, and computerized axial tomography seem to be of very limited value in diagnosis or assessment.

b) Cytology

Material for examination may derive from sputum, trap specimens and brush smears during bronchoscopy or needle aspiration of either lung parenchyma or pleural effusion. The value depends on the suitability of the specimen and the experience of the cytologist. Thus, early morning specimens are more likely to contain cells, while examination of saliva is a waste of time. Positive yield is higher with central tumours than with peripheral growths, yet even in the latter positive results in the region of 60%–90% may be obtained by increasing the number of samples of true sputum (HINSON and KUPER 1963; GRUNZE 1966; FISCHNALLER 1980).

c) Bronchoscopy

This is absolutely essential in diagnosis, particularly when a lung resection is contemplated. Generally, no patient is too old or too ill for bronchoscopy and contraindications are few; that is, disorders involving the larynx (tuberculosis, bilateral laryngeal palsy); it is unwise to take biopsies when a coagulopathy exists. The purpose of bronchoscopy is twofold; first, to confirm or establish the diagnosis and, second, to determine operability and decide what type of operation is possible. Both the rigid and the flexible fibre optic instruments should be used, as each complements the other. The examination should always be conducted in a methodical fashion, both bronchial trees being examined. Bilateral carcinomas or other pathological conditions have been encountered on the presumed healthy side. Resection is technically impossible, if there is: paralysis of one of the vocal cords, usually the left; involvement of the lower end of the trachea or origin of the main bronchi by carcinoma; or a rigid and widened main carina (in young patients determined efforts at radical extirpation might exceptionally be attempted). The assessment of operability must naturally be carried out by the surgeon. If no pathological changes are seen with the conventional bronchoscope, the fibre optic instrument can then be passed through the rigid tube, so that the segmental orifices of the second and third order can be visualized. This instrument can also be guided under fluoroscopic control to more peripheral lesions to obtain brush biopsies for cytology. LYALL et al. (1980) report a 30% improvement in the detection rate of carcinoma by the fibre optic brush cytology method when compared with biopsies obtained by the conventional bronchoscopic method.

d) Mediastinoscopy

This investigation is of proven value in the diagnosis of intrathoracic diseases, especially those associated with mediastinal lymphadenopathies. In cases of bronchial carcinoma it will detect mediastinal lymph node involvement and is, therefore, used in the preoperative assessment. A positive mediastinal lymph node biopsy is a contraindication to a thoracotomy in the elderly. Mediastinoscopy has increased the resectability rate to 95% when used regularly and has therefore saved many patients from unnecessary thoracotomies (NOHL-OSER 1979). It is a minor operation with a low complication rate and there is really no more of a contraindication to mediastinoscopy than to bronchoscopy; it should precede the latter so as to avoid anaesthetic difficulties due to intrabronchial bleeding after biopsy.

e) Percutaneous Lung Biopsy

In the diagnosis of suspected peripheral growths, aspiration needle biopsy, using image intensified fluoroscopy, has gained wide popularity. SAGEL (1978), reporting on 1,211 aspiration biopsies, was able to demonstrate malignant cells in 96% of patients with malignant disease. He used an 18 gauge modified Turner aspirating needle with a sharp outer cannula, but this was followed by a pneumothorax in 25% of cases. This could be dangerous in a patient with limited respiratory reserves, unless rapidly dealt with. The complication is reduced by using a two-needle technique. An outer needle (18 gauge) is made to strike the lesion first, so that a second needle (22 gauge) can be inserted through it; multiple aspirations can then be performed. The only problem which might cause concern is a negative biopsy in the presence of a lesion which clinically has the characteristics of malignancy.

f) Pleural Biopsy

The recognition of malignant cells in pleural fluid is difficult, as mesothelial cells are easily mistaken for malignant ones. Furthermore, gelatinization of the aspirated fluid must be prevented (3.8% sodium citrate), as no cells are found in jellied fluid. The fluid is centrifuged and its sediment examined. More reliable results are obtained from a pleural biopsy. This can be done under local anaesthesia, using a needle of the type developed by ABRAMS (1958), which with its side hole is wedged against the pleura to cut off a small piece of tissue with the inner sliding cannula. With this simple method, a positive biopsy was obtained in 60% –70% of cases with malignant effusion (HANSON and PHILLIPS 1962). An even better method of obtaining a good tissue sample is to perform a thoracoscopy under general anaesthesia, introducing Carlen's mediastinoscope through the chest wall (MAASSEN 1972). A double-lumen endotracheal tube, with which the lung can be collapsed, facilitates taking of biopsies under direct vision from several sites which look abnormal. An effusion in the presence of a bronchial carcinoma is not always a sinister finding, as it sometimes accompanies complete collapse of a lung or lobe, but a positive biopsy is a definitive contraindication to surgery.

g) Exploratory Thoracotomy

There remain those very rare instances where every investigation has failed to confirm malignancy yet clinical suspicion remains. In these circumstances a thoracotomy must be undertaken, provided that the patient is fit for it. With the chest open, a frozen section will clinch the diagnosis and the appropriate surgical steps are taken.

5. Assessment

Operability in lung cancer depends on: (a) the local and general extent of the disease; (b) the general health of the patient; and (c) the respiratory reserves. In the assessment attention must be paid to:

1. Bronchoscopic operability, as already described
2. Evidence of intrathoracic spread which constitutes a contraindication to surgery
   a) Mediastinal lymph node metastases (mediastinoscopy)
   b) Superior vena cava obstruction (venography if necessary)
   c) Recurrent laryngeal nerve paralysis (indirect laryngoscopy or bronchoscopy)
   d) Phrenic nerve paralysis (screening of diaphragm)
   e) Dysphagia due to oesophageal involvement (barium swallow)
   f) Pleural involvement (pleural biopsy, as already described)
   g) Extensive chest wall invasion in an elderly patient
3. Extrathoracic spread which denotes automatic inoperability
   a) Supraclavicular nodes
   b) Haematogenous metastases, e.g. liver (radioactive liver scan, ultrasound), brain (electroencephalography, brain scan), bone (radiography, bone scintigraphy)
4. General condition and diagnosis of concomitant disease, e.g. heart disease, diabetes, metabolic, hepatic or renal disease
5. Respiratory function

The first three points are self evident, but the last two are especially important in the elderly patient and will now be dealt with in greater detail.

a) General Condition

Age plays an important role in selection and will be discussed later; however, the chronological age may not correlate with the physiological one. The adage, which OSLER and MCCRAE (1908) attributed to Cazalès, "a man is as old as his arteries" remains true and applies especially to mental alertness. The onset and progress of cerebral arteriosclerosis can be judged best by close relatives and friends. It is, therefore, of great advantage to interview someone who has daily contact with the patient. A senile, uncooperative patient is at high risk. Intermittent claudication, cerebrovascular accidents and angina pectoris are manifestations of arteriosclerosis. A recent cerebrovascular accident is a contraindication to surgical treatment.

A quick screening assessment should include the three most important spheres of function: (a) the cardiopulmonary system, essential for adequate circulation and supply of oxygen; (b) the organs maintaining the "milieu intérieur", e.g. liver, kidneys, alimentary tract, suprarenals etc.; and (c) metabolism and its disorders, i.e. protein, fat and carbohydrate metabolism as well as water, electrolyte and acid–base balance.

b) Heart and Circulation

Mild symptoms of angina pectoris or a history of a single incident of myocardial infarction with no subsequent symptoms, does not increase the operative risk greatly. Persistence of symptoms, however, is evidence of reduced cardiac reserves and makes operation inadvisable. Uncomplicated intermittent claudication is not a contraindication.

The patient with cor pulmonale is in grave danger (MITTMAN 1961).

Controlled atrial fibrillation is not a contraindication to surgery nor are many arrhythmias which can now be controlled by cardiac pacing. A correlation between premature contractions and increased operative risk was found by WANG and HOWLAND (1958) and even more recently most of the arrhythmias were presumed to be sequelae of previous myocardial infarction (KUTSCHERA 1980). They are now believed to be caused by degenerative changes (Lenègre's, disease) and are, therefore, not necessarily associated with cardiomyopathy. Cardiac pacing has changed the outlook and the availability of demand pacemakers has overcome the initial disadvantages of pacing. Complete heart block and many other bradycardias without permanent atrioventricular heartblock are now amenable to this form of treatment (HAYWARD 1981). It has been of great benefit to geriatric patients, so that controlled arrhythmias can no longer be considered a contraindication to essential surgical treatment. Hypertension by itself need not cause concern, but associated arterial and kidney disease must be excluded (fundi and renal function).

c) Respiratory System

The main ventilatory changes occurring in old age (BATES et al. 1971) are a fall in vital capacity (VC) and maximum voluntary ventilation (MVV), while the residual volume (RV) and functional residual capacity (FRC) increase, so that the residual volume/total lung capacity ratio (RV/TLC) increases from a normal value of 20% to 35%–40% (COMROE et al. 1962). Blood gas analysis also shows that the partial oxygen pressure PaO_2 in arterial blood is dependent on height and weight and falls steadily with age, while $PaCO_2$ is not affected. This proves that the diffusing capacity is not appreciably altered with age (ULMER et al. 1976).

Table 2. Lung function limits for lung surgery (pneumonectomy)

Lung volumes	
Vital capacity VC	$>45 \times$ K ml (K = height in cm minus 100)
Forced expiratory volume in 1 s FEV_1	$>30 \times K$ ml/s
FEV_1/VC	$>$ 0.6
Maximum voluntary ventilation (MVV)	$>50\%$ of predicted value
Residual volume/total lung capacity (RV/TLC)	$>$ 0.5
Airway resistance (RAW)	$<$ 6 mmH_2O/s
Blood gases	
PaO_2	>70 mmHg (9.3 kPa)
$PaCO_2$	<43 mmHg (5.7 kPa)

Thus, most changes can be explained by the loss of elastic recoil of the lung, leading to an increase in lung volume and unstable ventilation, especially in the dependent parts of the lung.

A rough clinical estimate of the patient's lung function will already have been made during the clinical examination. A long-standing history of shortness of breath before the onset of the disease is significant. Obesity, fishmouth puffing, barrel-shaped chest, poor chest expansion and gross kyphosis are important and may make the need for further lung studies unnecessary. On the other hand, a 70-year-old man, who is jogging regularly and is not breathless when made to run up two flights of stairs, must be deemed fit.

Lung function studies nowadays are expected to produce predictive data about the prospects of success of a planned operation. This information is based on ventilation studies, blood gas analysis, ergometry, pulmonary haemodynamic investigations and regional perfusion and ventilation studies, using a ^{133}Xe scan. These methods can differentiate between the various causes of a given abnormality, such as hypoxaemia.

The following data are routinely recorded and give a rough indication of whether the respiratory function is adequate for lung surgery. The limits set by various authors regarding operability vary, but the spirometric lung volumes, given in Table 2, are those for a pneumonectomy (VON WICHERT 1981). Lower limits would be acceptable for more conservative resections. Other criteria of significance are: (a) failure of improving lung volume values with bronchodilators; (b) grossly abnormal ventilation–perfusion scintigraphy; and (c) electrocardiographic changes, e.g. cor pulmonale. Generally speaking, hypoxaemia at rest is a high risk factor in thoracic surgery, especially when hypercapnia, i.e. raised $PaCO_2$, is also present.

d) Kidney

Generalized arteriosclerosis may also affect the renal vasculature. The glomerular filtration rate is considerably reduced in old age, so that, according to GESSLER (1973), the filtration of the kidney in a healthy 85-year-old man is half that of a 20-year-old. The kidneys share with the lungs the function of maintaining the acid–base balance. When lung function is temporarily diminished in the postoperative period an additional burden is placed on the kidneys' reserves. Moreover, where there is renal impairment, renal failure may follow any major surgical procedure, especially when a period of hypotension occurs, resulting in renal ischaemia with consequent tubular dysfunction. For these reasons, the utmost caution is indicated when lung surgery is contemplated in the presence of bilateral parenchymal renal disease, such as glomerular nephritis or the nephrotic syndrome. Renal function can be monitored preoperatively relatively simply by urine analysis and by determining the blood urea and serum creatinine. The creatinine clearance test is done in borderline cases.

e) Liver
Routine investigations include alkaline phosphatase, serum proteins, serum electrophoresis and the aminotransferases SGOT and SGPT. The serum proteins give an indication of the general health of the patient and a level of under 6 g% suggests either liver metastases or an underlying liver complaint such as cirrhosis. Uncomplicated cirrhosis without ascites or episodes of bleeding is not a contraindication to operation, especially when the levels of serum albumin are above 3 g%, while the gamma-globulin proportion is 30% and the serum bilirubin not above 1.2 mg%. Patients with low serum protein levels have a low resistance to infection and are prone to thromboembolic complications. Should preoperative hyperalimentation with high protein intake not succeed in restoring these levels to normal within a short time, operative surgery is inadvisable.

f) Metabolism
The only metabolic diseases which are met fairly often in old people, are diabetes and gout. Uncomplicated diabetes under good control is not a problem. However, if there are vascular complications or diabetic nephropathy, it is a different matter. Gout in the elderly, including the drug-induced variety, for instance by thiazides, can also cause renal damage. The high complication rate and mortality in obese patients should be remembered. Apart from these metabolic diseases, the blood picture (haemoglobin and haematocrit) needs checking, so that any existing anaemia can be treated preoperatively. Rapid transfusion at the time of operation causes oedema of the lungs in old people.

g) Summary
The contraindications to operative treatment of lung cancer may be summarized as follows:

1. Anatomical
   a) Local spread, making operation technically impossible
   b) Systemic dissemination of tumour
2. Functional – extent of operation incompatible with the function of:
   a) Lung
   b) Heart and circulation
   c) Kidney
   d) Liver
   e) Brain
   f) Metabolism

   and because of

   g) General condition, e.g. age, weakness, cachexia, obesity.

6. Preoperative Treatment

This should be as short as is reasonable, lest complications associated with hospitalization occur. Some preoperative measures can be undertaken before admission. Once in hospital, the patient should be up and dressed before the operation and encouraged to walk about for most of the day. The following measures to improve the patient's condition may be indicated:

1. Smoking should be strongly discouraged
2. Bronchial infection is treated with the appropriate antibiotic
3. Bronchodilators may be given for obstructive airway disease
4. Steam inhalations are given to loosen sticky secretions
5. All patients above the age of 65 years are digitalized
6. Cardiac failure is treated by diuretics
7. Physiotherapy in the form of breathing exercises and postural drainage is of real benefit and gives an opportunity to establish psychological rapport with the patient
8. Any existing anaemia is corrected

7. Choice of Operation

Carcinoma of the lung can be excised by:

1. Standard pneumonectomy (simple extrapericardial)
2. Extended pneumonectomy (radical intrapericardial)
3. Lobectomy
4. Lobectomy with sleeve resection of the main bronchus
5. Segmentectomy
6. Wedge resection

The type of operation depends on: (1) the extent of the growth; and (2) the general condition of the patient, both of which will have been determined by preoperative assessment. The influence of age on the operative mortality is generally known. Thus, KUTSCHERA (1980) reports a mortality of 44% in patients over the age of 70 years. It has become apparent, however, that less radical operations carry a lower mortality without prejudice to the patient's prospects, so that FLAVELL (1962) could write: "It is foolish to carry out extensive extirpations and either kill the patient or render life intolerable for want of breath." BATES (1970) reported a mortality of 23% for pneumonectomy in those over 70 years of age, while for lobectomy or segmentectomy it was only 12.7% and the 5-year survival rate was nonetheless over 10% in these elderly patients.

The value of sleeve resection, whereby upper lobe tumours, involving also the main bronchus, can be excised with preservation of the remaining lobes, is well recognized (PAULSON and SHAW 1955; JOHNSTON and JONES 1959; REES and PANETH 1970). This entails an anastomosis of the uninvolved lobe or lobes to the main bronchus or trachea at a higher level. This method of conserving healthy lung tissue is obviously of special value in the elderly and those patients with limited cardiopulmonary reserves. An infinite variety of these so-called bronchoplastic procedures exists. The author (NOHL-OSER et al. 1982) described a tracheobronchoplastic procedure which makes it possible, under special circumstances, to excise right upper lobe tumours invading even the trachea, while preserving the middle and lower lobes. JENSIK et al. (1979) convincingly showed the amazingly good results which can be obtained in very old people by conservative surgery. This type of surgery has, however, limited application, because only early growths confined to a segment or, at the most, a lobe can be treated in this way. In this respect, early diagnosis is all important and is well shown by a review of a large series of U.S. Army personnel treated surgically for lung cancer. In this organization, where regular medical supervision resulted in early diagnosis and operation, the remarkable 5-year survival rate of 49% was achieved. JENSIK et al. (1979) reports on a series of 168 patients with peripheral stage I carcinoma treated by segmentectomy only. Almost 30% of these patients were over 70 years old, yet the surgical mortality was only 1.8% and the overall 5-year survival rate 53%. Apart from definite improvements in preoperative assessment, better postoperative care and a change of policy towards more conservative operations, no significant advances in operative techniques have taken place in the last 30 years.

The recent introduction of cryoanalgesia (MAIWAND and MAKEY 1981), however, must be considered an advance in the postoperative management. The intercostal nerves supplying the thoracotomy area are frozen under direct vision at the time of operation. It is an effective method of controlling thoracotomy pain, resulting in early mobilization of the patient, better respiratory ventilation, easier expectoration and lower incidence of complications, such as thromboembolism. It is too early to say whether the consequent reduction in postoperative morbidity will result in extending the indications for operation in the elderly in the future.

8. Postoperative Management

The postoperative period following pulmonary surgery may be uneventful or can be very stormy. Apart from haemorrhage, bronchospasm, sputum retention, pulmonary collapse and cardiac arrhythmias, there are the more serious complications peculiar to lung resections, such as persistent pneumothorax, empyema and bronchopleural fistula. For the sake of brevity, it must be asserted that the postoperative management can only be carried out safely by staff specially trained in the surgical care of cardiothoracic patients. The great majority of patients do not need nursing in an intensive care unit. Elderly patients, especially, do not react well psychologically to being nursed in an intensive care unit or in a single room.

It might be useful to mention here some of the hazards to which the elderly are especially prone in the postoperative period.

1. Postoperative respiratory failure, resulting from an imbalance of ventilation–perfusion in the lung is not uncommon. Serial blood gas analysis is the only reliable means by which to detect early respiratory failure. Simple hypoxaemia may respond to administration of humidified and warmed oxygen, remembering that PaO_2 levels are lower in old age, but if hypercapnia is also present then artificial ventilation becomes necessary.

2. Intravenous fluids should be restricted in old people to avoid oedema of the lung through overloading the circulation. Careful maintenance of the fluid balance is essential; an indwelling urinary catheter makes it possible to monitor

urinary output accurately and in the elderly male patient will circumvent urinary retention, which is so often caused by confinement to bed. Oral fluids can usually be commenced 12 h after operation.

3. Thromboembolism – it is now common practice (WESSLER 1980; DARK 1981) to give subcutaneous heparin prophylactically to all patients over the age of 40 years. A dose of 5,000 U is given 2 h before the operation and then a similar dose every 12 h after surgery. Early mobilization also helps in promoting venous circulation.

9. Palliative Treatment

Unfortunately, many patients present themselves rather late and are not in good enough physical shape to be suitable for surgery. In these, radiotherapy can undoubtedly be useful in the palliation of symptoms, such as haemoptysis, cough, dyspnoea or pain. The value of radiation therapy for superior vena caval obstruction and skeletal metastases is well known. More controversial is the question of attempting to cure the patient by radical radiation. The high dose of radiation required to achieve long-term control can cause serious complications, such as spinal cord damage and radiation fibrosis of the lung with consequent right heart failure. It is very doubtful in any case whether an elderly patient, deemed unsuitable for surgery, will be fit enough for this form of treatment.

Chemotherapy with cytotoxic drugs is also of little value in palliation. The only tumour which responds to this treatment is the small cell carcinoma, but the side effects of these drugs on the already sick patient are such that the morbidity of this regime far outweighs the advantages obtained.

Finally, it is worth mentioning that severe hypertrophic pulmonary osteoarthropathy, caused by right-sided tumours, can be miraculously relieved by a right vagotomy, carried out from the neck through a mediastinoscope (YACOUB 1966). Unfortunately, this cannot be done on the left side for anatomical reasons, and would require a left thoracotomy.

10. Summary

It is possible to treat lung cancer surgically in the elderly with a low operative mortality and have them live their allotted span of life in comfort. Careful assessment of both the disease and the general condition of the patient is essential. Moreover, the disease must be in its early stages, so that the resection can be kept within the limits of the patient's respiratory reserves. Any deviation from these stringent precepts is bound to end in disaster.

III. Empyema

A purulent pleural effusion is by definition an empyema. There are many conditions, which may be complicated by an empyema, but it would serve no useful purpose to enumerate them all. In the elderly the chief cause is infection in the lung, usually in the form of pneumonia. It is, however, important to remember that with advancing age carcinoma of the bronchus becomes a common condition, often presenting as a febrile chest illness. Examination of the sputum for malignant cells and bronchoscopy are, therefore, essential to exclude underlying malignancy.

The diagnosis is made on clinical grounds and radiographic evidence, but above all by awareness of its possible existence. It is confirmed by needle aspiration. The causal organism may not be identifiable, because antibiotic treatment has often been given in the early stages of a pulmonary infection. An empyema is considered to be acute when the history of the illness is of short duration, but is termed chronic when persisting over 2–3 months. The most important causes of a chronic empyema are failure to recognize an acute empyema or imperfect treatment in the acute stage. Less common causes are undiagnosed chronic lung disease (lung abscess, bronchiectasis, tuberculosis, bronchial carcinoma) and foreign bodies (war shrapnel, rib sequestrum, retained drainage tube or swab). A "silent" form of empyema has been reported (SAHN et al. 1973) during long-term steroid treatment and also in rheumatoid arthritis (JONES et al. 1971).

An undrained empyema may be complicated by a bronchopleural fistula or by an empyema necessitatis. In the former complication there is the danger of aspiration pneumonia or even drowning in pus, while an empyema necessitatis results from pus tracking through the rib cage and presenting itself as a fluctuating swelling under the skin. Both complications demand urgent treatment.

1. Treatment

The choice of treatment depends on the stage which the empyema has reached, whether it is acute with thin or thick pus, or chronic, and also on the patient's age and clinical state.

2. Acute Empyema

Aspiration and instillation of antibiotics may be successful in the early stages when the pus is still thin and remains thin. This treatment must be carried out every other day with full radiographic control. On each occasion, all fluid is removed, followed by instillation of the appropriate antibiotic, which is also given systemically in high dosage. Expansion of the lung is further encouraged by physiotherapy.

This form of treatment must be abandoned either when aspiration becomes difficult, because the aspirating needle becomes blocked by thick pus or when the fever does not subside or the radiograph shows multiple fluid levels due to loculation. In any case, it should be discontinued if pus continues to form after 14 days. The alternative form of treatment in the elderly is drainage by intercostal tube or rib resection. Decortication, that is excision of the empyema, although a very effective method, is a major undertaking and is not advisable in the frail or elderly.

3. Intercostal Drainage

Before the operation, the most dependent part of the empyema cavity is determined by instillation of 2–3 ml radiopaque dye into the empyema cavity and taking radiographs in two projections. The whole procedure is best carried out under local anaesthesia with the patient in the sitting position; this will prevent sudden flooding of the bronchial tree by pus, should a bronchopleural fistula be present. We prefer to use a large trocar and cannula through which the intercostal catheter is introduced, in preference to the plastic catheters with aluminium trocar that are now commercially available. We have seen some very serious complications, such as transfixion of the lung and even the heart, following the use of these trocar-mounted catheters.

The catheter is connected to an underwater seal bottle and physiotherapy is started as soon as possible to encourage lung expansion. In a few patients, this form of treatment will achieve complete obliteration of the empyema cavity and, therefore, a cure. More often, however, the pus becomes thick and blocks the tube and rib resection and drainage becomes necessary.

4. Rib Resection and Drainage

This can be done under local or general anaesthesia, employing a double-lumen endobronchial tube to isolate the affected side and thus prevent spillage into the bronchial tree. A short length of rib is removed over the lowest point of the empyema cavity, removing at the same time a small portion of the thickened empyema wall for histological examination. This investigation sometimes reveals an unknown underlying pathology, such as tuberculosis or neoplasm. The fibrinous contents of the empyema are removed and a large-bore tube is inserted. Postoperative management must be carried out by the surgeon in charge, lest careless aftercare should result in a chronic empyema. Progress is supervised by serial sinograms, which outline the empyema space and give information about its shape and size and its relation to the tube. The commonest and most disastrous mistake is to remove the drainge tube too soon or let it fall out without replacing it immediately. An empyema tube track tends to close within hours. The tube is only removed when the pleural space has become completely obliterated and this may take weeks. This does not, however, mean that the patient has to be kept in hospital for all that time.

During the first few days after the operation, the drainage tube is connected to an underwater seal bottle. This "closed" drainage facilitates the collection of considerable amounts of pus and encourages early expansion of the lung by reestablishing a negative intrapleural pressure. A special carrier for the underwater seal bottle allows early mobilization of the patient. "Closed" drainage is converted into "open" drainage, when the daily discharge is less than 100 ml. Dressings are applied over the cut end of the tube, which is held in place by a safety pin, fixed to the skin by adhesive strapping.

The patient may now be allowed to go home. A nurse needs to attend daily to change dressings and ensure that the tube remains securely fixed. Supervision as already indicated is carried out at fortnightly intervals on an outpatient basis and later by monthly visits until the tube can be removed.

IV. Spontaneous Pneumothorax

Rupture of a bleb is the commonest cause of a spontaneous pneumothorax in the young. In the elderly, especially those who suffer from chronic bronchitis and emphysema, persistent coughing and associated bronchospasm may cause rupture of a bulla. At any time, the small bronchopleural fistula, which caused the airleak, may become valvular and cause an increase in the size of the pneumothorax or even a tension pneumothorax. The rapid buildup of intrapleural pressure can cause alarming cardiorespiratory embarrassment and calls for urgent relief. If a life-threatening situation exists and no suitable instruments are available, a large-bore needle pushed into the chest will bring instant relief.

The generally accepted treatment for all but the shallowest of pneumothoraces is intercostal drainage and suction in the first instance. In old people, with already diminished respiratory reserves, the risk of a tension pneumothorax makes it necessary to treat *every* pneumothorax by intercostal tube. However, a pneumothorax must be distinguished from a large emphysematous bulla, because insertion of a catheter into a bulla may result in a tension pneumothorax. A rare cause of pneumothorax is underlying malignancy, which should be apparent on the chest radiograph.

The safest site for inserting an intercostal catheter is the fourth intercostal space in the midaxillary line, directing the trocar and cannula upwards, so that the tip of the catheter comes to lie in the apical region. The catheter is connected to an underwater seal bottle, whose exit tube in turn is connected to a suction pump. The suction must, however, be adequate to cope with the volume of air expelled, otherwise air will escape around the tube and surgical emphysema will develop. Daily chest radiographs are necessary to check on satisfactory lung expansion. The drain remains in place until no further air escapes on coughing or suction for at least the previous 24 h and the chest radiograph shows that a pneumothorax is no longer present.

Recurrence of a pneumothorax unfortunately occurs in about 20% of conservatively treated cases and in these some form of pleurodesis is necessary. In fit and young patients this is best achieved by a pleurectomy with closure of the fistula, but in elderly patients with sometimes grossly impaired respiratory function, a thoracotomy is not feasible and in these insufflation of iodized talc (SENGUPTA 1963) is advised. This procedure is best done under general anaesthesia. We use two trocars and cannulae, inserting one near the apex and the other lower down. About 10 g iodized talc (formula: iodine 50 mg, absolute alcohol 5 ml, talc 100 g.) is blown into the pleural cavity with a special insufflator.

The other cannula allows the air to escape, but can also be used for the introduction of a thoracoscope, if so desired. After insufflation of the powder, two intercostal catheters are introduced through the cannulae, which are removed over the catheters. Each drainage tube is then connected to a separate underwater seal bottle to which suction is applied. This procedure sometimes causes excruciating pain, for which the patient must be given powerful analgesics, such as morphine. If marked respiratory depression results, blood gas analysis will indicate whether temporary mechanical ventilation for 12–24 h is necessary. In grossly emphysematous patients, suction may have to be continued without a break, day and night, for weeks rather than days. In the author's experience, and contrary to customary belief, an intercostal catheter can be left in place for long periods without the risk of infection.

V. Emphysematous Cysts

Surgical treatment of emphysematous bullous disease is problematic, especially as the disease is usually bilateral. The assessment and selection for surgery of patients with bullous emphysema is difficult and the indications for excision of an emphysematous cyst are especially limited in the old age group. Preoperative investigations must include the usual routine respiratory function tests, which are supplemented by lung section radiography and lung perfusion and ventilation scan. The following criteria must be satisfied:

1. The patient suffers from progressive dyspnoea.
2. The bulla is well demarcated and occupies more than one-third of the hemithorax and there is evidence of recent enlargement with compression of the lung.
3. Chronic bronchitis, as evidenced by repeated chest infections and wheeziness, should not dominate the clinical picture; cor pulmonale or signs of cardiac failure following myocardial ischaemia are definite contraindications to surgery.

Surgery on giant bullae also presents problems for the anaesthetist. There is the very real risk of a buildup of tension within the cyst during induction of anaesthesia, which will not only compress the lung still further, but could cause rupture and a tension pneumothorax. The operation itself should aim at conservation of lung tissue and a lobectomy should be avoided. Large cysts are excised and obliterated, while smaller cysts are simply ligated or oversewn.

VI. Retrosternal Goitre

With the passing of time, goitres become nodular and undergo colloid degeneration. This causes enlargement of the gland, which often extends downwards into the superior mediastinum. Very old people are not infrequently affected. Although the lungs are not directly involved, the retrosternal prolongation of a goitre into the chest can cause respiratory symptoms through pressure on the trachea. There may be wheezing, shortness of breath and frequent respiratory infections, thus simulating chronic bronchitis. Haemorrhage into the retrosternal portion of the gland may cause sudden stridor, which could become potentially dangerous. For these reasons a retrosternal goitre should be removed. It is an operation which does not entail great risks to the elderly patient and, as great benefit may be conferred, it should be recommended without hesitation.

The majority of retrosternal goitres can be excised through the neck by the conventional cervical collar incision. The vessels to the gland are dealt with first in the usual manner and the retrosternal prolongation is then delivered into the neck by sweeping the index finger gently around the gland behind the manubrium. It is rarely necessary to split the sternum.

VII. Chest Trauma

The elderly pedestrian is especially prone to road accidents. Although the incidence of serious chest injuries is known to be greater in car passengers (Pribilla 1972), pedestrians may, nevertheless, sustain multiple injuries, of which head and chest injuries are the most lethal. The outlook for old people is poor. A combination of instability of the chest wall (fractured ribs, sternum), contusion of the lung, intrabronchial bleeding, oedema of the lung and entry of air, blood or both into the pleural cavity is often present and causes gross disturbances in the ventilation: perfusion ratios of the lung and changes in the physiological dead space. Hypoxaemia rapidly ensues, followed soon by respiratory acidosis. Anoxia as a result of airway obstruction is the immediate threat to life and a clear airway must be established immediately by simply extending the head, lifting the jaw forwards and introducing an oropharyngeal airway. Tracheal intubation is necessary in the deeply unconscious patient.

A chest radiograph, preferably in the upright position, and blood gas analysis are urgently required on admission to hospital. Once a good airway has been established, attention is directed to those conditions, which are most likely to embarrass cardiorespiratory function.

1. A pneumothorax and/or haemothorax requires an intercostal drain. Blood loss into the pleural cavity can then be measured hourly in the underwater seal bottle.
2. Humidified oxygen is given through a face mask.
3. To combat "shock", an intravenous infusion is started through which any medication may be given. A word of caution is indicated here; in old people who already have an impaired circulation, oedema of the lung ensues easily and they are, therefore, very vulnerable to overtransfusion. Hence, intravenous fluids must be restricted to less than 1,000 ml during resuscitation and 50 ml/h thereafter. Blood loss as measured in the underwater seal bottle is replaced by whole blood or plasma and crystalloid solutions are avoided at all costs.
4. A bronchoscopy may be necessary to remove inhaled vomit or blood.
5. Pain, which makes adequate breathing and the coughing up of secretions difficult, must be controlled by analgesics, local analgesic block or inhalation of analgesic mixtures of nitrous oxide/oxygen (Entonox). It is important to remember that the efficacy of a drug depends on its absorption, metabolism and excretion as well as end organ sensitivity. All these factors may be affected in old people. Thus, they become easily confused on sedation. The use of intrathecal morphine is attractive, but as this causes hypotension, it is better avoided.
6. Mechanical ventilation is required when the arterial blood gases are abnormal and this may have to be continued for a long time, when a flail chest (stove-in chest) causes respiratory insufficiency. Long-term ventilation calls for an elective tracheostomy. The disadvantage of prolonged artificial respiration in the elderly patient is the almost unavoidable complication of serious pulmonary infection, which carries a high mortality. Sometimes operative stabilization of the flail chest with wires or a steel bar is possible without too much trauma and this would then make long-term ventilation unnecessary.

B. Oesophageal Surgery

I. Introduction

Two of the few pleasures in life which can still be enjoyed in old age, are drinking and eating. One would, therefore, assume that a distressing symptom like dysphagia would make people seek early medical advice. This is not so; many patients put up with dysphagia until drinking becomes almost impossible. Dysphagia is often the main reason for advising surgical treatment in oesophageal disease and it often afflicts the aged. It is, however, very important not to forget that difficulty in swallowing in old people may also be caused by neuromuscular disorders, which involve the pharynx and, therefore, interfere with deglutition. Brainstem lesions, such as the posterior inferior cerebellar artery syndrome and pseudobulbar palsy, are common causes. Other neuromuscular diseases such as demyelinating disorders, myasthenia gravis and extrapyramidal diseases are also known to affect deglutition (SILBIGER et al. 1967). A history of difficulty in swallowing liquids, especially when they come up through the nostrils, is very suggestive of neuromuscular incoordination and warrants a careful neurological examination.

1. Assessment

A thorough assessment of the patient is carried out as described in the section on pulmonary surgery, not forgetting, however, that a patient who has been starving for a long time, may be debilitated because of malnutrition, dehydration, cachexia, and anaemia. These sequelae of dysphagia may be reversible, so that further reassessment may be needed after the deficiency in nutrition and the dehydration have been corrected. Dysphagia is so distressing that the risk of any procedure to relieve it must be balanced against the patient's likely tolerance to it and also the nature of the underlying disease.

When suspecting neurological disease, special attention should be directed on the motility of the soft palate and pharynx and possible coarse fibrillation of the tongue should be looked for. Examination with the laryngeal mirror might show pooling of food and saliva in the pyriform fossa. This is a sign of physical obstruction. The possibility of cervical lymphadenopathy is also investigated.

2. Radiographic Examination

A lateral view of the soft tissues of the neck can be helpful, as it may show a widening of the prevertebral tissues at the level of about the sixth cervical vertebra (postcricoid carcinoma) or an abnormal configuration of the air shadows in the trachea and oesophagus. This view may also show osteophytes in the cervical spine, which make oesophagoscopy with the rigid instrument especially hazardous. Barium swallow and meal with the use of cineradiography and videotape recording are of great advantage. This investigation will detect any disorders of bolus transport in the upper food passage and show abnormal motility, distortions, herniations, and obstructions in the oesophagus. Barium studies are not so reliable in diagnosing gastro-oesophageal reflux. Prior knowledge of the presence of any of these abnormalities can be of immense value to the endoscopist, as this forewarns of possible hazards which may be encountered during endoscopic examination. Finally, a routine chest radiograph is essential to detect any cardiopulmonary disease, especially respiratory problems due to possible aspiration.

3. Endoscopy

This investigation gives essential information on any abnormalities of the mucosa and other conditions within the lumen of the oesophagus. It can be carried out with the rigid conventional oesophagoscope or the flexible endoscope. Both instruments have their advantages and disadvantages. With the rigid instrument, adequate biopsies can be taken and its large lumen makes removal of large amounts of food debris (as in achalasia) and also large foreign bodies, easy. Moreover, the pliability and extent of strictures during dilatation is better appreciated through the rigid endoscope. On the other hand, an arthritic cervical spine, gross kyphosis or spiky osteophytes make the use of the flexible fibre optic gastro-oesophageal endoscope desirable. This instrument also permits accurate inspection and biopsy of malignant lesions of the cardia as it can be passed into the stomach. Dilatations of strictures are carried out partly blindly, because a guide wire is passed under vision into the stomach first, over which progressively larger olive-shaped metal dilators (Eder–Puestow) are then passed.

The level at which abnormalities are found in always recorded. If a malignant lesion 15–30 cm from the incisor teeth is found, a bronchoscopy should follow the oesophagoscopy, so that any possible involvement of the tracheobronchial tree can be detected.

4. Manometry and pH Studies

These investigations were for a long time research tools. With the introduction of miniaturized electronic transducers, manometry has found greater clinical application. These facilities should, therefore, be available in any unit where oesophageal surgery is routinely undertaken. The principal merit of manometry lies in the exclusion or diagnosis of associated motility disorders, which may accompany or be confused with an incompetent cardia or gastro-oesophageal reflux. Thus gastro-oesophageal reflux is not infrequently found in association with achalasia, scleroderma or oesophageal spasm. Manometry, however, is not a reliable method of diagnosing gastro-oesophageal reflux by itself; this is much more accurately determined with pH electrodes. pH studies can be carried out in various ways, among them the acid perfusion test is particularly useful in distinguishing such nonspecific symptoms as epigastric pain or heartburn due to reflux from those caused by other conditions such as myocardial ischaemia, biliary tract disease and gastric or duodenal ulcer.

In conclusion, these tests have contributed greatly to a better understanding of the pathophysiology of oesophageal disease and have resulted in improved operative results. Their value in problematic cases is emphasized by PEARSON (1981), who recommends preoperative monitoring by manometry, pH studies and perfusion tests in the following circumstances:

1. Suspected primary motor disorder from clinical history
2. Chest pain of obscure origin
3. Dysphagia of uncertain origin
4. Gastro-oesophageal reflux persisting after presumably adequate surgical treatment
5. Peptic stricture – occasional identification of associated primary motor disorder (scleroderma, diffuse spasm)

II. Carcinoma of the Oesophagus

Carcinoma of the oesophagus is a disease of the sixth and seventh decades, afflicting men more often than women. It causes progressive dysphagia, a symptom so distressing that it cannot be ignored and calls for urgent relief, however difficult the circumstances may be.

1. Pathology

Malignancy arising in the oesophagus is usually a squamous cell carcinoma, which is a slow growing tumour. Recent investigations by cytological screening and endoscopic examination (YANG GUANREI 1982) have shown that it takes 3–4 years for a carcinoma in situ to grow to the advanced stage at which the patient complains of dysphagia. The course of the disease from then onwards until death occurs, however, averages only about 9 months. An adenocarcinoma involving the lower end of the oesophagus arises usually from the gastric mucosa. A few cases of adenocarcinoma arising at higher levels in the oesophagus derive from islands of ectopic gastric mucosa. The growth spreads locally, especially by submucosal lymphatic extension and to the regional lymph nodes. Haematogenous spread is rare.

Little is known of the causative factors. The disease is very much more common in Japan and China than in western countries, so that environmental factors and diet may conceivably play a role. An association between the Plummer–Vinson (Paterson–Brown–Kelly) syndrome and postcricoid carcinoma is recognized. A higher incidence of malignancy has also been recorded in achalasia, hiatus hernia with reflux oesophagitis and following caustic burns of the oesophagus. The most common sites of cancer are those where a transient delay in the passage of ingested material occurs, that is the level of the cricopharyngeus, the aortic arch and the cardia.

From the surgical point of view, it is customary to divide the oesophagus into three sections; the upper third extends from the pharynx to the thoracic inlet, the middle third from the thoracic inlet down to the level of the inferior pulmonary vein, while the remainder of the oesophagus down to the cardia constitutes the lower third.

2. Symptoms

Dysphagia overshadows everything else and is often accompanied by severe weight loss, in marked contrast to dysphagia caused by tight peptic strictures, where weight loss is rarely seen. The difference is thought to be due to the increased catabolism that is met in malignant conditions. Other symptoms are vague pain or discomfort, not accurately localized, regurgitation, cough and surprisingly infrequent vomiting.

3. Clinical Assessment

The routine assessment of the general condition of any elderly patient has already been detailed in the section on pulmonary surgery. In this group of patients, the usual physical examination, with a special search for dissemination of the disease, is followed by routine barium swallow and meal and endoscopy, as with any other oesophageal disease. During oesophagoscopy the proximal level and mobility of the growth is defined and more proximal mucosal "skip" lesions are excluded. Biopsy of the tumour will determine the histology and bronchoscopy under the same anaesthetic may reveal a left recurrent laryngeal palsy (lymph node involvement at aortic arch level) or tumour invasion, fistulae or extrinsic compression of the tracheobronchial tree in the presence of tumours situated in the upper half of the oesophagus.

If major surgery is contemplated a liver scan may exclude obvious metastases. The nutritional state is assessed by checking the serum proteins and electrolytes. Hypoproteinaemia, especially a reversal in the albumin : globulin ratio, tends to lower resistance to infection and impairs primary healing. Moreover, a blood count will show whether there is need for correction of any anaemia.

4. Preoperative Management

The condition of the patient and the surgical treatment selected will determine the amount of effort spent on preoperative preparation. If the decision goes in favour of a plastic tube to overcome an obstruction, no great preparation is necessary. Nutritional depletion in many patients has to be corrected by hyperalimentation, if major surgery is planned. The choice lies between enteral and parenteral feeding. The expense and potential complications of intravenous nutrition make the former method preferable. The use of radiopaque small-bore enteral feeding tubes, which are best passed under endoscopic guidance through the obstruction, in conjunction with a portable battery-operated pump, has made continuous drip feeding simple and reliable. The patient is hardly aware of the nasogastric tube and is fully mobile. The only disadvantage is that large feeding volumes may induce diarrhoea and this limits the number of calories which can be delivered daily. There are several, all similar, commercial enteral diets available. The frequent anaemia should be corrected, in the last resort by a blood transfusion. Intravenous feeding is carried out only during the immediate postoperative period, when no oral intake is permitted. At the start of the operation a central venous catheter (superior vena cava) is introduced through the internal jugular vein and a urinary catheter is inserted at the same time, so that a strict fluid balance can be kept.

Throughout the preoperative period the patient should be up and dressed for most of the day. Vigorous chest physiotherapy is started and any respiratory infections, which are sometimes due to nocturnal aspiration, are treated with the appropriate antibiotic.

5. Treatment by Resection

The choice of treatment depends on the location, extent and type of growth and the general condition of the patient. The possibilities of treatment are:

1. Resection of the growth and replacement of the oesophagus by a viscus (gastric tube, jejunal loop, colon)
2. Palliative bypass of an irremovable growth
3. Intraluminal prosthetic tubes
4. Radiotherapy

General experience is that resection of the growth is the best treatment if it is possible. The main object is to restore satisfactory swallowing and alleviate pain. The 5-year survival rate in large series, spanning all ages, is only 17% (DARK et al. 1981), but more important is that about 90% of patients undergoing resections had unobstructed swallowing throughout their subsequent survival (PAYNE 1979; DARK et al. 1981). Moreover, the chances of actually carrying out a resection at the time of exploration, the operative resection rate, is fairly high and constant in most series, averaging about 85%.

The operative mortality varies enormously, depending no doubt on the selection of patients and the experience in the surgical unit. Certainly oesophageal surgery is the province of the dedicated specialist surgeon rather than the occasional performer, and though there has been a decrease in the operative mortality in recent years, it is still about 16% over the age of 70 years (PAGLIERO 1979).

A great variety of operations for resection and replacement of the oesophagus have been evolved and the choice depends not only on the location of the growth, but also on the preference of the surgeon. In elderly patients most surgeons would probably agree that the stomach is nearly always the best viscus for oesophageal replacement. Mobilization of the stomach is easily and rapidly achieved by dividing the short gastric and left gastric vessels without jeopardizing its excellent blood supply. Moreover, it is nearly always possible to elongate it without tension, so that it can be brought well up into the neck. Finally, only one anastomosis is required and this without the attendant risk of wound contamination, which is liable to occur when a segment of colon is interposed.

The only disadvantage of bringing the stomach up into the chest is that it can cause troublesome reflux with peptic stricture formation at the anastomosis. This late complication is, however, rarely seen when the anastomosis lies above the level of the aortic arch. Few patients survive long enough to experience it. The various operative procedures most suitable for elderly patients for the resection of the growth at different sites will now be described (Fig. 2).

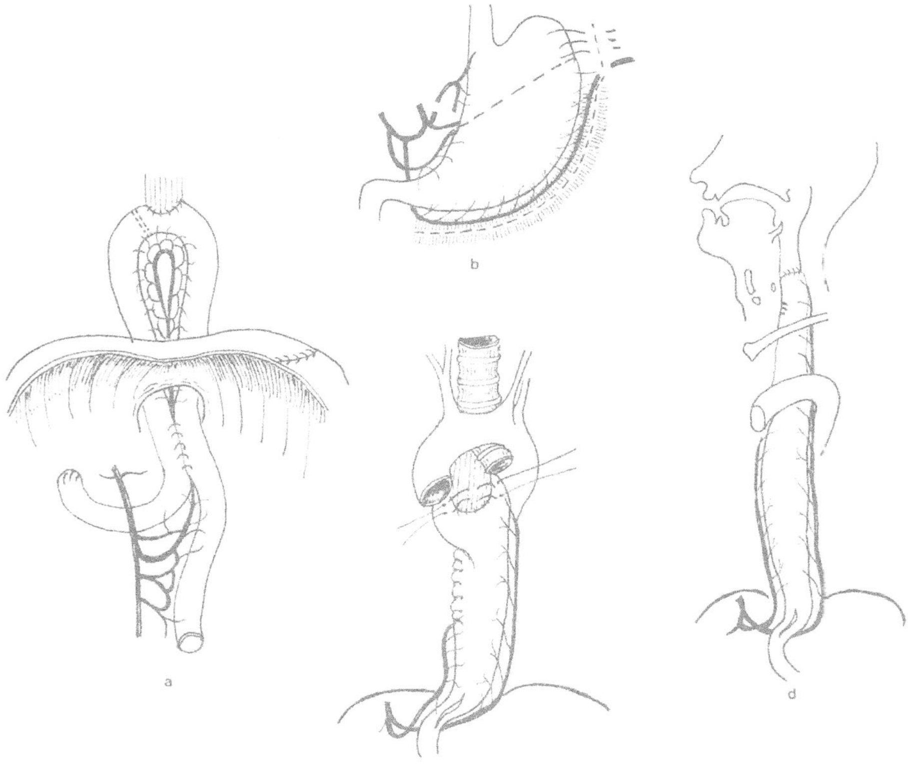

Fig. 2 a–d. Operations for carcinoma of the oesophagus in the elderly. **a** Loop oesophago-jejunostomy with entero-enterostomy and stapling of the afferent limb of loop after total gastrectomy. **b** Mobilisation of stomach, preserving the right gastric and right gastro-epiploeic vascular arcade along the greater curvature. **c** Oesophago-gastrectomy with anastomosis and fundoplication for tumours distal to the aortic arch. **d** 3-stage oesophagectomy with cervical oesophago-gastric anastomosis

a) Carcinoma of the Cardia

These are always radioresistant adenocarcinomas and metastasize early to the coeliac axis lymph nodes. The patient is prepared for a left thoracoabdominal approach, but to begin with only a small laparotomy incision, in line with the proposed thoracoabdominal incision, is made, so that a preliminary exploration of the abdomen can be carried out. If the lesion is found to be resectable, the incision is extended across the seventh costal cartilage and the left chest is entered along the seventh intercostal space. The diaphragm is opened by a peripheral circumferential incision parallel to its costal attachment, thereby avoiding interference with its nerve supply.A lower oesophagectomy together with a total gastrectomy and splenectomy is then carried out, dividing the oesophagus 8 cm above the lesion. This radical procedure is more expeditious than a partial gastrectomy and has a lower incidence of local recurrence of malignancy. Continuity is restored by a loop oesophagojejunostomy. Reflux of biliary and pancreatic secretions is prevented by an enteroenterostomy, at least 25 cm from the oesophagojejunal anastomosis, while at the same time the afferent loop is closed with staples just proximal to the oesophagojejunostomy (Fig. 2 a). This method virtually converts the loop into a Roux-en-Y type of loop without the tedious exacting vascular dissection which this entails.

b) Carcinoma of the Lower Third of the Oesophagus

In this situation (beyond 36 cm), a partial oesophagectomy combined with an upper partial gastrectomy is recommended. By means of automatic stapling device, the stomach is obliquely divided from the greater curvature towards the pyloric antrum (Fig. 2 b), retaining three-quarters of the greater curvature with its vascular arcade, but removing more than half of the lesser curvature. A gastric tube results, which can then be pulled up into the chest to be anastomosed by an end-to-side anastomosis to the oesophagus just below the aortic arch. The availability of a circular anastomotic stapler makes this anastomosis very much easier. A fundoplication around the anastomosis will lessen the tendency for reflux (Fig. 2 c).

c) Carcinoma of the Middle Third of the Oesophagus

For lesions in this location (24–36 cm), the well-established Ivor Lewis two-stage operation (LEWIS 1946) has stood the test of time. The first stage consists of an upper laparotomy during which the stomach is fully mobilized by dividing the left gastric, the left gastroepiploic and short gastric vessels, but preserving the vascular arcade along the greater curvature and the right gastric artery. Further mobilization of the stomach entails freeing the duodenum from its peritoneal reflexions (Kocher's manoeuvre). The hiatus is enlarged by dividing the crural sling and the lower oesophagus is bluntly mobilized by finger dissection from below. The first stage is concluded by carrying out a pyloromyotomy.

The second stage consists of a right thoracotomy through which the oesophagus and the growth are mobilized to well above the arch of the vena azygos. The previously mobilized stomach is pulled up into the chest and the oesophagus is divided and closed with a stapler at its junction with the stomach. The fundus of the stomach is anastomosed to the oesophagus just below the thoracic inlet. Some surgeons prefer to bring the stomach even higher up into the neck (third stage MCKEOWN 1979), because the incidence of anastomotic fistulae is lower and when it occurs the patient's chance of surviving this catastrophic complication is very much better (Fig. 2 d).

d) Carcinoma Above the Aortic Arch

A thoracic growth above the arch of the aorta or in the cervical portion of the oesophagus (upper third, above 24 cm) is resected, either by the three-stage procedure just mentioned, or a modification during which the oesophagus is divided from the mobilized stomach in the abdomen, which is then brought up into the neck substernally, where it is anastomosed to the oesophagus above the growth. The resection is then finally completed through a right thoracotomy.

e) Transhiatal Oesophagectomy Without Thoracotomy

This operative procedure has recently been advocated chiefly by ORRINGER and ORRINGER (1983), who advance some very cogent reasons for its adoption in the face of much criticism (SKINNER 1983). Its main advantage is the avoidance of a thoracotomy. Moreover, it can be carried out for a carcinoma at all levels, provided that a partial gastric resection has not been performed previously for peptic ulceration, because the stomach is used as a visceral substitute.

The first stage of the operation is carried out through an upper abdominal midline incision. The stomach is mobilized up to the oesophagogastric junction, as previously described, preserving the right gastric and gastroepiploeic vascular supply. A blunt dissection of the oesophagus is then continued upwards into the chest through the diaphragmatic hiatus. The next step is a collar incision in the neck, through which the upper oesophagus is mobilized by blunt finger dissection downwards into the mediastinum until the fingers of the hand through the hiatus meet the finger, introduced from above, inside the chest. The cardia can then be pulled up through the collar incision, so that an oesophagectomy with an anastomosis in the neck can be performed without opening the chest. The reader is referred to a detailed and profusely illustrated description of this operation by ORRINGER (1983).

The obvious advantage of this procedure is the elimination of a thoracotomy, which always causes so much respiratory embarrassment and for this reason should be seriously considered in elderly patients. The results of ORRINGER and ORRINGER (1983) in 143 patients are impressive. The operative mortality of 8% is low, considering that 19 patients were between the ages 70 and 79 years and five between 80 and 92 years. The major complication was a pneumothorax produced at the time of the operation, which was easily remedied by the introduction of an intercostal drain.

The main argument by the opponents of this procedure is that the blind mobilization in the chest does not achieve an adequate lymphatic clearence. The dismal 5-year survival rate of 6%, when the lymph nodes are involved (LI et al. 1981), makes this criticism irrelevant. Most resections for squamous cell carcinoma of the oesophagus ultimately prove to be palliative, with an occasional chance of cure as a bonus. Therefore, an oesophagectomy without a thoracotomy may well be the operation of choice in the elderly patient.

6. Postcricoid Carcinoma

Resection of this lesion in the elderly is not justified in the author's opinion for the following reasons:

1. It means a very mutilating operation, which entails a partial pharyngectomy, total laryngo-oesophagectomy, thyroidectomy and a block dissection of the cervical lymph nodes, restoring continuity by anastomosing either the stomach or colon to the pharynx.
2. An elderly patient finds oesophageal speech difficult to acquire.
3. The chances of survival, let alone the high operative mortality are dismal.

Most patients are, therefore, referred for radiotherapy, which at least does not carry such a high morbidity and mortality, though the cure rate is low.

7. Postoperative Management

The author is convinced of the value of heparinization to prevent postoperative thrombo-embolism. For that reason 5,000 U heparin are given 2 h before the operation and a similar dose is repeated every 12 h thereafter until discharge from hospital. The patient leaves the operating theatre with a nasogastric tube passed through the anastomosis, a central venous line (superior vena cava catheter) and a self-retaining catheter in the bladder. This ensures strict control over fluid balance, especially during the critical postoperative phase when all oral intake is avoided.

Fluid administration is as follows: dextrose/saline (0.18% NaCl and 4.3% Dextrose) is given throughout the operation at a rate of 2 ml/kg per 1 h. In addition, blood loss is replaced by whole blood and Hartmann's solution (compound sodium lactate intravenous infusion) is given (250 ml/h), while the serous cavities are exposed. We have often found that at the end of a sometimes prolonged upper abdominal dissection, a decrease in urinary flow can be reversed by increasing the osmolality with 500 ml plasma. A urinary flow of about 30 ml/h during the operation should be aimed at. The otherwise reduced urinary flow is corrected by increasing the fluid intake. Diuretics should only be administered as a last resort, because they tend to upset the electrolyte balance.

On return to the ward, the central venous line is connected to a manometer and blood is replaced as indicated by the central venous pressure reading. It is also our experience that the patient needs another 1 U plasma protein fraction in the first 24 h after operation to make up for the loss of serosanguineous fluids into the drainage bottles, as evidenced by the positive response in the lowered central venous pressure. Otherwise, the intravenous infusion of dextrose/saline, started in the theatre, is continued at a rate of 30 ml/kg for 24 h. This intravenous regime makes it absolutely essential to monitor carefully the serum electrolytes, urea, creatinine, and proteins. Haemoglobin and haematocrit estimations are also of value. The electrolytes are checked at least once a day, if normal, while the serum potassium may have to be estimated twice daily.

All our patients are ventilated artificially overnight after these big operations, because we have found that this lessens pulmonary complications, especially in the elderly, during the critical first 48 h. After extubation they are suitably postured, so that there is no risk of aspiration from the transposed stomach. The nasogastric tube is allowed to siphon into a bag.

Respiratory care in elderly patients is most important. Besides regular auscultation over the bases of the chest and a daily chest radiograph, blood gas analysis should be done on a regular basis. These measures should give early warning of pulmonary oedema. Basal crepitations, fluffy lung fields in the radiograph, and a low PaO_2 are the signs to observe. The treatment consists of small intravenous doses of frusemide and a very critical review of the fluid balance. Chest physiotherapy is started as soon as the patient can cooperate, but a word of warning is indicated. The aged patient must not be pushed to exhaustion by overenthusiastic physiotherapy and postural drainage is contraindicated, because of the danger of respiratory aspiration of gastric contents. Suction bronchoscopy under local anaesthesia for retained secretions is less distressing to the patient.

Nutrition in the immediate postoperative period is by intravenous hyperalimentation through the central venous line. Oral fluids in the form of sips of water are usually commenced 48 h after the operation and from then onwards the amount of fluids by mouth is progressively increased, adding milk to the feeds. At the end of the first week the patient is usually taking a minced diet and intravenous feeding can be discontinued.

8. Nonresectable Carcinoma

The patient may either be considered unfit for major surgery or the tumour may be irremovable. Under these circumstances the dysphagia may be relieved by passing a prosthetic tube (Mousseau–Barbin or Celestin) through the malignant stricture. These tubes may either be pushed or pulled through the obstruction. A laparotomy is necessary when the tube is being pulled into the stomach and this method would, of course, also be used when a carcinoma is found to be irremovable at operation. Most authors report a high mortality in the region of 30%–40%, for the pull-through procedure (PAGLIERO 1979; LISHMAN et al. 1980), although at the Mayo Clinic, Rochester, Minnesota, a mortality of only 10% in over 150 patients was recorded (PAYNE 1979). Pushing the tube through the malignant stricture avoids a laparotomy. For this purpose a special introducer for inserting a Celestin tube has been developed in Nottingham, England (ATKINSON et al. 1978). This consists of two flexible stainless steel tubes which, when locked together, grip the inside of the Celestin tube. The whole assembly is then pushed into the oesophagus over a guide wire, which had previously been passed into the stomach through the biopsy channel of a gastroscope. The actual intubation of the stricture is done under fluoroscopic control. Although this method is reported to have a lower mortality (LISHMAN et al. 1980), splitting of the oesophagus seems to be one of the major complications.

These tubes should never be used for benign strictures, as the consequences can be disastrous. Free reflux upwards through the tube will cause extensive oesophagitis, sometimes with severe haemorrhage, and in turn may result in further fibrotic narrowing.

Cervical lesions are not amenable to these tubes, as the funnel of the tube tends to obstruct the larynx or the tube rides up into the pharynx, nor can malignant tracheo-oesophageal fistulae be successfully managed by these means. Bypass procedures, using either stomach or colon and stapling the oesophagus above and below the growth, effectively stop the inhalation of food and saliva. Unfortunately nearly all patients who might benefit most are too ill for these major operations; elderly patients especially can hardly be expected to withstand such procedures.

9. Radiotherapy

Radiotherapy may be used palliatively for the relief of dysphagia. A treatment course lasts 2 weeks or so, given on a daily basis and is not a great strain even in the elderly. However, it is not very effective either. Radical radiotherapy is reserved for those reasonably fit patients who are deemed inoperable for reasons already stated. Treatment is given by supervoltage radiation on a daily basis for 5 or 6 weeks and a "tumour dose" of 5,000 cGy is aimed at. Treatment is arduous, but in successful cases dysphagia may be relieved early, although some patients develop fibrous strictures later, which can be difficult or even dangerous to dilate.

Attention to anaemia, malnutrition and infection (particularly lung infection) is at least as important as in surgical cases. Other complications include mediastinitis and oesophagobronchial fistulae. Though squamous carcinoma is radiosensitive and the radiotherapeutic treatment of postcricoid cancer is perfectly possible, results are poor and few large series can claim 5-year survival rates exceeding 20%. There is no evidence that cytotoxic drugs, either singly or in combination have any part to play in the treatment of oesophageal cancer.

III. Hiatus Hernia and Gastro-Oesophageal Reflux

Gastro-oesophageal reflux used to be considered synonymous with hiatus hernia. Although the two are frequently associated, one can occur without the other, and it is now generally accepted that they are separate entities. Hiatus hernia is a very common condition in western society.

There are two types of hiatus hernia. The far more common sliding type and the relatively rare paraoesophageal hernia. In the former, the gastro-oesophageal junction ascends through the hiatus into the chest and usually causes no symptoms, unless it is associated with abnormal reflux, when it may require treatment. In the paraoesophageal hernia the gastro-oesophageal junction remains in its normal position within the abdomen, but the stomach herniates alongside the oesophagus into a true peritoneal sac within the chest. Although a paraoesophageal hernia may cause no symptoms, it is potentially lethal, because of the high incidence of gastric obstruction, volvulus, infarction, and bleeding. At other times the intrathoracic gastric dilatation causes breathlessness and cardiac irregularities through pressure on the heart and lungs. The paraoesophageal hernia is more common in elderly people and should always be treated surgically, even in the absence of symptoms, for the reasons stated.

Gastro-oesophageal reflux, either of gastric or more rarely, biliary secretions, causes reflux oesophagitis, which is responsible for the symptoms of heartburn and regurgitation and the complications of bleeding, ulceration, and strictures. A review by NICHOLSON and NOHL-OSER (1976) of a large series of patients treated surgically for gastro-oesophageal reflux and its complications, revealed a significant increase in the incidence of severe oesophagitis and strictures with advancing age (Fig. 3). Strictures in the elderly are a difficult problem and if they are to be avoided, the earlier stages of severe oesophagitis, bleeding, and ulceration, must be detected by endoscopy and treated effectively. Too much reliance has been placed in the past on barium studies, which only show abnormal motility or narrowing of the oesophagus, which are already manifestations of established fibrosis. Unfortunately, there is a poor correlation between reflux symptoms and the severity of oesophagitis, so that some patients with marked symptoms may be found to have minimal mucosal changes, while in others, dysphagia is the first symptom. Strictures are also known to develop silently in bedridden patients or to follow prolonged nasogastric intubation.

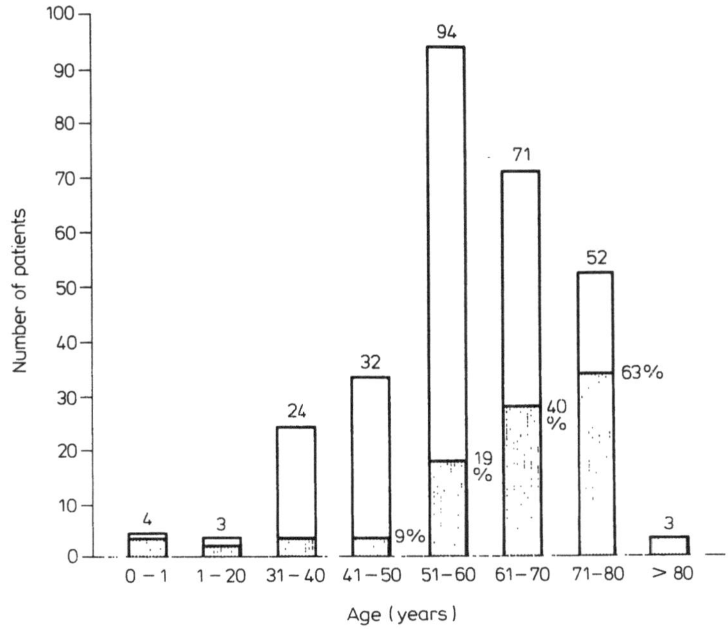

Fig. 3. Increasing incidence (*hatched areas*) of ulcerative oesophagitis or stricture formation with advancing age, as found on endoscopy in a series of 283 patients treated surgically for reflux oesophagitis

1. Management

Patients with persistent symptoms of reflux or dysphagia must be investigated by barium studies and endoscopy. The barium swallow and meal may reveal a hiatus hernia with or without reflux or a stricture. Endoscopy will detect the presence or absence of oesophagitis or a possible stricture. A biopsy must be taken whenever pathological changes are seen. Additional pH studies are necessary, should no abnormality by present to account for the symptoms. They will confirm and distinguish between acid and alkaline reflux, if present.

All other patients are treated on a strict medical regime, which cannot be detailed here. Only when troublesome symptoms persist after 6 months of rigorous medical treatment, should the possibility of surgery be considered. However, the investigations need repeating to ensure that reflux is actually the underlying cause. The long-term results of antireflux surgery have been disappointing in the past. Whether the new operative techniques, based on a better understanding of the pathophysiology, will be more successful remains to be seen. Moreover, the choice of operation depends on such factors as the presence of a stricture and its length, shortening and fixation of the oesophagus and possible associated motility disorders. Finally, the general condition of the patient will determine the most suitable operation.

2. Antireflux Fundoplication Operation

This type of operation is indicated in patients who either suffer from reflux and its complications or who have a paraoesophageal hernia. A variety of operations are in common use, of which the author prefers the Nissen fundoplication (NISSEN 1961), where the mobilized fundus of the stomach is wrapped around an intra-abdominal segment of the oesophagus. The long-term results of this operation depend on the success of restoring and maintaining a sufficient length of oesophagus in its normal intra-abdominal position. To achieve this without too much tension, it is often necessary to mobilize the oesophagus up to the aortic arch. This can only be done through a left thoracotomy. Before starting the fundoplication, a 50 Fr. Hurst–Maloney bougie is passed from above into the stomach. This will ensure that the fundoplication is not sewn too tightly around the oesophagus.

A high proportion (60%–70%) of strictures will resolve, after further reflux has been successfully prevented by this operation. On the other hand, a long stricture and a short oesophagus will make it impossible to bring the gastro-oesophageal junction down to its normal intra-abdominal position without tension. Moreover, with manifest perioesophagitis present, the fundoplication sutures are unlikely to hold in the oedematous tissues. Under such circumstances other steps have to be taken, which will be described presently.

IV. Strictures

The management of strictures causing significant dysphagia presents considerable problems, especially as some of these patients are in their seventh or eighth decade of life. It is desirable to avoid major surgery at that age. After a barium swallow and meal has shown the presence of oesophageal narrowing, the next step is evaluation by endoscopy. The stricture is dilated and several biopsies are taken from within the strictured area to determine whether the stricture is benign or malignant. The dilatation can be carried out with gum-elastic-tipped bougies (Chevalier Jackson) under direct vision through the rigid oesophagoscope or blindly with the Eder-Puestow metal olives passed over a guide wire, which was previously passed down the biopsy channel of a gastroscope. The author prefers the former method, because it allows an assessment to be made of the pliability and extent of the stenosis. Progressive dilatation with bougies up to 40 Fr. is usually possible.

This initial dilatation may relieve the dysphagia for more than a year in some patients, especially if they adhere conscientiously to the prescribed medical treatment. In many elderly or debilitated patients this dilatation is a valuable alternative to an operation where the risk is prohibitive, and it may be all that is necessary. More often dilatation will have to be repeated indefinitely, sometimes at 3- to 6-month intervals, and at other times longer intervals, and the patients must content themselves with living on semisolid diets. In others, however, the relief is only short-lived or may even fail altogether and in these, if the general condition allows, there is no other option but to operate.

A variety of operative methods, short of actual resection of the stricture, have been described. Dilatation and the abolition of reflux by fundoplication has already been detailed, when it was also pointed out that the operation is more likely to fail if the cardia cannot be restored to its position below the diaphragm. In the more advanced cases with long strictures and a shortened oesophagus, the Collis gastroplasty combined with a fundoplication is a widely favoured alternative (ORRINGER 1981). In this operation, the oesophagus is lengthened by fashioning a tube from the lesser curvature of the stomach with the aid of a stapler. It is an effective but complicated procedure, which carries a substantial morbidity and mortality in older people. For these reasons, the operation described by MILSTEIN (1975) is attractive, because of its simplicity and effectiveness. The technique is very briefly as follows. The fibrosed oesophagus is mobilized up to the aortic arch, the fundus of the stomach is freed as for a Nissen fundoplication. A vertical incision into the lumen, extending from the stomach across the stricture into healthy oesophagus above, splays out the strictured area, which is then closed transversely (Heineke–Mikulicz principle) with interrupted stainless steel wire sutures, starting on either side from the middle of the incision. Closure of this, seemingly gaping, fibrosed hole is unexpectedly easy, because on tying the sutures the redundant anterior gastric wall is drawn up and will close the gap without tension. A Nissen fundoplication within the chest, giving extra cover to the oesophagoplasty, completes the procedure. The only reservation about the long-term effect of this operation is that it creates an intrathoracic gastric pouch, with the possibility of further herniation and obstruction of the stomach. This can be avoided by enlarging the hiatus and suturing its margin carefully to the stomach.

The temptation of overcoming the obstruction by passing a tube (Celestin) through the narrowed segment, as is sometimes done for malignant strictures, must be resisted at all cost. The dire consequences of this action have already been discussed in Sect. B.II.8.

V. Neuromuscular Disorders of the Oesophagus

The passage of food from the mouth to the stomach depends on a well-coordinated neuromuscular mechanism. The initial phase of this swallowing process is highly complex and still ill understood. Motility disorders and incoordination of muscle contractions can involve the sphincteric mechanisms at either end of the oesophagus, while at other times a localized segment or the entire length of the oesophagus may show abnormal peristaltic activity. Moreover, abnormal muscle spasms can cause mucosal protrusions, forming diverticula. Any of these conditions may present themselves late in life and cause considerable distress, such as dysphagia or chest pain. The following conditions will be discussed:

1. Pharyngeal diverticulum (Zenker's pouch)
2. Intrathoracic oesophageal pulsion diverticulum
3. Achalasia of the oesophagus
4. Diffuse oesophageal spasm
5. Scleroderma

VI. Pharyngeal Diverticulum

This herniation of oesophageal mucosa at the back of the pharynx through a gap between the inferior pharyngeal constrictor muscle above and the cricopharyngeus muscle below (Killian–Jamieson dehiscence), is an acquired condition. Its incidence increases with age. The mucosal protrusion enlarges to form a pouch between the vertebral column and oesophagus, which compresses and deflects the oesophagus forward, thereby causing dysphagia. The entrance of the pouch lies above the cricopharyngeus, in direct line with the pharynx, so that an endoscope will always enter the pouch rather than the oesophagus, the opening of which lies anteriorly. Perforation during endoscopy is, therefore, a likely risk, especially if the existence of a pouch is unknown, because no barium study preceded this investigation. Moreover, food has a tendency to regurgitate up into the mouth or will sometimes spill over into the bronchial tree, because of this anatomical arrangement. A rare complication is the development of a squamous carcinoma in the diverticulum. Finally, a rather frequent association between gastro-oesophageal reflux and pharyngeal diverticulum has been noted (SMILEY et al. 1970).

1. Operation

This consists of two distinct steps. The first deals with the diverticulum, while the second consists of a myotomy of the cricopharyngeus muscle. Large diverticula are best excised, for which a 30-mm stapling device is a useful instrument. Before applying the stapler a 35 Fr. bougie is passed down into the oesophagus to prevent any narrowing at the level of excision. For small or medium pouches, a diverticulopexy, drawing the sac upwards and suturing it to the prevertebral fascia, will suffice.

The myotomy is carried out in the midline posteriorly, by carefully lifting the muscle off the mucosa with right-angled forceps and cutting it for a distance of at least 2 cm from the neck of the sac downwards. A transverse closure of the muscles after the myotomy will cover the mucosal repair of the diverticulectomy and prevent a postoperative fistula. As an extra precaution, a soft drain is passed down to the site of operation.

VII. Intrathoracic Oesophageal Pulsion Diverticulum

Another type of pulsion diverticulum is the epiphrenic variety, which tends to occur in the lower half of the thoracic oesophagus. These diverticula can occur at a higher level at or above the bifurcation of the trachea. They usually produce no symptoms and are found by chance during radiographic examination. Manometric studies show that the majority of epiphrenic diverticula have an underlying motility disorder, while some are associated with a hiatus hernia (PAYNE 1981). Operative treatment, however, is only indicated when the patient experiences significant symptoms, such as dysphagia or pain.

Full investigations by roentgenographic studies, manometry and endoscopy are necessary before surgery is undertaken. It is essential that the associated underlying abnormality is dealt with, and as it consists nearly always of muscular or organic obstruction distal to the diverticulum, a long myotomy must be combined with the excision of the diverticulum. A diverticulectomy without a myotomy is most likely to be followed by a sutureline leak and persistence of symptoms. A hiatus hernia or stricture, when present, should be dealt with at the same time. If a fundoplication is necessary, special care is needed to avoid nullifying the effect of the myotomy. The fundus of the stomach is, therefore, sewn loosely on either side to the muscles of the oesophageal wall, parallel to the myotomy opening, during the "wrap around" of the fundoplication. Moreover, a 50 Fr. Maloney bougie, passed into the stomach at the same time, will ensure that the fundoplication is not made too tight.

VIII. Achalasia of the Oesophagus

The aetiology of this disease is still unknown. It can occur at any age. It is important to appreciate that two distinct abnormal mechanisms are involved in this condition: (a) poor or absent oesophageal peristalsis; and (b) failure of relaxation (achalasia) of the lower oesophageal sphincter in response to deglutition. Operative treatment relieves only the obstructing element at the lower end and is, therefore, palliative.

In the early stages of the disease the body of the oesophagus looks relatively normal on the barium roentgenogram, but the oesophagogastric junction shows the characteristic "bird-beak" appearance with delay in the passage of the barium into the stomach. The appearance in the later stages is characterized by progressive dilatation of the oesophagus, until finally the classical megaoesophagus with its large sigmoid loop is seen. The liability to develop carcinoma later, in spite of successful treatment, is well known. The symptoms can be diverse; besides dysphagia, there may be dehydration, cough or choking due to respiratory aspiration, heartburn or pain as a result of retention oesophagitis. Sometimes bizarre habits are acquired to make the food go down, such as drinking copiously or performing the Valsalva manoeuvre.

1. Preoperative Oesophagoscopy

The purpose of this investigation is twofold. First, to empty the oesophagus of all retained fluid and food debris and second to inspect the sometimes voluminous oesophagus for possible carcinomatous changes. Induction of anaesthesia for this examination is fraught with the risk of aspirating fluid and decomposed food into the lungs. The anaesthetist must, therefore, take the necessary steps to avoid this mishap at all costs. Anaesthesia is started with the patient sitting well propped up. The cricoid cartilage is compressed firmly against the vertebral column, as soon as the injection of thiopentone is started, and this compression is not released until the endotracheal tube, with its cuff inflated, has been correctly positioned. Aspiration of the sometimes considerable amounts of food is facilitated by using a large-bore suction tube, while large food particles may need removal with forceps. Occasionally, food debris tends to cling to the inflamed oesophageal wall, making it impossible to get an adequate view of the mucosa, so that oesophageal lavage becomes necessary.

2. Treatment

It is generally agreed that the extramucous oesophagocardiomyotomy, commonly known as the modified Heller's operation, is the treatment of choice in this condition and should be carried out in the early stages of the disease. It has superseded every other form of treatment, including the forceful dilatation of the sphincter, using a hydrostatic bag. This latter method is not nearly as effective as the operation and is known to carry the risk of occasional oesophageal perforation by the dilator. Hydrostatic dilatation is, therefore, reserved only for the very frail patient, who would never tolerate an operation.

3. Preoperative Treatment

The need for preoperative treatment depends on the condition of the patient and the state of the oesophagus. Extreme malnutrition and dehydration must be corrected by hyperalimentation, as previously described, when the preoperative treatment of carcinoma of the oesophagus was discussed. A megaoesophagus is better treated by preliminary oesophageal lavage and should in any case be emptied before induction of anaesthesia.

The transthoracic approach gives the best access to the oesophagus, hiatus and stomach, so that an adequate myotomy can safely and neatly be carried out. Moreover, it makes it very much easier to perform an additional antireflux operation. The myotomy consists of a vertical incision through both the longitudinal and circular muscles of the oesophagus, until the mucosa pouts through between the margins of the incised muscles. The incision extends upwards over the dilated thick-walled portion of the oesophagus for a minimum distance of 3 cm and downwards to just beyond the oesophagogastric junction. The external identification of this junction is difficult. A few small veins traverse the organ at that point and serve as a reasonably satisfactory landmark. Some of these vessels must be divided and the consequent bleeding may be stopped by steady pressure with a swab, otherwise a suture/ligation with No 5–0 atraumatic nonabsorbable suture is indicated. Diathermy should never be used, as it can easily cause coagulation necrosis of the mucosa with dire results.

After completion of the myotomy a careful search is made for any remaining constricting circular muscle fibres. These tend to be especially adherent at the cardia and must be teased apart with the utmost gentleness to avoid the serious mishap of mucosal perforation. The dissection is completed by separating the muscular wall from the mucosa laterally on either side for about 1 cm. This releases the mucosa and prevents reapproximation of the incised oesophageal wall.

There is disagreement about the necessity of an additional fundoplication. The vast experience at the Mayo Clinic (Payne 1981) is that this is not necessary, provided that the myotomy is not extended beyond the cardia. There exists a great deal of uncertainty where this end point at the lower end of the myotomy incision should lie, to ensure that future reflux oesophagitis is avoided and yet the achalasia is adequately relieved. A collective series (Rees et al. 1970) showed that severe reflux oesophagitis remains the most notable complication, occurring in up to 25%–30% of patients. For this reason the author, in common with many others, carries out a routine fundoplication after completing the myotomy. The manner in which this is carried out without rendering the myotomy ineffective, has already been described when the treatment of intrathoracic oesophageal pulsion diverticulum was discussed.

IX. Diffuse Oesophageal Spasm

The cause of this primary motility disorder is also unknown. Pain, sometimes simulating angina pectoris, and dysphagia are the predominant symptoms. A barium swallow usually shows marked spasm of the whole oesophagus, the so-called corkscrew oesophagus. Occasionally a hiatus hernia, epiphrenic diverticulum or a hyperactive lower sphincter are associated with this disorder. On the other hand, the gastro-oesophageal junction relaxes in the usual manner in response to deglutition (FLYE et al. 1975). Radiographic examination and manometry determine the extent of involvement and surgical treatment will be based on the results of these investigations. Oesophageal pH studies will eliminate those patients in whom gastro-oesophageal reflux is the primary cause of the spasm. Otherwise, myotomy is the treatment of choice (LEONARDI et al. 1977) and as this may have to be done over a long stretch of the oesophagus, the operation is best carried out through the right chest. It is important not to extend the myotomy too far at the lower end and thus interfere with the lower oesophageal sphincter's function, which would inevitably result in reflux oesophagitis (PARIS et al. 1975).

X. Scleroderma

This condition is one of many connective tissue disorders not infrequently associated with oesophageal dysfunction (MUKHOPADHYAY et al. 1976). The histological features are muscle atrophy and fibrous tissue replacement, which results in diminished or absent peristalsis, loss of muscle tone and weak or absent lower oesophageal sphincter tone.

The oesophageal symptoms in these patients are mainly due to gastro-oesophageal reflux, with diminished peristalsis being a contributory factor responsible for delayed clearing of regurgitated gastric contents. This results in ulcerative oesophagitis and stricture formation in many patients. While scleroderma remains a systemic disease with involvement of the heart, kidneys and lungs, operative treatment should be considered in those patients in whom intensive medical therapy has failed and who are deemed fit for surgical interference (ORRINGER 1981). The choice of operation depends on whether there is oesophageal shortening and the presence or absence of a stricture. The management of these problems has been adequately dealt with when the treatment of reflux oesophagitis and strictures was discussed.

References

Abrams LD (1958) A pleural biopsy Punch. Lancet 1:30–31

Atkinson M, Ferguson R, Parker GC (1978) Tube introducer and modified Celestin tube for use in palliative intubation of oesophago-gastric neoplasms at fibreoptic endoscopy. Gut 79:669–671

Bates DV, Macklem PT, Christie RV (1971) Effects of age on pulmonary function. In: Ibid. Respiratory function in disease. Saunders, Philadelphia

Bates M (1970) Results of surgery for bronchial carcinoma in patients aged 70 and over. Thorax 25:77–78

Bignall JR, Moon AJ (1955) Survival after lung resection for bronchial carcinoma. Thorax 10:183–190

Comroe JH, Forster RE, Dubois AB, Briscoe WA, Carlsen E (1962) Pulmonary function pattern in the "Elderly Normal". In: Ibid. The Lung, clinical physiology and pulmonary function tests, 2nd edn. Year Book Medical Publishers, Chicago

Croft PB, Wilkinson M (1965) The incidence of carcinomatous neuromyopathy in patients with various types of carcinoma. Brain 88:427–434

Dark JF (1981) The complications of operations for lung cancer. In: Dyde JA, Smith RE (eds) The present state of thoracic surgery. The 5th Coventry conference. Pitman Medical, London

Dark JF, Mousalli H, Vaughan R (1981) Surgical treatment of carcinoma of the oesophagus. Thorax 36:891–895

Davis EW, Peabody JW, Katz S (1956) The solitary pulmonary nodule; a ten year study based on 215 cases. J Thorac Surg 32:728–770

Eckert P, Braun J, Hempel D (1979) Der Mensch im Alter: Aus der Sicht des Chirurgen. Chirurg 50:449–455

Fischnaller M (1980) Zytodiagnostik in der Pulmologie. In: Denk H, Sighart H (eds) Das Bronchuskarzinom heute. Holzhausens, Wien, p 112

Flavell G (1962) Conservatism in surgical treatment in bronchial carcinoma. A review of 826 personal operations. Br Med J 1:284–287

Flye MW, Sealy WC (1975) Diffuse spasm of the oesophagus. Ann Thorac Surg 19:677–687

Gessler U (1973) Akute und chronische Uraemie bei chirurgischen Erkrankten. Chirurg 44:401–407

Good CA, Wilson TW (1958) The solitary circumscribed pulmonary nodule. JAMA 166:210–215

Grunze H (1966) Derzeitiger Stand der Zytodiagnostik bei Erkrankungen des Thorax; 15jährige Erfahrung. Dtsch Med Wochenschr 91:1476–1483

Hanson G, Phillips T (1962) Pleural biopsy in diagnosis of thoracic disease. Br Med J 2:300–303

Harmer MH (1978) TNM Classification of malignant tumours, 3rd edn. Lederle, Fareham, UK

Hayward R (1981) Why do we pace. Br J Hosp Med 25:466

Hinson KFW, Kuper SWA (1963) The diagnosis of lung cancer by examination of sputum. Thorax 18:350–353

Jensik RJ, Faber LP, Kittle CF (1979) Segmental resection for bronchogenic carcinoma. Ann Thorac Surg 28:475–481

Johnston JB, Jones PH (1959) The treatment of bronchial carcinoma by lobectomy and sleeve resection of the main bronchus. Thorax 14:48–54

Jones FL, Blodgett RC (1971) Empyema in rheumatoid pleuropulmonary disease. Ann Intern Med 74:665–671

Kreyberg L, Liebow AA, Uehlinger EA (1967) Histological typing of lung tumours. World Health Organisation, Geneva

Kutschera W (1980) Die internistische Kontraindikation. In: Denk H, Sighart H (eds) Das Bronchuskarzinom heute. Holzhausens, Wien, p 168

Leonardi HK, Shea JA, Crozier RE, Ellis FH (1977) Diffuse spasm of the oesophagus, clinical, manometric and surgical considerations. J Thorac Cardiovasc Surg 74:736–741

Lewis I (1946) Surgical treatment of carcinoma of the oesophagus, with special reference to a new operation for growths of the middle third. Br J Surg 34:18–31
Li R, Lu Y, Chen H, Gu Y, Yang J, Hu J (1981) Late results of surgical treatment in oesophageal carcinoma and factors influencing prognosis. Chin Med J 94:729–732
Lishman AH, Dellipiani AW, Devlin HB (1980) The insertion of oesophago-gastric tubes in malignant oesophageal strictures: Endoscopy or surgery? Br J Surg 67:257–259
Lyall JRW, Summers GD, O'Brien IM, Bateman NT, Pike CK, Braimbridge MV (1980) Sequential brush biopsy and conventional biopsy: direct comparison of diagnostic sensitivity in lung malignancy. Thorax 35:929–931
Maassen W (1972) Direkte Thorakoskopie ohne vorherige oder mögliche Pneumothoraxanlage zugleich eine neue Methode der chirurgischen Pleura und Lungenbiopsie. Endoscopy 4:95–98
Maiwand O, Makey AR (1981) Cryoanalgesia for relief of pain after thoracotomy. Br Med J 282:1749–1750
McKeown KC (1979) Carcinoma of the oesophagus. J R Coll Surg Edinb 24:253–274
Milstein BB (1975) An operation for the treatment of intractable peptic stricture of the oesophagus. Isr J Med Sci 11:281–286
Mittman C (1961) Assessment of operative risk in thoracic surgery. Am Rev Respir Dis 84:197–207
Mukhopadhyay AK, Graham DY (1976) Esophageal motor dysfunction in systemic diseases. Arch Intern Med 136:583–588
Nicholson DA, Nohl-Oser HC (1976) Hiatus hernia: A comparison between two methods of fundoplication by evaluation of the long-term results. J Thorac Cardiovasc Surg 72:938–943
Nissen R (1961) Gastropexy and "fundoplication" in surgical treatment of hiatus hernia. Am J Dig Dis 6:954–961
Nohl-Oser HC (1979) The evolution and present status of mediastinoscopy. Endoscopy 11:1–4
Nohl-Oser HC (1980) The long-term survival of patients with lung cancer treated surgically after selection by mediastinoscopy. Thorac Cardiovasc Surg 28:158–161
Nohl-Oser HC, Fenn A, Dottori V (1982) Tracheo-bronchoplastic procedure in the treatment of advanced carcinoma of the right upper lung. Ann Thorac Surg 33:396–399
O'Keefe ME, Good CA, McDonald JK (1957) Calcification in solitary nodules of the lung. Am J Roentgenol 77:1023–1033
Orringer MB (1981) Surgical treatment of oesophageal strictures resulting from gastro-oesophageal reflux. In: Dyde JA, Smith RE (eds) The present state of thoracic surgery. The 5th Conventry conference. Pitman Medical, London, pp 83–94
Orringer MB (1983) Transhiatal oesophagectomy. In: Rob C, Smith R (eds) Operative surgery, alimentary tract and abdominal wall, vol 1, 4th edn. Butterworths, London, pp 192–203
Orringer MB, Orringer JS (1983) Esophagectomy without thoracotomy: a dangerous operation? J Thorac Cardiovasc Surg 85:72–80
Osler Sir W, McCrae T (1908) A system of medicine, vol 4. Oxford Medical Publications, London, p 430
Pagliero KM (1979) The problem of dysphagia. In: Vowles KDJ (ed) Surgical problems in the aged. Wright, Bristol, pp 51–67
Paris F, Benages A, Berengner J, Blasco J, Garrido B, Parsilla P, Ridocci MT, Carbonell C (1975) Pre- and post-operative manometric studies in diffuse esophageal spasm. J Thorac Cardiovasc Surg 70:126–132
Paulson DL, Shaw RR (1955) Bronchial anastomosis and broncho-plastic procedures in the interest of preservation of lung tissue. J Thorac Surg 29:238–251
Payne WS (1979) Palliation of esophageal carcinoma. Ann Thorac Surg 28:208–209
Payne WS (1981) Disorders of oesophageal motility. In: Dyde JA, Smith RE (eds) The present state of thoracic surgery. The 5th Conventry conference. Pitman Medical, London, pp 137–158
Pearson FG (1981) The significance of pressure measurements in the oesophagus. In: Dyde JA, Smith RE (eds) The present state of thoracic surgery. The 5th Coventry conference. Pitman Medical, London, pp 97–100

Pribilla O (1972) Datenverarbeitung und Dokumentation von tödlichen Verkehrsunfällen unter besonderer Berücksichtigung von Fußgängerunfällen. Arbeit Leistung 26:303–308

Pridun N (1980) Sicherung der Diagnose beim Lungenkrebs. In: Denk H, Sighart H (eds) Das Bronchuskarzinom heute. Holzhausens, Wien, p 129

Rees GM, Paneth M (1970) Lobectomy with sleeve resection in the treatment of bronchial tumours. Thorax 25:160–164

Rees JR, Thorbjarnarson B, Barnes WH (1970) Achalasia: results of operation in 84 patients. Ann Surg 171:195–201

Sagel SS, Ferguson TB, Forrest JV, Roper CL, Weldon CS, Clark RE (1978) Percutaneous transthoracic aspiration needle biopsy. Ann Thorac Surg 26:399–404

Sahn SA, Lakshminarayan S, Char DC (1973) "Silent" empyema in patients receiving corticosteroids. Am Rev Respir Dis 107:873–876

Sengupta A (1963) The treatment of recurrent spontaneous pneumothorax with iodine and talc poudrage. Br J Dis Chest 57:197–199

Silbiger ML, Pikielney R, Donner MW (1967) Neuromuscular disease affecting the pharynx, cineradiographic analysis. Invest Radiol 2:442–448

Skinner DB (1983) Comment on a paper by Orringer MB and Orringer JS, entitled "Esophagectomy without thoracotomy: a dangerous operation?" J Thorac Cardiovasc Surg 85:80

Smiley TB, Caves PK, Porter DC (1970) Relationship between posterior pharyngeal pouch and hiatus hernia. Thorax 25:725–731

Ulmer WT, Reichel G, Nolte D (1976) Die Lungenfunktionen, 2nd edn. Thieme, Stuttgart

Von Wichert P (1981) Preoperative general and function assessment. In: Nohl-Oser HC, Nissen R, Schreiber HW (eds) Surgery of the lung. Thieme, Stuttgart, p 15

Wang KC, Howland WS (1958) Cardiac and pulmonary evaluation in elderly patients before elective surgical operations. JAMA 166:993–997

Wessler S (1980) Low dose heparin reduces the incidence of post-operative pulmonary emboli and should be used routinely in general and thoracic surgery. In: Rapaport (ed) Current controversies in cardiovascular disease. Saunders, Philadelphia, pp 488–496

Willis RA (1960) Pathology of tumours, 3rd edn. Butterworths, London

Yacoub MH (1966) Vagotomy through mediastinoscopy for pulmonary osteoarthropathy. Br J Dis Chest 60:144–147

Yang Guanrei, Huang HE, Qui Sungliang, Chang Yuming (1982) Endoscopic diagnosis of 115 cases of early esophageal carcinoma. Endoscopy 14:157–161

Otorhinolaryngology

Otolaryngology in the Elderly

C. BECK

A. Introduction

The domain of otorhinolaryngology, like medicine of the rest of the human body, is subject to changes caused essentially by physiologic aging. Both genetic and environmental factors are likely to be involved. In our own specialty it is often better to speak of symptoms of or reactions to aging rather than of diseases of aging, for many of the manifestations do not amount to disease. The diseases that do occur are seldom peculiar to old age and are by no means characteristic of it. Their treatment does not differ fundamentally from that of the same diseases in other age groups. Without doubt, however, reactions to aging and diseases in old age can significantly impair function and quality of life, often presenting the old person with a difficult problem, depending of course on the great differences in attitudes between individuals and within individuals. The changes with aging to be described here are those specific to our specialty. The emphasis will be on etiology and pathophysiology in older people. The order followed will be that of the classical subdivisions of the specialty: the ear, the nose and its accessory sinuses, the pharynx, and the larynx.

No use will be made of statistics such as population age distributions and morbidities. Data from our specialty differ according to their origins from hospitals or specialist practices (PELLNITZ 1962; NOVOTNY 1969; MIKAT 1972; GOLEMANOV 1976; TZSCHOPPE 1976). Population age distribution and disease incidence are always changing. For example, in each subdivision of our specialty we are now seeing a significantly increased incidence of malignant tumors in younger people, whereas they used to be typical of the more elderly. In my opinion, therefore, statistical findings cannot throw any decisive light on the important facts, namely the pathophysiology of a symptom and its significance in the elderly.

B. Ear

I. Inner Ear

1. Presbycusis

Defective hearing is certainly the most obvious audiological feature of old age. The history is one of slowly progressive impairment of hearing and loss of ability to understand speech. The prevalence was first measured by ZWAARDEMAKER in

1891. Since then, intensive studies of the structural changes and their effect on function have been reported in a wealth of publications. The findings have been summarized and critically assessed in a survey made by HÜLSE and BOLL in 1979.

a) Morphological Findings

The morphological basis of presbycusis is degeneration of the sensory cells in the orgen of Corti, above all in the basal turn. Principally affected are the external hair cells (SCHUKNECHT 1955, 1964; FLEISCHER 1956; KIRIKAE et al. 1964; BREDBERG 1967; BELAL 1975; ANDERSON and MEYERHOFF 1982). Atrophy of supporting cells and secondary degeneration of auditory nerve fibers follow, with loss of neurons (SCHUKNECHT 1964; NOMURA and KIRIKAE 1968; JOHNSSON and HAWKINS 1972a). Also seen is increasing rigidity of the basilar membrane (DÖDERLEIN 1938; SCHUKNECHT 1964). The decisive factors seem to include areas of calcification, generalized thickening (MAYER 1920; CROWE et al. 1934; SAXÉN 1937), decreased concentration of substance (KRAUS et al. 1973), and deposition of neutral fats in the zona pectinata in the basal turn of the cochlea (NOMURA 1970).

The stria vascularis shows disintegration and thinning of its epithelium. Fibroblast density decreases. This is accompanied by increased cyst formation (FLEISCHER 1956, SCHUKNECHT 1964; JOHNSSON and HAWKINS 1972b; WRIGHT and SCHUKNECHT 1972). The cochlear blood vessels also show aging changes. The number of vessels is diminished, especially in the stria vascularis (JOHNSSON 1971; JOHNSSON and HAWKINS 1972b). The walls of the capillaries are markedly thickened and hyalinized, even to the extent of obliteration (SAXÉN 1973; JORGENSEN 1961; HANSEN and RESKE-NIELSEN 1965).

The most usual finding in the aging cochlea is the disappearance of ganglion cells from the spiral ganglion of the cochlear nerve. This decline in the number of nerve cells and their fibers begins at the basal end of the cochlea and advances towards the apex (SAXÉN 1937; FLEISCHER 1956; JORGENSEN 1961; HANSEN and RESKE-NIELSEN 1965; FLEISCHER 1972). Cell shrinkage and vacuolation are seen. Cytoplasm and nucleus are poorly stained and the nucleolus is absent. Ribonucleic acids are less abundant. The fundus of the internal acoustic meatus in elderly people undergoes progressive ossification in the vicinity of the tractus spiralis foraminosus (KROMPOTIĆ-NEMANIĆ 1968, 1969, 1971, 1972). It is postulated that bone apposition leads to degeneration of nerve fibers and compression of blood vessels. Changes are also found in the course of the auditory pathway. Investigations at this level, however, have been relatively few compared with studies of the cochlea. HANSEN and RESKE-NIELSEN (1963, 1965) and KIRIKAE et al. (1964) demonstrated vacuoles, pyknoses, and loss of ganglion cells in the ventral and dorsal chochlear nuclei, olive, quadrigeminal bodies, and medial geniculate body. ARNESEN (1982) estimated a loss of about 50% of the neurons in the dorsal and ventral cochlear nuclei of subjects with presbycusis as compared with the number of neurons expected to be present in normal subjects. Thinning of myelin sheaths and fragmentation of axons were found in the temporal lobes.

The structural changes of aging which cause senile deafness are found in all parts of the auditory pathway from the hair cells in the organ of Corti to the secondary receptor centers in the dominant cerebral hemisphere. On this basis attempts have been made to subdivide presbycusis according to the preponderant morphological changes. For example, SCHUKNECHT (1964) distinguishes four types, to each of which a distinctive pattern of audiological reactions can be ascribed:

1. Sensory presbycusis, in which atrophy of the organ of Corti and of the auditory nerve is predominant. Abrupt high frequency hearing loss is caused.
2. Neural presbycusis, in which nerve cells are lost along the auditory pathway. Impaired speech discrimination is the prominent feature.
3. Metabolic presbycusis, with atrophy of the stria vascularis. A flat hearing threshold curve is seen in the audiogram.
4. Mechanical presbycusis, caused by stiffening of the basilar membrane. The hearing threshold curves in the audiogram show continuous descent from low to high frequencies.

b) Impairment of Function

The morphological changes that have been described lead to impairment of hearing. Although this hase been the subject of numerous well-known studies using audiometry, including electric response audiometry, many details are still controversial. I therefore prefer to state the important facts and to avoid reference to obscure findings and conceptions. In pure tone audiograms the hearing threshold curves for both air and bone conduction slope downward at high frequencies, meaning that the deafness is sensorineural (e.g., BUNCH 1929; STEINBERG et al. 1940; GLORIG et al. 1957; BELAL 1975; FELDMANN 1981). Speech audiograms show that aging is accompanied by gradually increasing difficulty in distinguishing numerals.

Loss of speech discrimination is also evident in other respects. Thus, the predominant symptom of deafness in old age is a decline the inability to understand speech (ANDERSON 1982). Most affected are the consonants. Auditory aphasia results when the old person hears speech, but no longer understands it. Whether this loss of understanding of words with aging is entirely caused by a central nervous disorder preventing assimilation (BERGMANN 1971; JERGER 1973) or whether peripheral damage is contributory remains an open question. The ability to localize a source of sound is also lost (MATZKER 1958; FELDMANN 1981). This is attributed to physiologic senile degeneration of synapses and ganglion cells of the auditory pathway at the brainstem level.

According to studies by SATALOFF and MENDUKE (1957), CORSO (1959, 1963), and SCHMIDT (1967), hearing los with aging is not so great in women. HINCHCLIFFE (1959) suggests that this is because of differences between the sexes in their exposure to noise, whereas DIEROFF (1961) finds that in women the ear is less vulnerable to noise. Audiometric investigations – some of large populations – have resulted in the formulation of sets of standard average curves for separate age groups (STEINBERG 1940; WEBSTER et al. 1950; GLORIG et al. 1957; JATHO and HECK 1959; MANN and BECK 1978). Some of these sets differ greatly from the others. The curves now most relied on in the western world are those of GLORIG and NIXON (1962) and SPOOR and VAN LAAR (1967) (Fig. 1).

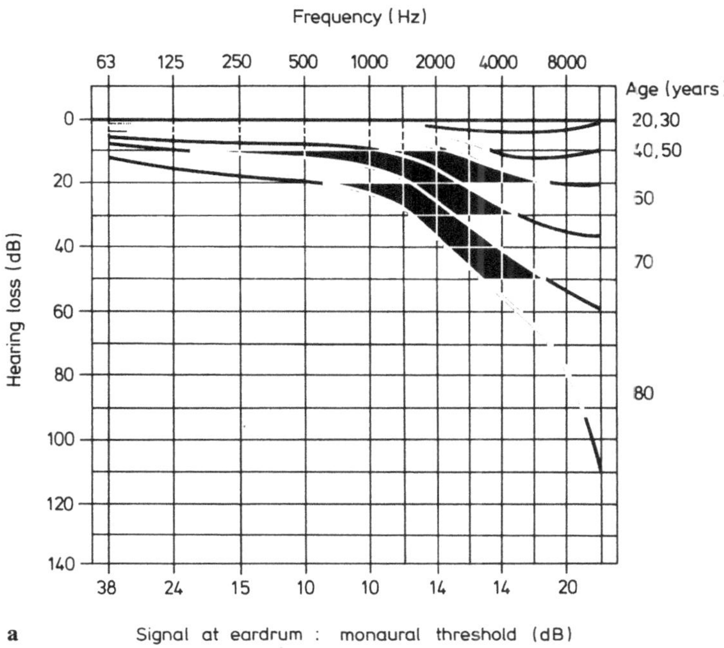

a

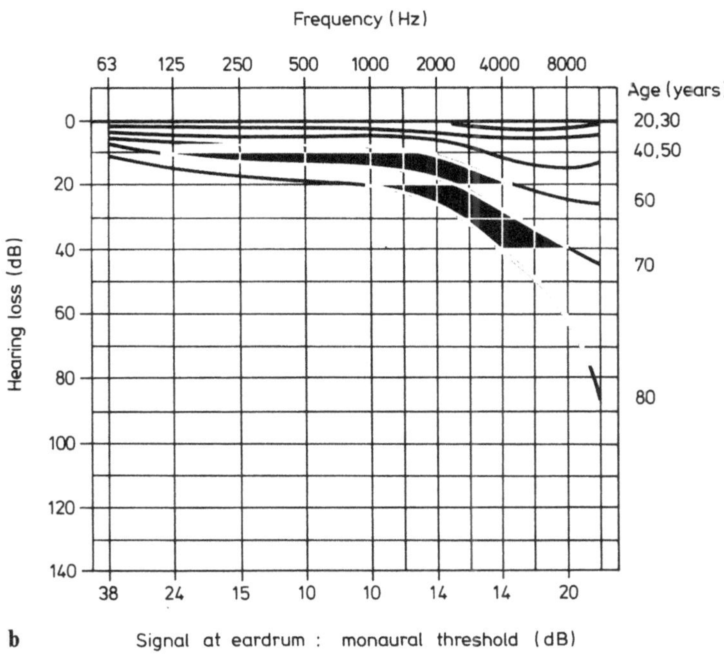

b

Fig. 1. a Mean hearing loss with aging in men **b** Mean hearing loss with aging in women (SPOOR and VAN LAAR 1967)

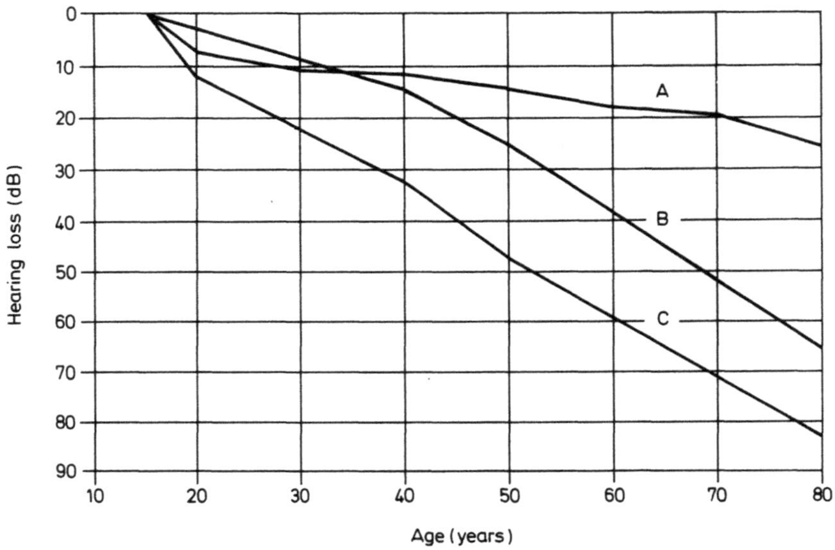

Fig. 2. Comparison of hearing levels at 6,000 Hz in different age groups among: primitive peoples (*curve A*); a rural population (*curve B*); and an industrial population (*curve C*) (PLESTER 1962)

c) Contributory Factors

Numerous audiometric studies of large groups of people make it evident that deafness with aging cannot be regarded simply as a physiologic occurrence and that the standard curves already referred to are not universally valid. For example, matched age groups in different groups of people exposed to different harmful noise levels have different hearing threshold curves. Socioacusis, hearing loss caused by environmental noise, at work and in everyday life, must help explain the differences. It must also help explain why aging urban and rural populations are not affected by hearing loss to an equal degree (Fig. 2; GLORIG et al. 1958; GLORIG and NIXON 1960, 1962).

Nutrition and mode of life must also affect the degree of deafness. Thus ROSEN and OLIN (1965) and ROSEN et al. (1970 a, b) showed in particular that a diet rich in saturated fatty acids leads to deterioration in hearing. Moreover, hypertension and coronary artery disease are also important (ROSEN et al. 1964 b). Noise and the so-called diseases of civilisation are therefore important factors. This assertion is supported by the results of hearing threshold studies in primitive peoples who are not exposed to noise, are free from diseases of civilization, and whose diet contains little or no fat. Good hearing in old age, with an only just demonstrable loss, hardly enough to call presbycusis, has been found in the Maba of the Sudan (PLESTER 1962; ROSEN et al. 1962, 1964 a), the Toda in southern India (KAPUR and PATT 1967), the Bantu and San in southern Africa (DICKSON 1968), and northern Cameroon tribes (SIMONETTA 1968). A critical review of the many studies of presbycusis, which is by no means an inevitable condition (BUNCH 1929), reveals many factors that contribute to its causation (see also ROSEN et al. 1964 a;

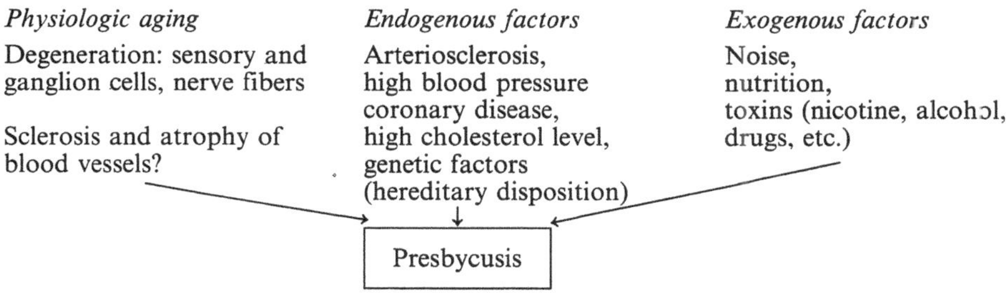

Fig. 3. Contributory factors in presbycusis

VON ARENTSCHILD 1972; BELAL 1975). The prime factor is physiologic aging of structures, undoubtedly influenced by genetic factors. In my experience presbycusis is often familial. Next in importance are influences of civilization, such as noise, diet, toxic agents (tobacco, alcohol, pharmaceuticals), and the diseases caused by these agents (Fig. 3). The morphological substrate is the whole auditory tract, from the hair cells to the cerebral cortex, but the changes in the different sections are variable in degree. The functional effect is a sensorineural hearing loss, most pronounced for high frequency sounds, affecting both ears equally, and slowly increasing.

d) Consequences of Presbycusis

The consequences of deafness in old age do not differ fundamentally from those of deafness in young people. Deafness is a handicap, which causes psychologic problems and interferes with social relationships. The deaf person feels isolated and excluded from society, and these feelings lead to increasing self-isolation and loss of confidence. Then come a sense of inferiority, distrustfulness, and even depression. Conflicts with family and neighbors become unavoidable. The older deaf person will experience all this to a greater extent, because general deterioration of brain function due to aging will be another important factor. Ability to communicate becomes significantly impaired (BECK 1970; BOONE et al. 1982). Conversations with groups of friends are avoided; theater and lecture visits cease. When traveling, failure to understand announcements at rail stations and air terminals causes problems. The feeling of isolation increases.

e) Treatment

The problems described are imperative reasons for therapeutic action. Metabolism in the inner ear can be improved by giving preparations that promote blood flow. Vitamin preparations are also recommended. In other words, the medication routinely used in gerontology is helpful. More important ist the use of hearing aids. Their object is to make better use of remaining function and so to improve ability to communicate (VON ARENTSCHILD 1972; LUNDBORG 1976; NIEMEYER 1980). Careful selection of the best appliance available for the patient often produces good results (Fig. 4), although the proportion of these decreases from the seventh decade (SILVERMAN and DAVIS 1970). The changes in the central ner-

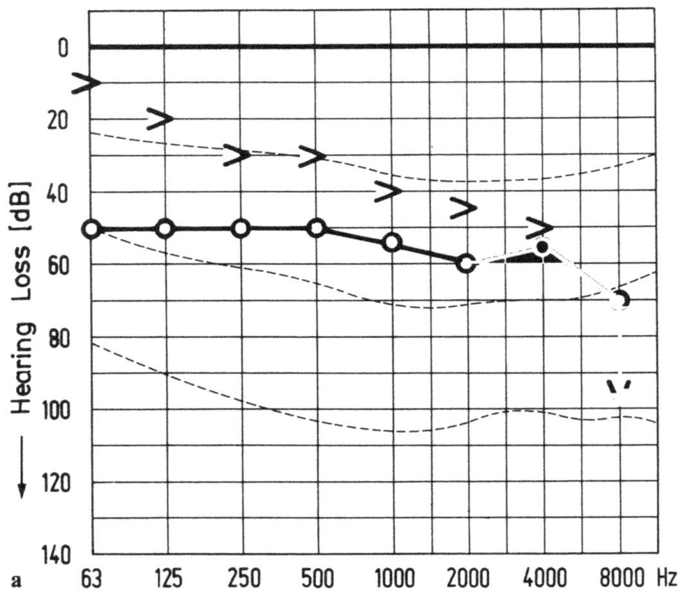

a

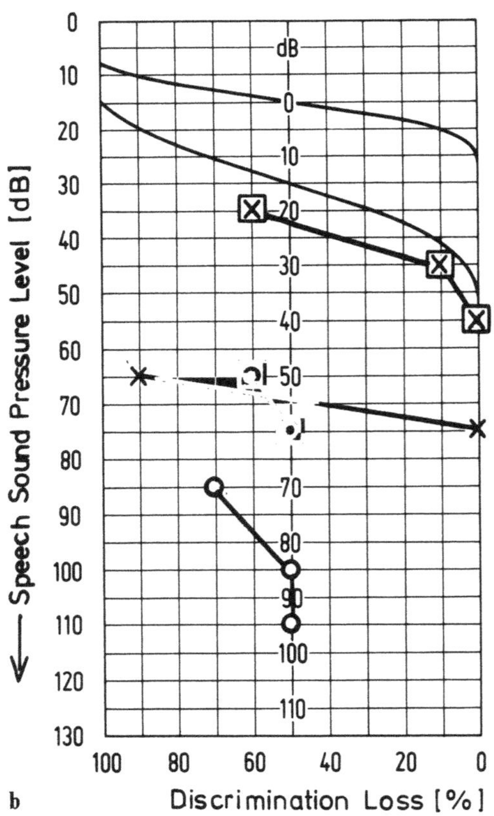

b

Fig. 4a, b. Inner ear deafness in an 85-year-old patient. **a** pure tone audiogram; **b** speech audiogram shows significant improvement in hearing with use of hearing aid. Symbols in *boxes* with hearing aid; *unboxed* symbols without hearing aid; *circles* refer to words; *crosses* refer to numerals vous system and the sensitivity to loud noise are hindrances to the successful use of hearing aids. Even so, the fitting of a hearing aid should always be given a trial (BECK 1968).

2. Vertigo in the Elderly

Structural changes associated with aging are also seen in the vestibular system (JOHNSSON and HAWKINS 1972a; BABIN and HARKER 1982). Loss of type I sensory cells in the saccule is particularly marked. The ampullary crests are scarcely affected. Cysts which appear in the neuroepithelium are considered to be evidence of senile degeneration (ROSENHALL 1974), as is a reduction in the number of afferent fibers. Degeneration of otoconia is also seen.

Whether these aging degenerative changes in the peripheral vestibular system have a key role in the causation of disturbances of balance is undecided, inasmuch as peripheral excitability also changes (ROSSBERG 1964; BRUNNER and NORRIS 1971; LAAN and OSTERVELD 1974; GRAMOWSKI 1976). Senile vertigo, which is experienced by 40%–50% of old people (ANDERSON and MEYERHOFF 1982), is probably most often caused by vascular damage in the vicinity of the brainstem (ČERNÝ 1965; GERLINGS 1966; SCHÖDER 1976).

II. External and Middle Ear

The pinna of the external ear becomes noticeably larger with aging (PELLNITZ 1962; FLEISCHER 1967). This is the result of an increase in the intercellular substance of its cartilage. In addition, there is increased growth of hair in the external acoustic meatus, particularly in men. A reduced amount of cerumen is produced because the glands atrophy (NOVOTNY 1969). A chronic nodular chondrodermatitis commonly affects the ears of old people (Fig. 5). The nodule, 3–6 mm in diameter, is extremely tender. The right pinna is the more commonly affected, as most elderly people sleep on the right side to relieve pressure on the heart. Surgical removal is indicated.

A frequently seen abnormality is a sclerosis of the tympanic membrane in which the number of elastic fibers decreases with age, being replaced by collagen fibers. A socalled arcus senilis around the periphery of the membrane is produced is lipid or calcium deposits. Arthritic changes are seen in the incudomalleolar and incudostapedial joints (ETHOLM and BELAL 1974; BELAL 1975). The articular cartilage becomes narrow, hyalinized, and calcified. The changes in the articular surfaces affect both ears symmetrically and are more pronounced in the incudomalleolar joint. Men and women are equally affected. In old age the annular ligament of the stapes loses some of its elastic fibers, shrinks, and undergoes calcification (GLANINGER 1961; CHLÁDEK 1966; BOLZ and LIM 1972; DORSCHNER and LEUTERT 1976). These changes cause increasing loss of elasticity in the system formed by the tympanic membrane and the auditory ossicles. This reduced elasticity increases acoustic impedance (VON WEDEL and OPITZ 1978), but does not cause any hearing loss (FLEISCHER 1967, 1972; ETHOLM and BELAL 1974).

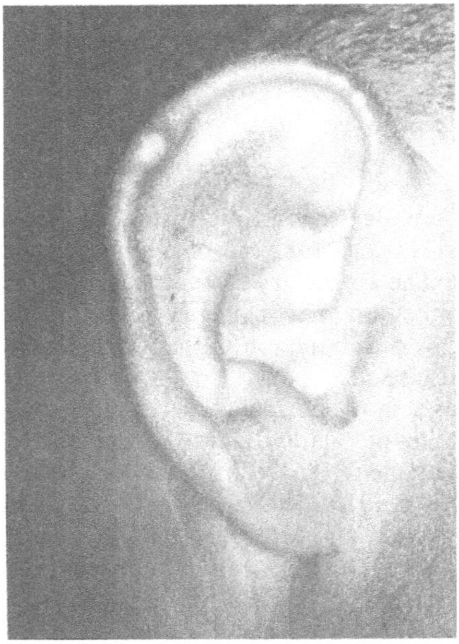

Fig. 5. Chronic nodular chondrodermatitis of the helix

C. Nose and Paranasal Sinuses

I. External Nose

Often seen in the later years of life is some drooping of the tip of the nose, the result of loss of elasticity in the cartilage and of senile bony involution of the upper jaw (WISSNER 1970; KROMPOTIĆ-NEMANIĆ et al. 1971). Instead of being downy, the hair in the vestibulum of the nose becomes bristly, especially in older men. Senile keratoses are often seen on the nose. These small warty swellings or uneven patches of skin appear after 50 years of age. Frequently, only the tip or the bridge of the nose is affected. Malignant change is possible.

A conspicuous appearance of the body of the nose is that of rhinophyma (bulbous nose, potato nose; Fig. 6). This is seen almost exclusively in old men. The skin of the cartilaginous part of the nose at first coarsens and assumes a gradually deepening blue–red colour. The ultimate result may be large bulbous excrescences that can interfere with breathing and eating. Rhinophyma is of seborrheic origin and is said to be related to acne rosacea.

II. Mucosa of Nose and Paranasal Sinuses

In children the nasal mucosa is deep red. In elderly people the colour changes to yellowish grey-blue (ZARITZKY 1936). Probably one of the reasons for this change is thickening of the tunica media of the small arteries. These are supplied by the

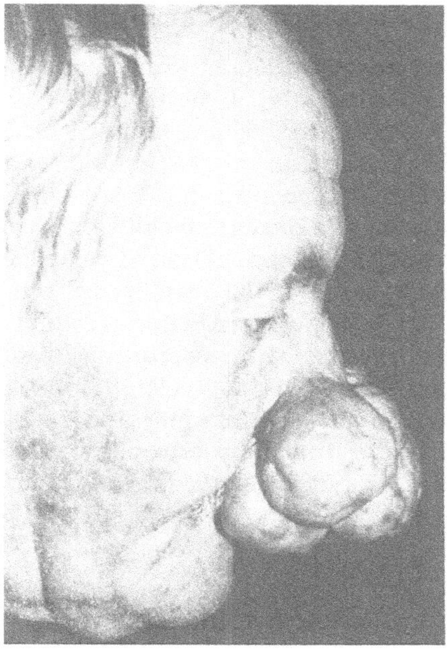

Fig. 6. Rhinophyma

maxillary artery and are part of the extracranial arterial network. In addition, the larger arteries, derived from the ethmoidal artery, are subject to thickening of the intima and thinning of the internal elastic membrane. Fibrotic changes cause involution of the cavernous tissue and its plexus of veins. The tissue loses its porosity, can no longer fill with blood, and consequently retains little ability to swell (ZARITZKY 1936; ZAOLI 1961). The vascular changes are articularly marked in the olfactory region (NAESSEN 1971). In advanced age the mucosa often atrophies. The mucus-secreting glands and goblet cells are reduced in number. Metaplasia of the cylindrical epithelium to squamous epithelium is seen in the mucosa of the nasal conchae (ZARITZKY 1936). The number of pigment granules in the supporting cells is increased (NAESSEN 1971).

The number of mast cells, which have a role in reconstruction and scavenging processes in the connective tissue of the nasal mucosa, is reduced. Parallel with the fall in the number of mast cells, the content of mucopolysaccharides decreases and that of amyloid and para-amyloid increases (BARONE and ZILIOTTO 1970). With increasing age, there is also a fall in the enzyme content of the nasal mucosa (BORGO and CONTI 1965). Opinions differ as to the consequences of these mucosal changes. MAGOMEDOV (1973) does not believe that they impair function in any way, but BRUK and GOLDMAN (1969) consider sinusitis to be relatively frequent in older people. The opinion of NOVOTNY (1969) that nasal polyps are more frequent in old age is one that we cannot share. Our own observations indicate that the functional impairment caused by the mucosal changes often leads to the classical complaint of atrophic rhinitis or to paroxysmal production of watery mucus.

III. Olfactory Impairment

Impairment of olfaction with aging has long been recognized (ZWAARDEMARKER 1895; SAWAKI et al. 1959; BOCCUZZI 1962; ISHIHARA and KOMATSU 1966; ROUS 1969; STRAUSS 1970; ZILSTORFF 1972; ROSEBURG et al. 1976; THUMFART et al. 1980). A raised olfactory threshold for all odors can invariably be demonstrated in healthy old people. The loss of smell is gradual and often unnoticed (SPECHT 1924). Suggested causes include increased tissue rigidity, reduced cell wall diffusion potential, degeneration of nerve cells and fibers, and decline in the number of blood vessels in the olfactory epithelium (ISHIHARA and KOMATSU 1966; NAESSEN 1971). Appositional bone growth, causing narrowing of the openings in the cribriform plate with consequent atrophy of nerve fibers, has also been argued (KROMPOTIĆ-NEMANIĆ 1969, 1972). Importance must also be attached to such changes in the olfactory bulb and tract as atrophy of nerve cells, loss of nerve fibers, and astroglial hypertrophy with the appearance of amyloid bodies (SMITH 1942; LISS and GOMEZ 1958; ISHIHARA and KOMATSU 1966).

IV. Epistaxis

Epistaxis is common and usually trivial, but it can endanger life and even prove fatal. This particularly applies to old people, in whom epistaxis affects men more than women. The age distribution curve of ambulant patients treated for nosebleeds of every possible etiology and degree of severity has a conspicuous peak among young people. However, in the age distribution curve of patients with severe epistaxis requiring inpatient treatment, children and juveniles are almost unrepresented. This curve reaches its peak in later life, between 50 and 70 years (FELDMANN 1973). Severe epistaxis is thus a geriatric problem (HARA 1962). Foremost among its causes are hypertension, correlated with age, and atherosclerosis (HARA 1962; NOVOTNY 1969; FELDMANN 1973). Another is Rendu–Osler disease, the only hemorrhagic condition that becomes worse with increasing age (GASTPAR 1969). The treatment of epistaxis does not differ fundamentally from that in younger patients. The full range of rhinologic treatment, including surgery, often has to be employed.

To sum up, the changes in the nose and paranasal sinuses that occur with aging include senile involution and degeneration, but these usually fall short of real disease. They scarcely affect function and quality of life, especially in the many old people who are almost unaware of any loss of sense of smell. The exceptions are rhinophyma, which, besides being disfiguring, can interfere with breathing and food intake, and severe epistaxis, which can endanger life.

D. Pharynx and Salivary Glands

I. Mucosal Changes

Changes in the pharyngeal mucosa and lymphoid tissue ring with aging are sparsely documented. Between 70 and 90 years of age, the pharyngeal mucosa often shows thickening and epithelial metaplasia. The connective tissue becomes fibrotic. Neutral polysaccharides are deposited in the deep glands. The lipid content of the mucosa and glands is diminished. The cholinesterase level does not change with increasing age, but the levels of cytochrome oxidase and adenosine triphosphatase decrease. All this is evidence of reduced activity of oxidative and energy-producing processes in old age (CONTI et al. 1965). The changes described are particularly marked in chronic pharyngitis, which is often seen in the elderly in its atrophic form (MAURER 1978). During the course of life the function and form of Waldeyer's tonsillar ring undergo change. Tissue proliferation in the first 3 years of life causes an increase in volume. The lymph follicles increase in number and size. The pharyngeal tonsil reaches its maximum size in early childhood. After this it begins to atrophy. After puberty it can rarely be detected (BECK 1966 b). By this time the palatine tonsil has attained its greatest size. Its involution begins by the age of 20 years, by which time the lingual tonsil has reached its greatest extent. The whole pharyngeal lymphoid tissue ring atrophies progressively from the age of 40 years (STROHM 1978). The microscopic changes taking place in the palatine tonsil have been described as hypotrophy and hypoplasia of the lymphocytic components, fibrosclerotic metaplasia of vessels and reticulum, and thickening of the epithelium (BERGGREN and HELLMANN 1930).

II. Loss of Taste

The size of the tongue increases with aging and it exhibits tortuous dilated veins both, sublingually and at its base. The area of cornified epithelium increases. Fissures and papillary hyperkeratosis make their appearance (BALOGH 1960; HERRMANN 1967; BREUSTEDT and HÖCKER 1978). Very noticeable are reduction in the number of taste buds and an accompanying flattening (AREY et al. 1935; BOURLIERE et al. 1958; BRUCHMÜLLER et al. 1976; BREUSTEDT and HÖCKER 1978). The histologic appearance is that of a hydrotropic change in the taste cells, with cystic degeneration and pyknoses (KRANZ et al. 1968). The structural changes cause a considerable loss of taste in old people (BOURLIERE et al. 1958; BERNDT et al. 1966; HERRMANN 1967; ROLLIN 1975; THUMFART et al. 1980). Sweet and sour tastes are the most affected. The taste threshold for saltiness is not affected. Often the perception of bitter tastes is even heightened. Loss of taste caused by the changes of aging is less pronounced in women than in men (BOURLIERE et al. 1958; HERRMANN 1967; FIKENTSCHER et al. 1976, 1977). Accompanying the reduction in taste in old age, a reduction in tactile sensation is observed (HERRMANN 1967).

III. Salivary Glands

The salivary glands also undergo senile involution, particularly evident as lipomatosis in the parotid, mainly as sclerosis in the others (RAUCH 1959; WATERHOUSE et al. 1973; VOGT et al. 1976). The parotid gland commonly shows loss of parenchyma (RAUCH 1959; WATERHOUSE 1973). Histologic preparations show large areas in which very little glandular tissue is present. Fatty tissue is seen in its place (Fig. 7). This fatty infiltration can be so exaggerated by alcohol abuse in elderly men that the parotids become obviously swollen. The submandibular and

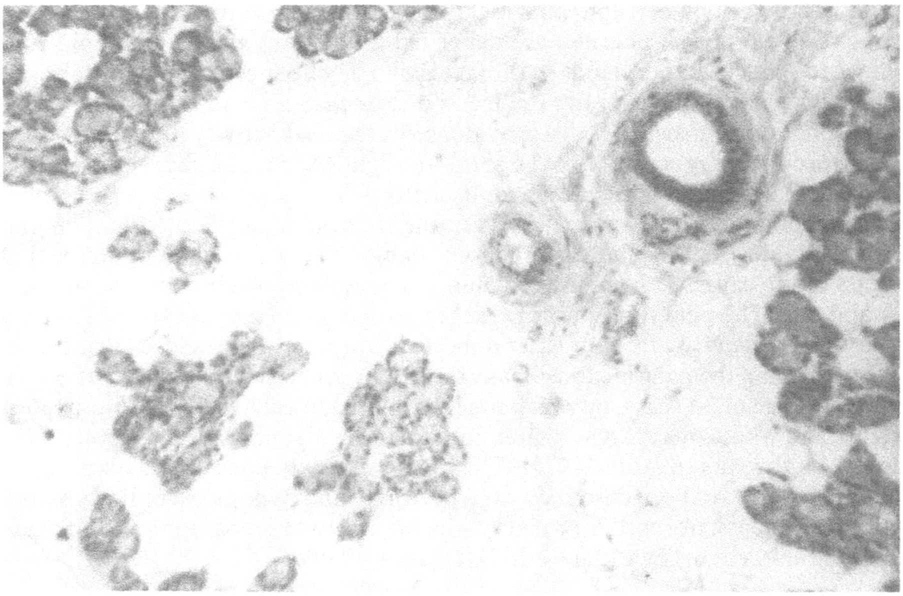

Fig. 7. Senile atrophy of the parotid gland. Parenchyma largely replaced by fatty tissue. Hematoxylin–eosin × 30

sublingual glands also show some loss of parenchyma and at the same time an increase in fatty tissue. Their main features, though, are scar formation in the parenchyma, obstructive changes in the duct system, and signs of chronic inflammation, which is at first pericanalicular (RAUCH 1959; SCOTT 1976, 1977). These changes may cause hardening and slight enlargement of the glands. The changes in the parenchyma cause the resting secretion of saliva to diminish. This leads to xerostomia, a condition that is more pronounced in women than in men (BERTRAM 1967; ENFERS 1968; VOGT et al. 1976). In addition, the saliva of both sexes has an increased total protein content and an increased sodium content in old age (VOGT and SEMMANN 1970). Independently of the structural changes, the submandibular gland often appears enlarged in people over 50 years old (Fig. 8). This is a normal feature of age, the gland standing out more clearly because of decrease in connective tissue elasticity and slackening of the skin (SCOTT 1960). This change is less evident in the parotid and sublingual glands because of their firmer muscular and fascial fixation.

These changes in the pharynx and salivary glands cause irksome symptoms, but not illness. The impairment of taste is certainly troublesome, as is the common complaint of dryness of the mouth associated with decreased saliva production. In our patients, just as we have not found diseases of the tonsils to become more frequent with increasing age, so too we have failed to find any increased frequency of disease of the parotid gland, either acute or chronic inflammation. Here, as in the ear and nose, the main effect of senile changes is a deterioration in the quality of life.

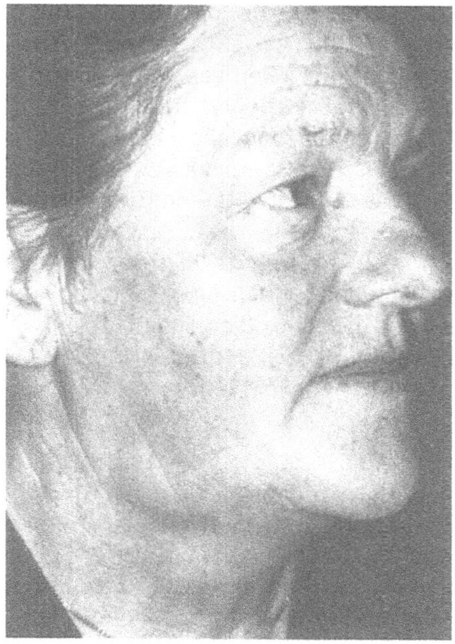

Fig. 8. Prominence of the submandibular gland as a physiologic feature of aging

E. Larynx

I. Morphological Findings

1. Macroscopic Changes

In the course of life, the larynx changes its anatomic relation to the vertebral column. Originally at the level of the third and fourth cervical vertebrae, it descends with advancing years to the level of the sixth and seventh. This descent is explained by senile atrophy of the supporting muscles and connective tissue (MOSER 1948). It can make tracheotomy much more difficult (BECK 1966, 1979). When the larynx of an old person is examined with the laryngeal mirror its interior spaces appear to be enlarged. This is because of atrophy of the soft parts which bound them. The significantly narrowed vestibular folds permit more of the vocal fold surfaces to be seen. The entrance to the sinus of the larynx looks wider and more open (KOFLER 1932). The aging epiglottis becomes increasingly yellowish in color and more rigid (OSTERLAND 1962). In men, its size and weight increase; in women, they decrease (PELLNITZ 1961; OSTERLAND 1962). This sex-specific structural change in the course of life may be attributable to hormonal influences.

2. Histologic Findings

a) Laryngeal Cartilages

Histologic examination of the cartilage of the epiglottis reveals extensive degeneration of cellular and elastic elements. The end products of this degeneration are taken up by the ground substance and cause it to increase in volume and density (PELLNITZ 1961; OSTERLAND 1962). Also be to found after the fifth decade, though infrequently, is calcification in the cartilage of the epiglottis (OSTERLAND 1962; PANTOJA 1968, HOMMERICH 1972).

The other laryngeal cartilages invariably become ossified, to a greater degree in men. Ossification begins in the thyroid cartilage at about 20 years of age, next affects the cricoid, and then from the third decade onward occurs in the arytenoid cartilages, but not as a rule in their vocal processes. There is much individual variation in the pattern of ossification. Generally, the bone formation proceeds in a caudocephalad direction. Islands of bone usually appear first in the inferior processes of the thyroid cartilage. The ossification is true new bone formation, i.e., endochondral ossification (RONCALLO 1948; GRIEBEL 1952; LEOPOLD and JAGOW 1961; PANTOJA 1968; HOMMERICH 1972; STROHM 1978).

b) Mucosa

Changes dependent on aging are also seen in the interior of the larynx. Normally, the vestibular folds and the walls of the sinus of the larynx are lined by ciliated epithelium, whereas the vocal folds are covered by thickened squamous epithelium provided with papillae. The configuration of the squamous epithelium and the expanse of the cylindrical epithelium now begin to differ from those found in the larynx during youth. Additional changes are involution of elastic tissue, combined with an increase in the calibers of venules and lymph vessels, and an increase in the amount of fatty tissue in the submucosa (KOFLER 1932). With increasing age, the mucosal epithelium becomes thinner, with loss of its papillae (KOFLER 1932; RICCI 1935; NOELL 1962; GUERINO and MILAZZO 1965; TRIANFIDI et al. 1972; LEUTERT 1976; HONJO and ISSHIKI 1980). The cells are irregularly arranged and often have poorly staining nuclei. The submucosa often shows splintering of elastic fibers and infiltration by fatty tissue. The vestibular folds are no longer uniformly covered by stratified ciliated epithelium; squamous epithelium is found in its place, either in patches or as a complete layer (RUCKES and CAUSÉ 1964). The number of seromucous glands is significantly diminished in old people (RUCKES 1964; TRIANFIDI et al. 1972). This reduction is accompanied by suppression of secretion, distension of gland lumen, concretion formation, and epithelial desquamation and cornification. The mucus produced is viscid. Because of this and the inadequacy of the amount produced, it can no longer fully perform its protective function. The resulting desiccation and crust formation cause unpleasant feelings in the larynx (STROHM 1978). The amount of fatty tissue in the margins of the folds increases with age. This produces a "vicarious" growth which occurs independently of the nutritional state of the rest of the body. It may even be seen in patients with fatal wasting diseases (STROHM 1978).

c) Vocal Folds

The main composition of the stratified noncornified squamous epithelium does not change with increasing age, but the total height of the epithelium decreases. The 8–12 layers of cells seen in middle age will be reduced to 6–8. This change is associated with flattening of papillae, especially over the vocal process of each arytenoid cartilage. The epithelium becomes less closely bound down to the vocal ligament (LEUTERT 1964; GUERINO and MILAZZO 1965). The few mucous glands of the vocal fold epithelium exhibit the same changes as those in the epithelium of the vestibular folds (KOFLER 1932; HOMMERICH 1972; STROHM 1978).

In old people, edema formation is often observed in the connective tissue layer (NOELL 1962; HONJO and ISSHIKI 1980). Connective tissue structures are regularly altered with age. A proportion of the elastic fibers show band-like broadening and disintegration with plaque formation (LEUTERT 1964, 1976). Electron microscopic studies of the phenomenon (HOMMERICH 1972) indicate that it is attributable to a change in the collagenous cement substance, which undergoes hardening and increased polymerization. The result is degeneration of elastic or collagen fibers, as demonstrated in aging connective and supporting tissue by LINDNER (1981) and in the vessel walls of aged animals by SEYDEWITZ and STAUBESAND (1983). More recent electron microscopic studies, in different age groups, of biopsies from the vocal folds (BECK and STAUBESAND 1984) have shown textural abnormalities of collagen fibrils in old people. These are characterized mainly by the appearance of individual dysplastic elements, by the more frequent occurrence of microfibrils arranged in parallel, and by whorls of fibrillary material (amianthoid fibers; Fig. 9). These changes are undoubtedly relevant to the vocal impairment of old age.

It has been recorded that aging of the musculature in the neighborhood of the vocal folds is accompanied by generalized reduction of fiber size. LEUTERT (1964) found that fiber diameter decreased from a maximum of 50–20 μm. Another sign of aging of the musculature is an increase in lipofuscin content. Hyalinosis and fibrosis are seen in the larger arteries, while the intima becomes thicker and the quantity of elastic fibers in the media increases. Thickening of the basement membrane of the muscle capillaries is observed. The muscle wasting that occurs can hence be explained by nutritional disturbance.

II. The Voice in Old Age

It might be thought that these aging changes in the larynx, especially in its epithelium, could contribute to the genesis of cancer, although other factors, such as exposure to external and internal irritants, would be more important. It is certain, however, that the changes in the larynx are largely responsible for deterioration in the voice with aging. The characteristic voice of old age is the outcome of a complex process in which central and peripheral involutionary changes work together. The change in vocal function is caused by physiologic involution of the central nervous system, changes (including degeneration) in the larynx and its supporting structures, and alteration in the elasticity of the thorax. Shifts in hormonal balance are also important.

The main characteristics of the voice in old age have been described in numerous studies (KOFLER 1932; STERN 1932, SHIPP and HOLLIEN 1960; HECKER 1969, BÖHME 1969; HABERMANN 1972; HOLLIEN and SHIPP 1972; GOLEMANOV and POPOVA 1976; HONJO and ISSHIKI 1980). These characteristics are described in the following paragraphs.

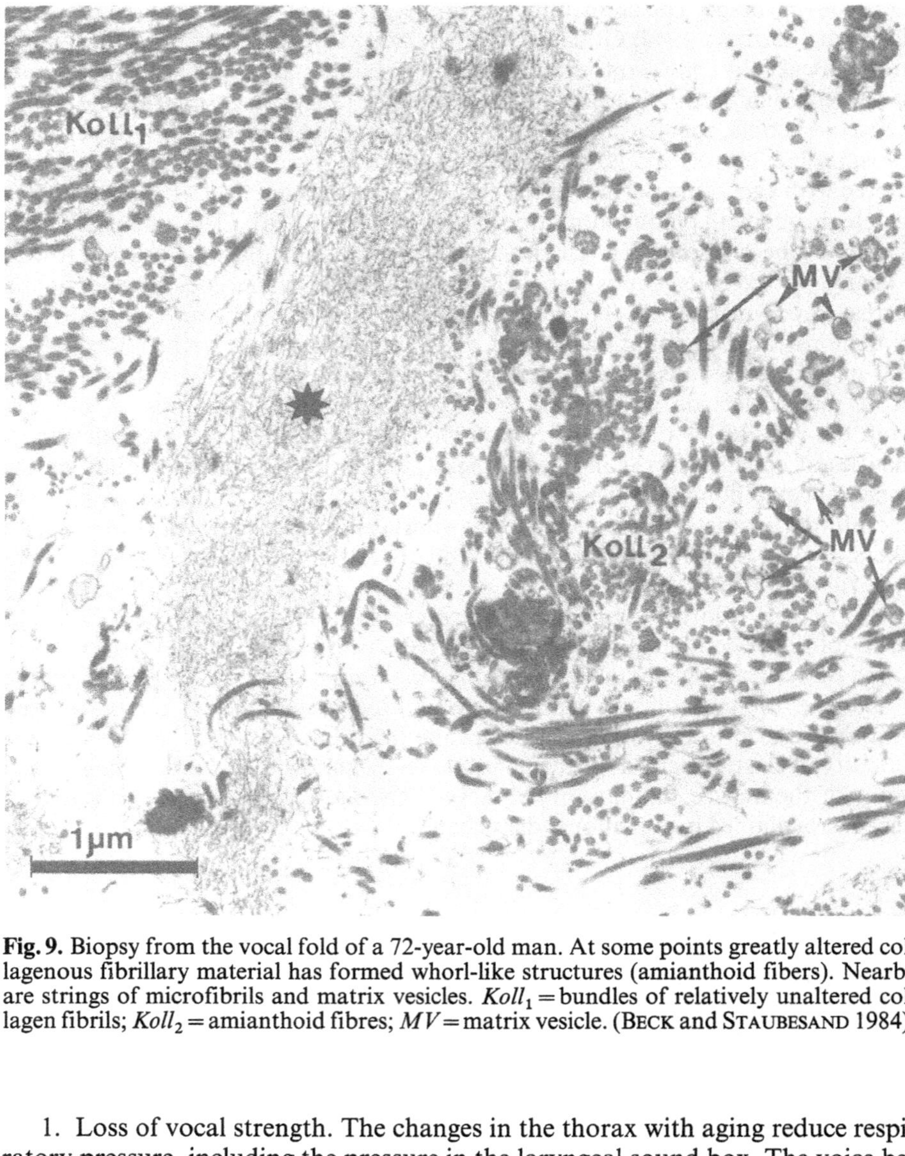

Fig. 9. Biopsy from the vocal fold of a 72-year-old man. At some points greatly altered collagenous fibrillary material has formed whorl-like structures (amianthoid fibers). Nearby are strings of microfibrils and matrix vesicles. $Koll_1$ = bundles of relatively unaltered collagen fibrils; $Koll_2$ = amianthoid fibres; *MV* = matrix vesicle. (BECK and STAUBESAND 1984)

1. Loss of vocal strength. The changes in the thorax with aging reduce respiratory pressure, including the pressure in the laryngeal sound box. The voice becomes soft and thin.

2. Change in vocal range. In women, there is relative lowering of the pitch of the voice (within its total range) so that the voice becomes deeper. In men, the range of pitch increases and the voice becomes higher; high-pitched tones are more frequently used in speech, to the extent of the senile descant voice being reached.

3. Impairment of vocal quality. The voice loses its beauty and is often colorless, flat, brittle, or tremulous. Because of the changes in the central nervous sys-

tem there is lack of the coordination required to maintain the same tension in the two vocal folds. The voice becomes shaky and the length of time a given note can be held is reduced.

4. Decrease in resonance. The loss of elasticity in the larynx and senile muscle atrophy in the pharynx cause impairment of resonance and of accuracy of tone.

5. Loss of fullness (chest voice). Atrophy of the vocal muscles causes incomplete closure of the glottis. With defective apposition of the vocal folds, the production of a proper chest voice is impossible.

6. Phonasthenia. The carrying power of the voice is diminished, phonation becomes sibilant, and habitual coughing is common.

It is rare for all or even most of these features to be found in one and the same person. Individual variations in onset are considerable, and chronologic and biologic ages can be strikingly different. Old people vary in their perception of aging of the voice. Many are hardly aware of it and do not regard it as a disorder or handicap. One good reason for this is that aging of the voice, unlike presbycusis, has little effect on the ability to communicate. However, for a performing artist, especially a singer, an aging voice often means the end of a career.

The treatment of vocal disorders caused by aging is problematic. Besides geriatric treatment, including medicinal, low frequency electrical stimulation can be tried. Results are inconclusive.

F. Therapeutic Aspects

I. Conservative Treatment

The conservative treatment, especially medicinal, of ear, nose, and throat diseases in the elderly does not differ from that in younger people. An often worthwhile additional measure in the old is to prescribe drugs that improve the blood supply to the cerebrum and inner ear, thus improving their metabolism, with the object of activating central processes and producing a general strengthening effect. It is also sensible to administer hormones, a combination of androgens and estrogens being particularly effective. Vitamins are also to be recommended. We have found the combination of vitamins A and E beneficial to patients with presbycusis and also to those with nasal, pharyngeal, and laryngeal geriatric symptoms. In many cases of presbycusis, the provision of a hearing aid is important. This question is discussed in Sect. B.I.1.e. For disorders of the voice in elderly people, the use of low frequency electrical stimulation may be tried in addition to the medication stated.

II. Ear, Nose, and Throat Operations in the Elderly

1. General Aspects

In our specialty, every disease in the elderly that requires surgical treatment is also encountered in younger people. The indications and operative techniques do not differ from those in younger patients, and so a detailed account is unnecessary.

An essential question is the endurance of the elderly person, in which respect biologic and chronologic age may by no means correspond. Many of the organs of an old person exhibit degenerative changes. They also show damage caused by past illnesses. The important parameters in all specialized surgical disciplines are the pathophysiologic features in relation to the overall state of the aged individual, the effects of the underlying disease, and the patient's reaction to the surgical operation.

Operations in our specialty are noted for their extremely low risk of thrombosis. The main reason for this must be that the patient can get up very soon after operation. Also very limited in number are other postoperative complications, such as bronchopneumonia. In addition, the good blood supply to the head and neck favors early and sound healing, even after extensive operations. The healing capacity after major tumor operations in the elderly is just as good as in younger people. With adequate care over the indications and the assessment of each patient as a whole, there need be no misgivings about major head and neck surgery in the elderly (LOEBELL and OTTO 1958; BECK 1966a; FENDEL 1976). Admittedly, some authors report a complication rate slightly above that in young people (APPAIX et al. 1960; LOEWY and HUTTNER 1966).

2. Specialized Aspects

It was the opinion of ROSENWASSER (1964) that stapedioplasty and tympanoplasty ought not to be performed in the very elderly, because the great sensitivity of the aged labyrinth makes sensorineural damage likely. Experience has shown, however, that there is no fixed age limit for stapes operations (PLESTER 1972; RIBARI 1976; WEYMAR et al. 1976). Furthermore, otosclerosis in the old is no different histologically or functionally from otosclerosis in the young (JORGENSEN et al. 1976). Nor is there any universal age limit for tympanoplasty, although caution is advised in patients above 60 years of age (PLESTER 1972; FEMENIČ and SUBOTIČ 1976). In deciding whether to operate to improve hearing, a decisive consideration is the patient's mental adaptability (in other words, biologic age). The provision of a hearing aid is certainly to be preferred if the prognosis is doubtful.

Another problem is cosmetic surgery in advanced age. Naturally, the majority of all cosmetic operations are on the face, the important visible part of the human body. The great question in our specialty is that of cosmetic surgery on the nose. In old people, this must be preceded by the most cautious deliberation, but there are circumstances in which it is appropriate (WEBSTER 1967; KÜHL 1968; BLOOM 1970, MENNIG 1976; STROHM 1978).

Another much discussed subject is that of tonsillectomy in the elderly. It is often recommended that patients over 50 years of age should not have this operation (JACKSON and JACKSON 1947; PREOBRAZENSKY 1974). Our experience and that of others is different (FALCAO 1951; SUZUKI and KAITO 1958). We have looked at the medical histories of 149 patients over 50 years of age who had tonsillectomies in the Ear, Nose, and Throat Hospital, Freiburg im Breisgau, West Germany, between 1 May 1970 and 30 April 1975 (BECK 1977). The oldest of these patients was aged 75 years (Fig. 10). The indications were no different from those in younger people. The study showed the healing potential and the compli-

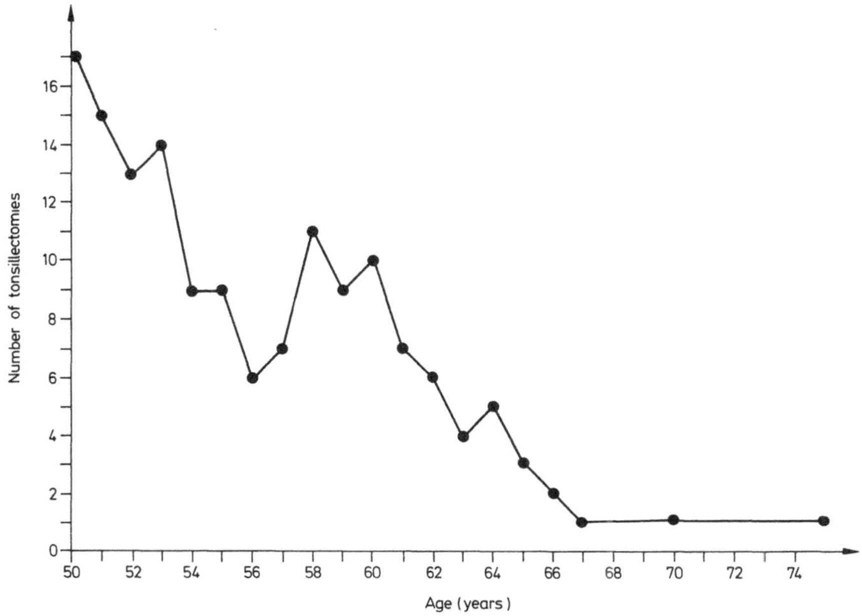

Fig. 10. Age distribution of 149 patients aged 50 years and over who had tonsillectomie between May 1970 and April 1975. (BECK 1977)

cation rate to be the same in young and old. Provided the indication is correct, tonsillectomy is justified even in later life.

G. Malignant Ear, Nose, and Throat Conditions in the Elderly

An account of relevant malignant conditions has been deliberately omitted from previous sections for two reasons. As already mentioned, malignant growths, especially in the oropharynx and larynx, are now seen much more frequently in young people than they were 10 years ago. For a 40-year-old to develop carcinoma of a tonsil or the larynx is no rarity. Consequently, I can no longer regard malignant conditions as being typical of old age. Second, their treatment in the old is not significantly different from that in the young. The therapy embarked upon depends on the extent of the tumor and the endurance of the patient, as in the case of a young person.

In my view it is the aftereffects of treatment that present our cancer patients with their great problem, much more serious in the older patient than in younger ones. Every operation for a malignant tumor in our specialty is potentially disfiguring or even multilating. Examples are the possible loss of an eye, the nose, part of the upper or lower jaw, the palate, or the tongue. Even tracheostomy may be necessary. Surgical scars on the face or neck may not always be possible to conceal. Many of these operations cause restriction or loss of vital functions such as eating or speaking. Irradiation of the head or neck has major systemic effects. The usually intense irradiation reaction in the outer skin and especially the oral and pharyngeal mucosa is responsible for pain and difficulty in eating. Severe dryness of the mouth often persists for a long time. This all means problems during reintegration in the family and society after discharge from hospital. The patient has to find a new mode of living, as otherwise there will be some risk of isolation. Consequently, in our specialty the decisive factor in the older cancer patient should be the extent of interference with function, which inevitably means a change in life-style and impairment of the quality of life, compared with which the therapeutic measures themselves retreat into the background.

H. Concluding Remarks

Apart from a few conditions such as rhinophyma and senile warts which are almost exclusively confined to the elderly, none of the abnormalities that we encounter in our specialty can be regarded purely as those of physiologic aging. They are caused by the wearing out of structures, and they have burdensome effects such as deafness, dry mouth, dry nasal mucosa with crust formation, and impairment of the voice. Treatment can seldom be more than symptomatic, but the alleviation of symptoms must be attempted. It is most important to preserve the ability to communicate, and this is impaired more by deafness than by aging of the voice. Preserving this ability prevents isolation of the old person and preserves the quality of life.

References

Anderson R, Meyerhoff W (1982) Otologic manifestation of aging. Otolaryngol Clin North Am 15 (2):353

Appaix A, Pech A, Rouvier P, Raybaud A (1960) La chirurgie des vieillard en ORL. J Fr Otorhinolaryngol 9:941

Arentsschild O v (1972) Das alternde Ohr: Funktionelle Aspekte. HNO 20:108

Arey LB, Tremaine M, Monzujo F (1935) The numerical and to pographical relations of taste boods to human circumvallate papille throughout the life span. Anat Rec 64:9

Arnesen A (1982) Presbyacusis – loss of neurons in the human cochlear nuclei. J Laryngol Otol 96:503

Babin R, Harker L (1982) The vestibular system in the Elderly. Otolaryngol Clin North Am 15 (2): 387

Balogh K (1960) Die physiologischen Veränderungen der Zunge beim Vorgang des Alterns. Österr Z Stomatol 57:71

Barone L, Ziliotto G (1970) La mucosa nasale nel vecchio. Riv Anat 36:274

Beck C (1966a) Hals-Nasen-Ohrenerkrankungen im Alter. In: Heilmeyer L, Holtmeier H, Schubert R (eds) Geriatrie. Thieme, Stuttgart, p 167

Beck C (1966b) Morphologisch-klinische Untersuchungen zur verzögerten Involution der Rachenmandel. J Laryngol Otol 45:769

Beck C (1968) Die Versorgung der Altersschwerhörigkeit als soziale Aufgabe. Akt Probl Geriatrie, Vol 1/140. Steinkopff, Darmstadt

Beck C (1970) Umweltprobleme für den schwerhörig alten Menschen. Aktuelle Probleme der Geriatrie, Geropsychologie, Gerosoziologie und Altenfürsorge, Vol 3/17. Steinkopf, Darmstadt

Beck C (1977) Tonsillektomie im Alter. Arch Otorhinolaryngol 215:147
Beck C (1979) Tracheotomia superior, media and inferior? Laryngol Rhinol Otol (Stuttg) 58:48
Beck C Staubesand J (1984) Das Kollagen der Stimmlippe im Alter. Arch Otorhinolaryngol 239:129
Belal A (1975) Presbyacusis: physiological or pathological. J Laryngol Otol 89:1011
Berggren S, Hellmann T (1930) Die chronische Tonsillitis. Ein Beitrag zur Lösung des Tonsillenproblems. Acta Otolaryngol [Suppl] 12:1
Bergmann M (1971) Hearing and aging; implications of recent research findings. Audiology 10:164
Berndt H, Gerhardt H, Wagner H (1966) Zur klinischen Elektrogustometrie. Die Abhängigkeit der Geschmacksschwelle vom Alter. HNO 14:340
Bertram U (1967) Xerostomia. Acta Odontol Scand [Suppl] 49
Bloom S (1970) Rhinoplasty in adolescence. Arch Otolaryngol 92:66
Boccuzzi V (1962) Fenomeni di senescenza nell' olfatto. Boll Mal Orecch 80:654
Böhme G (1969) Stimm-, Sprach- und Hörstörungen. Fischer, Jena
Böhme G, Hecker G (1970) Gerontologische Untersuchungen über Stimmumfang und Sprechstimmlage. Folia Phoniatr (Basel) 22:176
Bolz E, Lim D (1972) Morphology of the stapedio-vestibular joint. Acta Otolaryngol (Stockh) 73:10
Boone D, Bayles K, Koopmann Ch (1982) Communicative aspects of aging. Otolaryngol Clin North Am 15(2):313
Borgo M, Conti A (1965) La mucosa nasale respiratoria nella senescenza. Minerva Otorinolaryngol 15:177
Bourliere F, Cendron M, Rapaport A (1958) Modification avec l'âge des senils gustatifs de perception et de reconnaissance aux saveurs sallée et sucrée chez l'homme. Gerontologia 2:104
Bredberg G (1967) The human cochlea during development and aging. J Laryngolotol 81:739
Breustedt A, Höcker M (1978) Zungenveränderungen bei alten Menschen. Zahn Mund Kieferheilkd. 66:589
Bruchmüller W, Fikentscher R, Roseburg B (1976) Histologische Untersuchungen zur Altersdegeneration der Geschmacksknospen in den Wallpapillen des Menschen. In: Kaiser-Meinhardt I, Wendler J (eds) Geriatrische Aspekte in der HNO-Heilkunde. Thieme, Leipzig, p 189
Bruk A, Goldman I (1969) Otorhinolaryngological diseases in aged and senile persons. Vest. Otorinolaringol 31:32
Brunner A, Norris T (1971) Age-related changes in caloric nystagmus. Acta Otolaryngol [Suppl] 282
Bunch C (1929) Age variations in auditory acusty. Arch Otolaryngol 9:625
Cerný L (1965) Gleichgewichtsstörungen im Alter. Prakt Lék 45:344
Chládek V, Zelenka J (1966) Ligamentum annulare in old age. Cesk Otolaryngol 15:332
Conti A, Borger M, Perani G (1965) Die Pharynxschleimhaut im Alter. Histochemische und histoenzymologische Untersuchungen. Arch Ital Otol 76:551
Corso J (1959) Age and sex differences in pure tone thesholds. J Acoust Soc Am 31:498
Corso J (1963) Age and sex differences in pure-tone thresholds Survey of hearing levels from 18–65 years. Arch Otolaryngol 77:385
Crowe SJ, Guild SR, Polvog LM (1934) Observations of the pathology of the high-tone deafness. Bull Johs Jopkins Hosp 54:315
Dickson R (1968) The normal hearing of Bantu and Bushmen. J Laryngol Otol 82:505
Dieroff HG (1961) Zur geschlechtsunterschiedlichen Lärmfestigkeit. Arch Ohren Nasen Kehlkopfheilkd 177:282
Döderlein W (1938) Über Presbyakusis. Arch Ohren Nasen Kehlkopfheilkd 295
Dorschner W, Leutert G (1976) Über die funktionelle Struktur des Ligamentum annulare stapedis und deren altersabhängige morphologische Veränderungen. In: Kaiser-Meinhardt I, Wendler J (eds) Geriatrische Aspekte in der HNO-Heilkunde. Thieme, Leipzig, p 58

Enfers B (1968) The parotid and submandibular secretion in man. Acta otolaryngol (Stockh) [Suppl] 274
Etholm B, Belal A (1974) Senile changes in the middle ear joints. Ann Otol Rhinol Laryngol 83:49
Falcao J (1951) Le facteur „âge“ dans l’amygdalectomie. Ann Otolaryngol Chir Cervico fac 68:374
Feldmann H (1973) Nasenbluten als Notfallsituation. Laryngol Rhinol Otol (Stuttg) 52:314
Feldmann H (1981) Die Schwerhörigkeit des alternden Menschen. Dtsch Ärztebl 44:2067
Femenič B, Subotič R (1976) Zu den Tympanoplastikindikationen im Senium. In: Kaiser-Meinhardt I, Wendler J (eds) Geriatrische Aspekte in der HNO-Heilkunde. Thieme, Leipzig, p 247
Fendel K (1976) Einige Probleme der Alterschirurgie im Hals-Nasen-Ohren-Fach. In: Kaiser-Meinhardt I, Wendler J (eds) Geriatrische Aspekte in der HNO-Heilkunde. Thieme, Leipzig, p 236
Fikentscher R, Roseburg B, Spinar H, Bruchmüller W (1976) Zur geschlechtsspezifischen Altersabhängigkeit des Geschmacksvermögens. In: Kaiser-Meinhardt I, Wendler J (eds) Geriatrische Aspekte in der HNO-Heilkunde. Thieme, Leipzig, p 184
Fikentscher R, Roseburg B, Spinar H, Bruchmüller W (1977) Geschmacksverlust im Alter; Geschlechtsunterschiede. Clin Otolaryngol 2:183
Fleischer K (1956) Histologische und audiometrische Studie über den altersbedingten Struktur- und Funktionswandel des Innenohres. Arch Ohren Nasen Kehlkopfheilkd 170:142
Fleischer K (1965) Altern und Gehör. MMW 107:1238
Fleischer K (1967) Das alternde Ohr. Aesth Med (Berlin) 16:95
Fleischer K (1972) Das alternde Ohr: Morphologische Aspekte. HNO 20:103
Gastpar H (1969) Der Morbus Osler als haemorrhagische Diathese im höheren Lebensalter. Arch Ohren Nasen Kehlkopfheilkd 194:279
Gerlings PG (1966) Dizziness in older persons. Ear Nose Throat 45:49
Glanninger J (1961) Untersuchungen zur Festigkeit der Gehörknöchelchen und ihrer Gelenke. Monatsschr Ohrenheilkd 95:353
Glorig A, Nixon J (1960) Distribution of hearing loss in various population. Ann Otol Rhinol Laryngol 69:497
Glorig A, Nixon J (1962) Hearing loss as a function of age. Laryngoscope 72:1596
Glorig A, Wheeler D, Quiggle R, Grings W, Summerfield A (1957) 1954 Wisconsin state fair hearing survey: statistical treatment of clinical and audiometric data. American Academy Opthalmology and Otolaryngology and Research Center subcommittee on noise in industry, Los Angeles
Glorig A, Grings W, Summerfield A (1958) Hearing loss in industry. Laryngoscope 68:447
Golemanov W (1976) Das geriatrische operative Krankengut der Universitäts-HNO-Klinik und des Instituts für Endokrinologie, Gerontologie und Geriatrie der Medizinischen Akademie in Sofia. In: Kaiser-Meinhardt I, Wendler J (eds) Geriatrische Aspekte in der HNO-Heilkunde. Thieme, Leipzig, p 40
Golemanov W, Popova M (1976) Sonographische Untersuchungen der Greisenstimme. In: Kaiser-Meinhardt I, Wendler J (eds) Geriatrische Aspekte in der HNO-Heilkunde. Thieme, Leipzig, p 155
Gramowski K (1976) Experimentelle vestibuläre Prüfung bei älteren Normalpersonen. In: Kaiser-Meinhardt I, Wendler J (eds) Geriatrische Aspekte in der HNO-Heilkunde. Thieme, Leipzig, p 148
Griebel C (1952) Der gesunde und der kranke Kehlkopf im Röntgenbild. Thieme, Stuttgart
Guerino M, Milazzo F (1965) Studio istomorfologica della mucosa laryngea umana normale in soggeti di diversa età. Arch Ital Otol 76:656
Habermann G (1972) Der alternde Larynx: Funktionelle Aspekte. HNO 20:121
Hansen C, Reske-Nielsen E (1963) Pathological studies in perceptive deefness. Four patients with persbyacusis. Acat Otolaryngol [Suppl] (Stockh) 188:327
Hansen C, Reske-Nielsen E (1965) Pathological studies in Presbyacusis. Arch Otolaryngol 82:115

Hara HJ (1962) Severe epistaxis. Arch Otolaryngol 75:258
Hecker G (1969) Gerontologische Untersuchungen über Stimmumfang, Sprechstimmlage und Kehlkopfossifikation, Medizinische Dissertation, Leipzig
Herrmann H (1967) Zungenbefunde bei Personen verschiedenen Alters. Dtsch Zahnärztl Z 22:318
Hinchcliffe R (1959) The threshold of hearing as a function of age. Acoustica 9:303
Hollien H, Shipp T (1972) Speaking fundamental frequency and chronologic age in wales. J Speech Hear Res 15:155
Hommerich K (1972) Der alternde Larynx: Morphologische Aspekte. HNO 20:115
Honjo J, Isshiki N (1980) Laryngoscopic and voice characteristics of aged persons. Arch Otolaryngol 106:149
Hülse M, Boll B (1979) Literatur-Dokumentation zur Pressbyacusis. Bundesanstalt für Arbeitsschutz und Unfallforschung, Forschungsbericht 222, Wirtschaftsverlag NW, Bremerhaven
Ishihara M, Komatsu A (1966) The senile olfactory sense. Proc. 8th internat congr ORL, Tokyo, p 515
Jackson C, Jackson L (1947) Diseases of the nose, ear and throat. Saunders, London
Jatho K, Heck K (1959) Schwellenaudiometrische Untersuchungen über die Progredienz und Charakteristik der Altersschwerhörigkeit in den verschiedenen Lebensabschnitten. J Laryngol Otol 38:72
Jerger J (1973) Audiological findings in aging. Adv Otorhinolaryngol 20:115
Johnsson L (1971) Degenerative Veränderungen im alternden Innenohr, mit besonderer Berücksichtigung der vasculären Veränderungen, im Flächenpräparat der menschlichen Cochlea dargestellt. Arch Ohren Nasen Kehlkopfheilkd 200:318
Johnsson L, Hawkins J (1972a) Sensory and neural degeneration with aging, as seen in microdissections of the human inner ear. Am J Otol 81:179
Johnsson L, Hawkins J (1972b) Strial atrophy in clinical and experimental deafness. Laryngoscope 82:1105
Jorgensen M (1961) Changes of aging in the inner ear. Arch Otolaryngol 74:56
Jorgensen M, Bretlau P, Chevance L, Cousse J (1976) Die Otosklerose im Alter. In: Kaiser-Meinhardt I, Wendler J (eds) Geriatrische Aspekte in der HNO-Heilkunde, Thieme, Leipzig, p 69
Kapur Y, Patt A (1967) Hearing in Todas of South India. Arch Otolaryngol 85:400
Kirikae I, Sato T, Shitara T (1964) A Study of hearing in advanced age. Laryngoscope 74:205
Kofler K (1932) Histopathologische Veränderungen am Alterskehlkopf. Mschr Ohrenklinik 66:148
Kranz D, Bernd H, Wagner H (1968) Untersuchungen zur Altersveränderung der Geschmacksschwelle. Arch Otorhindaryngol 192:258
Kraus H, Fietzek J, Frommeyer F, Rüter U (1973) Interferometrische Richtmessungen zur Frage der Alterung der Basilar- und Tectorialmembran des Meerschweinchens. Arch Otorhinolaryngol 204:115
Krompotić-Nemanić J (1968) Presbyacusis and retrocochlear structures. Audiology 7:446
Krompotić-Nemanić J (1969) Presbyacusis, Presbystasis and Presbyosmia as consequence of the analogous biological process. Acta Otolaryngol (Stockh) 67:217
Krompotić-Nemanić J (1971) A new concept of the pathogenesis of Presbyacusis. Arch Otolaryngol 93:161
Krompotić-Nemanić J (1972) Über die Morphologie des inneren Gehörgangs bei der Altersschwerhörigkeit. HNO 20:246
Krompotić-Nemanić J, Kostović J, Rudan P, Nemanić (1971) Morphological and histological changes responsible for the droops of the nasal tip in advanced age. Acta Otolaryngol (Stockh) 71:278
Kühl M (1968) Chirurgisch-Kosmetische Indikation in Jugend und Alter. Aesthet Med (Berlin) 17:251
Laan F, Osterveld W (1974) Age and vestibular function. Aerospace Med 45:540
Leopold D, von Jagow G (1961) Das Röntgenbild des Kehlkopfes, eine Möglichkeit zur Altersbestimmung, mit Ergebnissen eines Blindversuchs. Beitr Gerichtl Med 21:181

Leutert G (1964) Über die histologische Biomorphose der menschlichen Stimmlippe. Gegenbauers Morphol Jahrb 106:11
Leutert G (1976) Die altersabhängigen morphologischen Veränderungen des menschlichen Kehlkopfes. In: Kaiser-Meinhardt I, Wendler J (eds) Geriatrische Aspekte in der HNO-Heilkunde. Thieme, Leipzig, p 49
Lindner L (1981) Zur Entwicklung und Alterung von Binde- und Stützgeweben. Anat Anz 75:61
Liss L, Gomez F (1958) The nature of senile changes of the human olfactory bulb and tract. Acta Otolaryngol Stockh 67:167
Loebell H, Otto K (1958) Greisenchirurgie in der HNO-Heilkunde. Z Laryngol Rhinol Otol Ihre Grenzgeb 37:54
Loewy A, Huttner D (1966) Head and neck surgery in patients past 70. Arch Otolaryngol 84:523
Lundborg T (1976) Die Hörgeräteversorgung im Alter und die damit erreichten Verbesserungen im Kommunikationsprozeß. In: Kaiser-Meinhardt I, Wendler J (eds) Geriatrische Aspekte in der HNO-Heilkunde. Thieme, Leipzig, p 129
Magomedov G (1973) Function of the nasal carvity in persons of senil age in Dagestan. Vestn Otorinolaringol 3:49
Mann W, Beck C (1978) Ein Beitrag zur Altersschwerhörigkeit. Laryngol Rhinolotol (Stuttg) 57:352
Matzker J (1958) Beruht die Altersschwerhörigkeit auf peripheren oder zentralen Veränderungen. Arch Ohren Heilkd 171:371
Maurer H (1978) Entzündungen des Rachens. In: Berendes J, Link R, Zöllner F (eds) HNO-Heilkunde, 2nd edn, vol 3/4. Thieme, Stuttgart
Mayer O (1920) Das anatomische Substrat der Altersschwerhörigkeit. Arch Ohrenheilkd 105:1
Mennig H (1976) Ästhetische Gesichtschirurgie in vorgerücktem Alter. In: Kaiser-Meinhardt I, Wendler J (eds) Geriatrische Aspekte in der HNO-Heilkunde. Thieme, Leipzig, p 231
Mikat B (1972) Altersstrukturen und Diagnosen von HNO-Patienten. HNO 20:334
Millazo F, Guerino M (1965) Recenti acquisizion sul rapporto fra modificazioni della mucosa laryngea nella senilita estati di precancerosi. Arch Ital Otol 76 Suppl 47
Moser F (1948) Pharynxdilatationen, ihr Krankheitsbild und ihre Ursachen. J Laryngol Otol 27:260
Naessen R (1971) An enquiry of the morphological characteristics and possible changes with age in the olfactory region of man. Acta Otolaryngol (Stockh) 71:49
Niemeyer W (1980) Die Schwerhörigkeit des alten Menschen und ihre prothetische Versorgung. In: Berendes J (ed) Aktuelle Probleme der HNO-Heilkunde. Deutscher Ärzteverlag, Köln-Lövenich, p 37
Noell G (1962) Zur Frage der altersbedingten Veränderungen der Larynxschleimhaut. Arch Otorhinolaryngol 179:361
Nomura Y (1970) Lipidosis of the basilar membrane. Acta Otolaryngol (Stockh) 69:352
Nomura Y, Kirikae J (1968) Presbyacusis. A histological-histochemical study of the human cochlea. Acta Otolaryngol (Stockh) 66:17
Novotny O (1969) Die Hals-Nasen-Ohrenkrankheiten im Greisenalter. Enke, Stuttgart, pp 448–481 (Handbuch der praktischen Geriatrie, vol 39
Osterland R (1962) Untersuchungen des menschlichen Kehldeckels unter besonderer Berücksichtigung der regressiven Veränderungen. Dissertation, Berlin
Pantoja E (1968) The laryngeal cartilages. Arch Otolaryngol 87:416
Pellnitz D (1961) Über den durch das Altern bedingten Gestaltswandel der menschlichen Epiglottis, Arch Ohrenheilkd 178:350
Pellnitz D (1962) Die Bedeutung von Ohrmuschel- und Nasenwachstum für die Indikationsstellung kosmetischer Operationen. Arch Ohrenheilkd 180:387
Pellnitz D (1972) Geriatrische Probleme in der Hals-Nasen-Ohrenheilkunde. HNO 20:97
Plester D (1961) Audiometrische Untersuchungen bei einem Naturvolk. Arch Ohren Heilkd 180:765
Plester D (1972) Das alternde Ohr. Chirurgische Aspekte. HNO 20:216

Preobrazensky N (1974) Angina und chronische Tonsillitis. Hippokrates, Stuttgart
Ptacek P, Sander E (1966) Age recognitions from voice. J Speech Hear Res 9:273
Rauch J (1959) Die Speicheldrüse des Menschen. Thieme, Stuttgart
Ribari O (1976) Otoskleroseoperationen bei Patienten in höherem Lebensalter. In: Kaiser-Meinhardt I, Wendler J (eds) Geriatrische Aspekte in der HNO-Heilkunde. Thieme, Leipzig, p 259
Ricci C (1935) Osservazioni istopathologiche nella larynge nella senes cenza. Arch Ital Anat Istol Pat [Suppl] 6:385
Rollin H (1975) Funktionsprüfungen und Störungen des Geschmackssinnes. Arch Otorhinolaryngol 210:165
Roncallo P (1948) Researches about ossification and conformation of the thyroid cartilage in man. Acta Otolaryng (Stockh) 36:110
Roseburg W, Fikentscher R, Spinar H, Bruchmüller W (1976) Zur Altersabhängigkeit des Geruchsvermögens. In: Kaiser-Meinhardt I, Wendler J (eds) Geriatrische Aspekte in der HNO-Heilkunde. Thieme, Leipzig, p 191
Rosen S, Olin P (1965) Hearing loss and coronary heart disease. Arch Otolaryngol 82:236
Rosen S, Bergmann M, Plester D, El-Mofty A, Satti M (1962) Presbyacusis study of a relatively noce-free population in the Sudan. Ann Otol 71:727
Rosen S, Plester D, El-Mofty A, Rosen HV (1964a) High frequency audiometry in presbyacusis. A comparative study of the Mabaan tribe in the Sudan with urban population. Arch Otolaryngol 79:18
Rosen S, Plester D, El-Mofty A, Rosen HV (1964b) Relation of hearing loss to cardiovascular disease. Trans Am Acad Ophthalmol Otol 68:434
Rosen S, Olin P, Rosen H (1970a) Dieatary prevention of hearing loss. Acta Otolaryngol (Stockh) 70:242
Rosen S, Preobrazensky N, Khechinashvili, Glzunov J, Kipshidze N, Rosen H (1970b) Epidemiologic hearing studies in the USRR. Arch Otolaryngol 91:424
Rosenhall U (1974) Epithelial cyste in the human vestibular apparatus. J Laryngol Otol 88:105
Rosenwasser H (1964) Otitic problems in the aged. Geriatrics 19:11
Rossberg G (1964) Die Altersabhängigkeit der vestibulären Leistungsfähigkeit. Ein Beitrag zur Regulationsfunktion des Vestibularsystems. Arch Ohrenheilkd 181:457
Rous J (1969) The effect of age on the function capacity of semell analyses. Cesk Otolaryngol 18:248
Ruckes J (1964) Dyschylie und Mikrolithiasis im menschlichen Taschenband in Abhängigkeit vom Lebensalter. Z Laryngol Rhinol Otol Ihre Grenzgeb 43:207
Ruckes J, Causé A (1964) Über Ausdehnung und Vorkommen von Plattenepithel am menschlichen Taschenband. Z Laryngol Rhinol Otol Ihre Grenzgeb 43:197
Sataloff J, Menduke H (1957) Presbyacusis. Trans Am Acad Ophthmalol Otolaryngol 61:141
Sawaki S, Fujiste S, Shitare T, Yoneyama F (1959) Geriatrics in otolaryngolog. Statistic studies on 376 japanese elderly individuals. J Otorhinolaryngol Soc Jpn 62:1589
Saxén A (1937) Pathologie und Klinik der Altersschwerhörigkeit. Acta Otolaryngol (Stockh) [Suppl] 23
Schmidt P (1967) Presbyacusis. Audiology [Suppl] 6:1
Schöder HJ (1976) Zur Reaktionsweise des Vestibularsystems im Alter. In: Kaiser-Meinhardt I, Wendler J (eds) Geriatrische Aspekte in der HNO-Heilkunde. Thieme, Leipzig, p 152
Schuknecht H (1955) Presbyacusis. Laryngoscope 65:402
Schuknecht HF (1964) Further observations on the pathology of Presbyacusis. Arch Otolaryngol 80:369
Scott J (1960) Prominence of the submaxillary glands in the aged. J Am Geriatr Soc 8:53
Scott J (1976) The incidence of focal chronic inflammatory changes in human submandibular salivary glands. J Oral Pathol 5:334
Scott J (1977) Quantitative age changes in the histological structure of human submandibular salivary glands. Arch Oral Biol 22:221

Seydewitz V, Staubesand J (1983) Kalzifizierung der Arterienwand als Alterungsprozeß. Elektronenmikroskopische und biochemische Untersuchungen am Modell der Vitamin-D_3-Überdosierung. Akt Gerontol 13:115–118
Shipp T, Hollien H (1960) Perception of the aging male voice. J Speech Hear Res 12:703
Silverman S, Davis H (1970) Counceling about hearing aids. In: Davis H, Silverman S (eds) Hearing and deafness, 3rd edn. Holt, Rinehart and Winston, New York
Simonetta B (1968) Sulla presbiacusi in tribu africane in alto primitive. Minerva Otorinolaryngol 18:101
Smith C (1942) Age incidence of atrophy of olfactory nervs in man. A contribution ot the study of the process of aging. J Comp Neurol 77:589
Specht F (1924) Störungen des Riechvermögens. In: Denker A, Kahler O (eds) Handbuch der HNO-Heilkunde, Vol 5. Springer, Berlin Heidelberg New York, p 673
Spoor A, van Laar F (1967) Presbyacusis. Audiology Suppl 1
Steinberg J, Montgomery H, Gardner M (1940) Results of the worlds fair hearing tests. J Acoust Soc Am 12:291
Stern H (1932) Über einige Ursachen und Folgen der Alterserscheinungen in der Stimmgebung. Monatschr Ohrenheilkd 66:1143
Strauss EL (1970) A study olfactory acuity. Ann Otol 79:95
Strohm M (1978) Hals-Nasen-Ohrenkrankheiten im Alter. Z Gerontol 11:107
Suzuki K, Kaito H (1958) Chronic tonsillitis and tonsillectomy in the advanced age group. Otorhinolaryngol Tokyo 3:55
Thumfart W, Plattig KH, Schlicht N (1980) Geruchs- und Geschmacksschwelle älterer Menschen. Z Gerontol 13:158
Trianfidi J, Kaliteevsky P, Zinchenko V (1972) The state of the mucous membrane of the larynx in the aged. Vestn Otorinolaringol 34:97
Tzschoppe A (1976) Der alternde Mensch in der Hals-Nasen-Ohrensprechstunde. In: Kaiser-Meinhardt I, Wendler J (eds) Geriatrische Aspekte in der HNO-Heilkunde. Thieme, Leipzig, p 35
Vogt K, Semmann W (1970) Zur physiologischen Beeinflussung der Gesamtproteinsekretion der großen Kopfspeicheldrüsen durch Tageszeit, Alter und Geschlecht. J Laryngol Rhinol 49:612
Vogt K, Meyer P, Kleber R, Tietz W (1976) Funktionelle Veränderungen der Speicheldrüsen des alternden Menschen und Möglichkeiten zu ihrer Therapie. In: Kaiser-Meinhardt I, Wendler J (eds) Geriatrische Aspekte in der HNO-Heilkunde. Thieme, Leipzig, p 280
Von Wedel H, Opitz H (1978) Funktionelle Auswirkungen des Alterungsvorganges auf das Mittelohr. Laryngol Rhinol Otol (Stuttg) 57:152
Waterhouse J, Clinsholm, Winter R, Patel M, Yale R (1973) Replacement of functional parenchymal cells by fat and connective tissue in human submandibular glands: an agerelated change. J Oral Pathol 2:16
Webster G (1967) Random reflections on rhinoplasty. Plast Reconstr Surg 39:147
Webster J, Himer H, Lichtenstein M (1950) San Diego county fair hearing survery. J Acoust Soc Am 22:473
Weymar P, Mahler KF, Meyer E (1976) Ergebnisse der Stapes-Chirurgie im höheren Lebensalter. In: Kaiser-Meinhardt I, Wendler J (eds) Geriatrische Aspekte in der HNO-Heilkunde. Thieme, Leipzig, p 255
Wissner G (1970) Altersveränderungen von Gesichts- und Ohrmerkmalen. Anthropol Anz 32:157
Wright J, Schuknecht H (1972) Atrophy of the spiral ligament. Arch Otolaryngol 96:16
Zaoli G (1961) Sulla senescenza dell' aparato vascolare nasoparanasale. Minerva Otorinolaryngol 11:351
Zaritzky L (1936) Über Altersveränderungen der Schleimdrüsen des kavernösen Gewebes der Schleimhäute des Atmungsgebietes der Nase. Monatsschr Ohrenheilkd 70:1057
Zilstorff K (1972) Über Altersveränderungen des Geruchssinns. HNO 20:124
Zwaardemaker H (1891) Der Verlust an hohen Tönen mit zunehmendem Alter: ein neues Gesetz. Arch Ohrenheilkd 32:53
Zwaardemaker H (1895) Die Physiologie des Geruchs. Engelmann, Leipzig

Ophthalmology

Aging of the Eyelids

H. MEYTHALER

A. Significance of the Lid in Vision

The lid apparatus is an intricate and complex mechanism. Great functional and cosmetic importance is associated with the interaction of the lid, musculature, and tendon apparatus. Orbital mechanisms also play an important role, as in the case of the orbital fat changes and elasticity changes of the muscularis orbitalis caused by aging. The closure of the lid is a complex mechanism consisting mainly of four phases: first of all the palpebral portion closes followed by the nasal half in a windshield wiper motion (ROHEN 1958). This wipes the tear film, vital to the transparency of the cornea, from the upper temporal to the loser nasal section of the eye and into the canaliculi and lower lacrimal duct.

This whole mechanism is maintained by the complicated structure of the m. orbicularis oculi, the different sections of the muscle having different functional roles. Medially positioned is a strong band of collagen (ligamentum canthi internum) which functions as the origin of all the fibers of the m. orbicularis. The opening motion of the lid is mainly accomplished by two muscles, the m. levator palpebrae, innervated by the third cranial nerve and the sympathetically innervated m. tarsalis. The edges of the lid should under normal circumstances fit the bulbus snugly.

The skin of the eyelid itself is different in histologic structure from the rest of the skin: the epidermis is substantially thinner and the papillaries are only sparsely developed. The subcutis possesses a very delicate and loose collagen and elastic fiber network, explaining its tendency to edema. Actual fat tissue is not present, in its place, especially in the upper lid, are modified, holocrine sebaceous glands (meibomian glands), the secretion of which plays an important role in stabilizing the tear film. These glands are supplemented by apocrine sweat glands (Moll's glands), accessory tear glands (Krause's glands) and small sebaceous glands (Zeis's glands). The inner side of the lid is lined with conjunctiva, whose goblet cells deliver mucin, important for the consistency of the tear film. Destruction of the goblet cells results in ocular pemphigus and hence kerosis and subsequent blindness.

B. Lid Changes Caused by Aging

I. Senile Atrophy

Senile atrophy (Fig. 1) normally tends to begin after the age of 50 years, with slender individuals seemingly more susceptible. Loss of tone and atrophia cause the

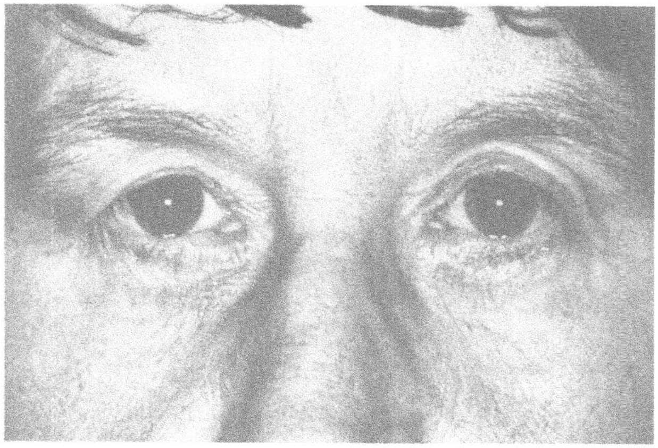

Fig. 1. Senile atrophy

development of small wrinkles, origining at the temporal section of the lids. The so-called crow's-feet wrinkles are located in the temporal periorbital region. Tarsal and marginal wrinkles are found mainly in individuals over 60 years of age in the lower lid regions (HEYDENREICH 1960). The essential pathologic anatomic cause, in addition to the thinning of the epidermis, is to be found in the atrophy of the collagen and elastic fibers. This mechanism is responsible for the typical appearance of aging skin of the lid. On the other hand, early loss of orbital fat helps the lid retain its smooth appearance.

II. Senile Pigment Abnormalities

The pink eyelid color of the adolescent changes over the years into a yellowish brown. This change is accelerated by increased actinic influences. Pigmented sebaceous keratosis and flat epithelial pigmentations are more frequent in older individuals. Malignity is not likely, with the exception of lentigo maligna. Furthermore, one finds in older people an increased number of yellowish nodes (colloid pseudomilium) varying from pinhead to pea size. There are hyaline degenerations of the collagen and elastic matrix of unknown cause (HEYDENREICH 1960). FAVRE and RACAUCHOT in 1937 originally presented a similar clinical picture of skin elastoidosis with black comedones and yellowish nodular, hemispherical cysts (see HEYDENREICH 1960). Males are predominantly affected. A pronounced colloidal degeneration of the superficial cutis is the main histologic finding.

III. Blepharochalasis

A diffuse atrophy of the elastic fibers of the upper lid leads to a slowly progressive sagging of the lids (Fig. 2), sometimes to such an extent that the skin fold covers the eyelash and on occasion even the pupil, causing a vision obstruction. The patients have a pronounced sad facial expression. Therapy is solely surgical and one should not spare any excessive lid skin. After a successful operation the patient's mental state improves.

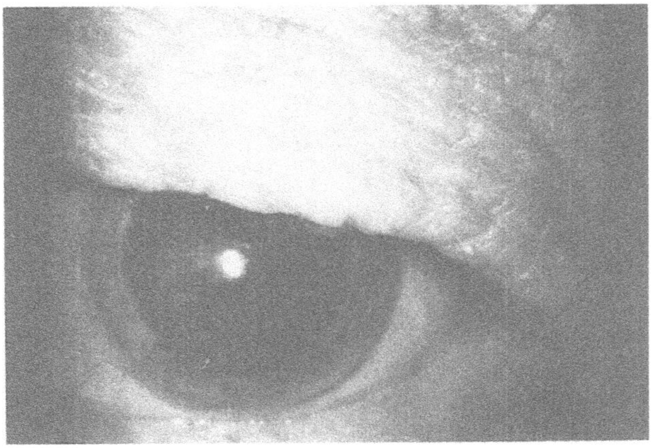

Fig. 2. Blepharochalasis

Excess lid skin is especially suited for covering defects present after the removal of malignant tumors. Diagnostically, one has to differentiate between the familiar blepharochalasis and Ascher's syndrome (combination of double lip and struma). SMITH (1964) observed in the aged a combination of blepharochalasis and prolapse of the tear gland.

IV. Bags Under the Eyes

Loss of elasticity of the collagen and elastic matrix of the lower lid leads to development of so-called bags unter the eyes. Their appearance before the age of 50 years necessitates the exclusion of a cardiac, nephrogenic, hematologic, or hepatogenic origin. When abnormally large their weight can cause the lid to sag, resulting in ectropion. Here again therapy is strictly surgical, but, unlike blepharochalasis, care should be taken not to remove too much skin, thus avoiding ectropion cicatriceum.

V. Fat Hernia

Orbital fat hernias, most often found bilateraly in the upper nasal region, are frequently mistaken for genuine tumors. Hereditary factors have been reported (SMITH 1964). The cause is a hernial weakness of the fascia tarso-orbitalis through which orbital fat presses into the underlying skin tissue of the upper lid.

VI. Senile Blepharophimosis

In old age, a decrease in size of the palpebral apertures, originating mostly from the temporal side, can be observed. In extreme cases, the outside edge of the cornea may be covered. The cause is slackening of the m. orbicularis and fascia tarso-orbitalis. Therapy is surgical.

VII. Seborrheic Dermatitis

Seborrheic eczema has its origin in a seborrheic diathesis (HEYDENREICH 1960) where body locations with multiple sebaceous and sweat glands are primarily affected. The efflorescences consist of reddish, flat singular foci, covered by small lamellated squamae and dark brown crusts. On the lid one mainly finds persistent blepharitis squamosa, with subsequent loss of the ciliae when transforming into blepharitis ulcerosa. After cure, the newly grown lashes are irregularly spaced and directed both inward and outward (trichiasis), causing chronic conjunctivitis by means of chafing. Much more menacing are cilia abrasion ulcers of the cornea. Treatment of seborrheic dermatitis is strictly conservative, local application of steroids has proven very successful. The trichiasis must be treated by cryoepilation.

C. Anomalies in the Position of the Lids Caused by Aging

I. Senile Ectropion

The lower lid begins to lose contact with the bulbus at the lower inner section of the ocular aperture (Fig. 3). The resulting eversion of the lacrimal point produces a disturbing epiphora, causing the patient constantly to wipe the tears away in a downward motion, this in turn producing an additional traction effect (wipe ectropion). In the course of weeks and months the lower lid turns outward, producing an epidermization of the delicate conjunctiva. This results in destruction of the goblet cells which are essential for mucin production. Senile ectropion is only seen in the lower lid, its main cause being the relaxation of the m. orbicularis and the l. canthi internum. Therapy is strictly surgical.

II. Senile Entropion

Much more frequent than senile ectropion is senile entropion (Fig. 4). The clinical picture being an inward curling of the lower lid with an apparent spastic component. This results in chafing of the ciliae on the bulbus, mainly of the cornea, leading to severe ocular complications. Individuals over the age of 70 years are predominantly affected. Formerly, a complex system of age-related changes to the lids and orbit were held responsible. More recent work, on the lower lid only, shows that the previous hypothesis of an abnormal muscle spasm can no longer be maintained (WINTER 1980); moreover, a shifting of the preseptal orbicularis fibers towards the lid margin was demonstrated. Aponeurosis of the lower lid also plays an important part: in the event of its becoming slack or dehiscent the lower tarsal margin also becomes loose. In addition, this process is favored by atrophy of orbital fat, caused by aging, and the resulting senile enophthalmos. Therefore, a disturbance of the equilibrium between the m. orbicularis and fascia tarso-orbitalis is present (ROHRBACH 1980). A further disadvantageous factor is chronic irritating conjunctivitis which can cause a shortening of the lower lid conjunctiva. Senile entropion is treatable only by surgery.

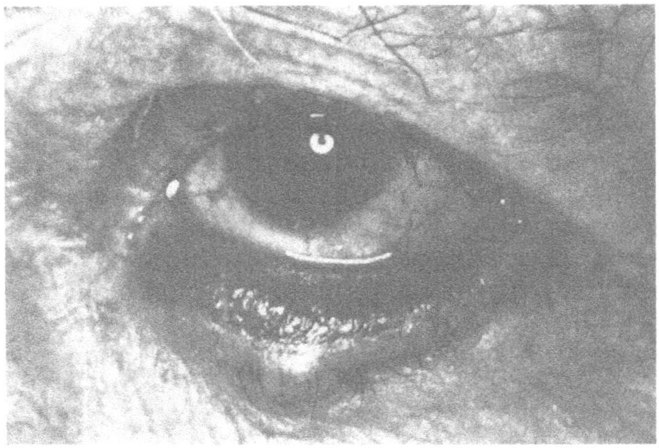

Fig. 3. Senile ectropion

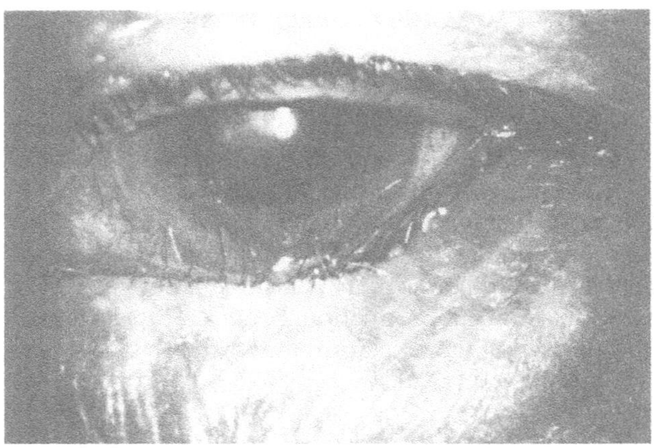

Fig. 4. Senile entropion

D. Motor Disorders of Lid Function Caused by Aging

I. Senile Ptosis

Senile ptosis (Fig. 5), mostly incomplete, is a very complex occurrence: besides the weakness of the m. levator palpebrae, the aging skin, with its fat hernias, plays a decisive role. Enophthalmos caused by fat atrophy in the orbit also contributes. In the event of a bilateral ptosis, a neurologic examination should exclude both the possibility of ophthalmoplegia progressiva and myasthenia gravis (Tensilon test).

E. Tumors of the Lid

Both benign and malignant skin tumors show a preference toward the aging skin of the eyelids.

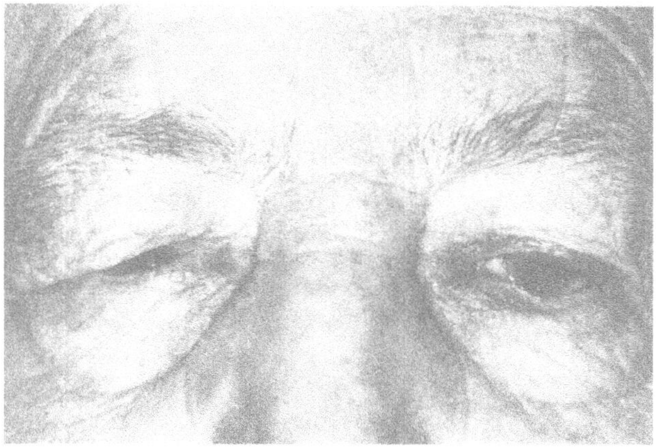

Fig. 5. Senile ptosis

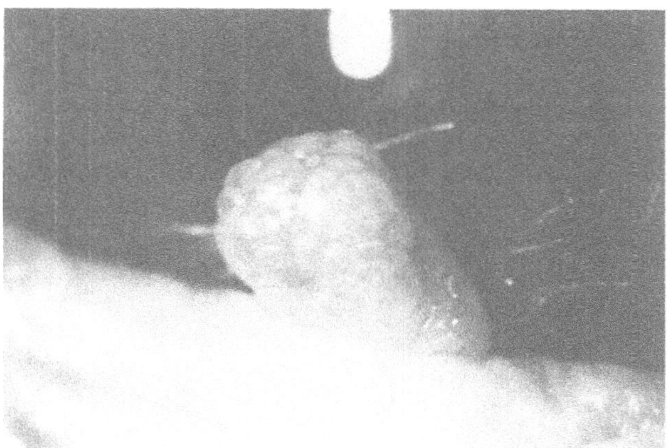

Fig. 6. Seborrheic keratosis

I. Pseudocancerous Lesions

By definition, pseudocancerous lesions of the skin are lesions that clinically, resemble carcinomas, but never turn into them. They are thus to be distinguished from precancerous lesions which often turn into malignant tumors. It is impossible to discuss here all the existing benign and malignant tumors of the lid, but seborrheic keratosis (Fig. 6) will be taken as representative of the pseudocancerous lesions. In the lid or periorbital region one mostly finds a pea-size, sharply bounded, brown-yellow tumor with a wart-like surface. The histology shows hyperkeratosis, papillomatosis, and a matrix proliferation of the basal cells. The inverted follicular keratosis shows all the clinical signs of seborrheic keratosis. A group of squamous cysts is found in the fine tissue structure, surrounded by acantholytic cells (squamous eddies). This is the cause of the frequent confusion with squamous cell carcinomas. The keratoacanthoma (Fig. 7) is a rapidly growing dome-like tumor with a keratin-filled crater. Contrary to the clinically similar basal cell carcinoma, one finds no significant atrophy of the epidermis. The keratoacan-

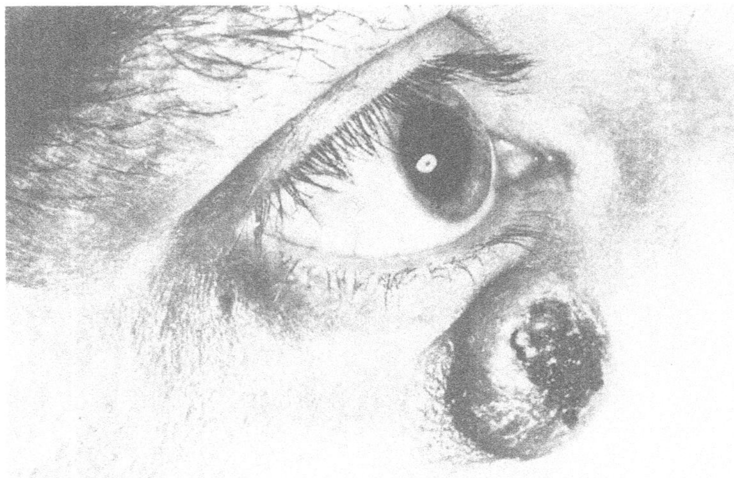

Fig. 7. Keratoacanthoma

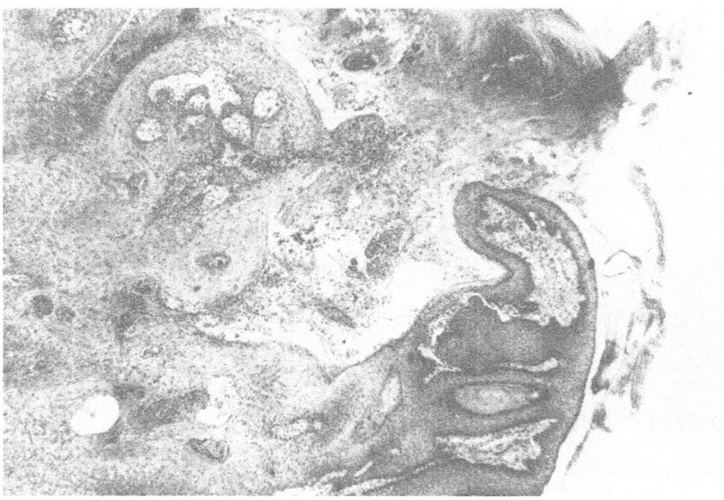

Fig. 8. Histologic findings in keratoacanthoma

thoma shows a pronounced tendency toward regression. The histologic picture (Fig. 8) is a keratin-filled crater with its margin inwardly inclined. Typical, besides acanthosis, is a normal maturing level of all the cells with signs of inverted follicular keratosis. This tumor represents a special form of pseudoepithelial hyperplasia.

II. Precancerous Lesions

A precancerous lesion not only looks similar to a carcinoma; without treatment it can transform into one, the prototype being senile actinic keratosis (sailors' skin). Multiple yellowish, flat or raised lesions with more or less dilated capillaries develop on the sun-exposed regions of the skin.

Signs of chronic inflammation as well as hyperkeratosis, parakeratosis, and acanthosis, with untypical cells in the deeper skinlevels are typical histologic findings. Mitosis is often seen. Cornu cutaneum located mainly on the lid margin is typical; atypical cells and mitosis at its base show imminent malignant development. Carcinoma in situ is more rarely found. Clinically, carcinoma in situ presents as a reddish, slightly raised, squamous alteration, hardly distinguishable from a pseudoepithelial alteration. Dyskeratosis (single cell squamous) is the pronounced cell arrangement. The nucleus–plasma relationship is tilted toward the nucleus. Mitosis is frequent.

III. Squamous Cell Carcinoma

Squamous cell carcinoma is diagnosed much too frequently (NAUMANN et al. 1980; BONIUK and ZIMMERMANN 1967; MEYTHALER 1973). The actual frequency of occurrence is between 3% and 5% of all malignant lid tumors. It is characterized by rapid development with its main location being the upper lid. On the lid, in terms of fine structure, the more benign and relatively more differentiated corneous types are found. In contrast to the benign pseudocancerous lesions, unregulated growth of tumor cells toward deeper skin layers is observed, the normal cell maturing process being lost. The tumor cells can be distinguished, depending upon differentiation through pleomorphy, polychromasy, and a multitude of atypical mitoses.

IV. Sebaceous Gland Carcinoma

Sebaceous gland carcinoma (Fig. 9) is the most frequent metastasizing tumor of the lid in central Europe (NAUMANN 1980). Most often it originates at the Meibomian gland of the upper lid, seldom from sebaceous glands of the caruncle. A circumscript madarosis and a noticeably yellow coloring of the tumor is typical. For differential diagnosis, it is important to note the characteristic feature of so-called pagetoid development in the epithelial of the conjunctiva, sometimes stretching from the lid margin, past the fornix, up to limbus. The accompanying blepharoconjunctivitis can sometimes obscure the picture of a malignant tumor. Fine structural growth can be either relatively distinct or infiltrative. The adenomatous structure (Fig. 10) of tumor cell formations enclosing necrotic areas is typical. Substantial pleomorphy of the tumor cells along with a large amount of atypical mitosis is pronounced. Staining of the fat produces intraplasmatic lipids.

V. Basal Cell Carcinoma

Basal cell carcinoma (Fig. 11) is the most frequent tumor of the eyelid and periorbital region (frequency ~90%). In a strict pathologic sense, basal cell carcinoma is considered to be semimalignant because of its inability to metastasize. On the

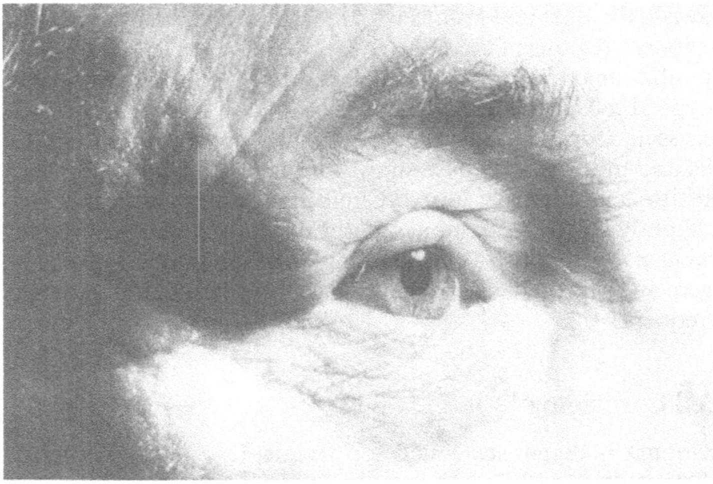

Fig. 9. Meibomian carcinoma

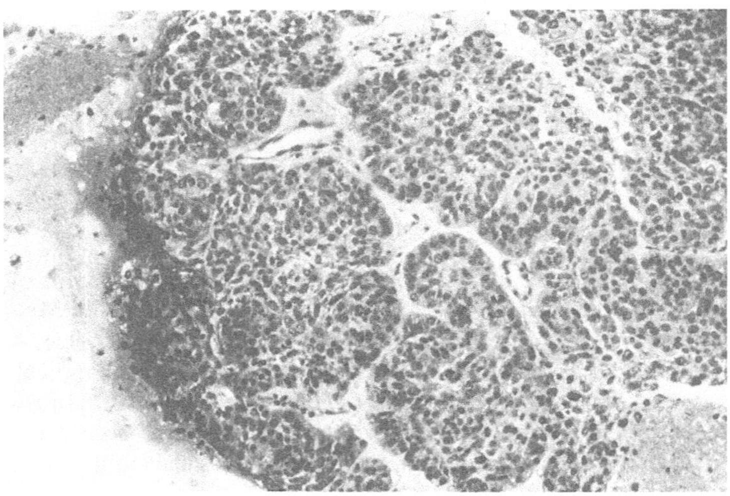

Fig. 10. Histologic findings in meibomian carcinoma

other hand, from a clinical point of view, its tendency towards aggressive, destructive growth determines its classification as a malignant tumor. Anamnesis over many years and solitary occurrence in aging skin are its signs, the favorite location being the lower nasal lid angle decreasing with more lateral location. Actinic keratosis is mostly the primary lesion. The nodular ulcerous type is the most frequent from, typically with its nacreous shine and visible capillaries through the atrophic skin. In the course of time, a central keratin-filled crater is formed under conditions of malnutrition, from which blood of fluid is discharged, often owing

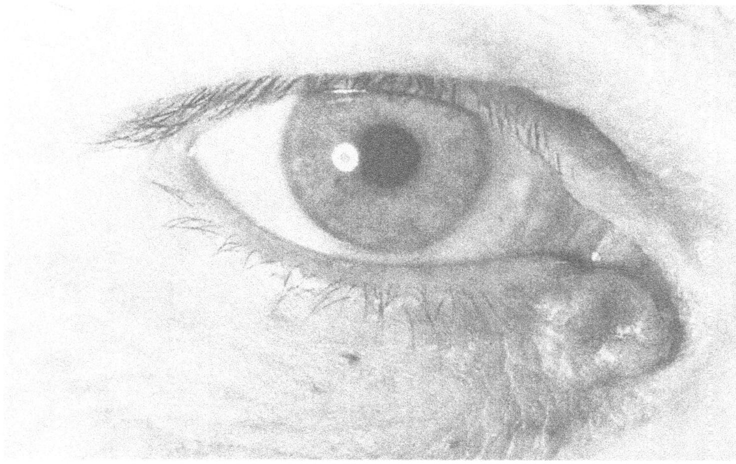

Fig. 11. Basal cell carcinoma

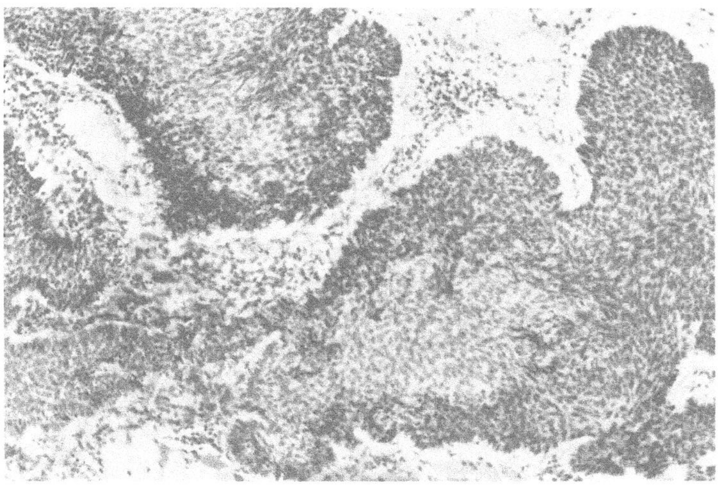

Fig. 12. Histologic findings in basal cell carcinoma

to mechanical irritation. Flat developing, fibrous basal cell carcinomas (ulcus rodens) are seen only after they begin to ulcerate. Large-scale destruction in the vicinity of the lid and periorbital region is called ulcus terebrans.

As a rule, histologic diagnosis presents no problem. The monomorphic cell picture (Fig. 12) with long oval or round tumor cells with deep basophilic nuclei and only little cytoplasm is typical. Intercellular connections are not observed. Marginal palisade arrangement of the narrow cells is indicative of a solid basal cell carcinoma. Epithelial pearls are not uncommon, occasionally leading to confusion with a corneous squamous cell carcinoma. As in all epithelial tumors they

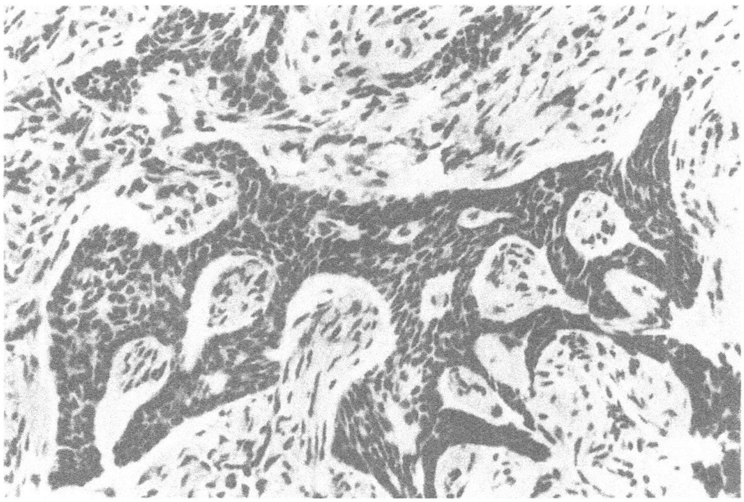

Fig. 13. Histologic findings in morphea-like basal cell carcinoma

have a tendency towards organoid differentiation, e.g., keratotosis or adenoid basal cell carcinoma. They are not as frequent and show a more benign type of behavior than that of the differentiation tumors (MEYTHALER 1973; WAGENMANN 1957). The surroundings are mostly distinctly bounded and show a more or less chronic inflammation toward the margin. Morphea-like basal cell carcinoma (Fig. 13) is one exception, having tumor formations out of fibrotically transformed mesenchyma, uncontrollably proliferating as small cords and cones into deeper layers, causing much trouble when one tries to excise the tumor out of healthy tissue. These patients should be closely checked postoperatively. Although a number of conservative treatments are listed (chemotherapy, X-ray, cryotherapy), we prefer surgical excision. This provides the only true means of control whether or not the excision was made in normal healthy tissue.

References

Boniuk M, Zimmermann LE (1967) Eyelid tumors with reference to lesions confused with squamous cell carcinoma. Arch Ophthalmol 77:29

Duke-Elder S (1974) The ocular adnexa, part I. Diseases of the eyelids. Kimpton, London

Favre M, Racauchot L (1937) Zit. in K. Velhagen: Der Augenarzt, vol 3. Thieme, Stuttgart–Leipzig 1960

Heydenreich A (1960) Krankheiten der Augenlider. In: Velhagen K (ed) Der Augenarzt, vol 3. Thieme, Stuttgart, pp 125–191

Kornzweig AL (1964) Lid affections of the aged. In: Fox SA (ed) Affections of the lids, vol 4. Little, Brown, Boston, pp 55–64

Kuper J, Müller N (1980) Zur Pathogenese und Kausalchirurgie des Entropiums senile durch en-bloc-Resektion. Klin Monatsbl Augenheilkd 176:1023

Meythaler H (1973) Zum Differenzierungsverhalten der Basaliome der Lider und ihrer Umgebung. Albrecht von Graefes Arch, Klin Ophthalmol 178:111–130

Naumann GOH (1980) Pathologie des Auges. Spezielle pathologische Anatomie, eds Doerr W, Seifert G. Springer, Berlin Heidelberg New York
Rohen J (1958) Anatomie des Auges. In: Velhagen K (ed) Der Augenarzt, vol 1. Thieme, Leipzig, pp 56–69
Rohrbach F (1980) Zur Korrektur des Entropium senile nach Schimek. Klin Monatsbl Augenheilkd 177:822–824
Schreck E (1977) Differentialdiagnose in der Ophthalmologie. Enke, Stuttgart
Smith B (1964) Common Degenerations of the lids. In: Fox AA (ed) Affections of the lids, vol 4. Little, Brown, Boston, pp 67–72
Wagenmann J (1957) Differenzierungspotenz der Basaliome in Bezug auf ihre Lokalisation. Dissertation, University of Tübingen
Winter N (1980) Senile Entropium-Genese und Therapie. Klin Monatsbl Augenheilkd 177:265
Yanoff M, Fine BS (1975) Ocular pathology. Harper and Row, New York

The Eye in the Aging Patient: Cornea

M. REIM

A. Structure of the Cornea

The cornea is the clear window in the eyeball by which pictures of the outside reach the inside of the eye. Owing to its curvature and smooth reflecting surfaces, it is part of the optical system of the eye. The transparent tissue of the cornea is void of blood vessels and therefore differs in structure, metabolism, and physiology from vascularized organs.

I. Epithelium

The surface is covered by 5–7 layers of nonkeratinizing squamous epithelium. The basal cells are arranged in a cylindrical pattern on the basement membrane, on top of which are cuboid, round, and polygonal cells of the intermediate layer. The surface is formed by flat cover cells with microvilli on the outside. They are covered with the tear film, imparting the smooth and reflecting aspect to the cornea. The top epithelial cells are scaled off and removed from the palpebral fissure by the efferent lacrimal canals.

II. Stroma

The largest part of the corneal thickness is composed of the stroma. Only 5%–10% of the stromal volume consists of keratocytes. The other 90% consists of extracellular material which is formed by regular collagen fibrils. These fibrils are evenly spaced by an interfibrillar matrix of proteoglycans. The lattice-like stromal structure of collagen fibrils 20–30 nm thick accounts for the transparency of this tissue. Close to the epithelium, the collagen fibrils are densely packed to form a smooth convex surface. The same condensation of proteins is found of the concave back of the cornea. It is microscopically homogeneous and is easily isolated as a glassy lamella. On the back of this layer, called Descemet's membrane, is the monolayer of the corneal endothelium.

III. Endothelium

Viewed from the back, the endothelium appears as a regular layer of hexagonal cells. The endothelial cells contain numerous mitochondria, an endoplasmic reticulum, and pinocytotic vesicles. They are tied together by zonulae occludentes. The endothelium acts as a diffusion barrier to keep the aqueous from entering the corneal stroma (ROHEN 1964).

IV. Metabolism

In all cells of the cornea, an active energy metabolism has been proven. The stromal substance is mainly synthesized by the keratocytes, but to a lesser degree also by the epithelium. The endothelium plays a major role in active transport. Unlike the epithelium, the endothelium can regenerate by mitosis only under certain circumstances, if at all (Reim 1972).

V. Physiology

The epithelium of the cornea forms a diffusion barrier to stop low molecular weight substances, water, foreign bodies, and microbes from penetrating the cornea. The epithelium can regenerate within 5–7 days, as shown by autoradiographic studies (Machemer et al. 1965). In this period, the basal cells divide by mitosis and migrate to the surface where they are desquamated. The endothelium controls the metabolism between cornea and aqueous by active transport and selective diffusion. The supply of nutrients such as glucose and amino acids occurs from the aqueous via the endothelium. Waste products like lactate diffuse in the opposite direction from the stroma through the endothelium into the aqueous. The marginal vessels that approach the limbus from the conjunctiva are of minor importance for the corneal supply of nutrients. The limbus, however, separating the corneal tissue from the blood system, is the location where many immunologic events take place. Furthermore, large molecules like albumin, plasma proteins, and lipoproteins that cannot penetrate the endothelium, diffuse from the limbal capillaries into the corneal stroma. Another important task of the endothelium is the active transport of bicarbonate and chloride ions from the corneal stroma into the aqueous. This mechanism keeps the corneal ground substance in a state of continuous dehydration. This gradient is important for the transparency of the stroma. Allowing water to enter the stroma freely will swell the interfibrillar matrix of proteoglycans and cause the collagen fibrils to separate and lose their regular lattice-like arrangement. The stroma will lose its transparency and the thickness will increase (Reim 1972, 1982).

B. Senile Changes of the Cornea

I. Clinically Visible Signs of Aging

1. Arcus Senilis

The arcus senilis is the most conspicuous sign of age. It is located at the edge of the cornea as a more or less circular, gray-white opacity. A small clear zone separates the arcus senilis from the limbus. While the peripheral borders of the arcus senilis are comparatively clear-cut, its central limits are less marked. To the center there is a wider zone of increasing transparency. The arcus senilis is most dense in the deeper layers of the stroma, where the opacification starts in most cases. It should be noted that the arcus senilis appears first under the upper and lower lid, if it is not a complete ring (Fig. 1). For the etiology of the arcus senilis see Sect. B.IV.3.

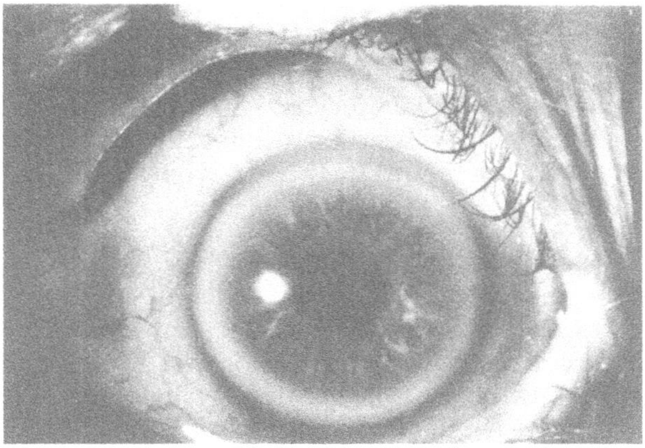

Fig. 1. Arcus senilis in the eye of a 75-year-old. There is a transparent zone between the ring-shaped gray opacification and the limbus. The limits of the arcus senilis are well defined to the periphery, but the transition to the clear center is gradual

2. Increased Shagreen of the Aged Cornea

In the outer layers of the aged corneal stroma, gray and white opacities can be seen with the slit lamp microscope, consisting of small gray streaks in otherwise clear tissue. This change is viewed as a condensation of the intracellular stromal matrix and is called shagreen because of its resemblance to the surface of leather. Its chemical composition is not known. It is possible that the chemical changes described in Sect. B.IV. may explain this condition in the cornea of elderly people.

3. Line of Stähli

This is a slightly curved brown opacity running across the center of the cornea and located in the upper stroma. It is hardly visible with the naked eye, but always with the slit lamp microscope. It mostly occurs in elderly people, but the etiology is not known. Sometimes a line of Stähli can be seen in younger people after keratitis.

4. White Limbus Girdle of Vogt

This typical aging change is an opacity in the palpebral fissure composed of shiny white crystalline deposits next to the limbus. Although it can be frequently found in elderly patients, there is little known about its chemical composition and electron microscopic structure (Fig. 2).

5. Cornea Guttata

Slit lamp examination with high magnification and oblique bright light reveals fine drop-like vesicles at the back of the cornea (Fig. 3). This is a frequent finding in the midperiphery of the cornea in older people. They are caused by focal prominences of thickened Descemet's membrane. For its ultrastructure see Sect. B.III. If the guttae in the endothelium become more numerous and cover the back of the cornea, the function of the endothelium to dehydrate the stroma will be im-

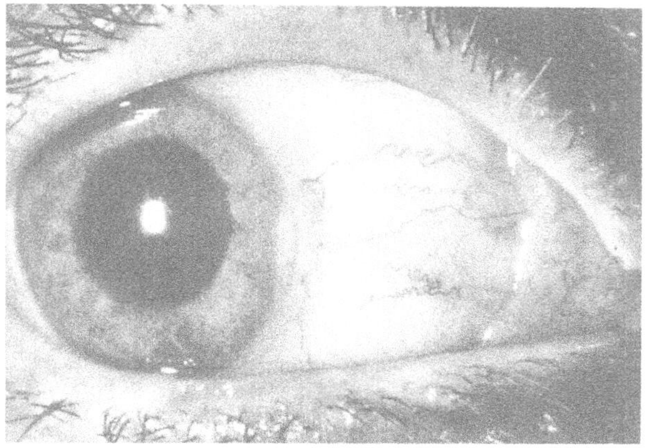

Fig. 2. White limbus girdle of Vogt. In the palpebral fissure adjacent to the limbus there is a shiny white crescent-shaped opacity of the cornea

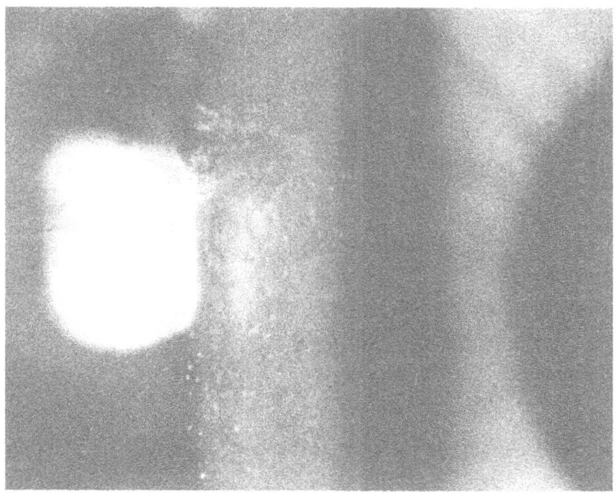

Fig. 3. Cornea guttata of a 60-year-old woman. From left to right, the reflex at the corneal surface, the small prominences of the guttae, and the blurred image of the eye can be distinguished

paired. Stromal and epithelial edema will follow, causing opacification of the cornea and marked decrease of visual acuity.

II. Clinical Changes Detectable by Special Techniques

1. Thickness of the Cornea

Owing to its lamellar structure and its firm mounting in the sclera, the cornea swells only in the direction of its thickness. There is a strong linear correlation between the water content and the thickness of the cornea. Therefore, in vivo measurement of the corneal thickness is a very precise measure of its water content (MISHIMA and HEDBYS 1968). Various authors (MARTOLA and BAUM 1968; KRUSE-HANSEN 1971) have shown that the central corneal thickness in humans is the same throughout life. Only the periphery gets slightly thinner. According

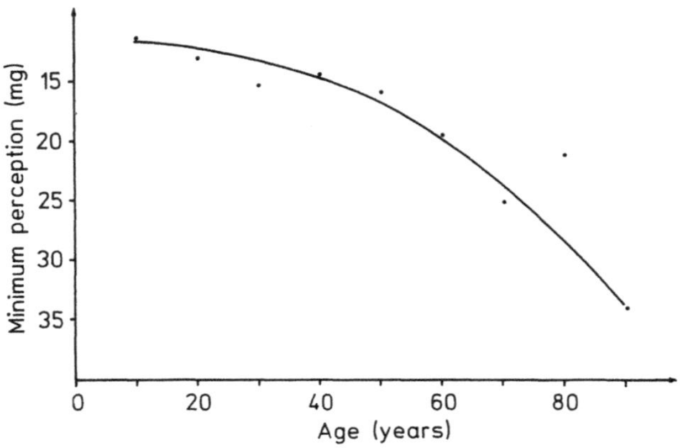

Fig. 4. Relation between corneal sensitivity and age. According to this study, sensitivity decreases with age. (BOBERG-ANS 1956)

to MARTOLA and BAUM (1968), the corneal thickness at the limbus decreases from 0.67 to 0.62 mm between the ages of 40 and 60 years. In 1976 EHLERS et al. found a corneal thickness of 0.54 mm in premature babies as compared with 0.52 mm in older children and adults.

2. Sensitivity of the Cornea

The threshold of sensitivity of the corneal surface is an important diagnostic criterion. It is measured with fine hairs or special stimuli. To define the threshold stimulus, the small surface area of the measuring device, its pressure on the cornea, and the speed of the impact are evaluated. BOBERG-ANS (1956) found an age dependence of corneal sensitivity (Fig. 4).

3. Specular Microscopy of the Endothelium

The development of specular microscopy by D. M. MAURICE (1968) made it possible to view the endothelium in vivo. With this method it is possible to photograph the outline of the endothelial cells, their size, and sometimes even the shadows of the nuclei. The pictures can be evaluated in terms of cell number per unit area, cell size, and cell defects.

a) Number of Cells

The introduction of clinically useful specular microscopes led to a great number of publications on the cellular aspects of the corneal endothelium. In 1978 STURROCK et al. counted the cell numbers in the central cornea and found a linear relationship between cell number and age. The coefficient of correlation in 67 people aged between 13 and 88 years was highly significant (Fig. 5). For the reduction in numbers of endothelial cells with age, OHLSEN (1979) specifies a coefficient of correlation of $r=0.59$, $P=0.01$, $N=76$. The variation, however, was similar to the study of STURROCK et al. (1978) 12%–16%. WILSON and ROPER-HALL (1982) reported similar results (Fig. 6).

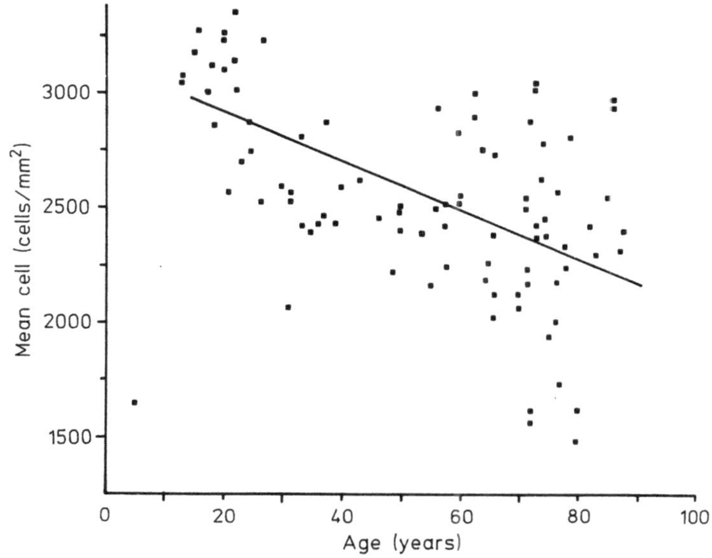

Fig. 5. Relation between endothelial cell count and age. Although the age dependence is obvious, there is no strong correlation owing to the large variation (STURROCK et al. 1978)

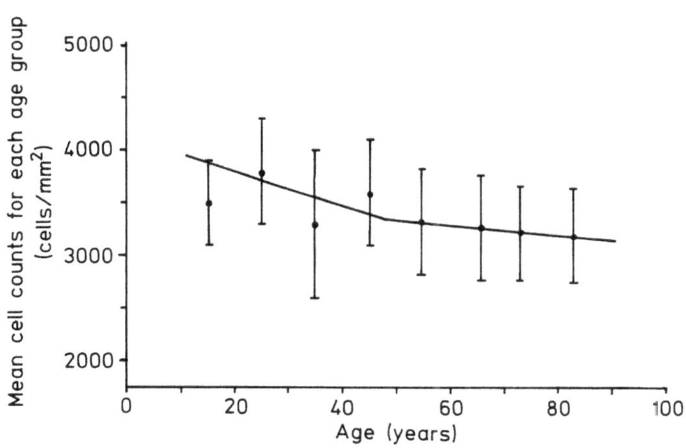

Fig. 6. Relation between endothelial cell count and age, demonstrating the large standard deviation. (WILSON and ROPER-HALL 1982)

b) Cell Distribution

LAING (1976), one of the first designers of a clinical specular microscope, could not demonstrate age dependence of the cell count, but did notice a variation of the cellular areas as viewed with the specular microscope. A similar study on the variation of cell size with age was published by WARING in 1981. Computer-calculated distribution curves of photographically measured endothelial cells of 71 patients aged between 12 and 79 years showed an obvious increase of variation

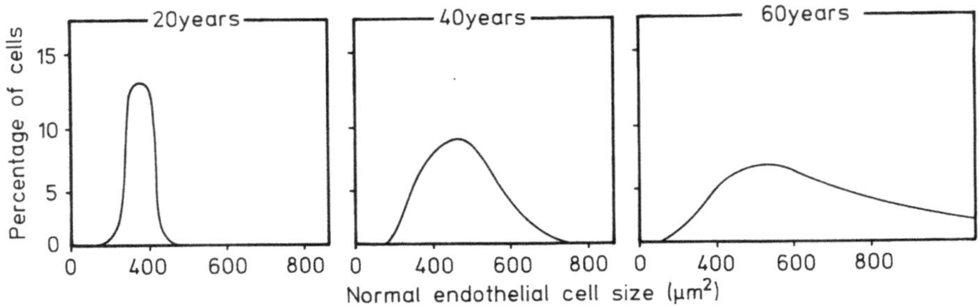

Fig. 7. Variation of cell size at various ages. In young corneas, cells are small and of similar size; with increasing age, cells vary considerably in size. (WARING et al. 1981)

of the area with age. The endothelial cell area of a 20-year-old varies between 200 and 400 µm, of a 40-year-old between 200 and 700 µm, and of a 60-year-old between 200 and 1,100 µm (Fig. 7).

According to these studies, a decrease of the endothelial cell count in the corneal center is statistically proven, but clinically only of minor significance because of its large variation. The age dependence of increasing variation applies only to eyes without accidental or surgical trauma. After contusion, perforation injuries, or intraocular surgery, even in younger people, not only the endothelial cell count decreases, but also clear differences in cell size can be shown.

4. Swelling Properties of the Stroma

Since the corneal swelling in vivo largely depends on the quality of the endothelial barrier function and its active transport of ions and water, the swelling property of the stroma in vivo cannot be examined in terms of age. In vitro, however, the swelling of the cornea can be assessed as a physical property if an excised cornea is placed in water. The thickness increases, the tissue gets turbid, and the weight increases in proportion to the water uptake. In this simple way physical and chemical properties of the macromolecular stromal substance can be measured. In an interesting study, BERAN (1981) was able to prove with a simple experiment that the swelling property of the human cornea decreases significantly with age (Fig. 8). Since in excised corneas the surfaces of the epithelium and endothelium can hardly play their physiologic role, the swelling property in vitro should largely depend on the water-binding properties of the collagen and/or the proteoglycans. The difficulties in measuring chemical changes of old age in macromolecules of the stroma are demonstrated in Sects. B.IV.1. and 2.

5. Regenerative Power of the Epithelium

Clinically, no weakness of the corneal epithelium in old people can be found, even epithelial defects seem to heal in elderly people as fast as in children. In animals MARRE (1967) was able to show, however, that regeneration of epithelial defects in old rabbits is significantly slower than in younger rabbits. Figure 9 shows, however, that the differences are too small to be detected in clinical routine.

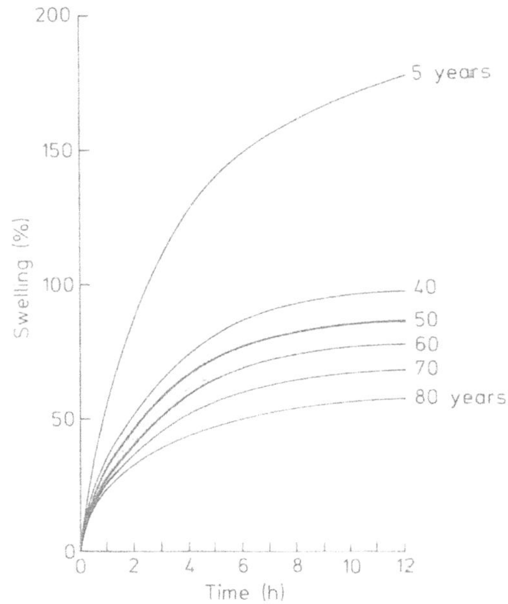

Fig. 8. Swelling property of the corneal stroma as a function of age. In old people, there is less stromal swelling than in children. (BERAN 1981)

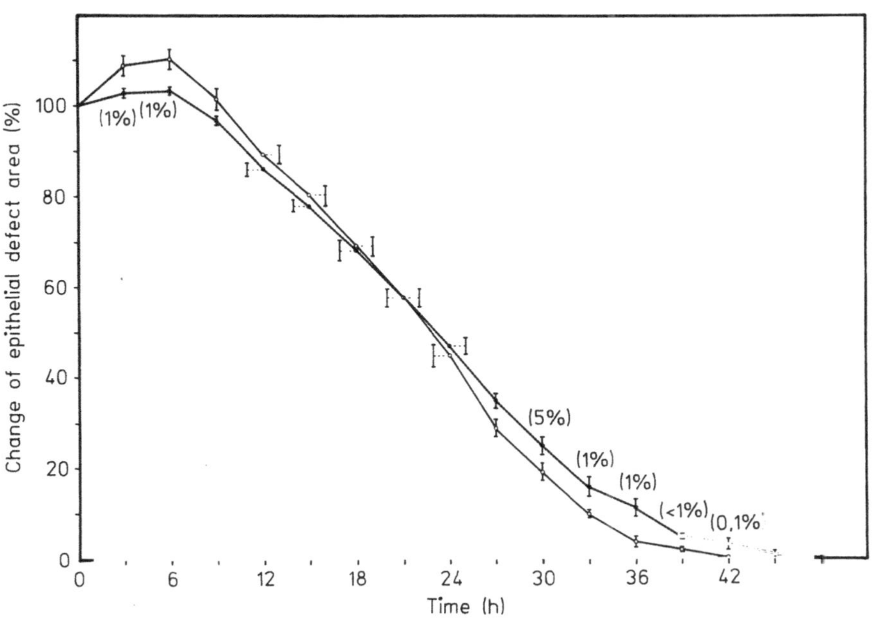

Fig. 9. Course of regeneration of the epithelium after corneal abrasion in young and old rabbits. The difference in speed of regeneration is statistically significant, but small; *t*-test significance levels (%) are shown in parentheses. (MARRE 1967)

6. The Endothelium in Old Donors

Long-term experience with corneal grafts as a routine operation has shown that the cornea of old donors healed as fast and clear as the cornea of younger people. Surgical experience confirms the results, experimentally found by BERAN (1981), that the cornea of older people does not swell as fast as the cornea of younger people. Because of this property, suturing of old corneas has been proven to be easier than handling younger corneas. Critical for the transparency of the graft is the endothelial cell count. Because of its large variation, however, there is always a risk of late decompensation of the cornea of older and younger donors. From the good results with old corneas as graft material, it can be concluded that functional defects of the cornea are not an inevitable consequence of aging.

III. Microscopic Changes in Old Age

1. Descemet's Membrane

The most striking change with age at the back of the cornea is cornea guttata. Microscopic and electron microscopic examination of such corneas shows wart-like excrescences and focal thickening of Descemet's membrane. Over these prominences of homogeneous proteins, the endothelial cells are attenuated. This can result in the decompensation of the endothelium if a great number of guttae is present. Microscopically, these focal thickenings of Descemet's membrane are termed Hassall–Henle bodies. In their book on the histology of the eye, HOGAN et al. (1971) show very impressive microscopic and electron microscopic pictures of these changes. They seem to be of the same material as Descemet's membrane. Descemet's membrane is to be conceived of as the true basement membrane of the corneal endothelium. In healing of corneal wounds that have led to a loss of Descemet's membrane, the formation of a new basement membrane can be seen that resembles the Descemet's membrane in every respect. From this it can be deduced that endothelial cells constantly produce the material for their basement membrane. Therefore, the thickness of Descemet's membrane increases continuously. Recently, ALVARADO and MURPHY (1982) measured an increase of 0.099 μm/year. In youth, the thickness of Descemet's membrane averages 4–6 μm, in older people, 14 μm. WORMER et al. (1979) examined in a histochemical study Descemet's membrane of cattle of different ages with alcian blue and $MgCl_2$. According to their results, a large part of the glycosaminoglycans in young animals consists of chondroitin sulfate. In older age, the inner zone of Descemet's membrane showed a staining indicating an increase of higher sulfated glycosaminoglycans, e.g., keratan sulfate or heparan sulfate. In this connection, it is suggested that with the constant flow of water during physiologic dehydration, glycosaminoglycans are carried from the stroma through the endothelium into the aqueous. Larger molecules like keratan sulfate are said to get caught in the dense collagen structure of Descemet's membrane. The same authors were able to prove by counting the nuclei that the cell count of the endothelium decreases significantly with age. This confirms the specular microscopic findings of Sect. B.II.3.

Table 1. Collagen fibril diameter and interfibrillar distance in the corneal stroma of a 17-year-old and a 63-year-old (POULIQUEN et al. 1984)

	Anterior	Middle	Posterior
Age (years)	Diameter of collagen fibrils (μm)		
17	21.6±0.14	21.0±0.14	21.9±0.09
63	19.6±0.14	20.6±0.15	21.3±0.16
	Interfibrillar distance (μm)		
17	43.5±0.35	44.2±0.29	43.7±0.24
63	38.5±0.34	41.9±0.37	44.1±0.42

2. Basement Membrane of the Epithelium

In the study of ALVARADO and MURPHY (1982), an increase of thickness with age was also proven for the basement membrane of the epithelium. While the thickness of the corneal epithelium itself staid the same at 54 μm in all ages, the basement membrane of the epithelium increased from 0.2 μm at 10 years to 0.6 μm at 90 years. At birth, the basement membrane of the epithelium appeared electron microscopically to be made of one single lamella. In older age, however, several fine layers superimposed in the basement membrane of the corneal epithelium could be differentiated.

3. Collagen Fibrils

ALVARADO and MURPHY (1982) found a constant thickness of Bowman's membrane and of the corneal stroma throughout life. Electron microscopically, the corneal stroma did not show any marked difference in the composition of the ground substance. KANAI and KAUFMANN (1973), however, were able to observe a decreased interfibrillar distance within the stroma in older age while the thickness of the fibrils staid the same.

Recently, POULIQUEN et al. (1984) reported data computed from the corneal stroma of a young and an old human individual, investigated with the electron microscope (Table 1). Their results clearly show that, in the corneal stroma, the diameter of the fibrils as well as the interfibrillar distance decrease with age.

However, based on his long-term experience in the field D. GRAF KEYSERLINGK (1983, personal communication) confirms that up to now there is no electron microscopic evidence of aging changes of the stroma. Therefore, in this context all findings must be judged with care because fixation of stroma can easily produce artifacts.

IV. Biochemical Changes in Old Age

1. Collagen

In many electron microscopic studies of the corneal stroma, it is repeatedly emphasized how even and homogeneous the collagen fibrils are at all ages. There-

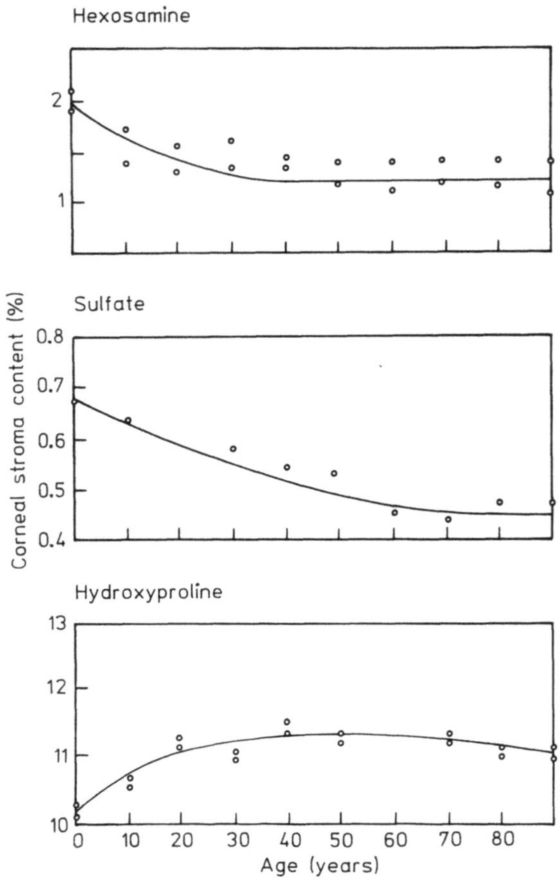

Fig. 10. Relation between hexosamine, sulfate, and hydroxyproline in the human corneal stroma and age. Decrease of hexosamine and sulfate and increase of hydroxyproline is evident. (BUDDECKE and WOLLENSAK 1966)

fore, it is not surprising that there are hardly any publications on the biochemical changes of the collagen matrix during aging. DARDENNE et al. (1968) were able to verify, by chemical analysis of cattle corneas, an increasing cross-linking of corneal collagen with age. A slight increase of hydroxyproline content was found by BUDDECKE and WOLLENSAK (1966) in 18 human corneas aged between 1 and 80 years (Fig. 10).

2. Glycosaminoglycans

Proteoglycans play an important role in the intercellular substance of the stroma because of the extremely regular and constant diameter of their molecules. Based on these properties, they seem to maintain the constant spacing between the collagen fibrils of the stroma to a great extent. While the chemical composition and special arrangement of the protein portion of the proteoglycans was discovered only recently (KELLER 1982), the glycosaminoglycan portion of the proteoglycans has been known for many years to show changes with age. ANSETH (1961) found that the chondroitin and keratan sulfate fractions in chicken and cattle change with increasing age. In calves, there was a glucosamine/galactosamine quotient of 1.2 and in older cattle of 1.8, indicating a relative increase of keratan sulfate over chondroitin sulfate. Analysis of different fractions revealed a decrease with age of the sulfate content in the condroitin fraction while there was an increase in the sulfate content of the keratan fraction. The studies of STUHLSATZ et al. (1974) also show that, in the cornea of older cattle as compared with calves, the content of keratan sulfate is higher than that of chondroitin sulfate and that the sulfation of the keratan fraction reaches higher values in older age.

In humans, the content of glycosaminoglycans and sulfates tends to decrease with age, as studies by BUDDECKE and WOLLENSAK (1966) suggest (Fig. 10). They found quite a constant relation between keratan sulfate and chondroitin sulfate in all age groups. Nevertheless, they considered the differences between newborn and old people remarkable. In newborn babies, they found very low sulfate content, but high values of chondroitin. In old age, the keratan sulfate content was highest with a high degree of sulfation. Compared with other glycosaminoglycan-containing tissues, the changes due to age in the cornea can be considered insignificant. BUDDECKE and WOLLENSAK (1966) also point at the relatively low metabolism of glycosaminoglycans in the cornea as described by DOHLMAN et al. (1965). According to the latter study the metabolism of radioactive sulfate, *N*-acetetyl-glucosamine, glucose, and galactose in the glycosaminoglycans of calves and older cattle were equally high. Apparently there was no age dependence in the metabolism of these substances.

STUHLSATZ and KELLER (1982) also discovered age dependence of the enzymes that help to synthesize glycosaminoglycans in the corneal stroma. Experimentally, a 2.6-fold activity of 3-phosphoadenylsulfate glucosaminesulfotransferase was found in the cornea of calves as compared with older cattle. With physiologic concentrations of the substrate, this enzyme proved to be seven times as high in the calf cornea. This finding could explain why there is a higher sulfation of condroitin in calf corneas than in those of older animals. An error in the transfer of information from the messenger RNA during the synthesis of specific enzyme proteins is discussed by STUHLSATZ (1974) as the cause for the decrease of the activity of glycosaminoglycansulfotransferase.

3. Lipids, Physical and Chemical Explanation of Arcus Senilis

Measurements of lipids in the cornea were described by ANDREWS (1962). He was able to detect all lipid fractions, although in lower concentrations, and in the arcus senilis, he found mostly cholesterol esters.

a) Lipid Spectra

In 1966 TSCHETTER published an analysis of lipid fractions of human corneas by means of gas chromatography. In nine eyes without arcus senilis aged between 40 and 72 years, he found 282–540 μg phospholipids in both corneas of one person, increasing with age. The content of cholesterol ranged between 64 and 360 μg. The higher values were found in older eyes. The glycerides in the human cor-

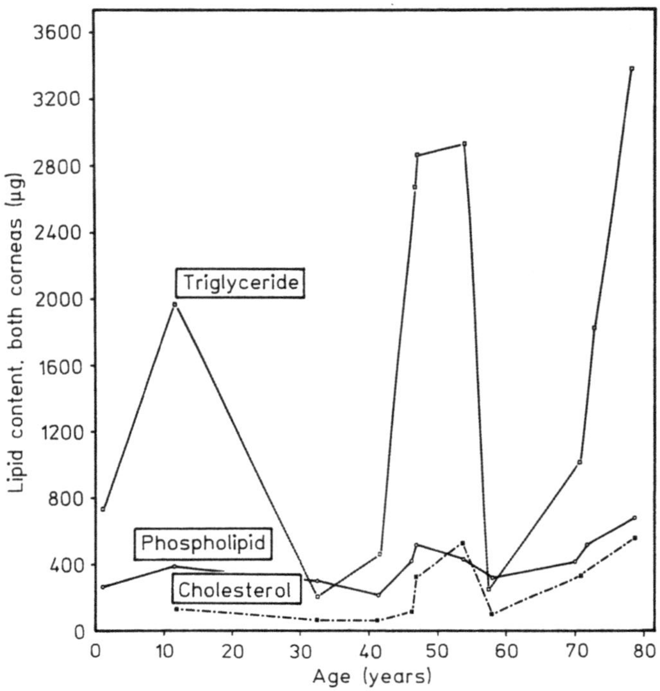

Fig. 11. Lipid content of the human cornea as a function of age. The *circled* values are very high and concern corneas with an especially marked arcus senilis. In general, there is a tendency to increasing corneal lipids with age. (TSCHETTER 1966)

nea weighed between 216 and 2,950 μg per cornea without any significant age dependence (Fig. 11). In one pair of corneas of a 45-year-old, 462 μg phospholipids, 553 μg cholesterol, and 3,044 μg glycerides were found. In one 70-year-old with a more pronounced arcus senilis the analysis disclosed 696 μg phospholipids, 607 μg cholesterol, and 3,517 μg glycerides. TSCHETTER (1966) also specified the chain length of the fatty acids of the corneal lipids, but there were neither remarkable values in the arcus senilis nor any age dependence.

b) Precipitation of Lipoproteins

Considering the etiology of the arcus senilis the study by POST (1966) is to be mentioned. In sophisticated experiments with gel difussion, the assumption was confirmed that the arcus senilis can result from precipitation of lipoproteins by the glycosaminoglycans in the cornea.

c) Arcus Senilis and the Blood Level of Lipoproteins

A correlation between the occurrence of an arcus senilis and hyperlipemia and hyperlipoproteinemia, respectively, has long been known. A good survey of the literature was published by THIEL et al. (1975). In this study of 60 patients with arcus

Table 2. Incidence of arcus senilis as a function of age (Jäger and Eisenhauer 1977)

Age (years)	11–20	21–30	31–40	41–50	51–60	61–70
Incidence (%)	17	75	87	82	90	100

senilis, a type II hyperlipoproteinemia was found. Jäger and Eisenhauer (1977) examined 63 patients with hyperlipoproteinemia type II. In young patients aged between 10 and 20 years, an arcus senilis was encountered in only 17%. In the higher age groups, the incidence of arcus senilis increased to 100% after the age of 60 years (Table 2).

According to these studies, the arcus senilis is a typical change of aging. If the arcus senilis is discovered at younger ages, a disorder of lipid metabolism must be suspected. According to Fielder et al. (1981), the arcus senilis starts in the warmer parts of the cornea, where it is also more pronounced. In this area the cornea is covered by the eyelids.

4. Metabolism

Changes due to age of low molecular weight substances and enzyme activities have not yet been described.

V. Diseases of the Cornea Not Specific for Old Age

H. J. Thiel (1981) names a number of entities typical of old age that cannot be considered physiologic:

Corneal ulcer
Marginal ulcer
Terrien marginal degeneration
Salzmann nodular degeneration
Viral keratitis
Pterygium
Mooren ulcer
Lipid keratopathy
Hyaloid degeneration of the cornea

References

Alvarado J, Murphy C (1982) Histological determination of the normal human corneal dimensions as a function of age. Invest Ophthalmol Vis Sci 22:37

Andrews JS (1962) The lipids of arcus senitis. Arch Ophthalmol 68:264–268

Anseth A (1961) Glycosaminoglycans in the developing corneal stroma. Exp Eye Res 1:116–121

Beran V (1981) Age and the swelling of the cornea. In: Trevor-Roper P (ed) The cornea in health and disease. Academic, London, pp 445–448

Boberg-Ans J (1956) On the corneal sensibility. Acta Ophthalmol (Kbh) 34:149–162

Buddecke E, Wollensak J (1966) Saure Mukopolisaccharide und Glykoproteine der menschlichen Cornea in Abhängigkeit vom Lebensalter und bei Keratokonus. Av Graefes Arch Klin Exp Ophthalmol 171:105–120
Dardenne MU, Iwangoff T, Diotallevi M (1968) Unterschiede im Verhalten des Kollagens der einzelnen Hornhautschichten mit zunehmendem Lebensalter. Ophthalmologica 156:385–393
Dohlman CH, Wortman B, Hultman S (1965) Incorporation of sulfate-S,N-Acetylglucosamin-1-C, Glucose-1-C, and Galactose-1-C into calf and beef corneal glycosaminglycan. Invest Ophthalmol 4:867–871
Duke-Elder (1965) Age changes of the cornea. In: Duke-Elder S (ed) System of ophthalmology, vol 8. Kimpton, London, pp 867–880
Ehlers N, Soerensen T, Brahmsen T, Poulsen EH (1976) Central corneal thickness in new borns and children. Acta Ophthalmol 54:285–290
Fielder AR, Winder AF, Cooke DE, Bowcock SA (1981) Arcus senilis and corneal temperatures in man. In: Trevor-Roper P (ed) The cornea in health and disease. Academic, London, pp 1015–1020
Hogan MJ, Alvarado JA, Weddell JE (1971) Histology of the human eye. Saunders, Philadelphia, pp 98–100
Jäger W, Eisenhauer GG (1977) Der diagnostische Wert des Arcus corneae als Hinweis auf Lipidstoffwechselstörungen. Klin Monatsbl Augenheilkd 171:321–330
Kanai A, Kaufmann HE (1973) Electron microscopic studies of corneal stroma. Aging changes of collagen fibres. Ann Ophthalmol 5:285–291
Keller R (1982) Zur Regulation der Biosynthese des cornealen Proteokeratansulfats. Dissertation University of Aachen
Kruse-Hansen F (1971) A clinical study of the normal human central corneal thickness. Acta Ophthalmol 49:82–89
Laing RA, Sandstrom MM, Berrospi AR, Leibovitz HM (1976) Changes in the corneal endothelium as a function of age. Exp Eye Res 22:587–594
Machemer R, Süchting P, Schuster R (1965) Die Einwirkung von Betastrahlen auf die DNS-Synthese und die Mitosetätigkeit am Epithel der Rattencornea. Av Graefes Arch Ophthalmol 168:489–501
Marre M (1967) Zur Altersabhängigkeit der Heilung von Hornhautepitheldefekten. Av Graefes Arch Klin Exp Ophthalmol 173:250–255
Martola EL, Baum JL (1968) Central and peripheral corneal thickness. Arch Ophthalmol 79:28–30
Maurice DM (1968) Cellular membrane activity in the corneal endothelium of the intact eye. Experientia 24:1094–1095
Mishima S, Hedbys BO (1968) Measurement of corneal thickness with the Haag Streit Pachometer. Arch Ophthalmol 80:710–715
Olsen T (1979) Non-contact specular microscopy of human corneal endothelium. Acta Ophthalmol 57:986–998
Post D (1966) Modellversuche zur Entstehung des Arcus lipoides corneae im Geldiffusionsversuch nach Ouchterlony. Av Graefes Arch Klin Exp Ophthalmol 170:123–136
Pouliquen Y, Patey A, Savoldelli M (1984) The use of covariance in the achievement of the characterisation of normal and keratoconus cornea. Ophthalmol Res (in press)
Reim M (1972) Warum ist die Cornea durchsichtig? Ber Zusammenkunft Dtsch Ophthalmol Ges 71:58–77
Reim M (1982) Die Bedeutung des Limbus für Ernährung der Cornea. In: Doden W (ed) Limbusprobleme, Studien zur Pathophysiologie des Limbus corneae. Enke, Stuttgart, pp 1–7
Rohen JW (1964) Das Auge und seine Hilfsorgane. Springer, Berlin Heidelberg New York (Handbuch der mikroskopischen Anatomie, vol 3/4)
Stuhlsatz HW, Muthiah P, Kaneko M, Momburg M, Greiling H (1974) Untersuchungen zur Struktur und Biosynthese der Cornea Proteoglykane des Kalbes und des Rindes. In: Platt (ed) Experimentelle Gerontologie. Fischer, Stuttgart, pp 117–131
Sturrock GD, Sherrard ES, Rice NSC (1978) Specular microscopy of the corneal endothelium. Br J Ophthalmol 62:809–814

Thiel HJ (1981) Altersveränderungen der Hornhaut. In: Francois J, Hollwich F (eds) Augenheilkunde in Klinik und Praxis. Thieme, Stuttgart, Chaps 2.2–2.10
Thiel HJ, Parwaresch R, Godt C (1975) Arcus corneae und Störungen des Fettstoffwechsels. Ber Rhein Westf Augenärzte 130:69–73
Tschetter RT (1966) Lipid analysis of the human cornea with and without Arcus senilis. Arch Ophthalmol 76:403–405
Vogt A (1930) Lehrbuch und Atlas der Spaltlampenmikroskopie des lebenden Auges. Springer, Berlin, pp 65–107
Waring III GO, Georgia A, Ford GE, Krohn M, Rosenblatt LS (1981) Individual corneal endothelial cell changes with age. A specular microscopic study. In: Trevor-Roper E (ed) The cornea in health and disease. Academic, London, pp 75–77
Wilson RS, Roper-Hall NJ (1982) Effect of age on the endothelial cell count in the normal eye. Br J Ophthalmol 66:513–515
Wormer W, Sames K, Rohen JW (1979) Histochemische Untersuchungen über Struktur und Altersveränderungen des Descemet'schen Membran beim Rind. Av Graefes Arch Klin Exp Ophthalmol 211:271–278

Age-Related Changes in the Anterior Segment of the Eye

J. W. ROHEN and E. LÜTJEN-DRECOLL

A. Introduction

In general, the tissues of the anterior segment of the eye undergo the same aging processes which take place in the organism as a whole. However, the special role of the eye as a device for optical function has led to the development of specialized mechanisms which, in some places, may also inhibit or even prevent common aging processes. This inhibition of age-related degeneration in certain constituents of the connective tissue may prevent early dysfunction in this important sensory organ. Such dysfunction may be more critical on the survival of the organism than comparable aging processes in the skin or bones; e.g., the maintenance of corneal transparency and a constant intraocular pressure are of fundamental biologic importance. The corneal transparency depends on a continuous process of dehydration and a certain degree of "nonaging" of the connective tissue found in the corneal stroma (cf. Sect. B. I). With respect to intraocular pressure maintenance, it appears that the age-related increase in outflow resistance is counteracted by a simultaneous decrease in aqueous formation. This may be the means by which the tissues of the ciliary body and the chamber angle maintain a fairly constant intraocular pressure during life. Similar interrelated processes may also develop at other sites of the eye (Fig. 1). Thus, aging in the eye cannot be considered an isolated, uniformly developing degenerative process. Rather, it is a complicated process of structural and biologic changes of interrelated functional systems whereby systems may compensate for changes occurring in a neighboring system and vice versa. We are far from a real pathologic or gerontologic understanding of such interrelations and functional mechanisms.

B. Cornea

The five-layer *epithelium* of the cornea has a very regular structure with a total thickness of about 50 μm. The surface of the superficial cell layer is covered with microplicae and microvilli which enable the tear film to remain attached to the eyeball. The turnover time of the corneal epithelium has been estimated to be 7–8 days (HANNA et al. 1961). It seems to become longer with increasing age.

The basal lamina and basement membrane of the corneal epithelium can clearly be differentiated from Bowman's membrane. They demonstrate the typical staining characteristics of subepithelial basement membranes (TENG and KATZIN 1953; CALMETTES et al. 1956; GRAUMANN and ROHEN 1958). In contrast, Bow-

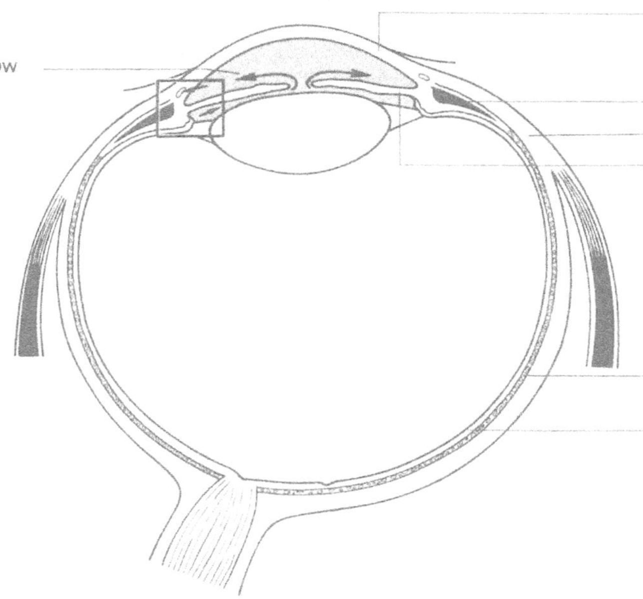

Fig. 1. Horizontal section through the human eye (schematic drawing). *Arrows* direction of aqueous flow; *rectangle* chamber angle region with anterior part of ciliary body and iris root

man's membrane is not a basement membrane, but rather a modified stroma layer. It is composed almost entirely of collagenous and other fibrils of connective tissue, which form a very tight, but irregularly arranged network. This network is embedded in a ground substance rich in acid glycosaminoglycans and glycoproteins. There are no cells and no elastic fibers within this layer. The border to the stroma layer is not distinct. Histochemically, a gradual change in staining characteristics can be seen.

I. Stroma

The corneal stroma is composed almost entirely of collagenous lamellae containing fibroblasts (keratocytes) and nonfibrillar interstitial substances. The 200–250 lamellae consist of densely packed collagenous fibers revealing a very regular pattern throughout the cornea (SCHWARZ 1972; BASHEY and KERN 1972). The parallel collagenous fibrils bundled within the lamellae are uniform in size and spacing. The interfibrillar spaces are filled with a cementing substance (matrix), which appears especially rich in glycosaminoglycans. The diameter of the collagenous fibrils remains relatively constant throughout life, varying between 210 and 360 Å (KAYES and HOLMBERG 1960; JAKUS 1961; SCHWARZ 1953, 1972; SCHWARZ and KEYSERLINGK 1969; SCHWARZ et al. 1966). Conversely, the collagenous fibers of the sclera gradually thicken with age (SCHWARZ et al. 1966; ROHEN and LÜTJEN-

DRECOLL 1981; LÜTJEN-DRECOLL et al. 1982). Although thickening of collagenous fibers does not necessarily mean "aging" of such fibrils (cf. VIIDIK 1979) there are also some other characteristics of corneal collagen which suggest that these fibrils remain in a relatively "young" stage.

SCHWARZ (1953, 1972) observed that the corneal collagenous fibrils always exhibit characteristics of "embryonic" or very young fibrils after the use of silver impregnation methods, so that the normal aging process seems to be inhibited in this type of tissue. This phenomenon can be considered to be of principal importance (cf. ROHEN and LÜTJEN-DRECOLL 1981), and raises the question of why the aging process of collagenous material of the cornea is slower or absent when compared with aging in the sclera or skin. The rapid thickening or ripening of the collagenous fibrils which occurs when the matrix is destroyed, e.g., following corneal wounds or during repair of this tissue (SCHWARZ and KEYSERLINGK 1969), strongly suggests that both the composition and the arrangement of the extracellular matrix are largely responsible for this "nonaging" of the corneal collagen.

The corneal stroma contains large amounts of glycosaminoglycans, which are specifically dehydrated by the underlying endothelial cell layer. This continual dehydration, the sequestration of the collagenous fiber bundles within a homogeneous mass of glycoproteins, and the low metabolic turnover rate of the stroma are clearly essential factors in the maintenance of corneal transparency. The net effect is that the extracellular material is kept in a relatively young stage of development, i.e., aging is nearly, or perhaps completely, arrested in this part of the eye. In this regard it is of interest that GREILING et al. (1976) did not find any of the age-dependent changes in the activity of certain enzymes of bovine cornea (glycosyltransferase, etc.) which are usually associated with aging processes in connective tissues.

Distinct from the nonaging of the corneal stroma, other ocular tissues clearly demonstrate age-related changes. After the age of 50 years, white deposits have often been observed which are located between the stromal lamellae of the ground substance of the most peripheral corneal stroma (within the limbus area at the border of the sclera). These deposits usually form a spherical ring near Bowman's layer and occur simultaneously in both eyes (arcus senilis, arcus lipoides, gerontoxon). They consist predominantly of cholesterol, phospholipids, and triglycerides (COGAN and KUWABARA 1959). The causes of these changes are not clear. Possibly, the mechanisms of the "nonaging" process in the central part of the corneal stroma are insufficient at its periphery, namely in the transitional zone of the limbus. This may be especially pronounced in cases of general metabolic disturbances, such as hyperlipoproteinemia (JAEGER and EISENHAUER 1977).

II. Descemet's Membrane

In complete contrast to the "nonaging" of the corneal stroma. Descemet's membrane which is often considered to be a basement membrane-like structure, changes substantially with age. This membrane gradually becomes thicker and also changes its chemical composition (DARDENNE et al. 1968; WORMER et al. 1979). According to BRINI (1957), the diameter of Descemet's membrane increases from 3.7 μm (0–10 years), to 4.7 μm (11–20 years), to 5.3–5.9 μm (21–80 years). Ho-

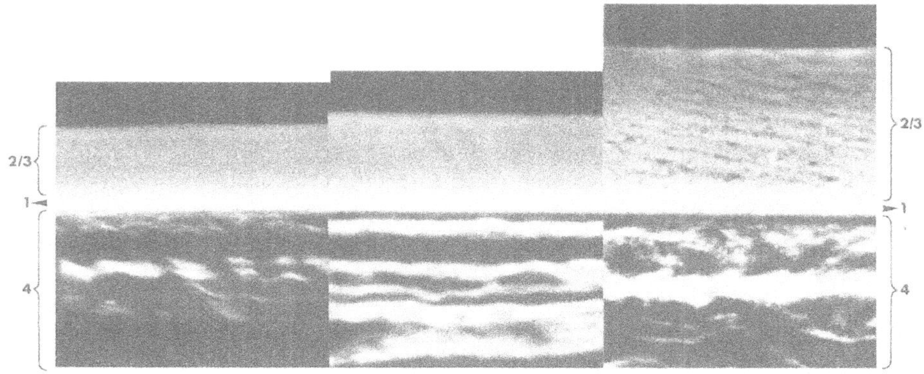

Fig. 2. Descemet's membrane of cows of different ages (1.5, 7 and 12 years; polarized light). 1 = zone 1; $^2/_3$ = zone 2 and 3, 4 = stroma corneae. Note the marked increase in the diameter of Descemet's membrane and the development of lamellation with age. × 960 (After WORMER et al. 1979)

GAN et al. (1971) stated that the thickness of this membrane increases to 10–12 μm during adult life.

Several studies have shown that Descemet's membrane is formed by a number of regularly arranged stratified layers (BAIRATI and GRIGNOLO 1954; JAKUS 1956, 1961; FEENY and GARRON 1961; KAYE and PAPPAS 1962; ROHEN 1964). With histochemical methods, Descement's membrane stained intensively with periodic acid–Schiff reagent, except for a small subendothelial line which revealed other staining characteristics (e.g., positive staining with alcian blue). This subendothelial layer could be separated completely from the remaining portion of the membrane (GRAUMAN and ROHEN 1958).

In a more recent histochemical study in cows of different ages, we showed that not only does the diameter of the entire Descemet's membrane increase (Fig. 2), but that the composition and distribution of glycosaminoglycans within this membrane change markedly with increasing age (WORMER et al. 1979). In contrast to younger age groups, the aged Descemet's membrane contains large amounts of alcian blue-positive material in its outer portions. Histochemical analysis showed that this material is probably heparan and/or keratan sulfate.

As a result of the aging processes, a characteristic lamellation of Descemet's membrane develops in higher age groups, ultimately leading to separation into three readily identifiable zones. Zone 1 borders on the stroma and usually appears as a thin line; its diameter does not change substantially with age. Zone 3 is located underneath the endothelium and thickens continuously with age. However, this zone does not stain intensively with alcian blue and seems to have an especially high content of sulfated glycosaminoglycans. The increasing incorporation of these substances in the outer layer of zone 2 may be one of the key factors involved in the thickening of Descemet's membrane as a whole.

These observations allow the tentative conclusion that the gradual accretion of mucoproteins within the outer part of Descemet's membrane may be a side effect of the continuous transport of fluid through the endothelial lining. In the course of stromal dehydration, the larger molecules may be retained within Descemet's membrane and thereby cause its age-dependent thickening. It then appears likely that the nonaging of the stroma is dependent on concomitant aging of its basal lamina, that is, one process takes place at the expense of the other. In persons over the age of 30 years, the outermost part of Descemet's membrane regularly shows periodic thickening, protruding into the anterior chamber (so-called Hassall–Henle warts). In these areas, atypical collagen, such as curly collagen, lattice collagen, or long spacing collagen, as well as irregular fissures filled with cytoplasmic processes or debris have been observed (FEENY and GARRON 1961; ROHEN 1962, 1964; JAKUS 1956, 1961). These seem to become more numerous in advanced age groups, although no quantitative evaluation has been performed to date.

The so-called Schwalbe's line does not develop from Descemet's membrane. This ring-like structure consists of equatorially arranged collagenous fiber bundles and ground substance which cover Descemet's membrane at its outermost periphery, thereby protruding into the anterior chamber. As far as is known, the formation of this tissue, which often contains atypical collagen and other atypical extracellular material, is not age-related.

III. Corneal Endothelium

A number of studies have been conducted on age-related changes in cellularity of this layer (BOURNE and KAUFMANN 1976; LAULE et al. 1978; BLATT et al. 1979; BIGAR 1982) In lower mammals (rabbits, rats, etc.), the endothelial cells located at the far periphery of the cornea are mitotically active throughout life (cf. ENKE and ROHEN 1983). After injury or cell loss, the peripheral cells begin to divide, usually beginning with amitotic divisions, which are followed by mitotic divisions. The newly formed cells then migrate into the wounded area, replacing the injured and nonviable cells (ENKE and ROHEN 1983).

In higher primates and humans, this regenerative capacity of the peripheral corneal endothelial cells seems to be lost. With increasing age, there is a loss of cellularity in this cell layer, which is no longer compensated by cell division, but rather by the spread of neighboring cells, which fill the gaps between the degenerated cells (KAUFMAN et al. 1966). In higher age groups, not only is the number of cells reduced, but also the shape and form of the cells appear irregular and uneven (Table 1). Between the normal cells, greatly enlarged, polygonal cells are seen, which often contain two or more nuclei (BIGAR 1982; ALVARADO et al. 1981).

Corneal dehydration results from an energy-consuming active transport of fluid out of the stroma. Experimental studies have shown that the endothelium of the cornea is essential for fluid transport and possesses the organelles and enzymes necessary to carry out this function. Two of these enzymes, namely Na^+, K^+-ATPase, and carbonic anhydrase, have been demonstrated histochemically whithin the corneal endothelium where they are found in larger quantities (for review see LÜTJEN-DRECOLL et al. 1981, 1983). The possibility of age-related changes in the amount of these enzymes in the endothelial cells has not been well explored.

Table 1. Cell density and cell area of human corneal epithelium in four different age groups (after BIGAR 1982)

Age (years)	2	6	50	101
Mean cell density (mm^{-2})	3.777	2.845	2.230	2.088
Mean cell area ± standard deviation (μm^2)	265 ± 61	351 ± 74	448 ± 130	479 ± 148

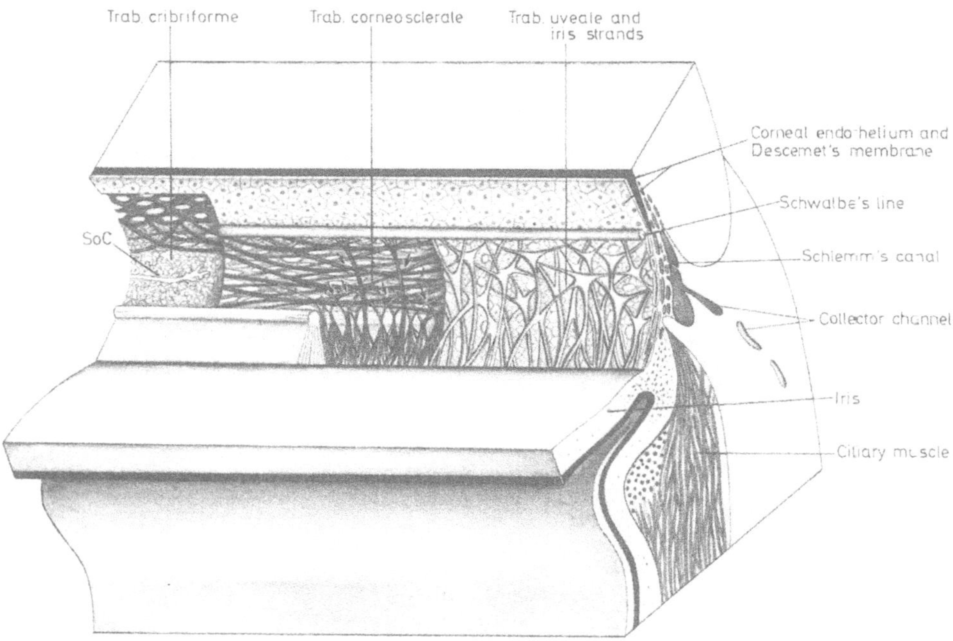

Fig. 3. Architecture of the trabecular meshwork in the human eye. *Arrows* anterior tendons of ciliary muscle. SoC = Sondermann's channel. (After ROHEN and UNGER 1959)

C. Trabecular Meshwork

In the human eye, the trabecular meshwork is located in front of Schlemm's canal and filters the aqueous humor. It consists of a complicated system of flat interlacing sheets, the so-called trabecular lamellae, and a somewhat more irregularly arranged connective tissue, rich in fibroblast-like endothelial cells underlying Schlemm's canal (Fig. 3). The aqueous humor passes through the intertrabecular spaces and enters the canal by way of small intracellular microchannels or vacuoles located within the endothelial lining of Schlemm's canal itself. Three portions of the trabecular meshwork may be distinguished: The outermost part, just underneath Schlemm's canal, is called the juxtacanalicular zone or cribriform layer. The central and largest portion is the corneoscleral meshwork and is arranged predominantly in sheet-like lamellae, completely covered by endothelial

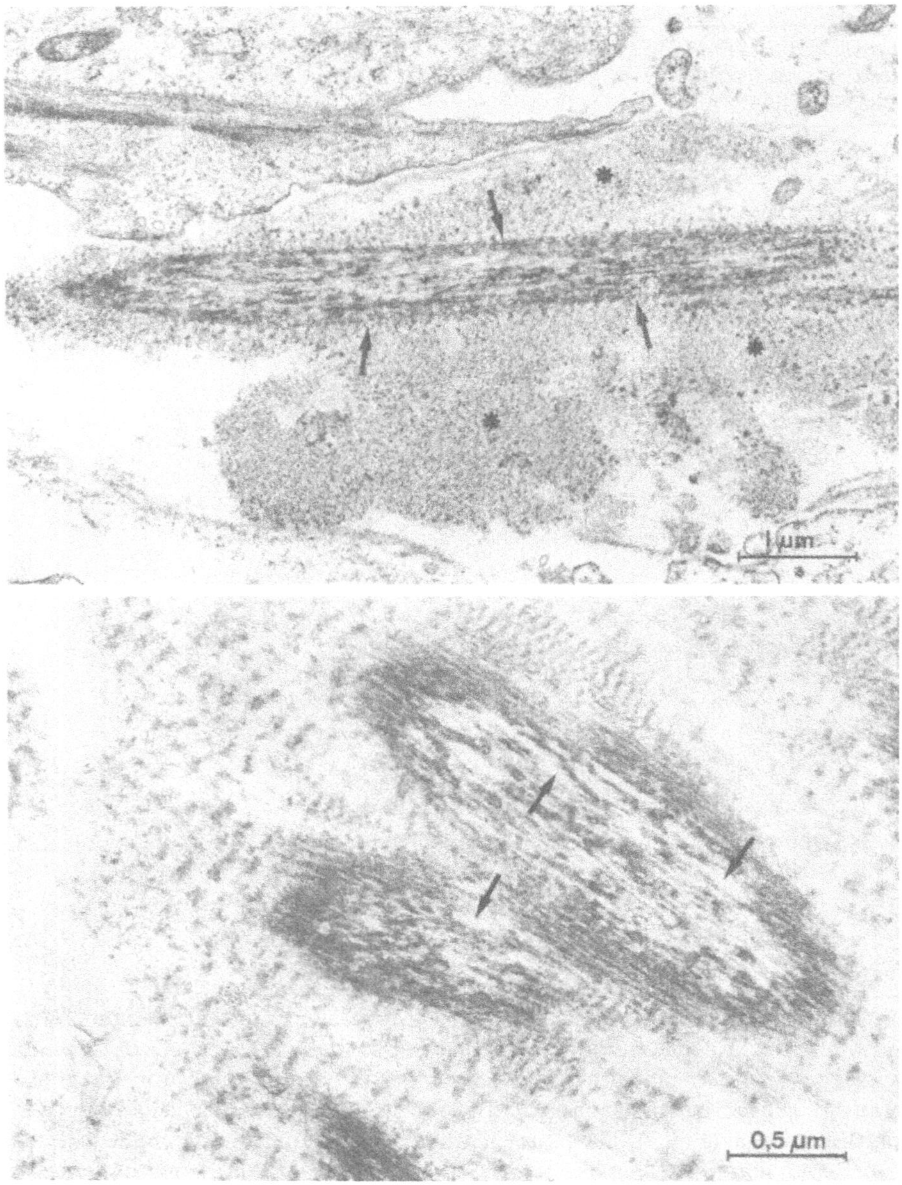

a

b

Fig. 4 a, b. Electron micrograph of sections through elastic-like fibers of the trabecular meshwork of a 66-year-old patient, **a** after incubation with alcian blue. Note the homogeneous sheath material (*asterisks*) surrounding the electrondense core of the elastic-like fiber (*arrows*); **b** after incubation with pancreatic elastase. Note, only the weakly osmiophilic strands within the fiber core are digested (*arrows*). (After LÜTJEN-DRECOLL et al. 1981) cells. The third portion, the uveal meshwork, consists of roundish, irregular tissue strands and comprises the innermost part of the trabecular meshwork. The central core of the trabecular lamellae consists of ground substance rich in glycosaminoglycans, collagenous and elastic-like fibers, and basement membrane material.

The diameter of the collagenous fibrils of the trabecular meshwork remains relatively constant throughout life, in contrast to the fibers of the scleral collagen. In the 6-year-old eye, the maximum diameter of the scleral collagen is 105 nm. In contrast, the diameter of the collagenous fibers in the cribriform and corneoscleral meshwork varies between 5 and 30 nm. There is no age-related increase in the thickness and appearance of the collagenous fibers in the trabecular meshwork. This is not so in the elastic material (ROHEN et al. 1981; LÜTJEN-DRECOLL et al. 1982).

Normal elastic fibers, such as seen in Bruch's membrane, consist of elastin which can be completely digested by pancreatic elastase, and are surrounded by a thin osmiophilic layer of specific fibrils embedded in a matrix. In the trabecular meshwork, however, elastase digests only small nonosmiophilic strands running within the center of the fiber (Fig. 4). The main body of the fiber is osmiophilic and resistant to elastase (LÜTJEN-DRECOLL et al. 1981). The elastic fibers of the trabecular meshwork are therefore specific fibers, which we call elastic-like fibers. The entire fiber is surrounded by a sheath, consisting of homogeneous material and very fine fibrils, which appear cross-banded with a periodicity of either 50 or 100–120 nm. This periodic material is embedded in glycosaminoglycans, mainly chondroitin sulfates (LÜTJEN-DRECOLL et al. 1981, 1982). The diameter of the central core of the elastic-like fibers remains constant throughout life, whereas the sheath thickness increases markedly with age. Mesurements based on cross sections have shown that in old eyes (older than 50 years) the thickness is nearly three times that of young eyes (2–20 years) (LÜTJEN-DRECOLL et al. 1982).

I. Trabecular Beams

The trabecular sheets are covered by a basement membrane-like structure which is continuous with Descemet's membrane (cf. ROHEN 1964; VAN DER ZYPEN 1971). This subendothelial membrane becomes intensely fluorescent with antibodies against collagen type IV or antilaminin. The most intense fluorescence is seen in the small zone immediately underneath the trabecular endothelial lining, which might be the true basal lamina. The innermost so-called glass-membranes and the central core of the trabecular beam show little or no fluorescence (LÜTJEN-DRECOLL et al. 1982). These results suggest that the homogeneous subendothelial membranes of the trabecular lamellae most probably consist of two different sheaths, a small subendothelial basal lamina and a thicker glass-membrane. With increasing age as well as in certain diseases (diabetes, chronic simple glaucoma), these membranes thicken substantially (Fig. 5). This thickening is primarily due to an increase in the glass-membranes as shown by immunofluorescent studies (RODRIGUES et al. 1976; LÜTJEN-DRECOLL et al. 1982). It often appears unevenly distributed, forming small dots or knots. Electron microscopically, the thickened membranes as well as the central core of the trabecular lamellae show clusters of long spacing or lattice (curly) collagen, which become especially numerous in old

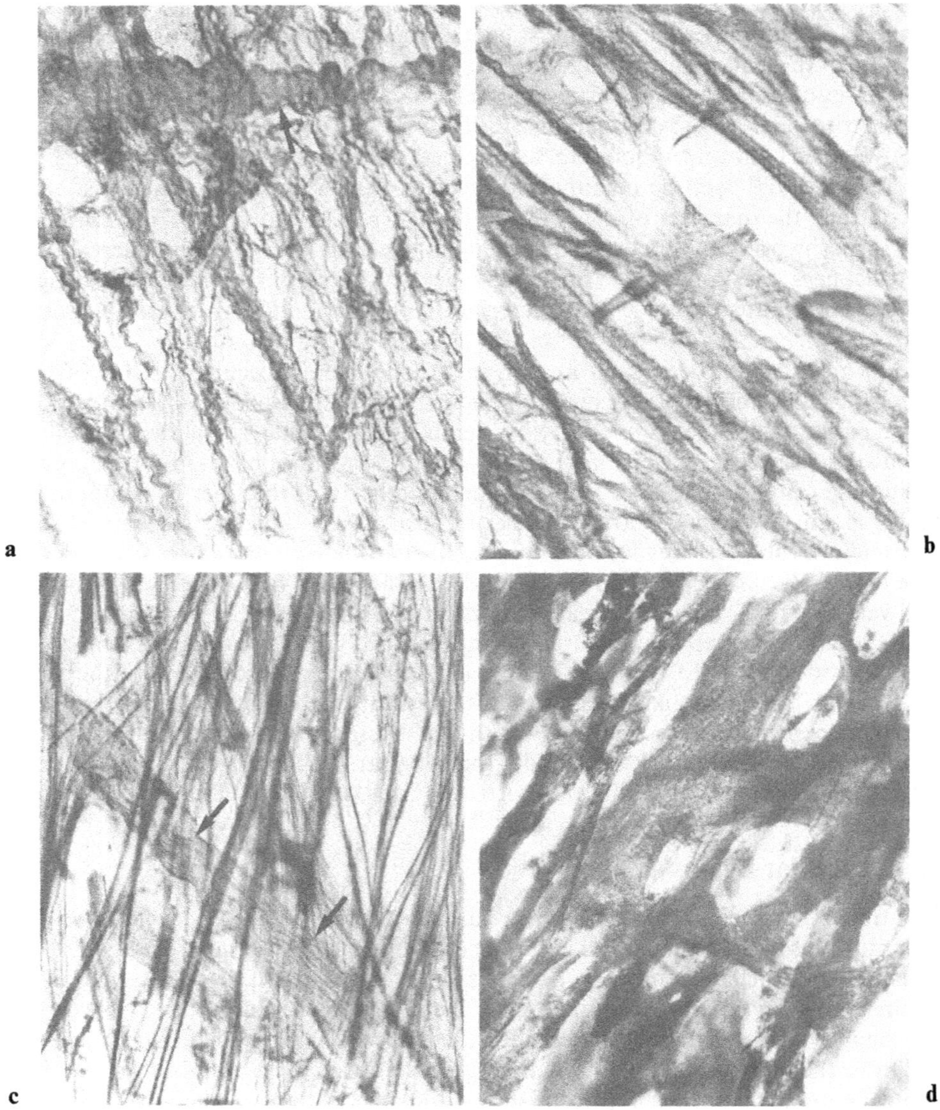

Fig. 5 a–d. Light micrographs of tangential sections through the human trabecular meshwork **a** newborn; **b** 1-year-old child; **c** 29-year-old adult; **d** 56-year-old adult. Note the increase in homogeneous material around the collagenous fibers with increasing age. *Arrows* = tendons of ciliary muscle. Gomori's stain, × 540

age (Fig. 6; LEESON and SPEAKMAN 1961; ROHEN and LÜTJEN-DRECOLL 1968, 1971; MCMENAMIN and LEE 1980; ROHEN 1982). A recent biochemical analysis of age-related changes in the composition of proteins extracted from the entire meshwork revealed that, by 80 years of age, nearly 40% of the protein-bound methionine is oxidized to methionine sulfoxide. This age-dependent accumulation of

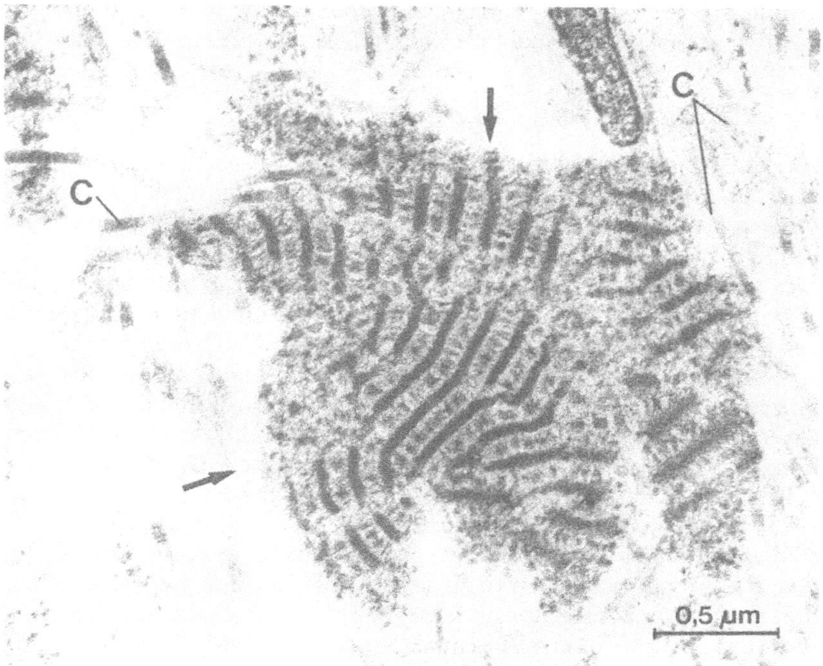

a

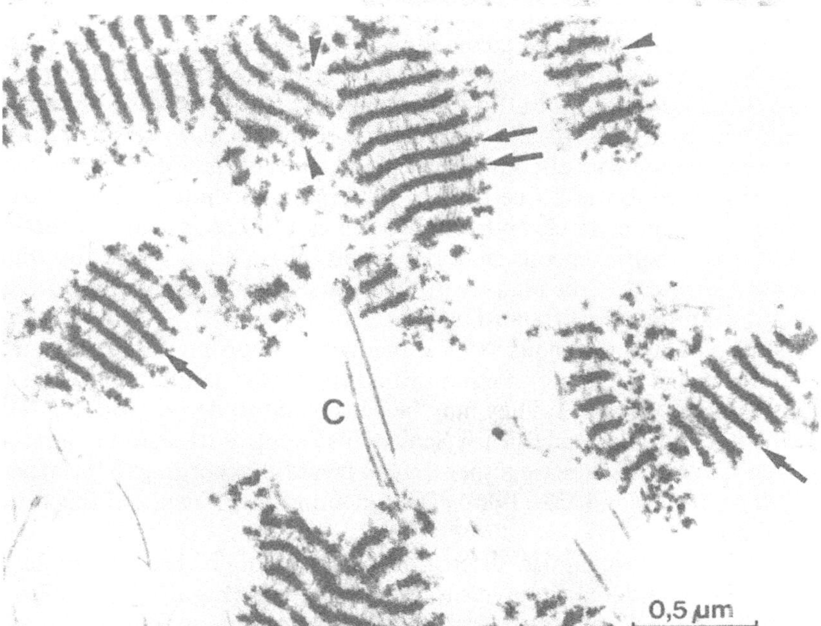

b

Fig. 6 a, b. Electron micrographs of so-called *Gitterkollagen*, i.e., curly or lattice collagen (*arrows*) found within the trabecular lamellae of a glaucomatous eye in a 79-year-old patient (*C* Collagenous fibers) **a** normal appearance; **b** after incubation with chondroitinase ABC and collagenase. The fine fibrils (*arrow-heads*) have been partly dissolved. (After LÜTJEN-DRECOLL et al. 1981) methionine sulfoxide may be related to the increase in lattice (curly) collagen or sheath material of the elastic-like fibers (HORSTMANN et al. 1983).

II. Cribriform Layer

Marked age-related changes are also observed within the cribriform layer of the trabecular meshwork. In contrast to the corneoscleral meshwork and the cornea, the extracellular material of the cribriform meshwork is completely immersed within the aqueous humor. This fluid perfuses the tissue and must therefore influence its structure. According to several authors, the extracellular material of the cribriform meshwork is the main source of resistance to aqueous outflow (BILL and SVEDBERGH 1972; LÜTJEN-DRECOLL 1973; see also ROHEN 1982).

In normal as well as in glaucomatous eyes of higher age groups, we found localized deposits of homogeneous or fine fibrillar extracellular material, which are generally located immediately underneath the endothelium of Schlemm's canal (Fig. 7). These deposits were initially called "plaques" (ROHEN and WITMER 1972; ROHEN 1982). Several other studies confirmed these findings (RODRIGUES et al. 1976; MCMENAMIN and LEE 1980; LEE et al. 1982). Further electron microscopic studies on tangential sections revealed that these "plaques", especially those of type III, are not plaques in the true sense of the word, but rather thickenings of the elastic-like fiber sheaths underneath Schlemm's canal and their connecting fibrils to the endothelium of the canal (ROHEN et al. 1981). With increasing age, and to a much greater extent in glaucomatous eyes, the amount of these deposits (type II and III) increases tremendously, thereby obstructing the pathways for aqueous outflow and reducing the diameter of the cribriform layer. This could lead to an elevation in outflow resistance, which in the case of chronic simple glaucoma might also result in an increase in intraocular pressure (ROHEN 1983). After incubation with chondroitinase ABC, most of these deposits were dissolved, with the exception of a fine fibrillar material immediately adjacent to the inner wall endothelium. If chrondroitinase AB is utilized instead of chondroitinase ABC, some homogeneous material is left surrounding these fine fibrils. This would indicate that the plaques of this area contain dermatan sulfates as well as chondroitin sulfates (LÜTJEN-DRECOLL et al. 1981).

Only the homogeneous "type I plaques", found predominantly underneath the endothelial lining of Schlemm's canal seem to be of different nature and origin (cf. ROHEN et al. 1981). They may be considered to derive from basement membrane-like material underneath Schlemm's canal. With age, the amount of this material seems to decrease rather than to increase, according to the measurements of MCMENAMIN and LEE (1980). The functional significance of this phenomenon is unknown.

There has been much discussion as to whether chronic simple glaucoma should be considered simply as a disease of aging (Fig. 8). The results of our ultrahistochemical studies on trabeculectomy specimens lead to the assumption that the structural changes within the trabecular meshwork of glaucomatous eyes are not solely due to pronounced aging processes, but rather to qualitative changes of the extracellular material and possibly also of cell functions, which differ from those found in the meshwork which is merely aged.

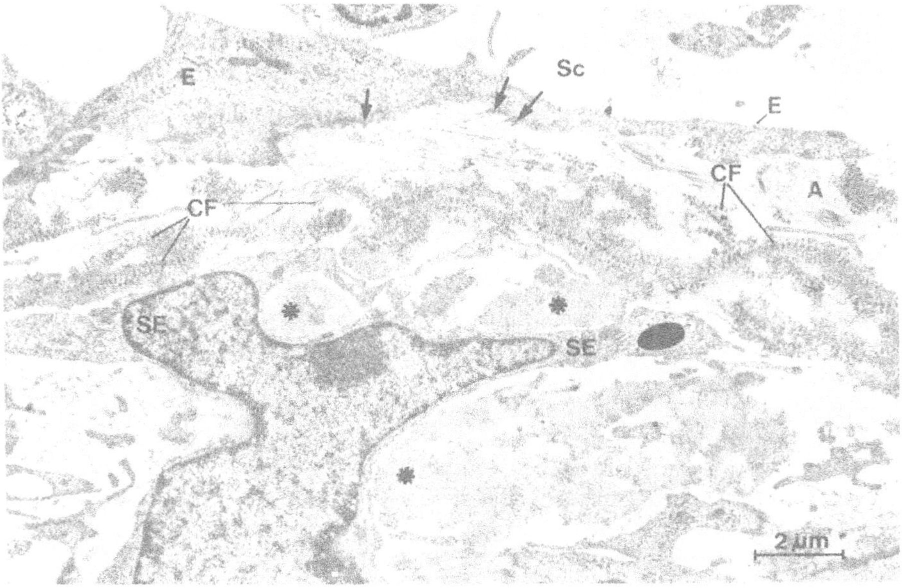

Fig. 7. Electron micrograph of an oblique tangential section through the inner wall of Schlemm's canal (*Sc*). Underneath the endothelial lining (*E*) of the canal, amorphous plaque material (*A*) and clusters of homogeneous plaques (*asterisks*) are seen. *CF* connecting fibers anchoring at the endothelium of Schlemm's canal (*arrows*); *SE* subendothelial cell (After ROHEN et al. 1981)

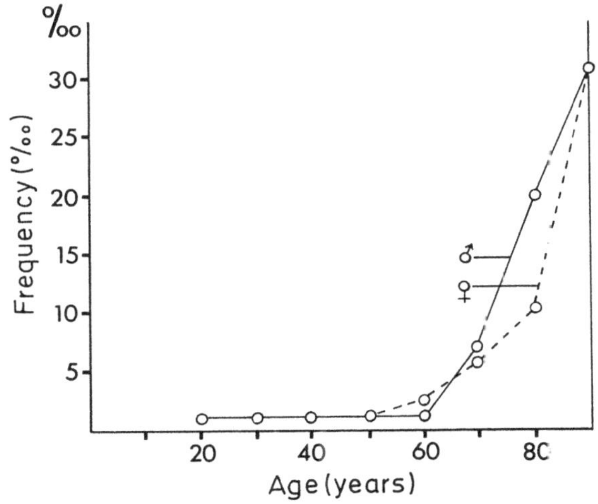

Fig. 8. Frequency of primary open-angle glaucoma in relation to age. (After ANDERSON 1958, cited by SACHSENWEGER 1971)

III. Trabecular Cells

One important function of the trabecular endothelial cells is phagocytosis. This capability is highly developed in these cells, endowing the trabecular meshwork with the noteworthy capacity for self-cleaning. This function seems to be of special importance for all biologic processes occuring in the trabecular meshwork

(ROHEN and UNGER 1959; ROHEN and VAN DER ZYPEN 1968; GRIERSON and LEE 1973, 1978; ROHEN and LÜTJEN-DRECOLL 1982). Phagocytic activity is also apparent in the macrophages or histiocytes often found within the intertrabecular spaces.

Several types of experiments yielding evidence of cellular activation were recently summarized by ROHEN and LÜTJEN-DRECOLL (1982). In these experiments, the cells covering the trabecular beams rapidly developed a great amount of rough endoplasmic reticulum and other cell organelles, thereby enlarging their cytoplasm and nucleus.

With increasing age, the activity of trabecular cells seems to be reduced. Trabecular meshwork cell cultures derived from human autopsy eyes do not exhibit an unlimited multiplication potential, but instead show a decline of proliferative activity which is positively correlated with the age of the donor eye (cf. GRIERSON et al. 1980). After "in vitro aging" of these cells (phase III cells according to Hayflick), a characteristic change in the synthesis of glycosaminoglycans was observed, involving a decrease in the production of hyaluronic acid and a concomitant increase in heparan sulfate synthesis (SCHACHTSCHABEL et al. 1981, 1982). It can be assumed that this change in glycosaminoglycan pattern during cell aging in vitro may also occur in vivo and be responsible for the age-related changes in the amount and quality of extracellular material deposited within the trabecular meshwork.

A recent quantitative analysis showed that, with increasing age, a decrease in cellularity of the meshwork occurs. According to ALVARADO et al. (1981), the cell number is a linear function of age, resulting from a loss of approximately 0.58% of cells per year. This change in cellularity parallels that seen in the corneal endothelium, implying that trabecular cells, like corneal endothelial cells, may have a limited regenerative capacity (GRIERSON et al. 1982).

D. Ciliary Body

The main functions of the ciliary body are accommodation and aqueous humor production. Both processes become markedly limited with increasing age, especially after the age of 50 years. The structures most important in the accommodation process are the ciliary muscle and the zonular apparatus. The ciliary processes which form the pars plicata, i.e., the anterior part of the ciliary body, are involved in aqueous formation (cf. REDDY 1982). The posterior part of the ciliary body, the pars plana, represents a transitional zone to the retina and choroid and is also the site of posterior zonular fiber fixation.

I. Ciliary Muscle

The ciliary muscle fills nearly the entire anterior portion of the ciliary body. The muscle consists of three portions (circular, radial, and longitudinal), which form

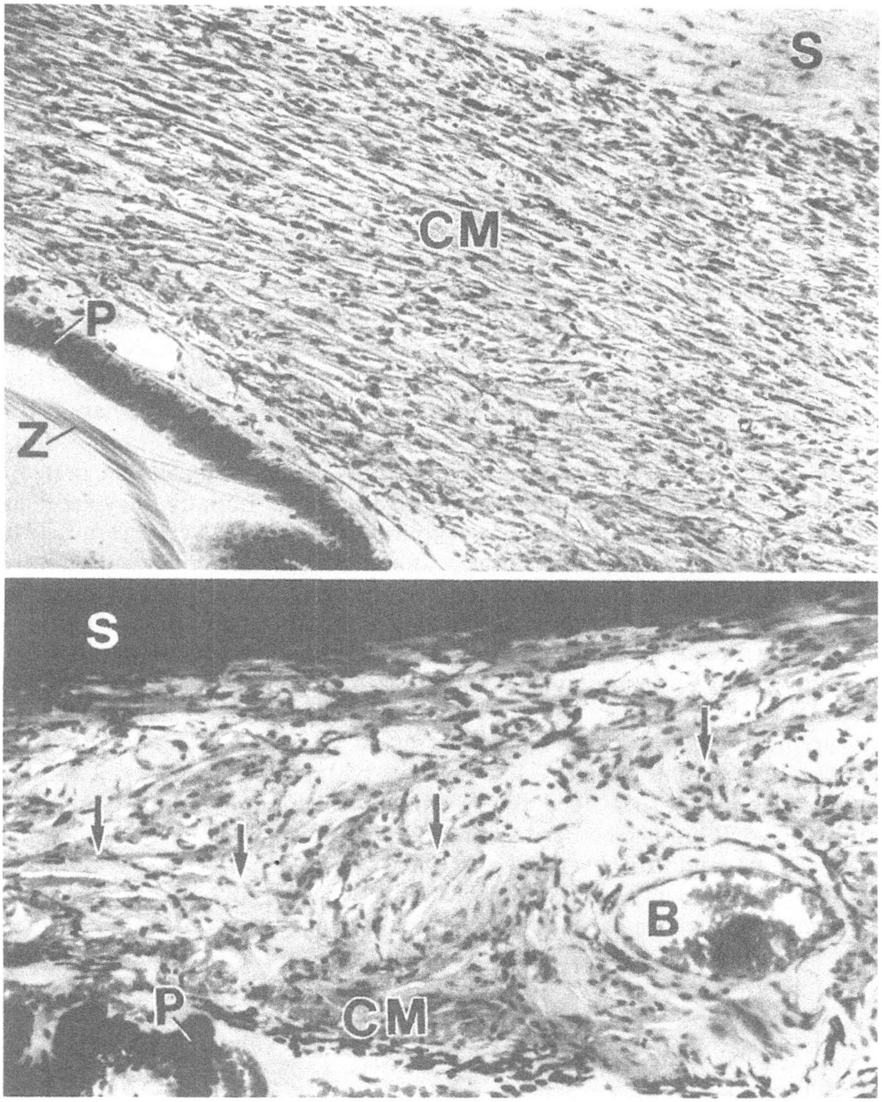

a

b

Fig. 9 a, b. Light micrograph of the ciliary muscle in a young and an old human eye. Note the increase of connective tissue, partly hyalinized (*arrows*), within the reticular portion of the aged ciliary muscle. *B* blood vessel; *CM* ciliary muscle; *P* pigmented epithelium; *S* Sclera; *Z* zonular fibers. **a** sagittal section, 20-year-old patient, HE × 160; **b** sagittal section, 62-year-old patient, HE × 208

a three-dimensional, very regular network with crossing angles increasing as one moves from the periphery to the core (ROHEN 1952, 1964). This muscle system is formed by smooth muscle fibers, which are grouped in bundles surrounded by a sheath of fibroblasts (ISHIKAWA 1962; ROHEN 1964; VAN DER ZYPEN 1967). These bundles interlace, and are separated by intermuscular tissue of collagenous and elastic fibers, ground substance, and free cells of connective tissue (fibroblasts, mast cells, macrophages, and occasionally also plasma cells). With age, an increasing number of muscle fibers degenerate especially within the circular portion, whereas the outermost longitudinal fiber bundles remain relatively unchanged, even at very advanced ages. Concomitant with the degeneration of muscle fibers, the intermuscular tissue is augmented and gradually becomes hyalinized, and the interstitial spaces become enlarged and filled with amorphous extracellular material and cellular debris (Fig. 9). R. STIEVE (1949) distinguished four stages in the aging process of the ciliary muscle: the first stage (0–21 years) is mainly progressive; the second (21–35 years) is considered the essentially functional stage in which the muscle reaches its full development; and the third stage (35–50 years) is already regressive, with an increase in the amount of connective tissue, especially at the roots of the ciliary processes, with the beginning of degeneration of muscle fibers. After the age of 55 years the degenerative changes dominate, and the muscle system gradually reaches its senile atrophic (fourth) stage.

Electron microscopically, structural changes of the ciliary muscle system are already visible between the 20th and 30th year of life. Initially, they are characterized by an increase in the amount of connective tissue between the muscle fiber bundles. There is an increase in fine granular or homogeneous material and irregularly arranged collagenous fibrils. The intermuscular fibroblasts appear activated, revealing an elaborate endoplasmic reticulum, many mitochondria, and ribosomes. After the age of 50 years many ciliary muscle fibers seem to degenerate, showing loss of myofilaments and inclusions of lipid droplets and lipofuscin granules (VAN DER ZYPEN 1970). In addition, lamellated bodies, matrix vesicles, and atypical collagenous fibers can be observed.

Recently, we found plaque-like deposits of extracellular material within the interstitial spaces of the aged ciliary muscle of normal and glaucomatous eyes similar to what has been described in the cribriform layer of the trabecular meshwork (ROHEN and SHIMIZU to be published). These deposits often contain cross-banded fibers showing a periodicity of 100–120 nm, resembling the curly or lattice collagen of the trabecular meshwork (ROHEN et al. 1981). We assume that these deposits also derive from the sheaths of elastic-like fibers, or are formed locally in an unknown manner.

II. Ciliary Processes

With increasing age, characteristic hyalinization of the connective tissue occurs within the ciliary processes. After the age of 50 years, especially at the tips of the ciliary processes, a thickening of the basement membranes can be observed (ROHEN 1964; YAMASHITA et al. 1960). Later (after 70 years), and to a much greater extent in certain diseases (diabetes, glaucoma), a great portion of the connective tissue of the ciliary processes becomes hyalinized (Fig. 10). These areas show a greater affinity for periodic acid-Schiff reagent and alcian blue, and often contain clusters of homogeneous material and cellular debris. Atypical collagen and fragmentation of fibrils are also found (cf. ROHEN 1964; VAN DER ZYPEN and RENTSCH 1971).

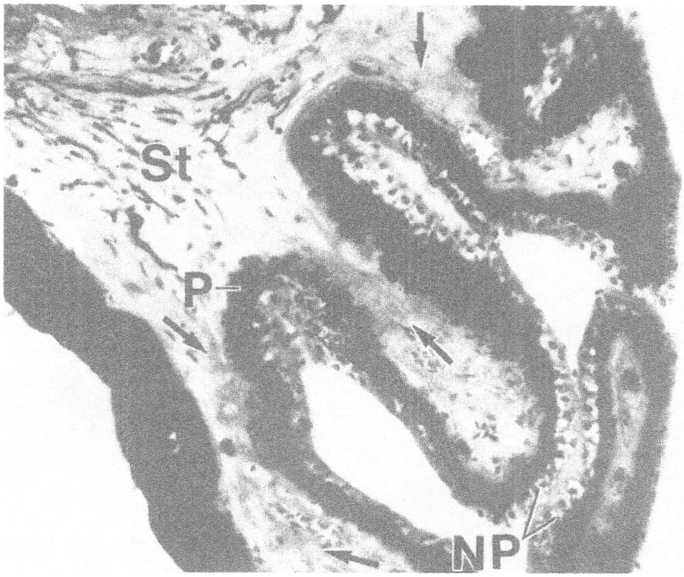

Fig. 10. Light micrograph of ciliary processes of an older eye, showing hyalinization of the connective tissue and thickening of basement membranes (*arrows*). *NP* nonpigmented epithelium; *P* pigmented epithelium; *St* stroma layer of ciliary processes. HE × 208

III. Ciliary Epithelium

The ciliary processes are covered by a two-layered epithelium. The outer layer is the pigmented epithelium, the inner layer the nonpigmented epithelium. Both layers are firmly attached at their apical regions by several types of junction, including puncta adherentia, desmosomes, and gap junctions (nexus) (RAVIOLA and RAVIOLA 1978; OBER and ROHEN 1979). In addition, there are many tight junctions (zonulae occludentes) mainly located at the apical part of the nonpigmented epithelial cells. Many investigators have shown the location of the blood–aqueous barrier to be at the level of these junctions (BAIRATI and ORZALESI 1966; OKISAKA et al. 1976; SHIOSE 1970; VEGGE 1971; SMITH and RUDT 1973, 1975; RAVIOLA 1977; RAVIOLA and RAVIOLA 1978).

Involutions of the cell membranes are present at the basal surface of both the nonpigmented and the pigmented epithelial cells as well as on the lateral side of the nonpigmented epithelium (interdigitations), which increase the cell surface and therefore might facilitate fluid transport or exchange. The nonpigmented epithelium appears especially rich in mitochondria. This fact suggests that this epithelium is actively involved in aqueous formation. More highly differentiated cells with an elaborate endoplasmic reticulum (fingerprints) and Golgi complexes are frequently distributed within the nonpigmented layer, but their function is unknown (cf. LÜTJEN-DRECOLL 1982).

With increasing age, the number of interdigitations and cell membrane involutions is reduced. Tiny cytoplasmic protrusions appear which gradually enlar-

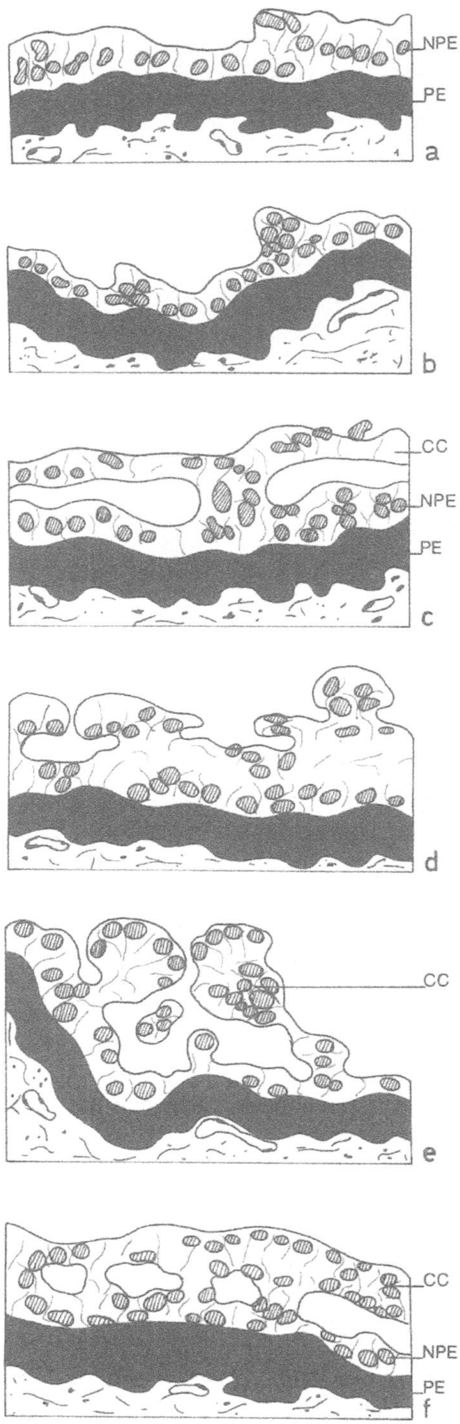

Fig. 11 a–f. Age-related changes of the ciliary epithelium in the human eye. *NPE* nonpigmented epithelium; *PE* pigmented epithelium; *CC* covering cells. **a** = 10 months; **b** = 2 years; **c** = 26 years; **d** = 33 years; **e** = 65 years; **f** = 71 years. (After ROHEN and ZIMMERMANN 1970)

Table 2. Incidence[a] of pars plana cysts in the human eye (After OKUN 1960)

Age (years)	Cysts	Incidence (%)
0–20	0	0
20–40	0	0
40–50	3	12
50–60	5	13
60–70	14	28
>70	18	34

[a] Incidence calculated as a percentage of eyes evaluated

ge and penetrate into the area of the internal limiting membrane. Finally, certain cells seem to migrate into this membrane, forming a layer of so-called covering cells inward of the nonpigmented epithelium (Fig. 11; ROHEN and ZIMMERMANN 1970). In advanced age, this development can be so pronounced that the impression of a "pseudoadenomatous hyperplasia" of the nonpigmented epithelial layer is given (cf. NAUMANN 1980). In contrast to these proliferative changes, the extent of which is regionally very different, degenerative changes also occur after the 30th year of life. These changes mainly involve the appearance of lipids, inclusions of pigment granules, and lamellated bodies within the cytoplasm of the nonpigmented epithelium. Conversely, the pigmented epithelium, especially at the tips of the ciliary processes, loses some of its pigment granules and gradually becomes depigmentated with increasing age. Structural irregularities at the border of the stromal layer have also been observed (VAN DER ZYPEN and RENTSCH 1971; LÜTJEN-DRECOLL 1982).

In the nonpigmented epithelium, mitochondria are more numerous in old age, whereas the other cell organelles are less numerous. In old age, the stromal layer and the basal lamina become much thicker, whereas the number of fenestrations in the capillary endothelium is significantly increased (HARA et al. 1977). The thickening of the basal laminae and the widening of the stromal layer of the ciliary processes in old age must make aqueous humor production more difficult. It could be that to compensate for this impairment, the ciliary processes develop more capillary fenestrations and the nonpigmented epithelium more mitochondria for the energy-dependent secretory processes. If so, one could consider this to be a similar mechanism to that discussed in Sect. B. III, where aging and nonaging processes compensate for each other.

At the orbiculus ciliaris (pars plana of the ciliary body) anomalies of the epithelial layers in the form of depigmentations, irregularities of layers and cell shape, and cysts of various sizes have often been observed (cf. ROHEN 1964).

From the analysis of about 500 autopsy eyes, OKUN (1960) found that the incidence of pars plana cysts increases with age (Table 2). Up to the age of 40 years, he found no cysts. It is not clear whether these changes are related to the functional decline of the accommodation system with age.

Pars plana cysts often develop between the pigmented and nonpigmented epithelium and contain large amounts of hyaluronic acid (FINE and ZIMMERMAN

1963). With increasing age, an increasing amount of iron deposits has been found in the nonpigmented epithelium of the pars plana (HAHN and TIMM 1976; BRYSON et al. 1966; YAMASHITA et al. 1960). The functional significance of these findings is not clear.

IV. Zonular Apparatus and Internal Limiting Membrane

The zonular fibers are closely attached to the internal limiting membrane of the ciliary valleys and the pars plana of the ciliary body. There are no direct connections with the tendons of the ciliary muscle or the membranes of the ciliary epithelial cells. Scanning electron microscopic studies (ROHEN 1979) revealed that two functionally different fiber groups exist: (a) the main fibers, which arise in the pars plana region and insert into the lens capsule; and (b) the span or tension fibers, which deviate from the main fiber system and insert mainly into the internal limiting membrane of the ciliary valleys. During accommodation, the ciliary muscle moves anteriorly and inwardly, thereby stretching the span or tension fibers. This action causes the anterior part of the zonula to relax and the anterior lens curvature to mold, increasing its refractive power. Since accommodation markedly decreases between the ages of 40 and 50 years, the zonula fiber system then serves only to retain the lens in place. One would therefore expect those fiber strands which are directly involved in the tissue displacement during accommodation to have largely degenerated after the age of 50 years.

Rarefaction of zonular fibers and structural changes in the architecture of the entire fiber system were indeed found by scanning electron microscopy. These studies were conducted following experimental "disinsertion" of the ciliary muscle in monkeys, after which retrodisplacement of the entire accommodation apparatus and a complete loss of accommodation was observed (KAUFMAN et al. 1979). Comparable changes of the zonular apparatus are also seen in higher age groups, in which the power of accommodation is greatly reduced (BORNFELD et al. 1974). According to these authors, zonular fibers inserting on the equator of the lens are found exclusively in the young eye. They disappear in old age. The number of zonular fibers at the pars plana and pars plicata of the ciliary body is also greatly reduced with increasing age. BORNFELD et al. (1974) also described polymorphous particles of an unknown nature measuring 3–30 μm, which were scattered over the entire zonule. In the infant eye, they were far more numerous than in the senile eye. During life, the insertion site of the zonular fibers at the anterior lens surface migrates centrally because of lens equator enlargement due to gradual thickening of the entire lens with age (BURKE and FARNSWORTH 1980).

Structural aging changes corresponding to the development and decline of the accommodation system also occur in the internal limiting membrane. During the first decade of life the internal limiting membrane, which originally appears as a thin monolayered basement membrane covering the nonpigmented epithelium, gradually becomes thicker, with development of small bridges and septa. This process starts at the ciliary valleys and proceeds posteriorly in the direction of the pars plana. The greatest diameter of this irregular membranous structure is always found in the ciliary valleys at places where the tension fiber system is affixed to the ciliary body (RENTSCH and VAN DER ZYPEN 1971; OBER and ROHEN 1979).

In higher age groups, many small electron-dense vesicles appear within the network of the internal limiting membrane, which originate either from the non-pigmented epithelium or the zonular fragments. In addition, cellular debris, lipid droplets, and vesicles of various sizes have been found (GÄRTNER 1965, 1970; RENTSCH and VAN DER ZYPEN 1971). After the age of 50 years, a number of free cells can bee seen embedded within the internal limiting membrane which seem to phagocytoze the particles irregularly distributed within it. Although no quantitative evaluations were made, we had the impression that these "cleaning processes", if any, become more active with increasing age. The origin of these cells is not known.

E. Iris

From a functional point of view, the iris can be divided into three principal layers: (a) the anterior border layer; (b) the stromal layer, which contains most of the blood vessels; and (c) the posterior layer, consisting of the iris muscles and the pigmented epithelium (ROHEN 1951).

The anterior border layer is not completely covered by endothelial cells. The surface cells resemble fibroblasts with long cytoplasmic processes radiating in all directions. Although the anterior border layer contains a greater amount of acid glycosaminoglycans, probably in the form of glycoproteins, there is no continuous barrier at the iris surface with the anterior chamber. Aqueous humor may therefore penetrate freely into or out of the iris tissue.

In the human iris, a continuously progressing reduction of connective tissue and ground substance is seen within the anterior border layer and the iris stroma, causing indentations, holes, fissures, and crypts on the surface layer (Fig. 12). Tissue reduction of this kind has not been observed in the iris of lower mammals, but develops slowly in higher primates and to a maximal degree in humans where it varies greatly between individuals (ROHEN and VOTH 1960).

In higher age groups the diameter of the entire organ decreases and the iris stroma becomes atrophic, leading to a reduction of iridic mobility. The aged patient is usually characterized by a miotic, relatively immobile pupil. The changes in mobility correlate with structure and quantitative changes of the collagenous fibers and ground substance deposited in the stroma or around the blood vessels. The iris stroma does not contain elastic fibers. The elasticity of the organ results from the organization of the tissue, especially from the blood vessels and their adventitial sheaths.

The collagenous fibers of the stromal layer show a precise pattern in the form of interlacing crossing bundles. This fiber lattice is capable of changing its angle according to the size of the pupil (ROHEN 1951, 1964). The blood vessels, which exhibit a corkscrew shape, are embedded in this fiber lattice, so that they can accommodate to the changes in pupillary size. The adventitial sheaths of the blood vessels are peculiar structures and very characteristic for the iris of the human eye.

The adventitial sheaths are several times larger than the vessel wall itself (see Fig. 12). They consist of an inner zone containing thin collagenous fiber (average diameter 30 nm) and an outer zone containing collagenous fibers of various thick-

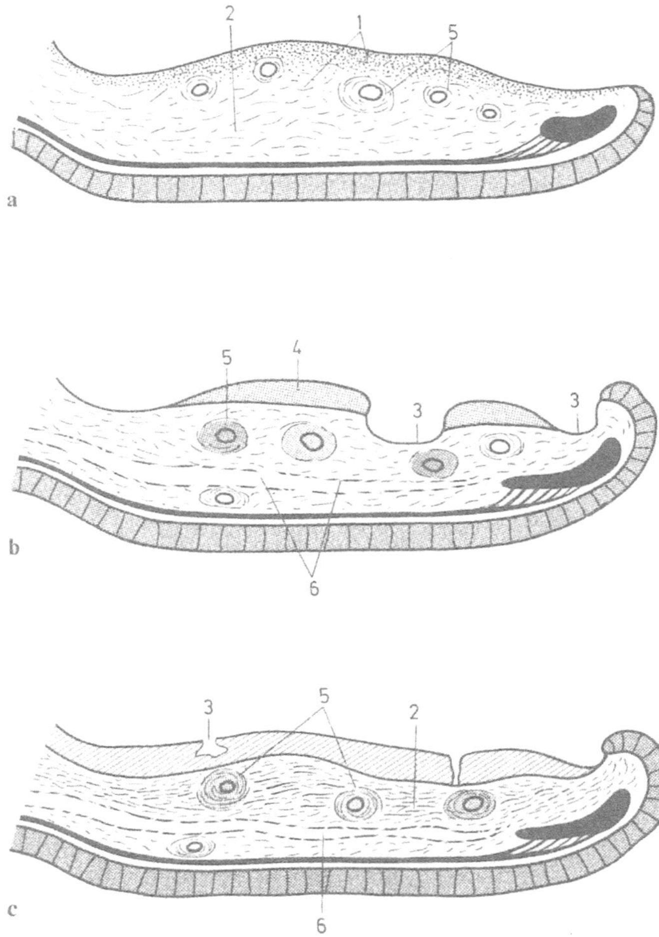

Fig. 12 a–c. Age-related changes in the structure of the human iris (schematic drawing). 1 = anterior leaf; 2 = stroma; 3 = crypts; 4 = zones of densification; 5 = adventitial sheaths of iris vessels; 6 = space of Fuchs. **a** = 0–28 years; **b** = 30–65 years; **c** = >65 years. (After OKAMURA and LÜTJEN-DRECOLL 1973)

nesses (diameter 30–120 nm). The age changes observed in the iris vessels include thickening of the basement membrane, enlargement of the inner zone, and a relative increase in the number of thicker fibers in the outer zone. There is probably a process of fiber formation and maturation in the adventitial sheaths, resulting in an increase in number and thickness of collagenous fibers correlated with age (OKAMURA and LÜTJEN-DRECOLL 1973). The fibers are embedded in a matrix rich in acid glycosaminoglycans, mainly hyaluronic acid and chondroitin sulfates. In the aging iris, a tendency toward a decrease in hyaluronidase-resistant glycosaminoglycans within the adventitial sheaths is noted. The opposite process takes place in glaucomatous eyes (SAMES and ROHEN 1978; SAMES 1979). In addition, the periadventital cellular layer, which separates the adventitial sheaths of the iris vessels from the stroma, becomes thicker with increasing age.

I. Anterior Border Layer

In the anterior border layer of the iris, distinct zones of cellular densification as well as zones of tissue disaggregation with endothelial defects at the iris surface develop progressively after the age of 50 years. In advanced age, the entire anterior leaf of the iris undergoes a marked cellular densification, while the stromal layer becomes increasingly atrophic. The crypts therefore appear shallower and the iridial vessels more prominent with increasing age. The anterior border layer also contains a great amount of acid glycosaminoglycans. In the aging iris, a decrease in hyaluronidase-resistant glycosaminoglycans in the vessel wall (as mentioned in Sect. E) and a concomitant increase in these substances in the anterior border layer was observed (SAMES and ROHEN 1978). Some parts of these glycosaminoglycans are probably keratan or heparan sulfate.

II. Pigment Epithelium

With age, the pigment epithelium gradually loses its pigment granules, causing this layer to become partially translucent (NORN 1971; DONALDSON 1974). At the pupillary margin, this degranulation can be very extensive, so that in some places only the cell borders are ophthalmoscopically visible (LATIES 1972). In advanced age, atrophy and partial degeneration of the smooth muscle fibers of both the sphincter and dilator muscles have been observed (cf. NAUMANN 1980). These phenomena can well explain the increasing rigidity and stiffness of the human iris with increasing age.

References

Alvarado J, Murphy C, Polansky J, Juster R (1981) Age-related changes in the trabecular meshwork cellularity. Invest Ophthalmol Vis Sci 21:714–727

Bairati A, Grignolo A (1954) Preliminary investigations of the submicroscopic structure of Descemet's membrane with the electron microscope. Boll Soc Ital Biol Sper 30:16

Bairati A, Orzalesi N (1966) The ultrastructure of the epithelium of the ciliary body. A study of the function complexes and of the changes associated with the production of plasmoid aqueous humor. Z Zellforsch Mikrosk Anat 69:635–658

Bashey RI, Kern HL (1972) Studies of collagen of bovine cornea. Ophthalmic Res 4:246–256

Bigar F (1982) Specular microscopy of corneal endothelium Dev Ophthalmol 6:1–94

Bill A, Svedbergh B (1972) Scanning electron microscopic studies of the trabecular meshwork and the canal of Schlemm. An attempt to localize the mean resistance to outflow of aqueous humor in man. Acta Ophthalmol 50:295–320

Blatt HL, Rao GN, Aquavella JV (1979) Endothelial density in relation to morphology. Invest Ophthalmol Vis Sci 18:856

Bornfeld N, Spitznas M, Breipohl W, Bijvank GJ (1974) Scanning electron microscopy of the zonule of Zinn. I. Human Eyes. Albert von Graefes Arch Klin Ophthalmol 192:117–129

Bourne W, Kaufman HE (1976) Specular microscopy of human corneal endothelium in vivo. Am J Ophthalmol 81:319
Brini A (1957) Le reseau trabeculaire de l'angle de la chambre anterieure. Etude histologique et histochimique. Ann Ocul (Paris) 190:755–777
Bryson JM, Wolter JR, O'Keefe NT (1966) Ganglion cells in the human ciliary body. Arch Ophthalmol 75:57
Burke PA, Farnsworth P (1980) Development of the human fetal lens. Invest Ophthalm Vis Sci (Suppl, ARVO, Orlando) p 116
Calmettes L, Deodati F, Flanel H, Bec P (1956) Etude histologique et histochemique de l'epithélium anterieur de la cornée et de ses basalés. Arch Ophthalmol (Paris) 16:481
Cogan DG, Kuwabara T (1959) Arcus senilis. Its pathology and histochemistry. Arch Ophthalmol 61:553
Dardenne MU, Iwangoff P, Diotallevi M (1968) Unterschiede im Verhalten des Kollagens der einzelnen Hornhautschichten mit zunehmendem Lebensalter. Ophthalmologica 156:385–393
Donaldson DD (1974) Transillumination of the iris. Trans Am Ophthalmol Soc 72:89
Enke P, Rohen JW (1983) Morphological studies on the regeneration of rabbit corneal endothelium under influence of corticosteroids. Albrecht von Grafes Arch Klin Exp Ophthalmol 220:19–24
Feeney ML, Garron LK (1961) Descemet's membrane in the human peripheral cornea. A study by light and electron microscopy. In: Smelser GK (ed) The structure of the eye. Academic, New York
Fine BS, Zimmerman LE (1963) Light an e.m. observations on the ciliary epithelium in man and rhesus monkey. Invest Ophthalmol 2:105
Gärtner J (1965) Elektronenmikroskopische Untersuchungen über Glaskörperrindenzellen und Zonulafasern. Z Zellforsch 66:737–764
Gärtner J (1970) Electron microscopic observations on the cilio-zonular border of the human eye with particular reference to the ageing changes. Z Anat Entwicklungsgesch 131:263–273
Graumann W, Rohen JW (1958) Chemohistologische Befunde am menschlichen Auge (Cornea, Sclera, Uvea). Z Mikrosk Anat Forsch 64:652–671
Greiling H, Driesch R, Momburg M, Jagdfeld R, Thomas J, Stuhlsatz HW (1976) Zur Alternsabhängigkeit der Glycosyltransferasen. In: Platt D (ed) Alternstheorien, 3rd Gießener Symposium. Schattauer, Stuttgart, pp 205–217
Grierson I, Lee WR (1973) Erythrocyte phagocytosis in the human trabecular meshwork. Br J Ophthalmol 57:400–415
Grierson I, Lee WR (1978) Further observations on the process of haemophagocytosis in the human outflow system. Albrecht Von Grafes Arch Klin Ophthalmol 208:49–64
Grierson I, Robins, E, Howes RC (1980) Preliminary observations in the human trabecular meshwork cells in vitro. Albrecht Von Graefes Arch Klin Ophthalmol 212:173–186
Grierson I, Wang Q, McMenamin PG, Lee WR (1982) The effects of age and antiglaucoma drugs on the meshwork cell population. New Perspectives in Ophthalmology. Research and Clinical Forums vol 4, no 5, pp 69–92
Hahn H, Timm G (1976) Untersuchungen zur physiol. Hämosiderosen des Auges. Folia ophthalmol 4:249
Hanna C, Bicknell DS, O'Brien JE (1961) Cell turnover in the adult human eye. Arch Ophthalmol 65:695
Hara K, Lütjen-Drecoll E, Prestele H, Rohen JW (1977) Structural differences between regions of the ciliary body in primates. Invest Ophthalmol Vis Sci 16:912–924
Hogan MJ, Alvarado JA, Weddell J (1971) Histology of the human eye. An atlas and textbook. Saunders Philadelphia
Horstmann HJ, Rohen JW, Sames K (1983) Age changes of proteins in the human trabecular meshwork. Mech Ageing Dev 21:121–136
Ishikawa T (1962) Fine structure of the human ciliary muscle. Invest Ophthalmol Vis Sci 1:587–608
Jaeger W, Eisenhauer GG (1977) Der diagnostische Wert der Arcus corneae als Hinweis auf Lipoidstoffwechselstörungen. Klin Monatsbl Augenheilkd 171:321

Jakus MA (1956) Studies on the cornea. II. The fine structure of Descemet's membrane. J Biophys Biochem Cytol (Suppl) 2:241

Jakus MA (1961) The fine structure of the human cornea. In: Smelser GK (ed) The Structure of the eye. Academic New York

Kaufman HE, Capella MS, Robbins JE (1966) The human corneal endothelium. Am J Ophthalmol 61:835

Kaufman PL, Rohen JW, Bárány EH (1979) Hyperopia and loss of accommodation following ciliary muscle disinsertion in the cynomolgus monkey. Invest Ophthalmol Vis Sci 18:665–673

Kaye GI, Pappas GD (1962) Studies on the cornea. I. The fine structure of the rabbit cornea and the uptake and transport of colloidal particles by the cornea in vivo. J Cell Biol 21–457

Kayes, J, Holmberg A (1960) The fine structure of Bowman's layer and the basement membrane of the corneal epithelium. Am J Ophthalmol 50–1013

Laties AM (1972) Specific neurohistology comes of age: A look back and a look forward. Invest Ophthalmol Vis Sci 11:553

Laule A, Cable MK, Hoffman CE, Hanna C (1978) Endothelial cell population changes of human cornea during life. Arch Ophthalmol 96:2031

Lee WR, Grierson I, McMenamin PG (1982) The morphological response of the primate outflow system to changes in pressure and flow. In: Lütjen-Drecoll E (ed) Basic aspects of glaucoma research. Schattauer, Stuttgart, pp 123–140

Leeson TH, Speakman JS (1961) The fine structure of extracellular material in the pectinate ligament (trabecular meshwork) of the human iris. Acta Anat 46:363–379

Lütjen-Drecoll E (1973) Structural factors influencing outflow facility and its changeability under drugs, a study in macaca arctoides. Invest Ophthalmol Vis Sci 12:280–294

Lütjen-Drecoll E (1982) Functional morphology of the ciliary epithelium. In: Lütjen-Drecoll E (ed) Basic aspects of Glaucoma research. Schattauer, Stuttgart, pp 69–88

Lütjen-Drecoll E, Lönnerholm G (1981) Distribution of carbonic-anydrase in the rabbit eye. Invest Ophthalmol 21:782–797

Lütjen-Drecoll E, Futa R, Rohen JW (1981) Ultrahistochemical studies on tangential sections of the trabecular meshwork in normal and glaucomatous eyes. Invest Ophthalmol Vis Sci 21:563–573

Lütjen-Drecoll E, Dietl T, Futa R, Rohen JW (1982) Age changes of the trabecular meshwork: a preliminary morphometric study. In: Hollyfield JG (ed) Structure of the eye, IV. Symposium. Elsevier North Nolland, Amsterdam, pp 341–348

Lütjen-Drecoll E, Lönnerholm G, Eichhorn M (1983) Carbonic anhydrase in the human and monkey eye by light and electron microscopy. Albrecht von Graefes. Arch Klin Ophthalmol 220:285–291

McMenamin PG, Lee WR (1980) Age-related changes in extracellular materials in the inner wall of Schlemm's canal. Albrecht von Graefes Arch Klin Exp Ophthalmol 212:159–172

Naumann GOH (1980) Pathologie des Auges. In: Doerr W, Seifert G, Uehlinger E (eds) Spezielle pathologische Anatomie, vol 12. Springer, Berlin Heidelberg New York

Norn MS (1971) Iris pigment defects in normals. Acta Opthalmol (Copenh) 49:887

Ober MJ, Rohen JW (1979) Regional differences in the fine structure of the ciliary epithelium related to accommodation. Invest Ophthalmol Vis Sci 18:655–664

Okamura R, Lütjen-Drecoll E (1973) Elektronenmikroskopische Untersuchungen über die Altersveränderungen der menschlichen Iris. Albrecht von Graefes Arch Klin Ophthalmol 186:249–269

Okisaka S, Kuwabara T, Rapoport SI (1976) Effect of hyperosomotic agents on the ciliary epithelium and trabecular meshwork. Invest Ophthalmol Vis Sci 15:617–625

Okun E (1960) Pathology in autopsy eyes. Am J Ophthalmol 50:424–429 (part I), 574–583 (part II)

Raviola G (1977) The structural basis of the blood-ocular barriers. Exp Eye Res (Suppl) 25:27–63

Raviola G, Raviola E (1978) Intercellular junctions in the ciliary epithelium. Invest Ophthalmol Vis Sci 17/10:959–981

Reddy VN (1982) Biochemistry of aqueous humor. In: Lütjen-Drecoll E (ed) Basic aspects of Glaucoma research. Schattauer, Stuttgart, pp 89–112
Rentsch FJ, Van Der Zypen E (1971) Altersbedingte Veränderungen der sog. Membrana limitans int. des Ziliarkörpers im menschl. Auge. In: Bredt H, Rohen JW (eds) Ageing and development, vol 1. Schattauer, Stuttgart, pp 70–94
Rodgrigues MM, Spaeth GL, Livalingham E, Weinreb S (1976) Histopathology of 150 trabeculectomy specimens in glaucoma. Trans Ophthalmol Soc UK 96:245–255
Rohen H (1951) Der Bau der Regenbogenhaut beim Menschen und einigen Säugetieren. Gegenbaurs Morphol Jahrb 91:140–181
Rohen JW (1952) Der Ziliarkörper als funktionelles System Gegenbaurs Morphol Jahrb 92:415–440
Rohen JW (1962) Über das Lig. pectinatum der Primaten. Z Zellforsch 58:403–421
Rohen JW (1964) Das Auge und seine Hilfsorgane. In: Möllendorff W, Bargmann W (eds) Haut und Sinnesorgane. Handbuch der mikroskopischen Anatomie des Menschen, vol 3/4. Springer, Berlin Göttingen Heidelberg New York, pp 348–354
Rohen JW (1979) Scanning electron microscopic studies of zonular apparatus in human and monkey eyes. Invest Ophthalmol Vis Sci 18:133
Rohen JW (1982) The evolution of the primate Eye in relation to the problem of glaucoma. In: Lütjen-Drecoll E (ed) Basic aspects of glaucoma research. Schattauer, Stuttgart, pp 3–33
Rohen JW (1983) Why is i.o. pressure elevated in chronic simple glaucoma? Anatomical considerations. XXIV. Int Congr Ophthalmol, San Francisco, American Academy Ophthalmology 90:758–765
Rohen JW, Lütjen-Drecoll E (1968) Über die Altersveränderungen des Trabekelwerkes im menschlichen Auge. Albrecht von Graefes Arch Klin Ophthalmol 175:285–307
Rohen JW, Lütjen-Drecoll E (1971) Age changes of the trabecular meshwork in human and monkey eyes. In: Bredt H, Rohen JW (eds) Ageing and development, vol I. Schattauer, Stuttgart, pp 1–36
Rohen JW, Lütjen-Drecoll E (1981) Ageing and non-ageing processes within the connective tissues of the anterior segment of the eye. In: Müller WEG, Rohen JW (eds) Biochemical and morphological aspects of ageing. Abhandlung Akademie der Wissenschaften und Literatur, Mainz. Steiner, Wiesbaden, pp 157–174
Rohen JW, Lütjen-Drecoll E (1982) Biology of the trabecular meshwork. In: Lütjen-Drecoll E (ed) Basic aspects of Glaucoma research. Schattauer, Stuttgart
Rohen JW, Shimizu TS (to be published) Fine structure of ciliary muscle tips and outer wall of Schlemm's canal in normal and glaucomatous eyes. Albrecht von Graefes Arch Klin Ophthalmol
Rohen JW, Unger HH (1959) Zur Morphologie und Pathologie der Kammerbucht des Auges. In: Abh Mainzer Akad Wiss Lit Math Naturwiss, Kl 3. Steiner, Wiesbaden, pp 1–206
Rohen JW, Van der Zypen E (1968) The phagocytic activity of the trabecular meshwork endothelium. An electron microscopy study of the vervet (cercopithecus aethiops). Albrecht Von Graefes Arch Klin Ophthalmol 175:143–160
Rohen JW, Voth D (1960) Zur Irisstruktur der Primaten. Ophthalmologica 140:27–33
Rohen JW, Witmer R (1972) Electron microscopic studies on the trabecular meshwork in glaucoma simplex. Albrecht Von Graefes Arch Klin Ophthalmol 183:251–266
Rohen JW, Zimmermann A (1970) Altersveränderungen des Ciliarepithels beim Menschen. Albrecht Von Graefes Arch Klinik Ophthalmol 179:302–317
Rohen JW, Futa R, Lütjen-Drecoll E (1981) The fine structure of the cribriform meshwork in normal and glaucomatous eyes as seen in tangential sections. Invest Ophthalmol Vis Sci 21:574–585
Sames K (1979) Histochemical demonstration of acidic glycosaminoglycans in the cell nuclei of the iris and other tissues. Acta Anat 103:74–82
Sames K, Rohen JW (1978) Histochemical studies on the Glycosaminoglycans in the normal and glaucomatous iris of human eyes. Albrecht Von Graefes Arch Klin Ophthalmol 207:157–167

Schachtschabel DO, Wever J, Rohen JW, Bigalke B (1981) Changes in glycosaminoglycans synthesis during in vitro ageing of cultured WI-38 cells and trabecular meshwork cells of the primate eye. In: Müller WEG, Rohen JW (eds) Biochemical and morphological aspects of ageing. Steiner, Wiesbaden, pp 175–185

Schachtschabel DO, Rohen JW, Wever J, Sames K (1982) Synthesis and composition of GAGs by cultured human trabecular meshwork cells. Albrecht Von Graefes Arch Klin Ophthalmol 218:113–117

Schwarz W (1953) Elektronenmikroskopische Untersuchungen über die Differenzierung der Cornea- und Sklerafibrillen des Menschen. Z Zellforsch 38:78–86

Schwarz W (1972) Anatomie der Cornea. Ber Zusammenkunft Dtsch Ophthalmol Ges 69:12–18

Schwarz W, Keyserlingk G (1969) Elektronenmikroskopische Untersuchungen an humanen Hornhautnarben und an einem getrübten Hornhauttransplantat. Virchows Arch [Pathol Anat] 347:115–128

Schwarz W, Keyserlingk G, Graf D (1966) Über die Feinstruktur der menschlichen Cornea mit besonderer Berücksichtigung des Problems der Transparenz. Z Zellforsch 73:540–548

Shiose Y (1970) Electron microscopic studies on blood retinal and blood aqueous barriers. J J Ophthalmol 14:73–87

Smith RS, Rudt LA (1973) Ultrastructural studies of the blood aqueous barrier. 2. The barrier to horseradish peroxidase in primates. Am J Ophthalmol 76:937–947

Smith RS, Rudt LA (1975) Ocular vascular and epithelial barriers to microperoxidase. Invest Ophthalmol Vis Sci 14:556–560

Stieve R (1949) Über den Bau des menschlichen Ziliarmuskels und seine Veränderungen während des Lebens ... Anat Anz 97:69–79, Z Mikrosk Anat Forschg 55:3–88

Teng CC, Katzin HM (1953) The basement membrane of corneal epithelium. A perliminary report. Am J Ophthalmol 36:895

Van der Zypen E (1967) Licht- und elektronenmikroskopische Untersuchungen über den Bau und die Innervation des Ziliarmuskels bei Mensch und Affe (Cercopithecus aethiops). Albrecht Von Graefes Arch Klin Ophthalmol 174:143–168

Van der Zypen E (1970) Licht- und elektronenmikroskopische Untersuchungen über die Altersveränderungen am M. ciliaris im menschlichen Auge. Albrecht Von Graefes Arch Klin Exp Ophthalmol 179:332–357

Van der Zypen E (1971) Vergleichende licht- und elektronenmikroskopische Untersuchungen über die morphologischen Grundlagen der Liquor- und Kammerwasserzirkulation. Habil.-schr. Altern und Entwicklung 3. Schattauer, Stuttgart

Van der Zypen E, Rentsch FJ (1971) Altersbedingte Veränderungen am Ziliarkörper des menschlichen Auges. In: Bredt H, Rohen JW (eds) Ageing and development, vol 1. Schattauer, Stuttgart, pp 37–94

Vegge T (1971) An epithelial blood-aqueous barrier to horseradish peroxidase in the processes of the newt monkey (Cercopithecus aethiops). Z Zellforsch Mikrosk Anat 114:309–320

Viidik A (1979) Connective tissues – possible implications of the temporal changes for the ageing process. Mech Ageing Dev 9:267–285

Wormer W, Sames K, Rohen JW (1979) Histochemische Untersuchungen über Struktur und Alternsveränderungen der Descemetschen Membran beim Ring. Albrecht Von Grafes Arch Klin Ophthalmol 211:271–278

Yamashita T, Becker B, Cibis PA (1960) Histochemical studies of the primate ciliary body. Am J Ophthalmol 50:407

Aqueous Humor and Vitreous Production

K. GREEN, E. A. BALAZS, and J. L. DENLINGER

A. Aqueous Humor

I. Volume

The volume and physical dimensions of the anterior chamber have been well studied, reflecting the ease of determination by optical techniques and ultrasonography. Anterior chamber depth increases by about 50% between birth and 2 years of age and thereafter undergoes a slow asymptotic increase until the age of about 14 years as a result of flattening of the anterior lens surface (LARSEN 1971 a, b). The lens continues to grow (WEEKERS et al. 1966; SORSBY and LEARY 1970) which contributes to the decrease in both depth and volume of the anterior chamber with age.

Anterior chamber depth decreases by 0.013–0.014 mm/year (LINDSTEDT 1916; RAEDER 1922; ROSENGREN 1930; CALMETTES et al. 1958), 0.01 mm/year (WEEKERS et al. 1961; FONTANA and BRUBAKER 1980), 0.008 mm/year (WEEKERS et al. 1966), or 0.019 mm/year (HEIM 1941) after maturity of the eye (15–20 years; see Table 1). The average depth of the anterior chamber is 3.0–3.4 mm at 40 years (FONTANA and BRUBAKER 1980). Males have larger anterior chamber depths than females by an average of about 4% (STENSTROM 1946; FONTANA and BRUBAKER 1980). The relation of emmetropia to anterior chamber depth averages about 0.06 mm/D (FONTANA and BRUBAKER 1980) greater in myopia, although a lack of relationship to myopia has also been reported (CALMETTES et al. 1958). LINDSTEDT (1916), RAEDER (1922), and LARSEN (1971 a) found a correlation between anterior chamber depth and the degree of emmetropia as well as a change in depth with age. Myopia greater than 3–4 D has no effect on anterior chamber depth as a function of age (WEEKERS et al. 1961).

Disease-induced pathologic changes result in dimensions which deviate from those given (WEEKERS and GRIETEN 1961; WEEKERS et al. 1966; TOMLINSON and LEIGHTON 1973, 1974; LOWE and CLARK 1973). In open-angle glaucoma the anterior chamber depth is significantly shallower than in age- and sex-matched normal subjects (3.12 vs 3.40 mm). It appears, therefore, that disease processes affect the dimensions more than those changes caused by aging (TOMLINSON and LEIGHTON 1974). Anterior chamber volume decreases by between 1 and 2 μl/year (HEIM 1941; JOHNSON et al. 1978; FONTANA and BRUBAKER 1980; BRUBAKER et al. 1981; see Table 1), is 6% greater in males (FONTANA and BRUBAKER 1980), and is greater in myopia by 4–7 μl/D (HEIM 1941; FONTANA and BRUBAKER 1980).

Table 1. Anterior chamber characteristics as a function of age

Characteristic	Change	Reference
Volume	1–2 μl/year	HEIM (1941); JOHNSON et al. (1978); FONTANA and BRUBAKER (1980); BRUBAKER et al. (1981)
Depth	– 0.008 mm/year	WEEKERS et al. (1966)
	– 0.01 mm/year	FONTANA and BRUBAKER (1980); WEEKERS et al. (1961)
	– 0.013 mm/year	LINDSTEDT (1916); RAEDER (1922); ROSENGREN (1930); CALMETTES et al. (1958)
	– 0.019 mm/year	HEIM (1941)
Intraocular pressure	+ 0.09 mmHg/year	BRUBAKER et al. (1981)
	Increase with age, especially over 40 years	ARMALY (1965); BANKES et al. (1968); COLTON and EDERER (1980); HOLLOWS and GRAHAM (1966); KAHN et al. (1977); KATAVISTO and SAMMALKIVI (1964); BENGTSSON (1972)
Aqueous flow rate	– 0.003 μl min^{-1} $year^{-1}$	GOLDMANN (1951)
	– 0.015 μl min^{-1} $year^{-1}$	BLOOM et al. (1976)
	– 0.006 μl min^{-1} $year^{-1}$	BRUBAKER et al. (1981)
Aqueous humor	– 0.006 μl min^{-1} $year^{-1}$	BRUBAKER et al. (1981)
Formation rate	Statistically lower rates with increasing age	BRUBAKER et al. (1981); BECKER (1958); KUPFER (1973); GAASTERLAND et al. (1978)
Scleral rigidity	Reduction with age	ARMALY and SAYEGH (1970)
Outflow facility	Decrease above 40 years	BECKER (1958); GOLDMANN (1951); PRIJOT (1961); ARMALY and SAYEGH (1970); WEEKERS et al. (1956); HUGGERT (1957); GAASTERLAND et al. (1978)

II. Composition

Aqueous humor composition of adult humans is well documented (ALTMAN and DITTMER 1974; COLE 1978), but age variations have not been studied in detail. A reciprocity has also been found (HOCKWIN and KOCH 1978) wherein the lens can influence the chemical composition of the aqueous humor (KUCK and CROSWELL 1974; DE BERARDINIS et al. 1966), in the same manner as disturbances of aqueous humor composition can induce lens changes (KASKEL et al. 1975).

POHJOLA (1966) found a significant reduction of aqueous glucose concentration with age, as well as a decrease in the steady state ratio of aqueous:plasma glucose. Since plasma glucose did not change, the decreased concentration of glucose must reflect reduced solute entry into the aqueous. In bovine eyes, ISMAIL et al. (1977) found that glucose and fructose levels increased during the first year of life with a maximum at about 5 or 6 years, but galactose and inositol were constant. KUCK (1963) found that age did not affect rat blood or aqueous humor glucose or fructose, although O'BRIEN and SALIT (1931) found that cow aqueous humor glucose content was lower than in calves. Other age-related changes (not necessarily decreases) in human aqueous humor concentrations as well as blood: aqueous humor ratios have been noted for urea, glucose, phosphorus, calcium, and alkaline reserve (LE REBELLER et al. 1976). BRUUN LAURSEN (1972, 1973) found a decrease in pyruvate and an increase in citrate in oxen and rabbits. BRUUN LAURSEN and LORENTZEN (1974), however, found no correlation between age and pyruvate or citrate concentrations or between age and aqueous:plasma ratios of glucose, pyruvate, or citrate in humans. The number of samples per age group in the latter study was low and perhaps not representative of the spectrum of changes which may occur. Species differences evidently exist.

Further study is needed to elucidate the biochemical changes occurring in the aqueous humor with age, since they may relate to the morphological changes in the ciliary processes which offers a less leaky permeability barrier to the passage of molecules into the aqueous humor. It is unlikely that the ionic composition changes markedly, although some change might be predicted based upon the mode of aqueous entry into the eye (GREEN et al. 1978).

The aqueous humor contains a small amount of sodium hyaluronate (MEYER and PALMER 1934; BALAZS et al. 1959; LAURENT et al. 1969; BALAZS 1965; LAURENT 1981). The concentration varies between 0.3 and 4.0 µg/ml in adults of various species. In human aqueous humor obtained during cataract surgery, the hyaluronate content was 1.14 ± 0.46 µg/ml. Patients with diabetes and/or glaucoma did not show a significant difference (LAURENT 1982). The bulk of the hyaluronate in the aqueous humor originates from the vitreous. It has been suggested that some of the hyaluronate in the bovine aqueous humor originates from the corneal endothelium (LAURENT 1981). In the aqueous humor of the owl, where the hyaluronate concentration is much higher (BALAZS 1965), a decreasing concentration gradient exists from the endothelium towards the lens. This may also indicate production by the endothelial cells. The variation of hyaluronate concentration with age has not been studied extensively. It was found that in bovine embryos (5–9 months) the hyaluronate concentration is about 75% lower than in the adult. In human aqueous humor of patients between 50 and 90 years of age there was no significant difference (LAURENT 1982).

III. Intraocular Pressure

An increase in intraocular pressure occurs with age as measured in large populations with applanation tonometry (ARMALY 1965, 1967; BANKES et al. 1968; COLTON and EDERER 1980; HOLLOWS and GRAHAM 1966; KAHN et al. 1977; BRUBAKER et al. 1981; see Table 1). Most studies have found that higher intraocular pressures appear at the age of 40 years and increase with age (ARMALY 1965; COLTON and EDERER 1980). These similarities occur despite differences in sample population, inclusion and exclusion criteria, and procedures for tonometry. The increase in intraocular pressure with age is less when measured with Schiotz tonometry (HOLLOWS and GRAHAM 1966; GRAHAM and HOLLOWS 1964; KATAVISTO and SAMMALKIVI 1964; LEYDHECKER et al. 1958). Noncontact tonometry also indicated an increase in intraocular pressure in a 61–70 age group compared with 0–10 and a 21–30 age group (RICHTER et al. 1979). Intertwined with these determinations of intraocular pressure is the greater prevalence of glaucoma in the older population and, since intraocular pressure is one of the criteria for determining glaucoma, it is invariably included in such determinations. Indeed, a follow-up of the 5,941 persons in the population of the BANKES et al. (1968) study revealed 42 persons with chronic open-angle glaucoma and 10 with angle-closure glaucoma (WORTHEN 1978).

BANKES et al. (1968), ARMALY (1965), KATAVISTO and SAMMALKIVI (1964), and GANLEY (1980) found that the rise in intraocular pressure with age was greater in females than males, particularly over the age of 40 years. This was attributed to the onset of menopause in females and the hormonal changes which accompany this age-related phenomenon (ARMALY 1965, 1967). BANKES et al. (1968) found a correlation between intraocular pressure and different phases of the menstrual cycle with lowest pressures at days 21–24 and highest pressures at days 9–12. After menopause, the pressure was higher, even in the 40–49 age group.

BENGTSSON (1972) found a correlation between age and intraocular pressure, but the association between increased age and systemic blood pressure was strong. The age–intraocular pressure relationship was dependent on increased systemic blood pressure, although the relative frequency of persons with abnormally high intraocular pressures was increased between 65 and 79 years. This was associated with an increase in the prevalence of simple glaucoma with age. BRUBAKER et al. (1981) found a significant increase in intraocular pressure in subjects ranging from 20 to 83 years of age, with a change of +0.09 mmHg/year.

The variation between applanation and Schiotz tonometry may reflect changes in ocular rigidity (DUKE-ELDER 1968) and the need for a weight change with the Schiotz tonometer with an increased intraocular pressure (WORTHEN 1978). Schiotz tonometry is subject to several sources of error. Care should be given to interpretations of measurements with this instrument (KOLKER and HETHERINGTON 1970) as the readings can result in artificial bimodal distributions (HOLLOWS and GRAHAM 1966; COLTON and EDERER 1980).

From high intraocular pressures averaging 21.1 mmHg at age 0–1 year, a fall occurs to 15.7 mmHg at age 8–9 years (KORNBLUETH et al. 1964). These studies were made with the Schiotz tonometer where the possibility of variation in scleral rigidity has to be considered as a source of error. ARMALY and SAYEGH (1970) found, by comparison of applanation and Schiotz tonometry, a reduction in ocular rigidity after water drinking in all age groups, and a general reduction in ocular rigidity with age. ARMALY and SAYEGH (1970) also found an effect of age upon the response of applanation pressure to water drinking, a provocative test in glaucoma detection, with the mean increase in pressure caused by a standard water load increasing with age. The cup:disc ratio has also been found to increase with age (CARPEL and ENGSTROM 1981) from a value of 0.31:1 in the first decade to 0.44:1 in the eighth decade; this occurred irrespective of the intraocular pressure.

IV. Formation

Two approaches have been taken to study aging effects on the rate of aqueous humor formation. First, aqueous humor formation rate is calculated from tonometric and tonographic data, using either an assumed or measured value for episcleral venous pressure,

$$F = C(P_i - P_e)$$

where F is aqueous humor formation rate, C is total outflow facility, P_i is intraocular pressure, and P_e is episcleral venous pressure. The second approach has used fluorescein as a tracer for aqueous flow, using either intravenous (GOLDMANN 1951), or transcorneal (JONES and MAURICE 1966) administration.

BECKER (1958) analyzed the data from 909 normal eyes and concluded that the rate of aqueous humor formation was stable up to the age of 60 years with a significant decrease with increasing age beyond this age. In 244 eyes less than 40 years of age, a flow rate of 2.0 ± 0.05 μl/min was found, while in 347 eyes of the 41–60 age group the flow rate was 1.9 ± 0.04 μl/min and in 318 eyes at age greater than 60 years the flow rate was 1.2 ± 0.03 μl/min. SPURGEON et al. (1958), however, failed to substantiate BECKER's observations. KUPFER (1973) and GAASTERLAND et al. (1978) also used tonography and tonometry in groups of 10 subjects each of ages 19–23 and 50–81 years and 33 subjects aged 21 years and 18 subjects aged 62 years, respectively. In each study, a significant fall in aqueous humor flow rate was found, although GAASTERLAND et al. (1978) found significant differences only in right eyes.

GREEN et al. (1978) analyzed the GAASTERLAND et al. (1978) data using a mathematical approach based on models of BARANY (1963) and PEDERSON and GREEN (1973) in which the volume flows and underlying pressure differentials causing the flows can be calculated. The data were analyzed in two ways; both analyses indicated that aging changes were associated with a decrease in ultrafiltration. This statistical analysis indicates a marked aging change on the process of aqueous humor formation. The findings correlate with vascular changes occurring with aging, as well as morphological changes in the basement membrane of the ciliary processes.

Studies with fluorescein have indicated a significant fall in aqueous humor formation rate with age (BRUBAKER et al. 1981; see Table 1). GOLDMANN (1951) also found a significant fall with increasing age, and BLOOM et al. (1976) found a significant inverse relationship by multiple regression analysis. BRUBAKER et al. (1981) examined 151 eyes of 113 subjects by transcorneal iontophoretic application of fluorescein. The procedure for calculating aqueous flow rate was described by COAKES and BRUBAKER (1979). A small but statistically significant decrease occurred in aqueous humor formation rate, 0.006 μl min^{-1} year^{-1} or -2.4% per decade. The change in aqueous formation rate is small compared with that occurring in anterior chamber volume or intraocular pressure (BRUBAKER et al. 1981). There is a suggestion of a significant break in formation rate at or about 60 years of age, at which point the change becomes larger (BECKER 1958; BRUBAKER et al. 1981). The relatively small sample size of both studies preclude these changes assuming statistical significance, but are suggestive of a marked change in the stability of aqueous humor formation.

BRUBAKER et al. (1981) point out that assumptions are made that all of the aqueous humor flows through the anterior chamber and that diffusional loss to the iris is minimal compared with loss due to aqueous flow. GOLDMANN (1951) found a statistically nonsignificant 13% increase in iris permeability to fluorescein per decade and if the data of BRUBAKER et al. (1981) are corrected for this iris diffusibility factor, there is a 50% greater decrease of aqueous humor formation with age (3.8% per decade compared with 2.4% per decade). While the anterior chamber volume decreases with age, this reduction occurs faster than the reduction in aqueous flow rate, thus the turnover constant actually increases with age (GAASTERLAND 1981). Such a change may be nutritionally beneficial for the lens, cornea, and trabecular meshwork which are perfused by the aqueous humor.

VAN NEROM et al. (1981) studied the effect of aging on iris and ciliary body vessel permeability. Arm–iris circulation time, the time elapsed between injection via the antebrachial vein and the first appearance of fluorescein in the radial arteries of the iris, increased with age at a rate of 0.1 s/year. This finding is not unexpected since arterial circulation time decreases with increasing age. Arterial time, the time needed for the dye to reach the pupillary margin from the limbus significantly increased linearly with age at a rate of 0.07 s/year. Fluorescein leakage from the pupillary margin also increased with age, and of five eyes which showed significant leakage, four were patients older than 40 years. Increasing age was associated with increasing aqueous fluorescein concentration (slope = 20.3 mg ml^{-1} $year^{-1}$ which reflects an increase in permeability of both iris and ciliary body blood vessels to fluorescein, especially as it is known that aqueous formation decreases with age. VAN NEROM et al. (1981) found a significant correlation between hemoglobin A_{Ic} both age and aqueous fluorescein concentration; they suggested that increased glycosylation of specific membrane proteins may increase iris and ciliary body vessel permeability.

SCHWARZ and KERN (1980) found decreased filling of the retinal arteries, optic disc, and peripapillary choroid with age. Patients showed effects of both age and glaucoma on these characteristics with both factors decreasing the perfusion times, perhaps reflecting the greater incidence of elevated intraocular pressure with age. BOLES-CARENINI and CAMBIAGGI (1957) concluded that neither intraocular pressure, nor outflow resistance, nor yet the range of outflow facility was significantly changed with age. Further analysis (SPURGEON et al. 1958) comparing the change in intraocular pressure per decade with the closest decade revealed no differences, but the 30–49 age group was significantly different from the 70–92 age group in terms of the deviation of pressure, although the average pressures were the same. The calculated flow rate was significantly different between the 10–29 age group and the 50–69 or 70–92 age group. They concluded that the measured parameters do not change significantly with age.

The decline in aqueous humor formation with age may be associated with histologic changes occurring in the ciliary body. Alterations occur in the nonpigmented ciliary epithelium and the inner limiting membrane over both the pars plicata and pars plana (HOGAN et al. 1971). The cells of the ciliary process crests show only moderate changes, but the cells of the valleys and side walls of the processes develop irregularities of the basal cell surface, that is, the cell surface facing the posterior chamber. In the pars plana, cells become thinner and taller as the basal surfaces become irregular and form thin branching processes. The intercellular spaces widen along the lower two-thirds of the cells.

The changes in the inner limiting membrane with age involve some thickening above the crests of the ciliary processes and much greater thickening in the valleys. The crevices between the partially separated cells become filled with membrane. The spaces formed between the cells along their lateral sides become straighter and cause separation of the lateral interdigitations (HOGAN et al. 1971). FINE and ZIMMERMAN (1963) observed an acid mucopolysaccharide flocculent deposit in the widened intercellular spaces. MISSOTEN (1964) also found that the basement membrane (or inner limiting membrane) became thicker with increasing age as the result of laminae formation of basement membrane-like material which forms a reticular pattern. Granular material is found within the reticular meshwork similar to that seen in Bruch's membrane of the choroid during aging (HOGAN et al. 1971).

V. Outflow

BECKER (1958), GOLDMANN (1951), PRIJOT (1961), ARMALY and SAYEGH (1970), and WEEKERS et al. (1956) found a decrease in outflow facility with age in humans and HUGGERT (1957) obtained similar data in rabbits. Other investigators have found no change in outflow facility with increasing age (BOLES-CARRENINI and CAMBIAGGI 1957; SPENCER et al. 1955; SPURGEON et al. 1958; GRANT 1951).

BECKER (1958) divided his population into decades and, while finding little change in intraocular pressure with age, found that outflow facility declined steadily. At age 60 years, however, a marked change in calculated flow rate occurred. In enucleated normal perfused eyes, the outflow facility was also negatively correlated with age. These findings in living eyes were true of both normal and glaucomatous eyes. BECKER (1958) drew attention to atrophy of the ciliary body noted in elderly patients and correlated this with the change in aqueous flow rate. GAASTERLAND et al. (1978) found a decrease in total outflow facility with increasing age, which was caused by a reduction in both true outflow facility and pseudofacility, resulting in a minor increase in intraocular pressure (Table 1).

The perfusion studies (BECKER 1958) indicated that structural changes occur in the drainage channels of the eye as can be demonstrated histologically (TENG et al. 1955). In beef eyes, HUGGERT (1957) also found a greater number of smaller pores in eyes from older animals. BECKER (1958) noted that the decrease in aqueous volume and the rate of aqueous formation could lead to a maintenance of flow rate, despite the decline in outflow facility and anterior chamber volume. SPENCER et al. (1955) analyzed only 20 patients in each decade with tonography and concluded that no age-related change occurred, although above the age of 50 years there appeared to be a decrease in outflow facility.

SEGAWA (1979) studied morphological specimens of the trabecular meshwork with electron microscopy. As outflow facility declined with age, the amount of all measured morphological components increased. The thickness of the corneoscleral meshwork membrane and of the elastic fiber sheath of the corneoscleral meshwork increased significantly with age. Amorphous material underneath and within 10 μm of the trabecular wall endothelium also correlated with age, without being statistically significant. The positive correlation between the amount of polysaccharide and age suggests that the increase is due to inhibition of catabolism rather than overproduction (SEGAWA 1979). It is uncertain as to whether the increase in amorphous material is the cause of the increased resistance, or is generated by the decreased aqueous flow which occurs with aging. Since aqueous turnover is increased, it would appear that the derangement in the outflow system occurs before any decrease in perfusion of the meshwork.

McMENAMIN and LEE (1980) found that the percentage area of trabecular meshwork occupied by amorphous ground substance and fibrillar material decreased with age and the percentage area occupied by electron-dense material increased in an electron micrographic study. ROHEN and LÜTJEN-DRECOLL (1971) suggested that both the overall thickness of the inner wall of Schlemm's canal and the number of cell layers decreased with age.

FINE (1964) examined the anterior chamber angle of both humans and rhesus monkeys (Macaca mulatta) with light and electron microscopy. Changes found with open-angle glaucoma were considered to be an acceleration of normal aging processes of these tissues. The aging changes consist of increasing intermolecular and intramolecular cross-linking of the collagen fibrils with a concomitant loss of polysaccharide. FINE et al. (1981) presented histologic findings in aging normal and glaucomatous eyes, identifying two basic changes in the angle. First, a scleral spur forms from the scleral roll (FINE and YANOFF 1979) by a process of collapse and accretion of uveal meshwork concurrent with hyalinization (ROHEN and LÜTJEN-DRECOLL 1971) or atrophy of the ciliary muscle. The second process is proliferation of endothelial, and possibly juxtacanalicular, connective tissue into the lumen of Schlemm's canal (YANOFF and FINE 1975). When these aging changes become excessive or localized to one portion of the angle, other ocular glaucomatous changes can occur.

The trabecular sheets of the corneoscleral meshwork of older eyes have large deposits of collagen which are not found in young (0–10 years) eyes (HOGAN et al. 1971). The posterior portion of the uveal meshwork, prominent in children, is increasingly difficult to identify and demonstrate in older persons. Sheets of collagen and tropocollagen aggregates are found in the deep corneolimbal region of the drainage angle.

VI. Summary

The anterior chamber decreases in size and volume (1–2 μl/year) once maturity is reached, and is dependent on the refractive status of the eye since myopic eyes are deeper and hyperopic eyes shallower than emmetropic eyes. Disease states, such as open-angle glaucoma, cause alterations in the dimensions. Aqueous humor composition shows age-dependent changes in some organic compounds which reflect some interaction between the lens and aqueous humor.

Intraocular pressure increases with age, with an increasing occurrence of glaucoma. Outflow facility decreases with age and scleral rigidity increases. These age-associated events contribute to the rise in intraocular pressure, and since the major site of fluid outflow resistance appears to be the inner wall of Schlemm's canal, the morphological changes occurring in both the trabecular meshwork and

Schlemm's canal cause an increased resistance. More rapid changes result in glaucoma and reflect an acceleration of normal aging processes. Aqueous humor formation decreases with age, which should result in a fall in intraocular pressure, but intraocular pressure increases; thus, the other aging changes are more influential, particularly outflow resistance.

Fluid inflow may be reduced because of vascular or membrane changes. Vascular changes occur in the capillary bed supplying the site of aqueous humor formation. The basement membrane (inner limiting layer) of the ciliary processes thickens with age and the cellular elements of the ciliary processes change. The decrease in outflow facility is not caused by a reduction in flow rate inducing a grater buildup of material, but rather is due to a change in either secretion or catabolism of glycosaminoglycans and collagen in the matrix.

The culmination of this age-related phenomenon is open-angle glaucoma which is treated either medically or surgically. Medical treatment requires considerations of the other age-related changes (DANGEL and HAVENER 1981), where steroids, for example, may induce elevated intraocular pressure by alteration of the secretory pattern of the trabecular meshwork cells. Glaucoma medications should be used judiciously to reduce potential side effects, and the effects of systemically administered medications in the ophthalmic patient should be understood. Maculopathy can result from the use of epinephrine in elderly, aphakic patients after cataract surgery. Other systemic drug effects may be exacerbated in the elderly patient with vascular disease, hypertension, or coronary artery disease.

B. Vitreous

I. Structure

The vitreous is the transparent connective tissue matrix which fills the space bordered by the lens, ciliary body, and retina. The rheological state can be gel (gel vitreous) or liquid (liquid vitreous). The relative amount of gel and liquid varies both with species and with age. The volume of the liquid vitreous in human eyes increases from birth to adulthood and the structure and macromolecular composition changes considerably. During aging further changes occur which form the basis of some pathologic processes (BALAZS 1982). The sequence of changes occurring during aging of human vitreous is different from that in most animals, leading to pathologic conditions typical of the human eye.

The basic vitreous architecture is based on the intensity of light scattering. Thin (10–20 nm) but uniform unbranched type II collagen fibrils (MATOLSKY et al. 1951; MATOLSKY 1952; SCHWARZ 1951; GROSS et al. 1955) are responsible for light scattering, and their presence or absence as well as orientation determines the biomicroscope image. Dark areas, where light scattering is weakest, are regions where the fibrils are absent or very widely spaced (EISNER 1976) and are channels, lacunae, or pools of liquid vitreous (EISNER 1975, 1976; TOLENTINO et al. 1976). The opaque, more homogeneous, areas where scattering is stronger are vitreous gel, where collagen fibrils are randomly distributed (SNOWDEN and

SWANN 1980; BALAZS and DENLINGER 1979). Depending on the interfibrillar distance, or the fibril density, the gel is more, or less, rigid. In the periphery of the vitreous, close to the retina, ciliary body, and lens, the gel is denser than in the central region, even in those primates in which the bulk of the vitreous is liquid (BALAZS and DENLINGER 1979).

Accumulation and orientation of collagen fibrils in two-dimensional systems (fibers, tracts, or membranes) scatter light more strongly, but the difference originates from a variation in the distribution and orientation of the collagen fibrils (BALAZS 1982). The two most important topographic variations in network density are at the base and the center of the vitreous. The network is densest where thin fibrils condense to fibers (BALAZS 1961) at the vitreous base at all ages, and in young adults is least dense in the posterior central area.

While most of the gel vitreous is composed of a random collagen fibril network, some fibers are organized as parallel aggregated bands. Those fibers which can be seen fairly well in the living eye with slit lamp examination, especially in older adults (EISNER 1975; 1976; TOLENTINO et al. 1976), run from the base of the vitreous to the optic nerve head parallel with the retina. Other fibers cannot be detected with the slit lamp because the fiber orientation is parallel to the illumination. These fibers are attached to the posterior lens capsule and to the basement membrane covering the macular area, thus mechanical stress during surgical manipulation of the lens capsule can be directly transmitted posteriorly (BALAZS 1982). These stresses may cause pathologic changes in the posterior vitreous and macula (posterior vitreous detachment, macular edema, and cysts; IRVINE 1953; TOLENTINO and SCHEPENS 1965).

In the cortical, or outer, layer of the gel vitreous are the vitreous cells or hyalocytes. These are differentiated and highly specialized mononuclear phagocytes separated by 2–3 cell diameters, and their concentration varies with age and topography (SZIRMAI and BALAZS 1958; BLOOM and BALAZS 1965). They are not present behind either the lens or zonules and are responsible for hyaluronic acid synthesis (ÖSTERLIN and JACOBSEN 1968; FREEMAN et al. 1979). Hyalocytes can also function as phagocytes when inflammation, including hemorrhage, occurs in the vitreous (BALAZS 1968; GLOOR 1973).

Cloquet's canal is the remnant of an embryonic arteriole (hyaloid artery) which crosses the vitreous from the optic disc to the posterior pole of the lens, where it branches and provides the blood supply for the rapidly growing tissue. It has the fine structure of an arteriole and the characteristic multilayered, fenestrated sheets are typical of basement membranes produced by smooth muscle cells surrounding an arteriole. When circulation ceases after birth, the cellular elements disappear rapidly. Cloquet's canal then remains as an acellular skeleton made up of multilayered fenestrated sheets and collagen fibrils (BLOOM et al. 1980). In the young human eye, Cloquet's canal is dense and well defined. In adult eyes, the canal has relatively well-delineated superior and inferior "plicated membranes", which are the remnants of the basal lamina and the collapsed collagen filament structure of the arteriole wall, and become less distinguishable, especially in the center of the vitreous, as it becomes surrounded by increasing fibrous and laminar structures. The membranes show some dislocation (ascension phenomenon) following movement of the eye.

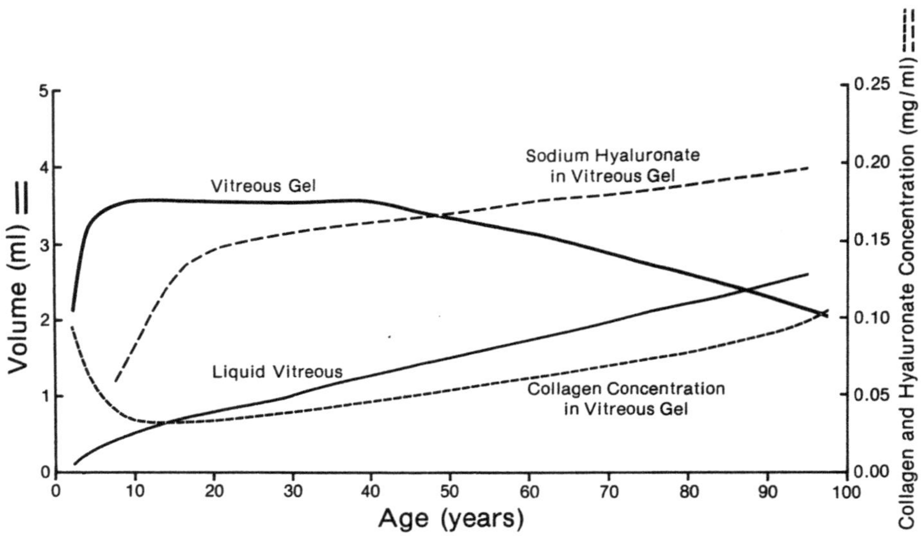

Fig. 1. Age-related changes in: vitreous gel volume (*upper full curve*); liquid vitreous volume (*lower full curve*); sodium hyaluronate concentration (*upper broken curve*); and collagen concentration (*lower broken curve*)

II. Composition

Liquid vitreous appears in the human eye after 4 years of age and after this time all postmortem human eyes contain at least 15% liquid vitreous. At maturity (14–18 years of age), about 20% of the total vitreous space is filled with liquid vitreous (FLOOD and BALAZS 1977). Liquid vitreous was found in only 9% of individuals under 20 years of age by slit lamp examination (EISNER 1975), but it is distributed in narrow channels within the gel, too small to be detected with the slit lamp. After 40 years of age, the liquid vitreous volume increases and channels fuse into larger pockets which are readily visible in the slit lamp. Between 40 and 84 years of age, 92% of all eyes axamined with the slit lamp show pockets or large pools of liquid vitreous (EISNER 1975). Studies of more than 1,000 postmortem human eyes between 20 and 97 years of age show that the liquid vitreous volume steadily increases after 40 years of age (Fig. 1). By the age of 80–90 years, over half the total vitreous volume is liquid (FLOOD and BALAZS 1979). Associated with the increase in liquid volume is a decrease in photoprotective enzymes and fluorescent chromophores (GIRSCH and ZIGMAN 1981).

The amount of gel vitreous also increases with age, reaching a plateau at about 10 years. At 40 years, as the second phase of liquid vitreous volume increase begins, the gel vitreous volume decreases, and persists during the remainder of life (Fig. 1). The basic difference between gel vitreous and liquid vitreous is that the latter does not contain collagen fibrils. The liquid vitreous is viscous because it contains sodium hyaluronate and, depending on the concentration of this substance, the viscosity of the liquid vitreous may be 2–4 times that of water or aqueous humor. Only the rhesus monkey has been found to have similar physical characteristics of the vitreous during aging (DENLINGER et al. 1980). Most other mammals including the most frequently used experimental laboratory animals (rabbit, rat, cat, dog) have very little or no liquid vitreous throughout life (BALAZS 1973).

1. Sodium Hyaluronate

A sodium hyaluronate molecular network fills the entire space between the collagen fibrils, consisting of spheroidal sodium hyaluronate molecules (molecular weight $2\text{–}4 \times 10^6$) with a diameter about ten times larger (200–300 nm) than that of the collagen fibrils. A single sodium hyaluronate molecule is made up of a long random coil of a thin (1–2 nm) polysaccharide chain and the space between the coils is filled with water. Because of the large hydrated specific volume of this polyanion ($V_o \sim 2{,}000$) and its random distribution and relatively low concentration, the light scattering is not sufficient for it to be seen with the biomicroscope. The sodium hyaluronate is produced by the hyalocytes (FREEMAN et al. 1979; JACOBSON 1976; HULTSCH and BALAZS 1973) embedded in the cortical gel vitreous and where the sodium hyaluronate concentration is highest (BALAZS 1954). The lare molecules slowly diffuse along a concentration gradient toward the anterior chamber, and leave the eye through the trabecular meshwork and Schlemm's canal. The turnover time (half-life) of these molecules in the eyes of two monkey species was found to be several months, indicating the slow diffusion of these molecules through the collagen fibrillar network (E.A. BALAZS, M.I. FREEMAN, F. REGNAULT, 1981, the Fate of Na-hyaluronate Injected into the Vitreus of Owl Monkey, unpublished data; DENLINGER 1982).

The sodium hyaluronate concentration in the gel vitreous is low at birth, but increases during vitreous growth (Fig. 1). When liquid vitreous appears, the sodium hyaluronate concentration is about the same in both the liquid and the gel. The sodium hyaluronate concentration in the liquid vitreous gradually increases and reaches adult levels by age 20 years. From 20 to 70 years of age, the sodium hyaluronate concentration remains the same in both gel and liquid vitreous. After 70 years of age there is a dramatic increase of the sodium hyaluronate concentration in the liquid vitreous, but not in the gel vitreous. Sodium hyaluronate has the same molecular size in old and young eyes, as well as in the liquid and gel vitreous (BALAZS and FLOOD 1978).

2. Collagen

The collagen concentration of the human gel vitreous decreases after birth, reaching its lowest level at the time when the eye is fully developed (Fig. 1). The total amount of collagen in the gel vitreous, however, does not change significantly, and the concentration decreases owing to an increase in the total gel vitreous volume. No collagen fibril synthesis or loss occurs during the growth of the eye and the parallel increase in vitreous volume. As the collagen matrix separates, the decreasing concentration of collagen fibrils imparts less rigidity to the gel vitreous. The collagen concentration in the gel vitreous increases over 50 years of age, thus the decrease in gel volume is due to collapse of the fibril network with a consequent increase in the liquid vitreous volume (BALAZS and FLOOD 1978).

III. Basement Membranes

In general, the entire basement membrane of the retina, which separates the glial cells (Müller cells) from the vitreous, becomes thicker during aging of the human eye (GÄRTNER 1965, 1970; RENTSCH and VAN DER ZYPEN 1971). The basement membrane bordering the vitreous at the ciliary body undergoes a different developmental and aging change. In the young human, the basement membrane over the nonpigmented epithelium is a single (40–50 nm) layer. This membrane becomes multilayered during maturation, forming a system of fenestrated sheets which extend into the vitreous. Vitreous fibrils are pushed back from the surface of the epithelium by this extensive reticular network. When the gel vitreous shrinks at 40–50 years of age, an extensive network of basement membrane covers the whole ciliary processes and later extends over the pars plana (RENTSCH and VAN DER ZYPEN 1971). The thickness of this membrane can be 4,000–5,000 nm after the age of 60 years (GÄRTNER 1970) and this thickening is a uniquely human phenomenon. The basement membrane is produced by lens cells, ciliary epithelia, and glial (Müller) cells (NEWSOME et al. 1976). The transformation of the basal lamina to a multilayered membranous network may be one of the contributing factors to the decline of accomodation in humans after 40–45 years of age (presbyopia) (BALAZS and DENLINGER 1982).

IV. Posterior Vitreous Detachment

Slit lamp examination of the living human eye reveals another aging change, posterior vitreous detachment (PISCHEL 1953; GOLDMANN 1962). It is assumed to be the separation of the cortical gel vitreous from the basement membrane. A thin layer of cortical gel may remain attached to the basement membrane, and a break in the vitreous could occur within the gel, creating a vitreoschisis (BALAZS 1973). One clinical investigation found a 20% frequency of posterior vitreous detachment between 54 and 63 years and a 49% frequency between 63 and 89 years (EISNER 1975). A higher (50%–65%) incidence in a population over 50 years of age has also been noted (PISCHEL 1953; FAVRE and GOLDMANN 1956).

Thickening of the posterior retinal basement membrane may be a prerequisite of some types of posterior vitreous detachment. Since this change in the physical characteristics of the vitreous occurs in most of the aging population and usually does not lead to any serious pathologic change or impairment of vision, it is considered a normal aging change. Support for this contention is given by the observation that 94% of individuals with senile nuclear opacities of the lens also have posterior vitreous detachment (ROSEN 1962). Posterior vitreous detachment, however, can occur at any age as a result of chronic intraocular inflammation, severe trauma, or perforating injury to the eye, and after chorioretinal degeneration as well as in aphakic or highly myopic young individuals.

These changes may encompass the entire range characteristic for aging of the human vitreous: thickening of the retinal basement membrane, an increase in the liquid vitreous volume, collapse of the gel, and aggregation of the collagen fibrils into large fibers. These changes occur in all aging human eyes, yet posterior detachment of the vitreous is not a universal phenomenon. Posterior vitreous detachment mainly occurs suddenly and spontaneously, often after a fall or blow to the head. The subjective symptoms are photopsia, metamorphosia, blurred vision, and moving opacities in the vitreous (floaters), which may be explained by the sudden collapse of the gel vitreous caused by a separation between the vitreous fibrillar network and the posterior basal lamina, or a schisis in the weaker precortical gel vitreous. Detachment is rarely complete at onset, especially in the macular and optic nerve area, where fibers of the contracting gel vitreous remain attached to the basal lamina of the retina and exert a mechanical pull.

Posterior vitreous detachment, as with other aging phenomena, may become a pathogenic factor in the development of hemorrhage, retinal tears leading to retinal detachment, and cystoid degeneration of the macula. In addition, the age-related changes typical of the posterior vitreous can trigger serious complications in eyes with diabetic retinopathy or with rhegmatogenous retinal detachment. Posterior vitreous detachment as an aging phenomenon appears unique to humans. The rhesus monkey vitreous is the only one described to date showing developmental and aging changes very similar to humans (DENLINGER et al. 1980). While rheological and biochemical studies show a striking similarity between this primate and the human, posterior vitreous detachment has not been observed in animals up to 21 years of age, but may occur in older animals.

The morphological and physical changes leading to posterior vitreous detachment are well understood. The arrangement of the collagen fibrils suspended in the viscoelastic sodium hyaluronate solution is altered, a process caused by the dislocation of the fibrils, but the cause is not known. Studies on the aging human vitreous (BALAZS and FLOOD 1978), showed that degradation and redistribution of sodium hyaluronate does not occur and no experimental evidence supports the concept of chemical changes in the collagen causing network contraction. The most probable explanation is that in young (less than 5 years of age) human vitreous a delicate balance exists between the noncross-linked collagen fibrils and the sodium hyaluronate molecules (BALAZS and DENLINGER 1982). The collagen network is fairly uniformly distributed in the nonviscous or low sodium hyaluronate concentration medium, but as the vitreous volume increases with growth of the eye, the distance between the fibrils increases because new fibrils are not formed. Sodium hyaluronate then enters the gel and stabilizes the more labile fibril network.

At full growth of the eye, the volume of the gel is at a maximum, as is the concentration of the sodium hyaluronate between the network-forming fibrils. This is already a precarious equilibrium, which creates small channels of liquid vitreous and, during aging, eye and body movements, as well as mechanical impacts on the head and eye, cause small but recurrent dislocations of the network, resulting in a decrease in gel volume and the formation of larger liquid vitreous pools. As the liquid vitreous reaches a certain volume and the attachements between the collapsed gel vitreous and the cortical gel or the posterior basement membrane are sufficiently weakened, a relatively small mechanical insult to the eye may trigger a sudden posterior vitreous detachment – the end point of normal vitreous aging. At this point either an uneventful continuation of the aging process or, in the presence of pathologic changes in the neighboring tissue, a major impairment of vision occurs (BALAZS and DENLINGER 1982).

V. Summary

Development of the vitreous is characterized by a slowly increasing concentration of sodium hyaluronate and a parallel increase in the gel volume (BALAZS and FLOOD 1978). New collagen fibrils are not formed, since the collagen concentration steadily decreases. Collagen fibrils are randomly distributed in the gel, thus fibers cannot be observed during the first decade. Vitreous volume doubles between birth and adulthood. The entire vitreous is a gel up to the age of about 4 years, but after this time liquid channels develop which represent up to 20% of the total vitreous volume of the adult eye. During the last phase of volume increase, fibril aggregation occurs and fibers are seen in the vitreous. Development of the vitreous ends when it reaches its maximum volume, the collagen concentration has reached a minimum in the gel and the sodium hyaluronate concentration, both in the gel and liquid vitreous, has reached a maximum.

From 45–50 years of age, liquid vitreous increases as a result of gel shrinkage or collapse (BALAZS et al. 1980). The sodium hyaluronate concentration and molecular size do not change until the age of 70 years. At that time in some normal human eyes, the sodium hyaluronate concentration increases considerably in the liquid vitreous (BALAZS and FLOOD 1978). The basal laminae adjacent to the peripheral retina undergo a steady thickening during aging (FINE and TOUSIMIS 1961). The thickness of the reticular multilayer basal laminar system at the ciliary body increases considerably between 50 and 90 years of age (BALAZS and DENLINGER 1982) reaching 4–5 μm after the age of 69 years (GÄRTNER 1965; RENTSCH and VAN DER ZYPEN 1971).

Another aging change is a separation of the posterior cortical gel vitreous from the retina (CAULFIELD 1964; PISCHEL 1953). The detachment can occur because the thicker basal lamina does not hold the collagen fibrils, and they in turn pull away from it. Alternatively, the thin cortical gel can separate from the rest of the gel, creating a vitreoschisis (BALAZS 1973) which would appear as a separation between the retina and vitreous. It occurs in 49% of the population between 63 and 89 years of age (EISNER 1975) and at 50%–65% frequency after the age of 50 years (PISCHEL 1953; CAULFIELD 1964). Posterior vitreous detachment can occur at any age after chronic intraocular inflammation, severe trauma, or injury to the eye, as a result of degenerative processes of the choriocapillary–pigment epithelial system (chorioretinal degeneration), or in aphakic or highly myopic eyes. It should be regarded as a symptom which is the result of, or develops in parallel with, thickening of the retinal basal lamina, the increase of liquid vitreous volume, and aggregation of collagen fibrils into large fibers.

The aggregation of collagen fibrils into fibers and the resulting tracts and strands in the vitreous produce another aging phenomenon appearing in parallel with the decrease (collapse) of the collagen fibrillar gel network. With posterior vitreous detachment this phenomenon reaches its most pronounced stage. The floaters, observed in most cases with posterior vitreous detachment, are aggregates of collagen fibrils which sometimes combine with the membranes of the Cloquet's canal. If they are in the central and premacular regions and move with the movement of the eye, they may cause symptoms or interfere with vision. Aging of human vitreous is very different from that of other mammals and most primates (BALAZS et al. 1980). The only similar aging process was observed in the rhesus monkey (DENLINGER et al. 1980) although posterior vitreous detachment was not found in this species.

Acknowledgements. This work was supported by U.S. Public Health Service grants EY 01413, EY 04558 (K.G.), and EY 01747 (E.A.B.). The secretarial assistance of Ilene Prior, Keely Daniel and Doris Garrett is gratefully acknowledged.

References

Altman PL, Dittmer DS (1974) Biology data book, 2nd edn, vol 3. Federation of American societies for experimental biology, Bethesda, Maryland

Armaly MF (1965) On the distribution of applanation pressure. I. Statistical features and the effect of age, sex and family history of glaucoma. Arch Ophthalmol 73:11–18

Armaly MF (1967) Age and sex correction of applanation pressure. Arch Ophthalmol 78:480–484

Armaly MF, Sayegh RD (1970) Water drinking test. II The effect of age on tonometric and tonographic measures. Arch Ophthalmol 83:176–181

Balazs EA (1954) Structure of the vitreous gel. Acta XVII Congress Ophthalmol 11:1019–1024

Balazs EA (1961) Molecular morpholgy of the vitreous body. In: Smelser GK (ed) The structure of the eye. Academic, New York, p 293

Balazs EA (1965) Amino sugar-containing macromolecules in the tissues of the eye and the ear. In: Balazs EA, Jeanloz RW (eds) The amino sugars: The chemistry and biology of compounds containing amino sugar. II-A Distribution and biological role. Academic, New York, p 401

Balazs EA (1968) The molecular biology of the vitreous. In: McPherson A (ed) New and controversial aspects of retinal detachment. Harper and Row, New York, p 3

Balazs EA (1973) The vitreous. Int Ophthalmol Clin 13:169–187

Balazs EA (1982) Functional anatomy of the vitreus. In: Jakobiec F (ed) Ocular anatomy, embryology and teratology. Harper and Row, Philadelphia, pp 425–440

Balazs EA, Denlinger JL (1979) Vitreous and join-comparative morphology and biochemistry. Atti Giorgio Ronchi 34:637–647

Balazs EA, Denlinger JL (1982) Aging changes in the vitreus. National Academy of Sciences, Washington D.C.

Balazs EA, Flood MT (1978) Age-related changes in the physical and chemical structure of human vitreous. Presented at the 3rd International congress of eye research, Osaka, Japan

Balazs EA, Laurent TC, Laurent UBG, De Roche MH, Bunney DM (1959) Studies on the structure of the vitreous body. VIII. Comparative biochemistry. Arch Biochem Biophys 81:464–479

Balazs EA, Toth LZ, Ozanics V (1980) Cytological studies on the developing vitreous as related to the hyaloid vessel system. Albrecht Von Graefes Arch Klin Ophthalmol 213:71–85

Bankes JLK, Perkins ES, Tsolakis S, Wright JE (1968) Bedford glaucoma survey. Br Med J 1:791–796

Bárány E (1963) A mathematical formulation of intraocular pressure as dependent on secretion, ultrafiltration, bulk outflow, and osmotic reabsorption of fluid. Invest Ophthalmol Vis Sci 2:584–590

Becker B (1958) The decline in aqueous secretion and outflow facility with age. Am J Ophthalmol 46:731–736

Bengtsson B (1972) Some factors affecting the distribution of intraocular pressures in a population. Acta Ophthalmol (Copenh) 50:33–46

Bloom GD, Balazs EA (1965) An electron microscopic study of hyalocytes. Exp Eye Res 4:249–255

Bloom GD, Balazs EA, Ozanics V (1980) The fine structure of the hyaloid arteriole in bovine vitreous. Exp Eye Res 31:129–145
Bloom N, Levene RZ, Thomas G, Kimura R (1976) Fluorophotometry and the rate of aqueous flow in man. Arch Ophthalmol 94:435–443
Boles-Carenini B, Cambiaggi A (1957) Are aqueous humor dynamics influenced by aging? Am J Ophthalmol 44:395–401
Brubaker RF, Nagataki S, Townsend DJ, Burns RR, Higgins RG, Wentworth W (1981) The effect of age on aqueous humor formation in man. Ophthalmology 88:283–288
Bruun Laursen A (1972) Citrate and pyruvate concentrations in bovine aqueous humor. Acta Ophthalmol (Copenh) 50:420–430
Bruun Laursen A (1973) Pyruvate and citrate concentrations in rabbit aqueous humor determined by an enzymatic procedure. Acta Ophthalmol (Copenh) 51:700–709
Bruun Laursen A, Lorentzen SE (1974) Glucose, pyruvate and citrate concentrations in the aqueous humor of human cataractous eyes. Acta Ophthalmol (Copenh) 52:477–489
Calmettes L, Deodati F, Huron H, Béchac G (1958) Etude de la profondeur de la chambre antérieure. Arch Ophthalmol (Paris) 18:513–542
Carpel EF, Engstrom PF (1981) The normal cup-disk ratio. Am J Ophthalmol 91:588–597
Caulfield JB (1964) Medical progress: Application of the electron microscope to renal diseases. N Eng J Med 270:183–194
Coakes RL, Brubaker RF (1979) Method of measuring aqueous humor flow and corneal endothelial permeability using a fluorophotometry nomogram. Invest Ophthalmol Vis Sci 18:288–302
Cole DF (1978) ciliary processes. In: Heilmann K, Richardson KT (eds) Glaucoma. Saunders, Philadelphia, p 44
Colton T, Ederer F (1980) The distribution of intraocular pressures in the general population. Surv Ophthalmol 25:123–129
Dangel ME, Havener WH (1981) Drugs and the aging eye. Geriatrics 36:133–140
De Berardinis E, Tieri O, Inglio N, Polzella A (1966) The composition of the aqueous humor of man in aphakia. Acta Ophthalmol (Copenh) 44:64–68
Denlinger JL (1982) Metabolisme de l'hyaluronate de sodium au niveau des tissus articulaires et oculaires. Doctoral thesis, Université de Lille, p 369
Denlinger JL, Eisner G, Balazs EA (1980) Age-related changes in the vitreus and lens of rhesus monkey (Macaca mulatta). Exp Eye Res 31:67–79
Duke-Elder WS (1968) System of ophthalmology, vol 4. The physiology of the eye and of vision. Mosby, St. Louis
Eisner G (1975) Zur Anatomie des Glaskörpers. Albrecht Von Graefes Arch Klin Ophthalmol 193: 33–56
Eisner G (1976) The anatomy and biochemistry of the vitreous body. Doc Ophthalmol Proc Ser 7:87–104
Favre M, Goldmann H (1956) Zur Genese der hinteren Glaskörperabnebung. Ophthalmologica 132:87–97
Fine BS (1964) Observations on the drainage angle in man and rhesus monkey: A concept of the pathogeneis of chronic simple glaucoma. Invest Ophthalmol Vis Sci 3:609–646
Fine BS, Tousimis AJ (1961) The structure of the vitreous body and the suspensory system of the lens. Arch Ophthalmol 4:95–110
Fine BS, Yanoff M (1979) Ocular histology. A text and atlas, 2nd edn. Harper and Row, Hagerstown
Fine BS, Zimmerman LE (1963) Light and electron microscopic observations on the ciliary epithelium in man and rhesus monkey. Invest Ophthalmol Vis Sci 2:105–137
Fine BS, Yanoff M, Stone RA (1981) A clinicopathological study of four cases of primary open-angle glaucoma compared to normal eyes. Am J Ophthalmol 91:88–105
Flood MT, Balazs EA (1977) Hyaluronic acid content in the developing and aging human liquid and gel vitreous. Invest Ophthalmol Vis Sci [Suppl] 16:67
Fontana S, Brubaker RF (1980) Volume and depth of the anterior chamber in the normal aging human eye. Arch Ophthalmol 98:1803–1808
Freeman MI, Jacobson B, Balazs EA (1979) The chemical composition of vitreous hyalocyte granules. Exp Eye Res 29:479–484

Gaasterland E (1981) Discussion of paper by Brubaker et al. (1981). Ophthalmology 88:287–288
Gaasterland DE, Kupfer C, Milton R, Ross K, McCain L, MacLellan H (1978) Studies of aqueous humor dynamics in man. VI. Effect of age upon parameters of intraocular pressure in normal human eyes. Exp Eye Res 26:651–656
Ganley JP (1980) Epidemiological aspects of ocular hypertension. Surv Ophthalmol 25:130–135
Gärtner J (1965) Beziehungen zwischen Fuundusdiagnostik und Elektronenmikroskopie, dargestellt am Beispiel der Glaskörperrinde in der Ora-Serrata-Gegend. „Netzhautablösung". Mod Probl Ophthalmol 5:154–169
Gärtner J (1970) Electron microscopic observations on the cilio-zonular border area of the human eye with particular reference to the aging changes. Z Anat Entwicklungsgesch 131:263–273
Girsch SJ, Zigman S (1981) Biochemical studies of vitreous relative to age. Invest Ophthalmol Vis Sci [Suppl] 20:139
Gloor PP (1973) Zur Entwicklung des Glaskörpers und der Zonula. III. Herkunft, Lebenszeit und Ersatz der Glaskörperzellen beim Kaninchen (Autoradiographische Untersuchungen mit ^{3}H-thymidin). Albrecht Von Graefes Arch Klin Ophthalmol 187:21–44
Goldmann H (1951) Abflussdruck, Minutenvolumen und Widerstand der Kammerwasser-Strömung des Menschen. Doc Ophthalmol 5:278–356
Goldmann H (1962) Senescenz des Glaskörpers. Ophthalmologica 143:253–279
Graham PA, Hollows FC (1964) Sources of variation in tonometry. Trans Ophthalmol Soc UK 84:597–613
Grant WM (1951) Clinical measurements of aqueous outflow. Arch Ophthalmol 46:113–131
Green K, Gaasterland DE, Milton R, Bowman K (1978) Influence of aging on aqueous humor production. Interdiscipl Top Gerontol 13:14
Gross J, Matoltsy AG, Cohen C (1955) Vitrosin: A member of the collagen class. J. Biophys Biochem Cytol 1:215–220
Heim M (1941) Photographische Bestimmung der Tiefe und des Volumens der menschlichen Vorderkammer. Ophthalmologica 102:193–220
Hockwin O, Koch HR (1978) Lens. In: Heilmann K, Richardson KT (eds) Glaucoma. Saunders, Philadelphia, p 67
Hogan MJ, Alvarado JA, Weddell JE (1971) Histology of the Human Eye. Saunders, Philadelphia
Hollows FC, Graham PA (1966) Intraocular pressure, glaucoma and glaucoma suspects in a defined population. Br J Ophthalmol 50:570–586
Huggert A (1957) An experiment in determining the pore-size distribution curve to the filtration angle of the eye. I. Acta Ophthalmol (Copenh) 35:12–19
Hultsch E, Balazs EA (1973) In vitro synthesis of glycosaminoglycans and glycoproteins in cells of the vitreous. Association for research in vision and ophthalmology, p 43
Irvine SR (1953) A newly defined vitreous syndrome following cataract surgery; interpreted according to recent concepts of the structure of the vitreous. Am J Ophthalmol 36:599–619
Ismail RM, Edelbi AH, Rösinger M (1977) Chemical composition of the aqueous humor of bovine eyes dependent on predetermined time upon removal. Albrecht Von Graefes Arch Klin Ophthalmol 202:55–62
Jacobson B (1976) Biosynthesis of hyaluronic acid in the vitreous. V. Studies on an particulate hyalocyte glycosyl transferase. Exp Eye Res 27:246–258
Johnson SB, Coakes RL, Brubaker RF (1978) A simple photogrammetric method of measuring aqueous humor volume. Am J Ophthalmol 85:469–474
Jones RF, Maurice DM (1966) New methods of measuring the rate of aqueous flow in man with fluorescein. Exp Eye Res 5:208–220
Kahn HA, Leibowitz HM, Ganley JP (1977) The Framingham eye study. I. Outline and major prevalence findings. Am J Epidemiol 106:17–32
Kaskel D, Scholz R, Hockwin O, Zeismer W (1975) Composition of aqueous humor and lens after carotid ligation. Ophthalmol Res 7:409–415

Katavisto M, Sammalkivi J (1964) Tonometry among persons over 40 years of age. Acta Ophthalmol (Copenh) 42:370–377

Kolker AE, Hetherington J (1970) Diagnosis and therapy of the glaucomas, 3rd edn. Mosby, St. Louis

Kornblueth W, Aladjemoff L, Magora F, Ben Dor D (1964) Intraocular pressure in children measured under general anesthesia. Arch Ophthalmol 72:489–490

Kuck JFR (1963) Sugar and sugar alcohol levels in the aging rat lens. Invest Ophthalmol (Vis Sci) 2:607–611

Kuck JFR, Croswell HH (1974) Lens as the chief source of fructose in rabbit aqueous humor. Ophthalmol Res 6:189–196

Kupfer C (1973) Clinical significance of pseudofacility. Am J Ophthalmol 75:173–204

Larsen JS (1971 a) The sagittal growth of the eye. I. Ultrasonic measurement of the depth of the anterior chamber from birth to puberty. Acta Ophthalmol (Copenh) 49:239–262

Larsen JS (1971 b) The sagittal growth of the eye. II. Ultrasonic measurement of the axial diameter of the lens and the anterior segment from birth to puberty. Acta Ophthalmol (Copenh) 49:427–453

Laurent TC, Barany EH, Carlsson B, Tidare E (1969) Determination of hyaluronic acid in the microgram range. Anal Biochem 31:133–145

Laurent UBG (1981) Hyaluronate in aqueous humour. Exp Eye Res 33:147–155

Laurent UBG (1982) Studies on endogenous sodium hyaluronate in the eye. Doctoral thesis, Acta Universitatis Uppsaliensis 428

Le Rebeller MJ, Crockett R, Maurain C, Sirieix F (1976) Nouvelle contribution à l'étude des composants de l'humeur aqueuse chez le sujet normal par utilisation des techniques d'analyses automatiques. Arch Ophthalmol (Paris) 36:749–764

Leydhecker W, Akiyama K, Neumann HG (1958) Der interokulare Druck gesunder menschlicher Augen. Klin Monatsbl Augenheilkd 133:662–670

Lindstedt F (1916) Über die Messung der Tiefe der vorderen Augenkammer mittels eines neuen, für klinischen Gebrauch bestimmten Instrumentes. Arch Augenheilkd 80:104–167

Lowe RF, Clark BAJ (1973) Posterior corneal curvature. Correlations in normal eyes and in eyes involved with primary angle-closure glaucoma. Br J Ophthalmol 57:464–470

Matoltsy AG (1952) A study on the structural protein of the vitreous body (vitrosin). J Gen Physiol 36:29–37

Matoltsy AG, Gross J, Grignolo A (1951) A study of the fibrous components of the vitreous body with the electron microscope. Proc Soc Exp Biol Med 76:857–860

McMenamin PG, Lee WR (1980) Age related changes in extracellular materials in the inner wall of Schlemm's canal. Albrecht Von Graefes Arch Klin Ophthalmol 212:159–172

Meyer K, Palmer JW (1934) The polysaccharide of the vitreous humor. J Biol Chem 107:629–634

Missoten L (1964) L'ultrastructure des tissus occulaire. Bull Soc Belge Ophthalmol 136:3–204

Newsome DA, Linesenmayer TF, Trelstad RD (1976) Vitreous body collagen. J Cell Biol 71:59–67

O'Brien CS, Salit PW (1931) The chemical constituents of the aqueous, vitreous and lens. A comparative study on animal eyes. Am J Ophthalmol 14:582–589

Österlin SE, Jacobson B (1968) The synthesis of hyaluronic acid in vitreous I. Soluble and particulate transferases in hyalocytes. Exp Eye Res 7:497–510

Pederson JE, Green K (1973) Aqueous humor dynamics: A mathematical approach to measurement of facility, pseudofacility, capillary pressure, active secretion and x_c. Exp Eye Res 15:265–276

Pischel DK (1953) Detachment of the vitreous as seen with slit-lamp examination. Am J Ophthalmol 36:1497–1507

Pohjola S (1966) The glucose content of the aqueous humor in man. Acta Ophthalmol (Copenh) [Suppl] 88:11–80

Prijot E (1961) Contribution a l'étude de la tonométrie et de la tonographie en ophthalmologie. Doc Ophthalmol 15:1–225

Raeder JG (1922) Untersuchungen über die Lage und Dicke der Linse im menschlichen Auge bei physiologischen und pathologischen Zuständen, nach einer neuen Methode gemessen. Albrecht von Graefes Arch Klinik Ophthalmol 110:73–108
Rentsch FJ, Van der Zypen E (1971) Altersbedingte Veränderungen der sogenannten Membrana limitans interna des Ziliarkörpers im menschlichen Auge. In: Bredt H, Rohen JW (eds) Altern und Entwicklung. Schattauer, Stuttgart, p 70
Richter S, Horn D, Bergknoff H (1979) A survey of intraocular pressures with emphasis on patients under ten years of age. Am J Optom Physiol Opt 56:193–196
Rohen JW, Lütjen-Drecoll E (1971) Age changes of the trabecular meshwork in human and monkey eyes. In: Bredt H, Rohen JW (eds) Ageing and development. Schattauer, Stuttgart, p 1
Rosen E (1962) Vitreous detachment. Associated nuclear sclerosis. Am J Ophthalmol 54:837–841
Rosengren B (1930) Studien über die Tiefe der vorderen Augenkammer mit besonderer Hinsicht auf ihr Verhalten beim primären Glaukom. Acta Ophthalmol (Copenh) 8:99–136
Schwartz B, Kern J (1980) Age, increased ocular and blood pressures, and retinal and disc fluorescein angiogram. Arch Ophthalmol 98:1980–1986
Schwarz W (1951) Die Gelbkörperfibrillen des menschlichen Glaskörpers. In: Verhandlungen der Anatomischen Gesellschaft auf der 49. Versammlung in Heidelberg. Fischer, Jena
Segawa K (1979) Electron microscopic changes of the trabecular tissue in primary open-angle glaucoma. Ann Ophthalmol 11:49–54
Snowden JM, Swann DA (1980) Vitreous structure. V. The morphology and thermal stability of vitreous collagen fibers and comparison to articular cartilage (type II) collagen. Invest Ophthalmol Vis Sci 19:610–618
Sorsby A, Leary G (1970) A longitudinal study of refraction and its components during growth. Medical research council, Special report ser 309, Her Majesty's stationary office, London
Spencer RW, Helmick ED, Scheie HG (1955) Tonography: Technical difficulties and control studies. Arch Ophthalmol 54:515–527
Spurgeon WM, Boles-Carenini B, Cambiaggi A (1958) Are aqueous humor dynamics influenced by aging? II. Am J Ophthalmol 46:845–855
Stenstrom S (1946) Untersuchungen über die Variation und Kovariation der optischen Elemente des menschlichen Auges. Acta Ophthalmol (Copenh) [Suppl] 26:1–103
Szirmai JA, Balazs EA (1958) Studies on the structure of the vitreous body. III. Cells in the cortical layer. Arch Ophthalmol 59:34–48
Teng CC, Paton RT, Katzin HM (1955) Primary degeneration in the vicinity of the chamber angle as an etiological factor in wide-angle glaucoma. Am J Ophthalmol 40:619–631
Tolentino FI, Schepens CL (1965) Edema of posterior pole after cataract extraction: a biomicroscopic study. Arch Ophthalmol 74:781–786
Tolentino FI, Schepens CL, Freeman HM (1976) Vitreoretinal disorders, diagnosis and management. Saunders, Philadelphia
Tomlinson A, Leighton DA (1973) Ocular dimensions in the heredity of angle-closure glaucoma. Br J Ophthalmol 57–475–486
Tomlinson A, Leighton DA (1974) Ocular dimensions and the heredity of open-angle glaucoma. Br J Ophthalmol 58:68–74
Van Nerom PR, Rosenthal AR, Jacobson DR, Pieper I, Schwartz H, Grieder BW (1981) Iris angiography and aqueous photofluorometry in normal subjects. Arch Ophthalmol 99:489–493
Weekers R, Grieten J (1961) La mesure de la profondeur de la chambre antérieure en clinique. Bull Soc Belge Ophthalmol 129:361–381
Weekers R, Watillon M, DeRudder M (1956) Experimental and clinical investigations into the resistance to outflow of aqueous humour in normal subjects. Br J Ophthalmol 40:225–233

Weekers R, Grieten J, Lavergne G (1961) Etude des dimensions de la chambre antérieure de l'oeil humain. Ophthalmologica 142:650–662

Weekers R, Luyckx-Bacus J, Weekers JF (1966) Etude ultrasonique des dimensions respectives des segments antérieur et postérieur du globe oculaire dans diverses affections génétiques. In: Oksala A, Gennet H (eds) Ultrasonics in ophthalmology: Proceedings on the Munster symposium. Karger, Basel, p 215

Worthen DM (1978) Intraocular pressure and its diurnal variation. In: Heilmann K, Richardson KT (eds) Glaucoma. Saunders, Philadelphia, p 54

Yanoff M, Fine BS (1975) Ocular pathology. A text and atlas. Harper and Row, Hagerstown, pp 594–598

The Eye in the Elderly: Lens

O. HOCKWIN and C. OHRLOFF

A. Introduction

The lens is a transparent, avascular structure with the following main characteristics:

1. The lens is part of the refraction system of the eye (Fig. 1). The total refraction of the human eye is about 59 D, the contribution of the lens being about 19 D (at rest).
2. During the first half of life, the lens is able to vary its refraction (accommodation) so that objects close to the eye are cleary seen. At maximum accommo-

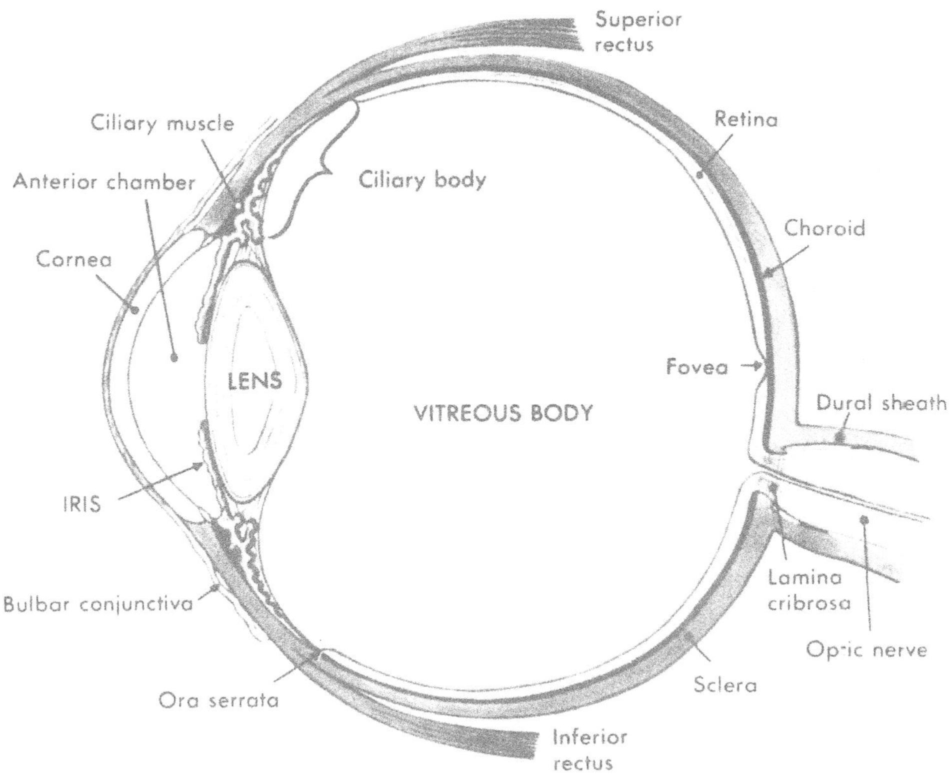

Fig. 1. Cross section through the human eye (STEIN and SLATT 1968)

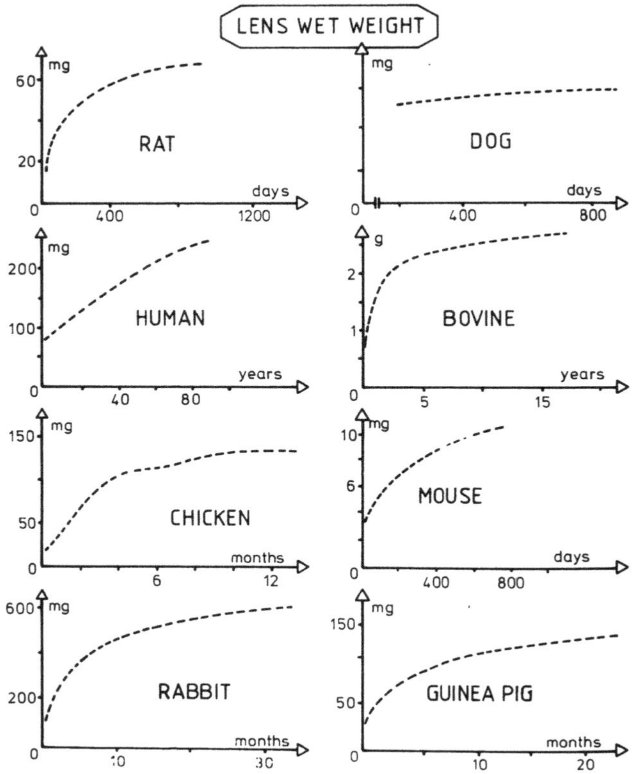

Fig. 2. Lens wet weight as a function of age (eight different species)

dation, total refraction is about 70 D since that of the lens is able to increase up to 30 D.

3. The lens, together with the zonula fibers, forms a diaphragm in the eye to maintain the form of the vitreous so that the latter cannot prolapse.

While Aulus Cornelius Celsus (ca. 25 B.C.–50 A.D.) was of the opinion that the lens is a crystal – and this is the origin of the term "crystalline lens" – we have learned in the meantime that it is by no means inorganic, but rather an organic structure with certain anatomic, physical, and biochemical properties.

With increasing age, the physical properties of the eye lens are subjected to characteristic alterations which also affect the process of vision. At about the fourth decade, the human lens loses its ability to modify its form, and thereby its ability to accommodate to different angles of focus (see Sect. C. VI). In advanced age, loss of lens transparency is frequently observed. In this case, visual acuity is limited by formation of cataracta senilis which finally leads to blindness. The so-called senile cataract is still one of the main causes of blindness among the world population.

During the last century, a flood of investigations on the processes of lens aging and on the age-related changes leading to senile cataract have been carried out.

In the beginning, such investigations were mostly based on clinical observations; for about 30 years, however, biologic and biochemical research on age-related lens changes has become more and more important (NORDMANN 1954, 1962, 1972, 1977; KUCK 1975; HOCKWIN 1971, 1978a, b, 1981; BLOEMENDAL 1981; DUNCAN 1981; AUGUSTEYN et al. 1979; AUGUSTEYN and COLLIN 1980). This is easily explained by the fact that the lens, on account of its pertinent properties with respect to anatomy and biochemistry represents a useful model for gerontologic research. Some of these properties are:

1. The lens consists mostly of anuclear cell fibers. New fibers are formed in the periphery, that is, at the lens equator; they elongate and lose their cell nucleus. Compared with other tissues, they are similar to erythrocytes (SRIVASTAVA 1980).
2. Protein synthesis only takes place during this phase of cell differentiation to lens fibers; thus, there is no renewal of protein in later life. Further, in the normal lens the protein is not proteolytically catabolized.
3. The lens grows during the entire life span so that new fiber layers continually cover the older ones, similar to the annual rings of a tree. Lens growth is closely correlated with age, therefore it is possible to evaluate the age of certain species from their lens wet weight (Fig. 2).

Since the lens normally does not release cells or fibers into its environment, it contains cells of all age periods. The lens nucleus, formed during the embryonic phase, corresponds to the age of the individual, while the lens cortex represents young tissue. Thus, the eye lens represents the only tissue in the human system that allows one to compare tissue of different age which are biologically identical.

B. Lens Structure

I. History of Development

Development and anatomy of the lens have been discussed in various detailed reports by, for instance, AMSLER et al. (1961), BARGMANN (1962), BRAUS (1960), CORDES (1957), DUKE-ELDER (1963), FISCHER (1938). The lens is of ectodermal origin. The first differentiation (3–4 weeks) can be observed in human embryos of about 4 mm as a round, disc-shaped epithelial thickening in the superficial ectoderm (Fig. 3). This thickening is induced by the optic vesicle, which is now at a more advanced stage of growth. Further cell growth in the approximately 5- to 6-mm-long embryo causes the lens disc to turn toward the eye cup and thus to form a shallow pit, the lens cavity, which gradually deepens. By means of further formation of the enveloping fold of ectoderm and lens cavity, the lens gradually narrows and finally closes. The vesicle disconnects in the 4-week-old embryo (approximately 8 mm). Shortly after disconnection, at about 10 weeks, a thin structureless lens capsule, analogous to the basal membrane of the epithelial tissue, is formed round the vesicle.

While the cells in the anterior hemisphere of the vesicle maintain their rather cubic form and are now called anterior lens epithelium, the cells of the posterior wall begin to lengthen in the direction of the anterior lens epithelium; they become

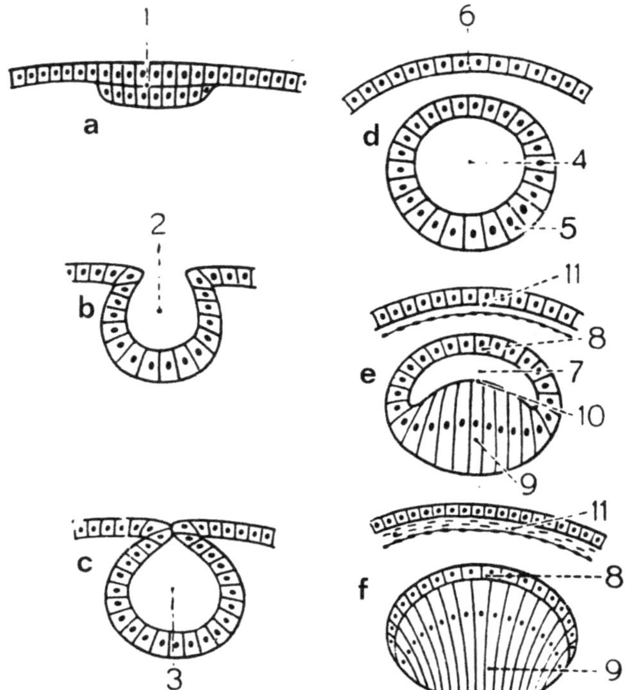

Fig. 3 a–f. Schematic representation of lens development **a** lens disc (plate); **b** lens cavity; **c** lens vesicle before ligation (or segmentation); **d** lens vesicle after ligation; **e** Differentiation of anterior lens epithelium and lens fibers; **f** after disappearance of the cavity in the vesicle, the lens fibers have grown toward the anterior lens epithelium. *1* = lens disc (plate); *2* = lens cavity; *3* = lens vesicle; *4* = cavity of lens vesicle; *5* = wall of lens vesicle; *6* = superficial ectoderm; *7* = lens cavity; *8* = anterior lens epithelium; *9* = lens fibers (primary); *10* = lens convolution; *11* = rudiment of cornea (AMSLER et al. 1961)

lens fibers and form a convex bulge. In approximately the sixth embryonic week, the lens fibers touch the anterior epithelium; the lens cavity disappears, and the lens becomes a solid body. At the same time, the cell nuclei of the lens fibers migrate forward and form a convex line called the nuclear bow (or arch). These fibers constitute the primary lens fibers which remain unchanged in the lens center over the whole life span, and which evidently constitute the transparent embryonic nucleus, the fibers extending from the posterior pole directly to the anterior pole. Relatively late, i.e., in about the third embryonic month, the fibers eventually lose their cell nuclei and their mitochondria.

The point of transition between the anterior lens epithelium and the lens fibers is called the lens equator. While the lens fibers are no longer capable of division after differentiation, the lens epithelium maintains its ability to divide and, in the equatorial zone, even its ability to differentiate to lens fibers. Therefore, in the zone of the lens equator, a continuous regeneration of cells, elongating to lens fibers, takes place (secondary lens fibers). These cells elongate in the direction of

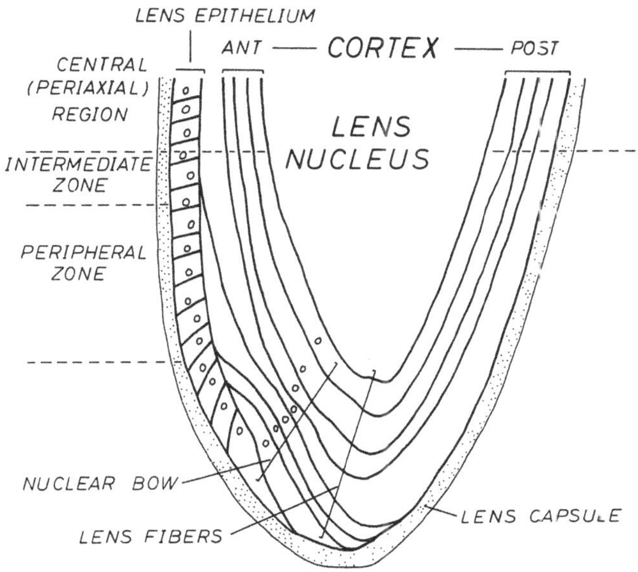

Fig. 4. Schematic representation of cross section through the lens, illustrating appositional growth (older, vertebrate lens). The new fibers form the cortical part and represent young tissue. The fibers formed during the embryonic, fetal, and postnatal phase (up to puberty) constitute the lens nucleus and represent old tissue.

the anterior pole as well as in the direction of the posterior pole of the lens (Fig. 4). In this manner, layer upon layer of newly generated fibers are formed (appositional growth). During differentiation, the secondary lens fibers also lose their cell nuclei and their cell organelles. The central part of the lens is composed of the oldest, anuclear cells and is called the nucleus lentis.

II. Anatomy of the Lens

The lens is a transparent, biconvex organ of relatively high elasticity, owing to the fact that the lens tissue is firmly enclosed in the lens capsule. If the capsule is removed, this elasticity is no longer present. The lens is kept in place by the ciliary body and is pressed to the iris from behind, without being actually connected with the latter (see Fig. 1). Thus, the anterior lens part adjoins the iris and the anterior chamber, the posterior part the vitreous, and the equatorial zone the posterior chamber. The lens surface is slightly curved while the curve of the posterior part is more pronounced. Both lens areas merge in a convex periphery, the lens equator.

The lens substance is surrounded by an elastic capsule of varying thickness. The anterior part of the capsule is thicker than the posterior part and thinnest in the region of the posterior pole. During aging, the capsule does not change in any remarkable way (Kobayashi and Suzuki 1975).

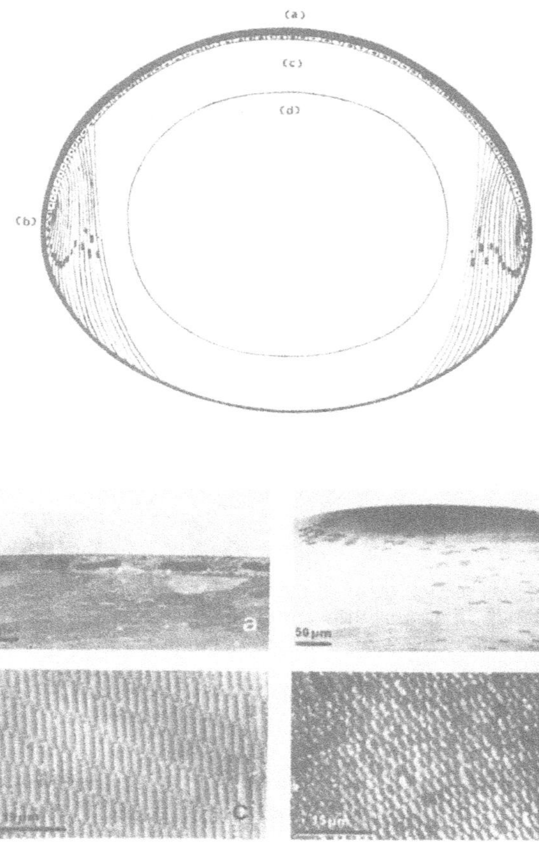

Fig. 5 a–d. Schematic representation of cross section through an older rat lens a epithelium and capsule or anterior cortex; b equator – transformation of epithelial cells to fiber cells; c anterior cortex; d lens nucleus (HARDING and DILLEY 1976)

III. Histology and Fine Structure of the Lens

The major part of the lens cortex and the lens nucleus consists of cell fibers. Light microscopy shows that the cortical fibers are hexagonal and 8–12 mm long, 5–7 µm wide, and about 3 µm thick (Fig. 5). As soon as new fibers are formed, the older fibers form the lower layers and lose their nucleus as well as their organelles, so that the typical lens fiber in the optically active part is anuclear. Electron microscopic examination shows that the cytoplasm of the fibers is amorphous, even at some distance from the equator. Here the double refraction of the lens indicates that in the cytoplasm a submicroscopic fine structure with characteristic configuration of the micelle prevails. The fibers are covered by a membrane and are joined by cytoplasm protrusions (invaginations) (Fig. 6).

The form of the fibers and the manner of their cross-linking changes in the deeper layers. The form of the fiber becomes less regular, the connections to other fibers increase and get less orderly, the cell membrane is in part no longer well preserved; however, single fibers are still visible. Total loss of cell membrane has been found only in pathologic lenses (KUWABARA 1975; HARDING et al. 1976).

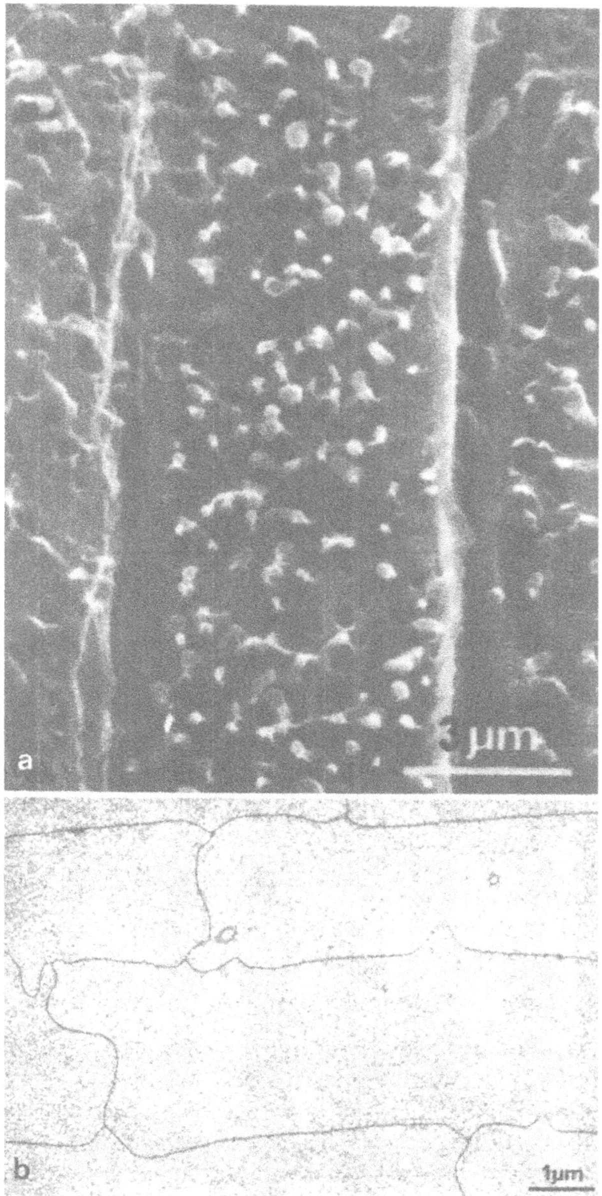

Fig. 6 a, b. Electron microscopic photographs of lens fibers from the anterior part of the superficial cortex (human, clear, young lens) **a** scanning, electron micrograph showing the large number of plasma protrusions and invaginations on the fiber surface (x 8,000); **b** cross section showing the invaginations, cell membrane and cytoplasm (x 13,000) (KUWABARA 1975)

C. Growth of the Lens

The lens grows throughout life, formation and apposition of lens fibers takes place even in old age. Thus, the anterior and the posterior cortex is formed round the nucleus (see Fig. 4). Since the lens does not shed any cells, the lens nucleus is as old as the individual.

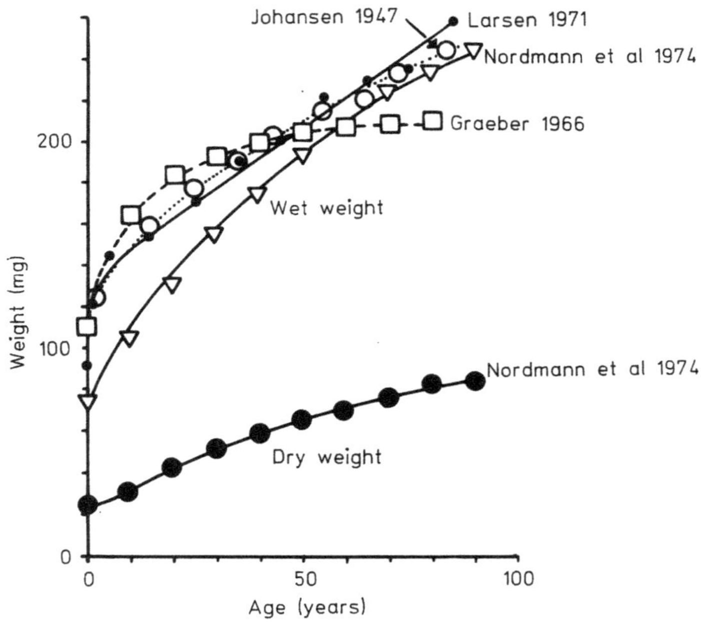

Fig. 7. Growth curve of human lens; dependence of wet weight and dry weight on age

I. Lens Weight

The continuous growth effects an increase in volume and weight during aging. At puberty, the neonatal lens weight is doubled, and at the age of 70 years, it is tripled. A definite logarithmic weight–age relationship can be determined for certain species, e.g., human, chicken, guinea pig, rabbit, rat, mouse, dog, and cattle (for review see HOCKWIN 1971; NORDMANN et al. 1974; see also Fig. 2). This correlation enables age determination of animal lenses to be carried out.

II. Lens Weight and Volume in Relation to Age

The graphs in Fig. 7 interpret some recent results from growth curves of human lenses. The data obtained by NORDMANN et al. (1974) resulted from enucleated eyes which had previously been subjected to slit lamp control, while the data of other investigators may have been influenced by postmortem changes.

The curve for dry weight of normal human lenses, as illustrated in Fig. 7 shows the constancy of the water content. It also illustrates the capacity of the lens to synthesize new proteins. Growth curves relating to lens volume show a pattern similar to that for lens weight (Fig. 8).

III. Specific Weight of the Lens

From data on lens wet weight and volume, information may be gained on the specific weight in relation to age. The values reported, however, are somewhat con-

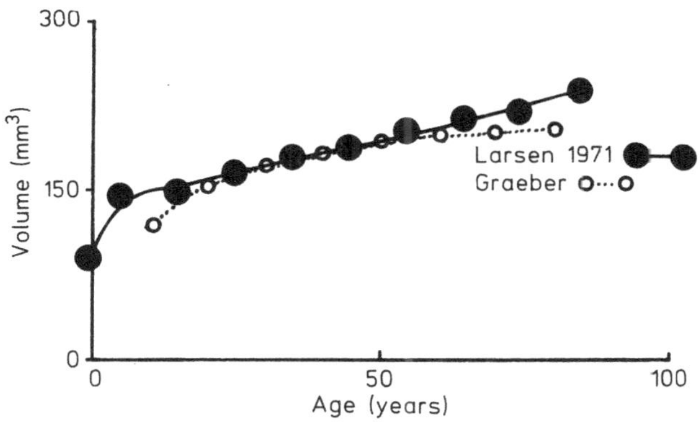

Fig. 8. Volume of human lens in relation to age

tradictory. While LARSEN (1971) and SCAMMON and HESDORFFER (1937) registered an increase, other results indicate constant values of about 1.08–1.09. The values calculated from the data on weight and volume reported by GRAEBER (1966) show that the specific weight decreases with advancing age. Investigations performed with bovine and rat lenses (SCHMUTTER 1961; HART and PECKHAM 1953) indicate that their weight: volume ratios are unrelated to age, except for the early postnatal phase.

IV. Diameter of Equator: Lens Thickness

Appositional growth determines the external dimensions (LARSEN 1971; SPRENGER 1966; WEEKERS et al. 1973). The frontal or equatorial diameter is subject to steady growth, accompanied by increased lens thickness. From 159 emmetropic eyes, WEEKERS et al. (1973) calculated a linear regression and the correlation coefficient of 43.5% shows that about half of the lens thickness is a function of age. SPRENGER (1966) found similar values; for the lens of a newborn infant, he extrapolated a value of 3.32 mm. However, the Sprenger curve of human lenses also suggests sex differences which had not been observed by Weekers. Female lenses are less thick than male lenses of the same age. Corresponding differences are also found for lens weight and volume (JOHANSEN 1947; HARDING et al. 1977). This has been confirmed with animals (cattle SCHMUTTER 1961; rats HOCKWIN 1978c; NORBY 1958; beagle dogs HOCKWIN et al. 1979b).

V. Lens Volume/Eye Volume

The larger space occupied by the older lens implies a decreased depth of the anterior chamber, and a decrease in length of the vitreous body. However, according to WEEKERS et al. (1973), there is no correlation between thickness and length of bulb which means that, in a hypermetropic eye, the lens takes up a proportionally larger space than in the myopic eye.

VI. Lens Biometry with Respect to Accommodation

The lens changes its form by accommodation. While it has been an established fact for more than a century that the increase in lens thickness through the accommodation process causes a decrease in the depth of the anterior chamber (VON HELMHOLTZ 1855; SAUNTE 1905), recent investigations with ultrasonic methods demonstrated that the posterior part of the lens also shifts in the direction of the vitreous body (LEPPER et al. 1980). This fact induced COLEMAN (1970) to reconsider the hypothesis of the accommodation mechanism, taking into account an active participation of the vitreous body.

D. Nutritional Supply of the Lens

Since the lens represents an exclusively epithelial tissue, there are no blood vessels. Only during the embryonic phase, i.e., the period of major growth, are there sufficient blood vessels in the immediate neighborhood, among them, from the beginning of the fifth embryonic week, the embryonic fibrous tissue which is rich in blood vessels, the tunica vasculosa. The part lying in the pupillary region is called the pupillary membrane. The arterial supply goes via the ciliary vessels and via the arteria hyaloidea which, coming from the retinal central artery, runs through the primary vitreous in the direction of the lens. The whole tunica vasculosa lentis is normally formed during the embryonic phase (about 8–9 months of pregnancy). Later, the lens is entirely dependent on supply by the aqueous.

I. Aqueous Humor Composition

The extensive investigations on the chemical composition of the aqueous humor (COLE 1970), performed to optimize media for the in vitro incubation of lenses, have evidently led to a disregard of the central role the lens plays in the chemical processes of the anterior eye segment. In general, both specialists in aqueous humor research and physiologists are of the opinion that aqueous humor dynamics are mostly a problem of reactions to aqueous humor formation and outflow. This approach led to studies on particular systems of the anterior eye segment. In these investigations, little attention has been paid to the fact that the aqueous, on its way from the site of formation, i.e., the posterior chamber, to the site of outflow, i.e., the chamber angle, passes certain substances to the surrounding tissues, taking up metabolic end products at the same time. Owing to this exchange of material, the concentration of a substance in the aqueous is the result of many dynamic equilibria, including flow equilibria, and subsequent reaction processes in the neighbouring compartments (HOCKWIN et al. 1978a).

II. Changes of Aqueous Humor Composition by the Lens

Various findings demonstrate the interrelation between the lens and its environment, especially in regard to the aqueous humor. MÜLLER (1939) found an increase in lactic acid in the aqueous humor of rabbits in the first stage of naphthalene-induced cataract. VARMA and REDDY (1972) reported changes in the content of phospholipids in rabbits with alloxan-induced diabetes.

III. Changes of Lens Properties by the Aqueous Humor

If the normal chemical composition of the aqueous humor is disturbed, e.g., by galactose feeding or by causing an amino acid deficiency, the effects of these interrelations are disclosed by changes in lens biochemistry. The same effect is produced by disturbances of the circulation following ligature of the common carotid artery, and is due to shifts in the metabolic conditions of all parts of the biologically open "anterior eye segment" system (KASKEL et al. 1975; SCHOLZ et al. 1976). Disturbances originating in the aqueous can also be induced by aqueous puncture, a procedure which leads to the detection of cataracts caused by a combination of subliminal cataractogenic effects (HOCKWIN 1969, 1980; HOCKWIN and KOCH 1975; KRETZBERG 1982; BARTOLIČ 1982).

Clinical experience with older patients, who show an increased tendency to formation of lens opacities following intraocular surgery with loss of aqueous humor, supports these findings. The frequently expressed opinion that lens opacities often follow filtering operations may well be explained by the same mechanism.

IV. Aqueous Composition in Aphakic Eyes

By investigating the aqueous humor of aphakic eyes, it is possible to estimate roughly the degree to which the lens is responsible for the concentration of certain aqueous substances. FISCHER (1931) and KUCK and CROSSWELL (1974) found a decrease in lactic acid concentration in the aqueous humor of aphakic eyes after intracapsular extraction. According to KUCK, the fructose content also decreases, approximating the values found in blood, while the concentration of glucose remains unchanged, which indicates that the fructose present in the aqueous is, for the greater part, provided by the lens. BITO et al. (1973) found an increase in glucose and calcium, and a decrease in lactic acid, ascorbic acid, and protein in the aqueous of aphakic eyes 70 days after extracapsular lens extraction.

V. Aqueous Composition and Age

The examples reported point out the chemical interrelations between the lens and its environment. In regard to the fact that the biochemical properties of the lens are strongly dependent on the age of the individual (HOCKWIN 1971, 1976), it has to be assumed that exchange processes are also subject to age-related changes. Various findings on changes in concentrations of important metabolic substances present in the aqueous, e.g., glucose, fructose, pyruvate, citrate, amino acids, and enzymes, indicate such an age dependence (BRUUN-LAURSEN and LORENTZEN 1974; ISMAIL et al. 1977; POHJOLA 1966).

VI. The Lens as Part of an Open Biologic System

The importance of the lens as part of the anterior eye segment does not rest merely on its physical properties. For rather a long time, studies on the chemical interrelations between this organ and its environment have been totally neglected, which may be due to the obsolete opinion that the lens is only a dead or, at most, bradytrophic structure, without any significant biochemical processes. NORDMANN and MÜLLER were among the first who, in the early 1930 s, were able to prove that the lens has its own individual and specific metabolism, which makes possible the synthesis of the rather organ-specific proteins during the entire life span, and provides the energetic conditions necessary to maintain its most important physiologic characteristic – transparency. Since then, biochemical investigations on the lens have been intensified and specialized. This, however, has certain disadvantages, and one should take care not to neglect or disregard the general aspect.

Several attempts have been made to analyze the individual biochemical processes within the aqueous in order to learn how far the contiguous tissues, as partners of the biologically open system, are involved in determining the concentrations of the substances in the aqueous. Among the numerous biochemical interrelations between the aqueous and the surrounding tissues of the eye, those involving the lens have been the first and most frequently investigated.

Simultaneous investigations in both systems on electrolyte dynamics between aqueous and lens have been done relatively often; here, however, in vitro investigations with aqueous substitutes have been given preference. The electrolyte ions themselves have no sequential reactions in the individual compartments, which might alter their properties. Therefore, changes in the factor responsible for the maintenance of equilibrium in the sample analyzed do not occur in this case. We may assume that our knowledge of the interrelations of ions (electrolytes) accounts for the conditions in situ.

Within the scope of investigations on electrolytes, the experiments on the dynamics of amino acids between aqueous and lens have been adapted to the methods applied. Here, too, in vitro investigations received priority (KINSEY 1957; KINSEY and REDDY 1963; KERN and HO 1973). In general, they show that concentrations of free amino acids are higher in the lens than in the aqueous. However, the fact that the free amino acids of the lens are further metabolized, as found by TRAYHURN and VAN HEYNINGEN (1973), and that they are further used for lens protein synthesis, has been totally neglected. WEBER (1961) showed certain interrelations which could be demonstrated by intravenous injection of ^{35}S-labeled methionine in blood, aqueous, lens, and even in lens epithelium and the deeper fiber layers at different times after injection (Fig. 9). This procedure not only gave an insight into transport dynamics, but also facilitated the calculation of half-life for the synthesis of the lens proteins, which, as regards the epithelium, lies within the range of a few hours. This span is surprisingly short and indicates a high rate of synthesis. Unfortunately, these experiments were never repeated, which may be due to the rather difficult experimental assay involved. With respect to carbohydrate and nucleotide metabolism KASKEL et al. (1975) have performed experiments with rabbits to demonstrate the biochemical changes in aqueous humor and lens composition after unilateral ligation of the a. carotis communis.

The results obtained indicate that this experimental model promises a much better treatment of the basic problem than the attempts at a mathematical approach, where the assumptions rarely meet the actual conditions. At the same time, the findings of KASKEL

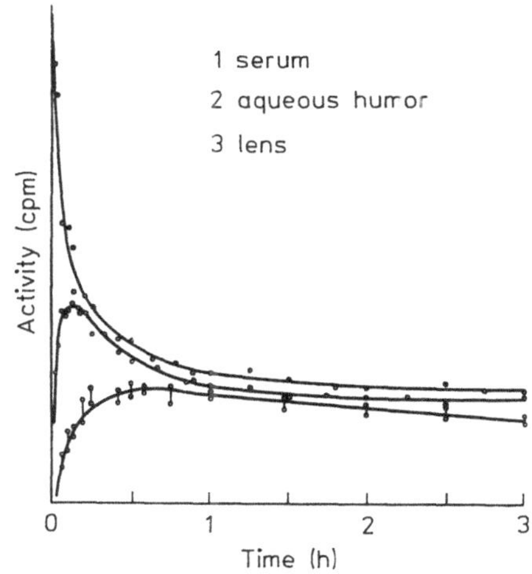

Fig. 9. Methionine-^{35}S in serum, aqueous humor, and lens of rabbits after intravenous injection, as a function of time (WEBER 1961)

et al. (1975) show clearly that one should not attempt to interpret physiologic and pathophysiologic findings on the intraocular fluid exchange without taking into account the biochemical conditions of open biologic systems if one wants to avoid the risk of misinterpretation.

E. Light Transmission of the Lens

I. Transparency for Visible and Ultraviolet Light

Light transmission is the most important factor in the optical function of the lens. In this respect the high protein content (35% of lens fresh weight) plays an important role. Within the intact fiber, the protein molecules have a high degree of spatial order. They are densely packed and there is little change in the density of the light scattering protein particles throughout the lens. This is the morphological and physical basis for its transparency.

The transmission characteristics (Fig. 10) of normal human lenses show certain changes with increasing age, as indicated by LERMAN and BORKMAN (1976). The data reveal that there is a relatively high ultraviolet (UV) transmission (300–400 nm) in young lenses. UV transmission drops markedly above 25 years of age. These data parallel the relative lack of fluorescent pigment in young lenses and their increase with aging. There is a concomitant decrease in the transmission of UV (300–400 nm) as well as an increase in color of the lens nucleus. The latter may account for the decreased transmission of visible light which is absorbed by the photochemically generated chromophores in the old lens (LERMAN 1980 b).

II. Disturbances of Transparency

Accumulation of water within the lens results in a decrease of transparency (development of turbidity). Localized alterations in the density of packing of the lens

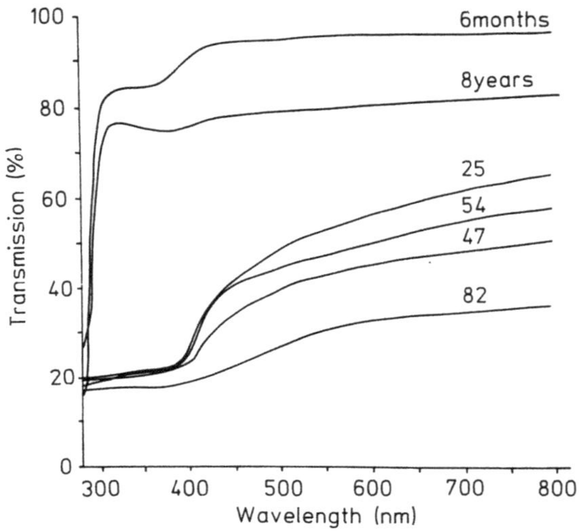

Fig. 10. Ultraviolet and visible light transmission of normal human lenses aged between 6 months and 82 years (LERMAN and BORKMAN 1976)

proteins, owing to significant configurational changes in proteins and/or aggregation developing in various portions of the lens (cortex), will also lead to changes in transparency as light scattering is increased. With increased protein aggregation, high molecular weight compounds are formed which have low water solubility, and a loss of transparency occurs, since most of the incident light is reflected (BENEDEK 1971; MILLER and BENEDEK 1973; LERMAN and HOCKWIN 1981; BETTELHEIM and BALAZS 1981). This shows that the transparency of the lens is dependent on the physicochemical state of its proteins.

III. Lens Fluorescence

Visible lenticular fluorescence was first described well over a century ago (REGNAULD 1858). Within the last decade, a significant revival of interest with respect to lens pigments and fluorescence has occurred owing to the utilization of more refined techniques in studies on whole lenses as well als protein extracts. Investigations by UV and visible transmission spectroscopy, fluorescence, and phosphorescence spectroscopy, electron spin resonance, and laser Raman spectroscopy have contributed much to our understanding of photochemical effects of UV radiation ($400 > \lambda > 295$ nm) on the ocular lens (LERMAN 1980 b).

IV. Applications of Scheimpflug Photography

1. Lens Photography

Lens photography according to the method of SCHEIMPFLUG (1906), with subsequent densitometric analysis, enables the application of an objective measurement procedure for lens transparency in vivo and for the detection and documentation of development and progress of lens opacities (BROWN 1973 b; NIESEL 1982; HOCKWIN et al. 1979 a; HOCKWIN and DRAGOMIRESCU 1982).

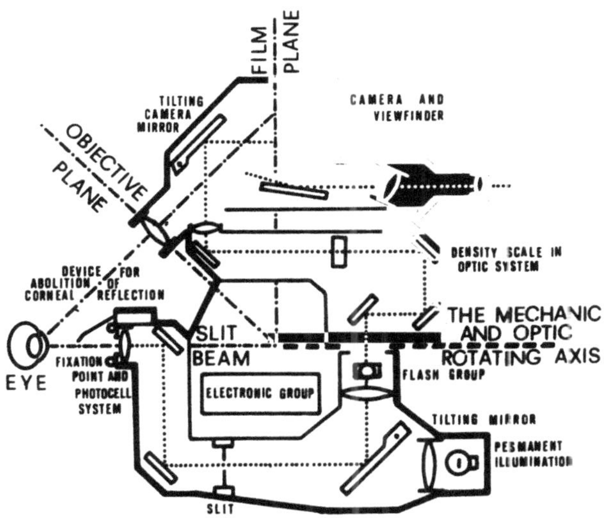

Fig. 11. Schematic section through the Topcon SL 45 camera, illustrating the Scheimpflug principle: film plane – objective plane – slit beam

Documentation of findings in the lens has always been rather difficult. So far, only written reports of drawings made by slit lamp microscopy have been used. Photographs of the findings obtained with this instrument could not be accurately evaluated because of the insufficient depth of field and the poor reproducibility of the method during follow-up examinations (HENDRICKSON and KOCH 1977).

In Scheimpflug photography, an image with sufficient depth of field can be obtained of an oblique object, if the plane of the object, the plane of the photographic objective, and the image plane meet at one point and the respective angles correspond (Fig. 11). NIESEL (1966a, b) and BROWN (1973a, b) developed this technique for investigations of the anterior eye segment, including the lens. DRAGOMIRESCU et al. (1978) designed an instrument which is now commercially available as the Topcon SL 45 (Topcon, Tokyo, Japan). The photographs taken with this instrument represent an accurate and complete record for the patient's file (Fig. 12). Figure 13 shows examples of various lenses.

LERMAN et al. (1981) incorporated special filters in front of the flash lamp, permitting photography not only in visible light, but also in UVA (320–400 nm) light. Special quartz-coated filters with a transmission between 320 and 380 nm thus enable an in vivo excitation of the chromophore groups in the lens and the photographs then show the emitted fluorescence. The authors found that results from evaluation by densitometric image analysis of these photographs correspond with certain properties found by in vitro fluorescence measurements of human lenses (LERMAN and HOCKWIN 1981).

2. Densitometric Image Analysis

Densitometric image analysis of the film negatives providing the necessary data (see Fig. 12) is more than a routine complement of the photographic procedure (HOCKWIN and DRAGOMIRESCU 1981a, b, 1982). A suitable means of evaluation is linear densitometry (Fig. 14). For this purpose, the part of the negative showing

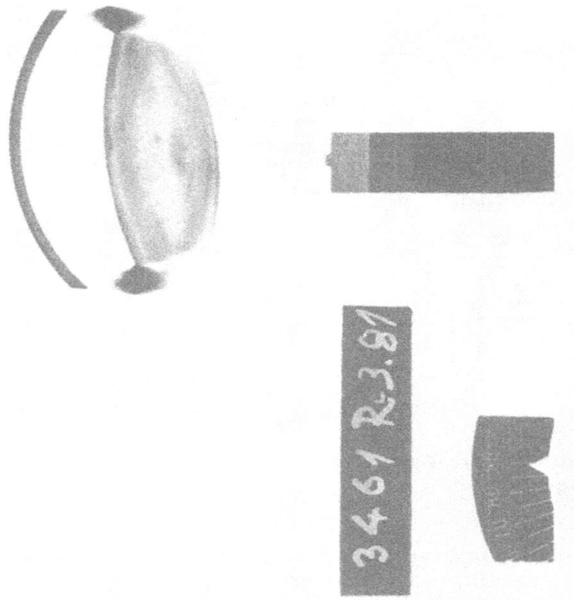

Fig. 12. Negative of a Scheimpflug photograph of the anterior eye segment by the Topcon SL 45 camera. On the right-hand side of the picture: five-step density scale, patient's identification, and camera position

the middle of the lens is led past the window of the densitometer and the variation in film blackening is registered by the monitor.

Figures 15 and 16 show the results obtained by microdensitometry for a normal lens (Fig. 15) and for a lens with changes in nucleus and subcapsular opacities which are more pronounced in the rear than in the front (Fig. 16). Both densitograms clearly show the lens structure. In the graphs, the single lens layers are demonstrated by different hatching. The Scheimpflug photos beneath the curves show that the intensity of the film blackening (corresponding to light areas on the positive) is indicated by the height of the densitometer deflection (y axis) which means that the transparency of the lens in question can be expressed quantitatively.

The densitograms were subdivided into a maximum of ten sections. These sections represent the morphological lens parts:

1. Anterior capsule
2. Superficial anterior cortex
3. Anterior cortex
4. Anterior cortex
5. Supranuclear region
6. Nucleus
7. Nucleus
8. Supranuclear region
9. Posterior cortex
10. Posterior capsule

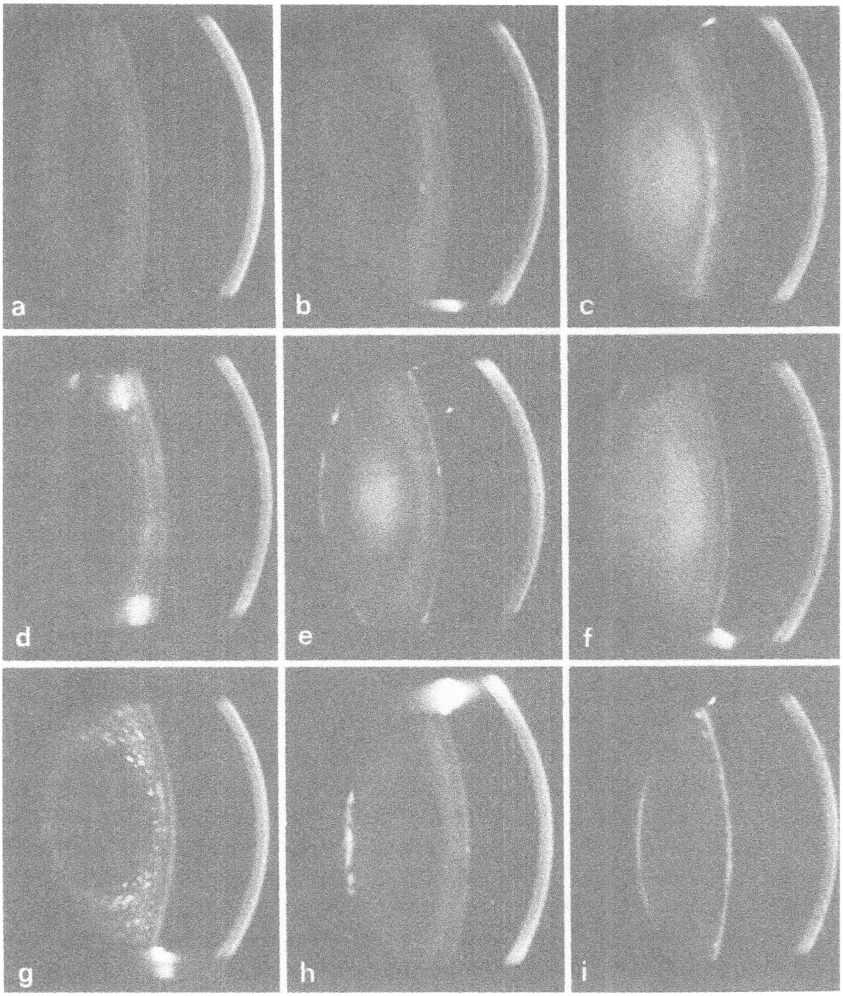

Fig. 13 a–j. Scheimpflug photographs of different lenses **a** 25-year-old normal lens; **b** 45-year-old normal lens; **c** 70-year-old lens showing increased light scattering of the deeper cortex and nuclear density; **d** 66-year-old lens with cataracta cuneiformis (wedge-shaped) and waterclefts; **e** 55-year-old lens with dense nuclear and superficial (subcapsular cortical) opacities; **f** 57-year-old lens with nuclear cataract; **g** 52-year-old lens with cataracta coronaria; **h** 35-year-old lens with subcapsular cortical cataract (induced by corticosteroid therapy); **j** 28-year-old lens with superficial cortical cataract and rather thin lens, corresponding to patient's age

Along the x axis, measurements of distances give values of cornea thickness, depth of anterior chamber, lens thickness, lens cortex, and size of nucleus (Brown 1973 a, b; Niesel et al. 1976). Evaluating the relative density by determining the height of the densitogram for certain characteristic lens layers, as reported by Niesel and Bachmann (1974), Niesel and Rokos (1976), and Niesel et al. (1976)

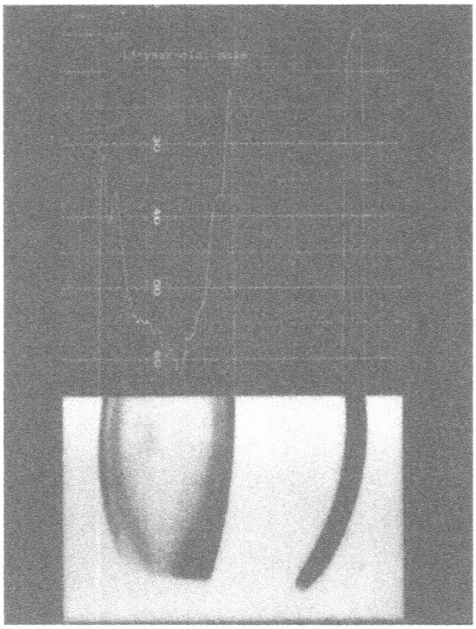

Fig. 14. Linear densitometry of a photograph of a normal lens (13-year-old volunteer). Densitometer deflection corresponds to areas of light scattering

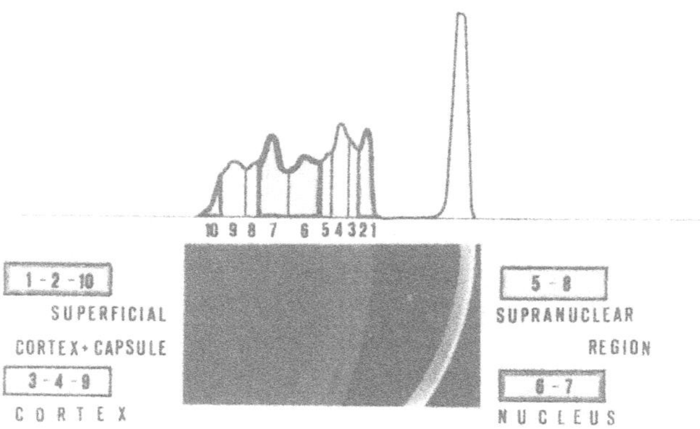

Fig. 15. Densitogram of a normal lens. The single lens sections are shown

is not the ideal method for assessing lens opacities which may not only increase in density during the test period, but may also show an increase in size of the affected area. The evaluations by HOCKWIN and DRAGOMIRESCU (1981 a, b, 1982) have therefore introduced the densitogram planimetry technique. This means that the area beneath the densitogram is included in the evaluation by a combined measurement of dimension (x axis) and density (y axis).

With a planimetry program available for the Bascom–Turner y–t recorder (Bryan-Southern Instruments, Newton, Massachusetts), the densitometer curve is followed and the planimeter values for the single lens sections read. The proportion of the lens section in relation to the total area representing lens density may thus be calculated.

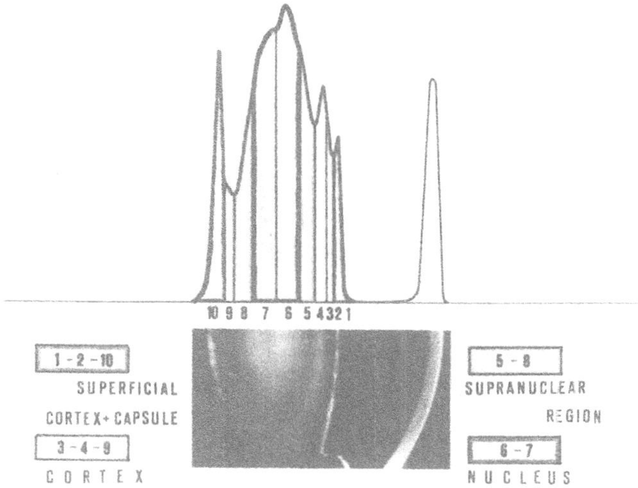

Fig. 16. Densitogram of a lens with nuclear and subcapsular opacity. The single lens sections are shown

3. Calculation of the Methodological Error

To determine the probable error of the method, several investigations have been performed. HOCKWIN et al. (1983) have investigated the possible error factors separately. The Scheimpflug camera (Topcon SL 45) is provided with an internal standard covering three or five density steps (see Fig. 12). The height of the steps is registered on the densitogram together with the densitogram of cornea and lens. In a previous test with 100 patients, these heights were measured (4 for each eye in 4 separate examinations = 3,200 photographs). The result was as follows:

$$x_1 = 24.0 \pm 1.01 \text{ mm}; x_2 = 57.0 \pm 2.4 \text{ mm}; x_3 = 107.0 \pm 4.5 \text{ mm}.$$

The coefficient of variation for all three standard density steps is about 4.2%. These coefficients involve the errors of the internal standard, quality of film, batch of material, flash lamp, and negative development. The image of the cornea of the patient's eye will naturally show hardly any change. The mean value of the height of the densitometer deflection for the cornea was calculated as 69.0 ± 4.26 mm. The coefficient of variation is 6.18%, representing the value for an external standard. If the cornea height is referred to height 2 of the five-step density scale (Fig. 17), the resulting quotient (from 39 photographs of 13 patients) is 0.94 ± 0.04. The coefficient of variation is about 3.7%, which means that the evaluation of the densitometer curve of the lens by planimetry (after setting the densitometer height for the cornea as the maximum deflection of the y–t recorder) corresponds to a correction of our internal standard (4.2%) (WINTER 1981).

For the calculation of the probable error in lens densitometry and planimetry, photographs of six volunteers (three examinations in three consecutive weeks) were used, taken at 0° and 180° camera positions, temporal and nasal, respectively; light incidence 12 h–6 h. As may be seen in Fig. 18, a coefficient of vari-

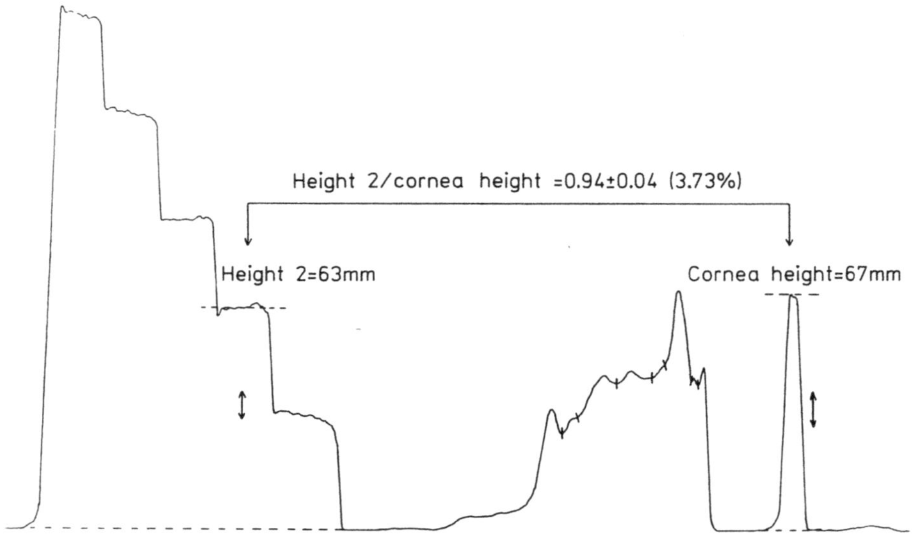

Fig. 17. The methodological error of the Scheimpflug method as calculated from the quotient internal standard/external standard (internal standard represented by second step of standard density scale; external standard represented by height of cornea deflection). Compared with other measuring procedures in the medical field, the methodological error is rather low (3.7%)

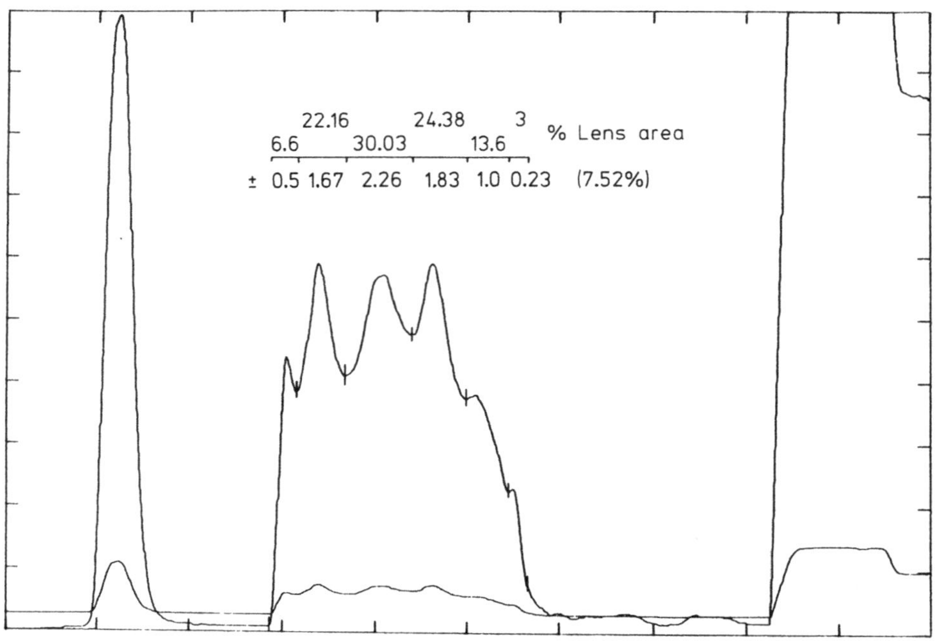

Fig. 18. Densitometry and planimetry of lens areas

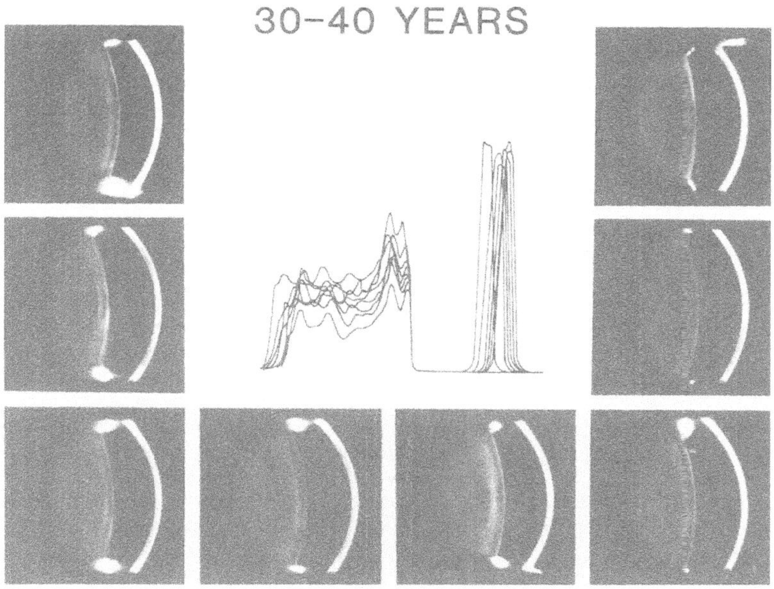

Fig. 19. Scheimpflug photographs of the anterior eye segment of normal volunteers. The densitograms of the individual lenses have been superposed. The graph shows that normal lenses of similar age are rather different which indicates the biologic individuality of lenses, the differences becoming more pronounced with increasing age (30 to 40-year-old lenses)

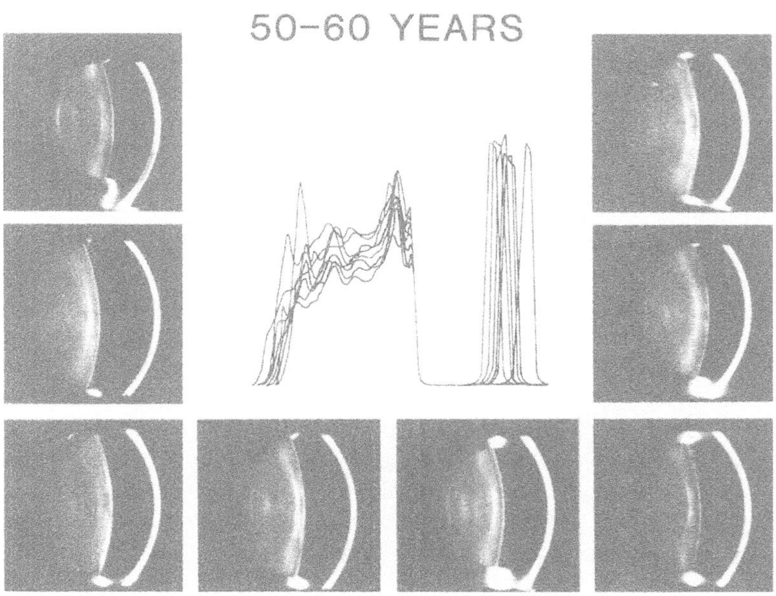

Fig. 20. See Fig. 19; (50 to 60-year-old lenses)

ation of 7.52% was obtained. Considering these calculations, we were sure that relatively objective data on lens transparency could be expected by the method involving Scheimpflug photography and densitometric image analysis. Owing to biologic individualities, however, the data were not as objective as expected, although the method as such is easily reproducible.

Professor H. Goldmann (former Director of the University Eye Clinic, Bern, Switzerland) is known as a keen and knowledgeable observer. He declared that the human lens may yield a great deal of information on the life history of the individual. The densitogram obtained by the slit lamp shows great individual differences of light scattering, dependent on the state of the proteins. Since the state of the proteins is not only a true criterion of age, but may also be modified by endogenous and exogenous influences, uniform light scattering and corresponding densitometer curves may scarcely be obtained from a group of age-matched persons. Investigations by HOENDERS and BLOEMENDAL (1982) and HOCKWIN (to be published, 1982 a, b) indicate that it must be expected that between older persons the differences in lens densitograms are more distinct than between younger persons. Figure 19 and 20 illustrate this fact. From the Scheimpflug photographs attached to each series of curves, it can be seen that they belong to normal lenses. Comparison of Fig. 19 with Fig. 20 shows the age difference of the two groups. Similar results have been reported by SASAKI et al. (1980). Besides the great individual variation, the general increase in age-dependent density can be observed by taking into account the densitometer deflection.

If one were to try to calculate mean values from the series of curves in Figs. 19 and 20, the rather high variations of the individual values would render such a group comparison nearly impossible (see WEIGELIN and HOCKWIN 1982).

F. The Lens and Aging

Developments in the field of medicine during the last decades have led to high life expectancy, particularly in the western world. This implies that the number of older patients has increased considerably which means that the age-related diseases leading to decreased visual acuity and blindness have also increased. Especially, senile macular degeneration of the retina and senile lens opacification, the so-called senile cataract, are among these diseases.

The eye is an organ which lends itself to age studies as no other organ in the human system does. Thanks to classical examination methods, it is possible to observe in vivo all parts of the eye at almost microscopic magnification (ophthalmoscope, slit lamp microscopy). Another generally known typical age criterion is the decreased accommodation ability of the lens, resulting in presbyopia. Presbyopia and cataract will be discussed in the following sections.

I. Presbyopia

Many people first become aware of the phenomenon of aging by changes in their sensory perceptions. Among those first noticed is presbyopia, occurring during the natural aging process where the lens loses its ability to accommodate.

The human eye is able to change its refraction (accommodation) in order to form a sharp image of near and distant objects. The mechanism of accommodation involves a change in the form of the lens, the latter becoming more rounded, which increases refraction.

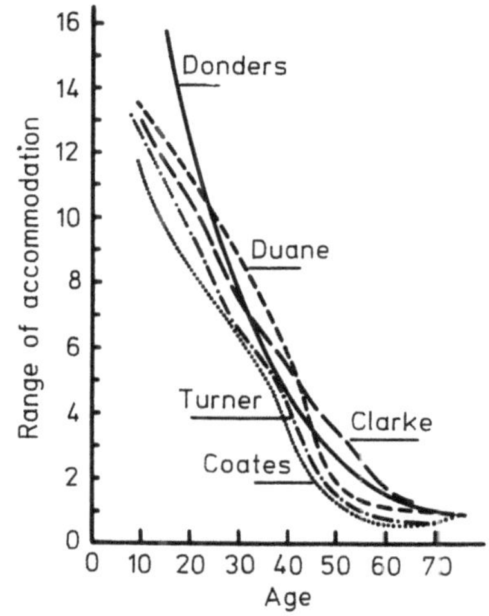

Fig. 21. Range of accommodation (as a function of age in human lenses. (For references BORISH 1970)

In this process, external as well as intracapsular (internal) accommodation plays a role.

External accommodation means a change of the lens form by the ciliary muscles aided by the zonula fibers and the lens capsule. VON HELMHOLTZ (1896) was one of the first to elucidate these interactions. In near vision, the ciliary muscle contracts and relaxes the zonula Zinnii. The elasticity of the lens (capsule) then increases the thickness of the lens in the direction of the eye axis. In distant vision, the ciliary muscle relaxes, effecting a tension of the zonula fibers and a flattening of the lens, particularly of the surface. The processes involved in accommodation in the lens were termed the "intracapsular accommodation mechanism" by GULLSTRAND (1911) who elucidated the phenomenon. However, he assumed a shift of the lens fibers themselves while VOGT (1922) assumed a shift of material within the lens fibers. MÜLLER (1938) thought that such intracapsular processes were due to contractile properties of the lens fibers and also dependent on lens metabolism. KLEIFELD (1954, 1956) and KLÉTHI and MANDEL (1965) were able to demonstrate in vitro that, during accommodation, energy-consuming processes take place and fiber shifts as well as shifts of material within the fibers occur. These findings are further supported by reports of KIBELAAR et al. (1980) who were able to determine actin in the lens cell fibers.

The maximum increase in refraction corresponds to the range of accommodation representing the difference (in diopters) of refraction between near point and far point. Figure 21 illustrates that the range of accommodation decreases linearly up to the age of 60 years, when it is practically zero. This means that the range of accommodation may be regarded as an index of the true age. BERNSTEIN and BERNSTEIN (1945) investigated the range of accommodation of various individuals of equal age and compared them with their life expectancy. They postulated a positive correlation between longevity and range of accommodation by which calculation of the biologic age would be possible. This, however, could not be verified. The age-dependent phenomenon of presbyopia has long been ascribed to the assumption that the nucleus of a normal lens gets harder (by loss of water) and thereby less elastic. This, however, does not hold true for the normal human lens (WEALE 1963; BARBER 1973). This wrong assumption has often led to the false concept that sclerosis is part of the normal aging process and that this leads to cataract formation. This version is often found in the ophthalmic literature and may be due to findings of advanced nuclear cataracts in animal lenses where hard (pathologic) nuclei were found. In human lenses, however, the same protein and water content is found in nucleus and cortex, independent of age (BARBER 1973; HOCKWIN et al. 1978).

Changes of the elastic properties which presumably lead to loss of accommodation are probably also due to changes in the capsule membrane and/or the cell membrane. Cross-linking of the lens cell fibers, for instance, is less well ordered and regular in the older lens and this might also cause a loss in elasticity (KOBAYASHI and SUZUKI 1975). Should intracapsular accommodation in vivo be dependent on metabolic conditions, it may be assumed that the decreased energy metabolism of the aging lens also affects accommodation.

II. Age Changes of Lens Transparency, Development of Lens Opacities

As already mentioned in Sects. E.I. and E.IV., the light transmission of the lens is closely dependent on age. This is due to increased light scattering caused by changes in protein structure accompanied by changes in packing density. Particular wavelengths may be affected rather differently by the distribution process, particularly if fluorescent chromophore groups are excited by the incident light (LERMAN 1980 b). The capacity of the lens to transmit light is not homogeneous. Scheimpflug photographs and densitometric image analysis curves (Sect. E.IV.) demonstrate by way of light scattering that, as regards the single lens sections, their transparency may be different (see Figs. 19 and 20).

Figure 22 demonstrates the transparency conditions in the previously mentioned ten lens sections of normal volunteers (three age groups). Light scattering of each section is expressed as a percentage of whole lens light scattering. The age-related increase in light scattering affects in particular the deeper cortical zone (sections 3 and 4) and the nucleus (sections 6 and 7).

The inhomogeneity of the transparency of single lens areas is shown by multiple linear densitometry of Scheimpflug photographs (Fig. 23). In this case, the sections were measured parallel to the optic axis and their densitometer curves jointed together. The alterations in transparency do not usually affect visual acuity. This is only the case if opacification or strong coloration of the lens substance is present, which is then called a cataract, and is the most frequent disease of the organ. An estimated 2 million people per year lose their visual acuity to some extent through this disease. This holds true particularly for older people and has led to the term cataracta senilis. However, to consider aging as such as the only causative factor does not seem justified (see Sect. G).

With respect to morphology, lens opacities show various forms and are localized at different sites. This is demonstrated in various atlases with detailed illustrations of the various forms of opacifications (VOGT 1921, 1931; KOBY 1924; MEESMANN 1927; DUVERGER and VELTER 1930; SAUTTER 1951), and need not be discussed here (for references see KOCH 1976). The factors leading to lens opacities are manifold and are described in the works mentioned.

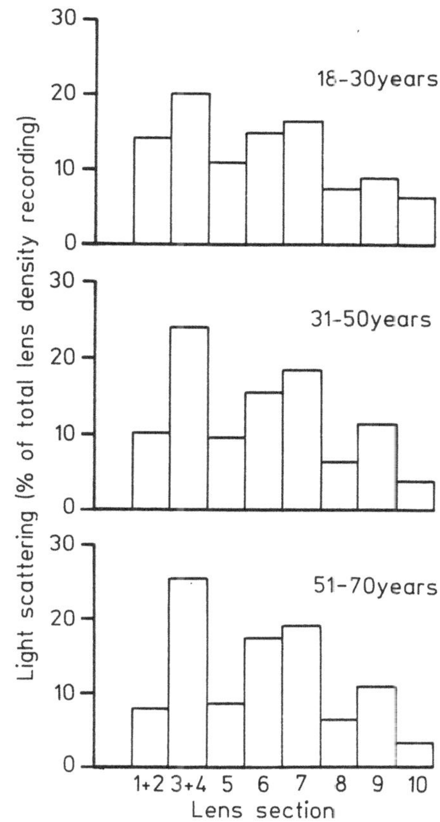

Fig. 22. Distribution of light scattering in single lens sections. Mean values of normal lenses (for details of lens sections see Fig. 15)

The opacifications discussed here may be located in the anterior or the posterior cortex or in the lens nucleus (Fig. 24). The process may finally result in total opacification (cataracta totalis). The question of the different sites of localization can only be elucidated by taking into account a multifactorial pathogenesis (see Sect. G). The opacities observed in the elderly are often located in certain lens areas (see the schematic compilation of BELLOWS 1981). In Fig. 25, Scheimpflug photographs are attached, illustrating the great variety of cataract types.

Depending on the localization and extent of change, the opacity may lead to decreased visual acuity and even to blindness of the affected eye. These disturbances may be explained by three different mechanisms (see Figs. 26, 27, 28, 29; KOCH 1976):

1. Any opacity is liable to decrease the optically active diameter, and has the effect of an aperture or diaphragm (Fig. 26 peripheral opacity; Fig. 27 central opacity).

2. Cataracts may cause light scattering at the borders of opacified areas, increasing the sensitivity of the eye toward light (Fig. 28 light scattering in cataracta stellata et coronaria).

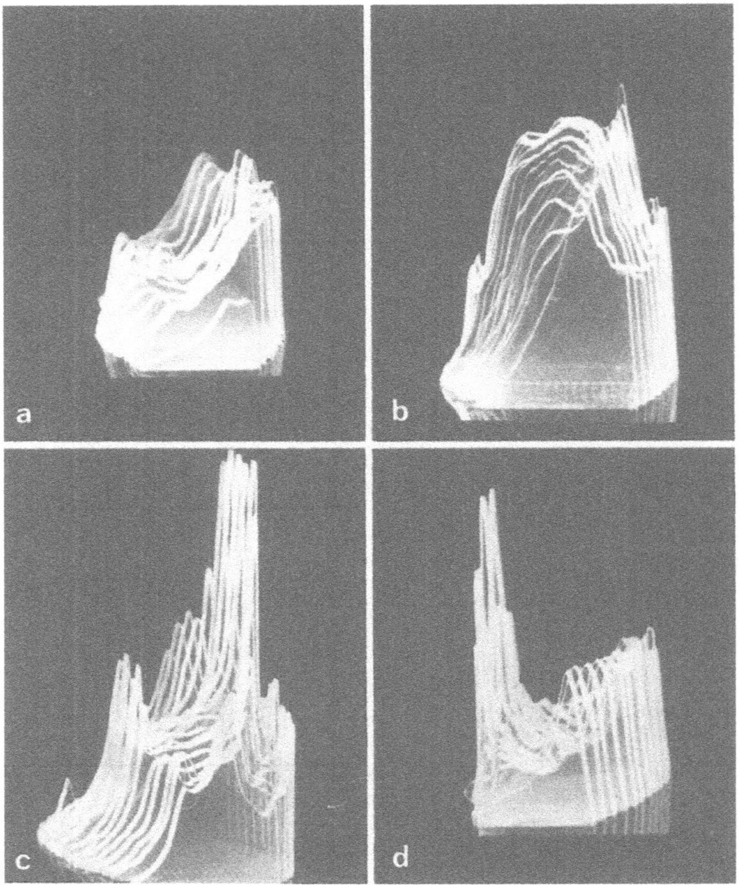

Fig. 23 a–d. Multilinear densitometry of Scheimpflug photographs of different lenses evaluated by Joyce Loebl 3 CS microdensitometer (window dimensions 50 × 500 μm). Beginning at the lens center, lens densitograms were taken every 0.5 mm (original size). By joining the single densitograms, a three-dimensional record of the lens density in the areas in question may be obtained **a** 25-year-old normal human lens; **b** nuclear opactiy and density of the anterior supranuclear region; **c** fusiform cataract opacity of the anterior deeper cortex; **d** posterior subcapsular cataract. In all pictures the anterior lens surface is on the right-hand side

3. Lens opacities may cause light absorption and may, with respect to wavelengths, be selective. In this case the opacified lens acts as a filter (gray or colored). This filter effect naturally leads to false color vision, as well as decreased contrast and resolving power (Fig. 29). This is most obvious in the case of alterations of the nucleus, where coloration of the central lens areas occurs (yellow-brown).

In general, all three mechanisms are involved in cases of decreased visual acuity. Depending on morphology and localization, one or another predominates.

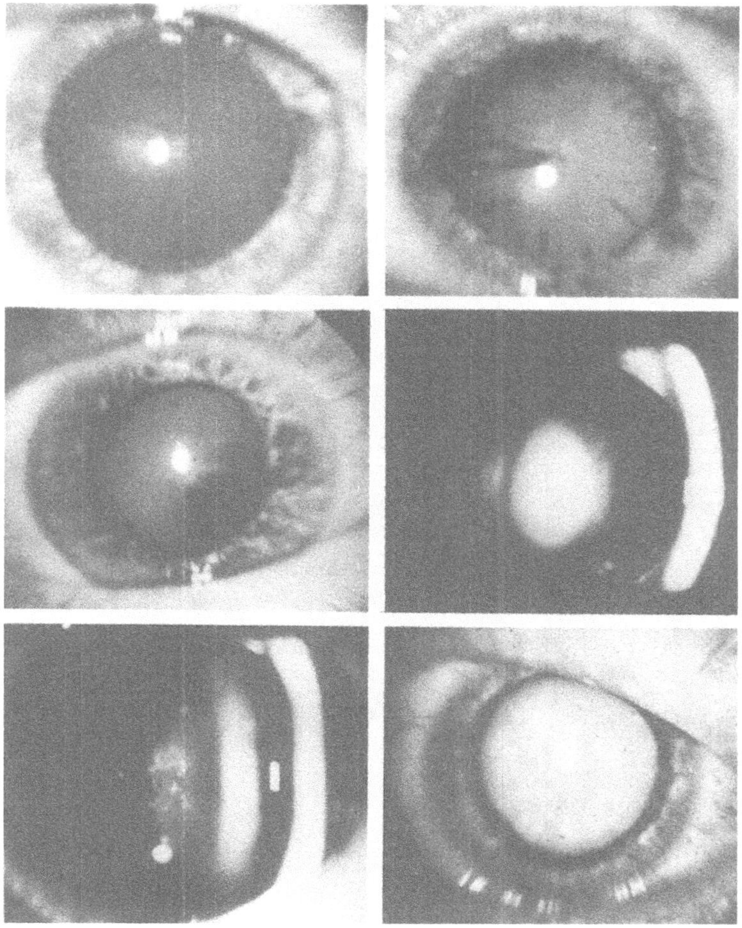

Fig. 24 a–f. Development of cataracta senilis **a** clear lens; **b** watercleft and fusiform opacity of the anterior lens cortex; **c** wedge-shaped opacification in the nasal lower quadrant of the anterior cortex (cataracta cuneiformis); **d** nuclear slerosis with brown coloration of the posterior nuclear and cortical parts; **e** subcapsular opacities of the posterior cortex; **f** complete opacification (cataracta totalis)

III. Age Changes of Biochemical Lens Properties

Reviews of age-related changes in lens biochemistry have been published by HOCKWIN (1971), NORDMANN (1972), BARBER (1973), KUCK (1975), HARDING and DILLEY (1976), BLOEMENDAL (1981), HOENDERS and BLOEMENDAL (1983).

Investigations of the last few decades have verified the presence of a lens metabolism by which substances are taken up from the aqueous and are utilized for the formation of lens substance and the maintenance of its structure (Table 1). Such investigations also showed the strong correlation between changes in metabolism and the pathogenesis of the

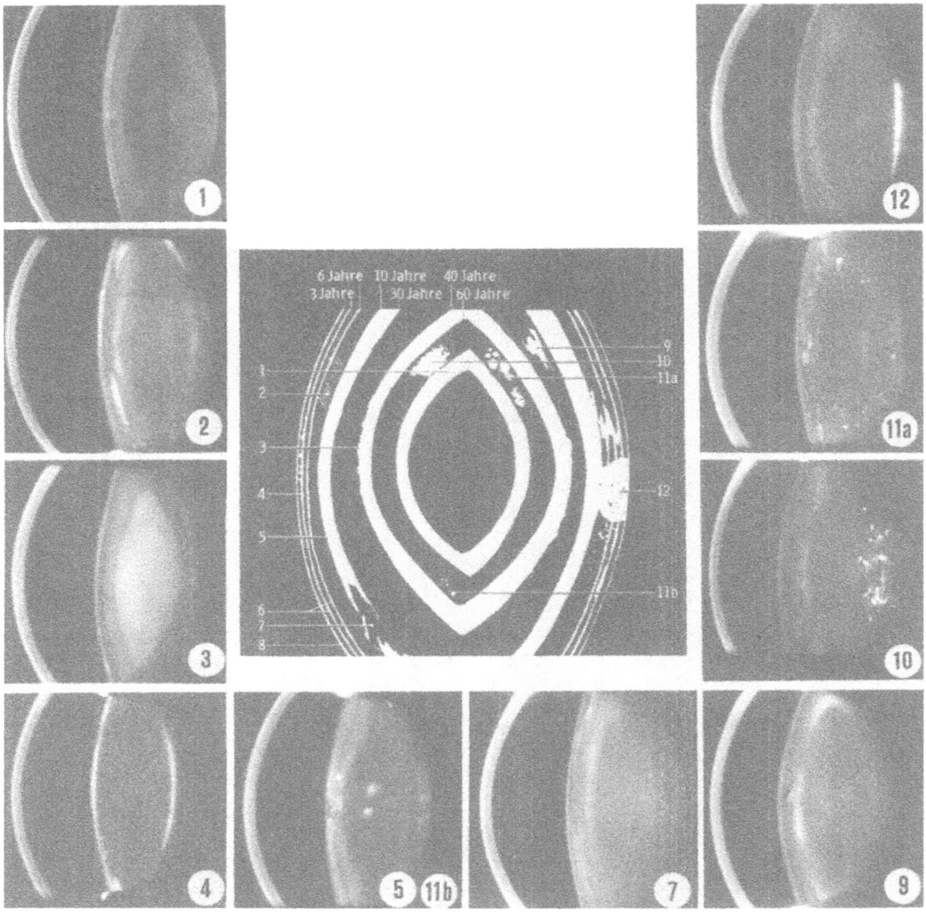

Fig. 25. Optic section through the lens, showing localization of lens opacities (BELLOWS 1981). Scheimpflug photographs of the different forms of opacities are attached. The numbers refer to the numbers in the schema. *1* = 25-year-old normal lens; *2* = lamellar clefts; *3* = aged nuclear region; *4* = subcapsular opacities; *5* = anterior zone of disjunction (and *11b* punctiform opacities); *6* = (striated capsule); *7* = waterclefts; *8* = (capsule surface); *9* = cataracta cuneiformis; *10* = cataracta dilaterata; *11a* = cataracta coronaria; *12* = posterior subcapsular cortical cataract

---

Fig. 26. Loss of visual acuity by cataract. Effect like an aperture diaphragm if opacity is situated peripherally. Experimental galactose-induced cataract (KOCH 1976)

Fig. 27. Loss of visual acuity by central opacity (incident light beam from above (dilated pupil) and from below (narrow pupil). Specimen of cataracta polaris anterior (KOCH 1976)

Fig. 28. Loss of visual acuity by cataract. Effect by light scattering (cataracta stellata et coronaria) (KOCH 1976)

Fig. 29. Loss of visual acuity by cataract. Filter effect (cataracta presenilis with nuclear sclerosis due to diabetes mellitus) (KOCH 1976)

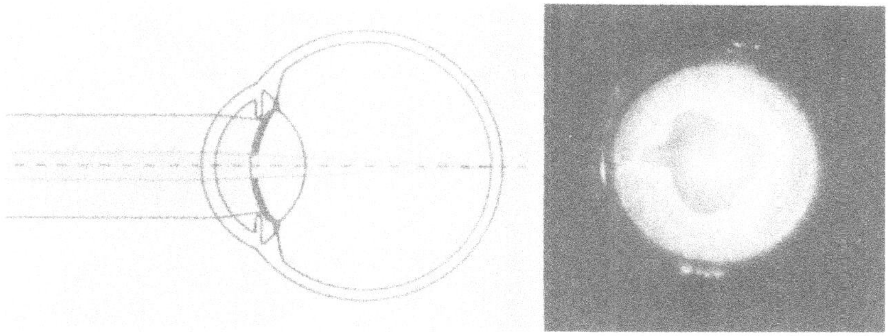

Fig. 26.

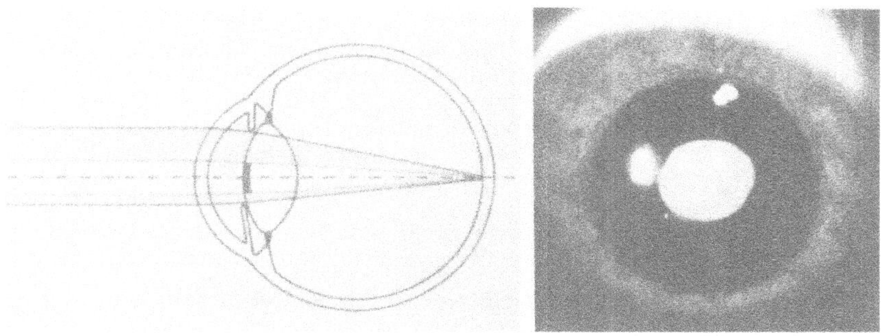

Fig. 27.

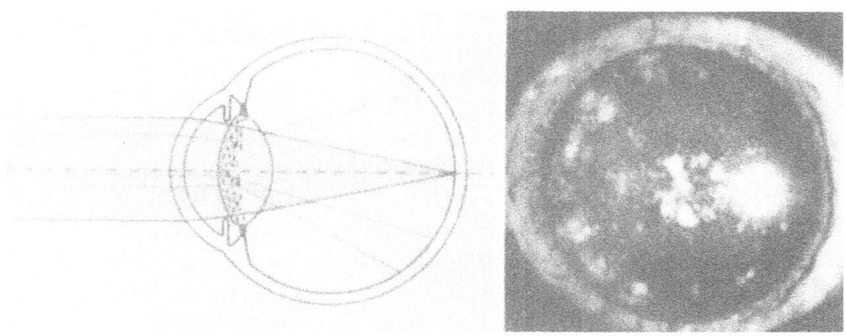

Fig. 28.

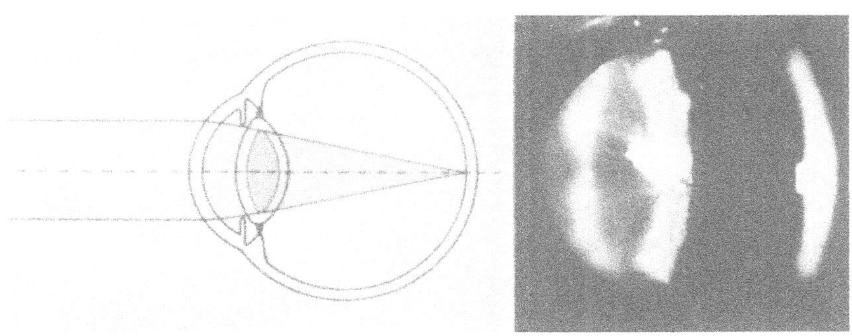

Fig. 29.

Table 1. Chemical composition of the vertebrate eye lens (estimated values)

67% Water + 33% Nonvolatile substances		
1.5%	Inorganic material (Na^+, K^+, Ca^{2+}, Mg^{2+}, Cl^-, PO_4^{3-})	
3%	Organic compounds (lipids, ascorbic acid, glutathione, creatine, urea, ATP, lactic acid, glucose...)	
0.5%	RNA, DNA	
95%	Protein:	crystallins (90%)
		+ membrane proteins
		+ cytoskeletal proteins
		+ enzymes

so-called cataracta senilis. This means that investigations of the causes of cataracta senilis involve the complex problems of causative factors and mechanisms of aging as such. Therefore, lens research is as important for clinical ophthalmology as it is for gerontologic problems. For such investigations the lens represents a perfect model since, owing to its appositional growth during the whole life span, it contains biologically identical tissues from different periods of life. It is therefore possible to separate the lens nucleus (old tissue) from the lens cortex (young tissue) for purposes of comparison (HOCKWIN and KLEIFELD 1965). Comparative investigations on species of different ages are also possible since for various species the determination of the lens fresh weight allows calculation of age (see Fig. 2).

In this respect it turned out rather early that comparison between young, clear lenses and old, opacified ones will not suffice, the crucial point is to gain insight into metabolic processes of aging, but still clear lenses. By experimental cataract research, we were able to find certain pieces of the puzle, representing a possible pathogenic cataractogenesis (HOCKWIN and KOCH 1976; HOCKWIN et al. 1976a). Among them are the accumulation cataract, i.e., a cataract induced by the additive effects of two noxae which, occurring separately, do not effect opacification (HOCKWIN and KOCH 1975). Further, artificial lens aging by X-irradiation (HOCKWIN 1961, 1962), cataracts induced by changes in the aqueous after unilateral ligature of the a. carotis communis (KOCH et al. 1974), or by influences of the protein metabolism through amino acid deficiency (lack of the essential amino acid tryptophan) (OHRLOFF et al. 1978; KOCH et al. 1982), also belong to the group of cataracts induced by additive factors.

Actually, there are already numerous results on energy metabolism, i.e., carbohydrate metabolism on the one hand, and protein metabolism on the other hand. The approaches of individual research groups may have favored one or the other metabolism for methodological reasons, nevertheless it is obvious that two different hypotheses have been pursued, assuming the primary cause to lie either protein metabolism or in energy metabolism and their respective changes (impairment).

1. Protein Metabolism

The lens protein content of 35% explains the fact that the lens proteins are one of the main target objects in lens research. Since the protein represents mostly structural protein in well-ordered form which guarantees the transparency of the lens, it is evident that the composition of the protein and its age-related changes

Table 2. Chemically or physically defined processes observed in lens proteins upon aging (postsynthetic alterations)

Formation of high molecular weight, eventually insoluble aggregates (superaggregation)
Formation of disulfide bridges and other covalent cross-links
Deamidation of Asn and Gln residues
Partial degradation of polypeptide chains at characteristic sites
Racemization of Asp residues
Nonenzymatic glycosylation
Photooxidation of Trp residues

are of great interest. Up to now, however, little is known of its spatial structure and its cross-linking (secondary, tertiary, and quarternary structure) in the lens. Detailed reports on the chemical composition of the primary structure of single lens crystallins and their respective age-related alterations, however, have already been published. In general, these concern differences in the composition of the water-soluble lens crystallins, α, β, and γ, and of the water-insoluble protein (albuminoid) between various regions of the lens (nucleus–cortex) as well as between lenses of different age. Two mechanisms exert their influence on the composition of the proteins: (a) changes in protein synthesis; and (b) changes after synthesis has been concluded (postsynthetic changes).

The synthesis of γ-crystallin, for instance, does not take place uniformly over the whole life span, but nearly exclusively in the embryonic and the young lens (FRANÇOIS and RABAEY 1956). In the older lens, it is therefore mainly found in the lens nucleus (KLEIFELD et al. 1956) which corresponds broadly to the embryonic lens. Also, the molecular weight of γ crystallin is different in bovine nucleus und lens (KABASAWA and KINOSHITA 1974). Isoelectric focusing also shows differences in the separation behavior and demonstrates clearly that more γ crystallin is found in the nucleus than in the cortex and that the fractions in nucleus and equator are not identical. The β crystallin fractions of low molecular weight (β_9–β_{12} in human and rat lenses, and slightly less in the bovine lens) are subject to a decrease which in the equator region might be due to synthesis (BOURS and HOCKWIN 1977).

On the other hand, protein changes after synthesis is complete (postsynthetic alterations) also happen during the aging process (Table 2). In this respect, the increase in water-insoluble protein as well as the increase in water-soluble, high molecular weight protein are of great importance. The water-insoluble protein, for instance, which is 5% of the total protein in humans and rats at birth, increases to 40% (human) and 50% (rat) with aging (Fig. 30; CLARK et al. 1969). This had also been found by JESS (1920) and KRAUSE (1934); other investigators (DISCHE et al. 1956; NEWSOM and HOCKWIN 1967; SPECTOR et al. 1971; VAN KAMP and HOENDERS 1973; BOURS and HOCKWIN 1977) have worked on the problem. In most cases, however, only studies involving relative comparisons of the water-soluble proteins were performed.

BOURS et al. (1978) then investigated the distribution of α_H, α_L, β_H, β_L, and γ crystallins, together with the water-insoluble protein in single lens areas as a function of age. They found that most of the low molecular weight α_L and β_L crystallin

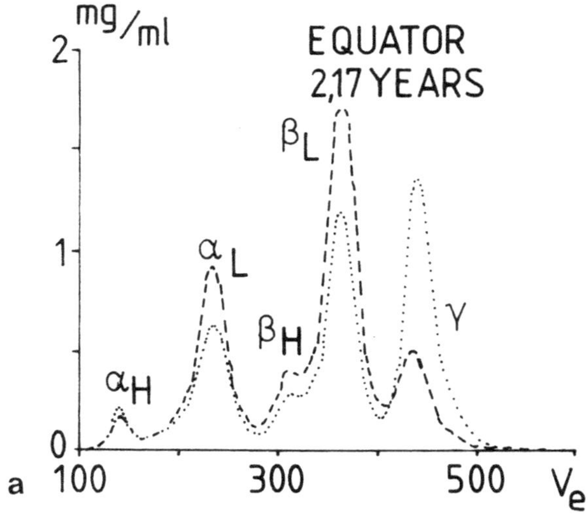

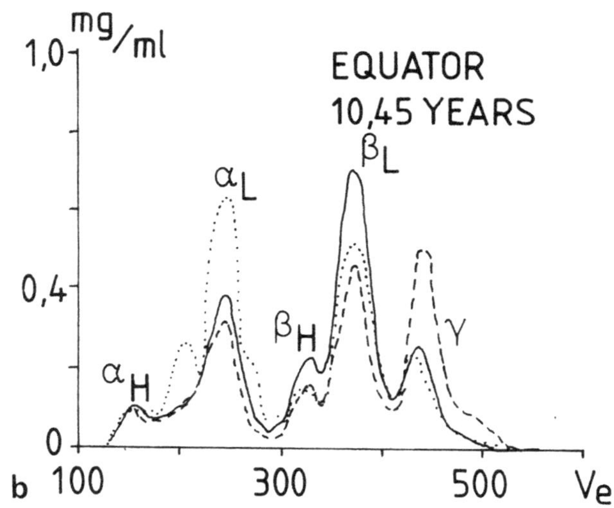

Fig. 30 a–d. Separation of water-soluble protein in equator and nucleus of bovine lenses by Sepharose 6B. *Full curves* extinction at 280 nm; *dashed curves* extinction at 260 nm; *dotted curves* protein according to the Lowry method. $\alpha_H = \alpha$ crystallin of high molecular weight, $1–5 \times 10^6$; $\alpha_L = \alpha$ crystallin of low molecular weight, about 80,000; $\beta_H = \beta$ crystallin of high molecular weight, 220,000; $\beta_L = \beta$-crystallin of low molecular weight, 80,000; $\gamma = \gamma$ crystallin, 20,000. The increase in high molecular weight crystallin in the nucleus of the lens is particularly pronounced. **a, b** equator; **c, d** nucleus (BOURS et al. 1978)

is present in the equator, i.e., 50% in the equator and 16% in the nucleus and that this proportion is independent of age. The high molecular weight α_H and β_H crystallin is found in highest concentration in the nucleus. It is known that the subunits of α_H and β_H crystallin are identical to those of the low molecular weight α_L and β_L crystallin (SPECTOR et al. 1971; HERBRINK and BLOEMENDAL 1974).

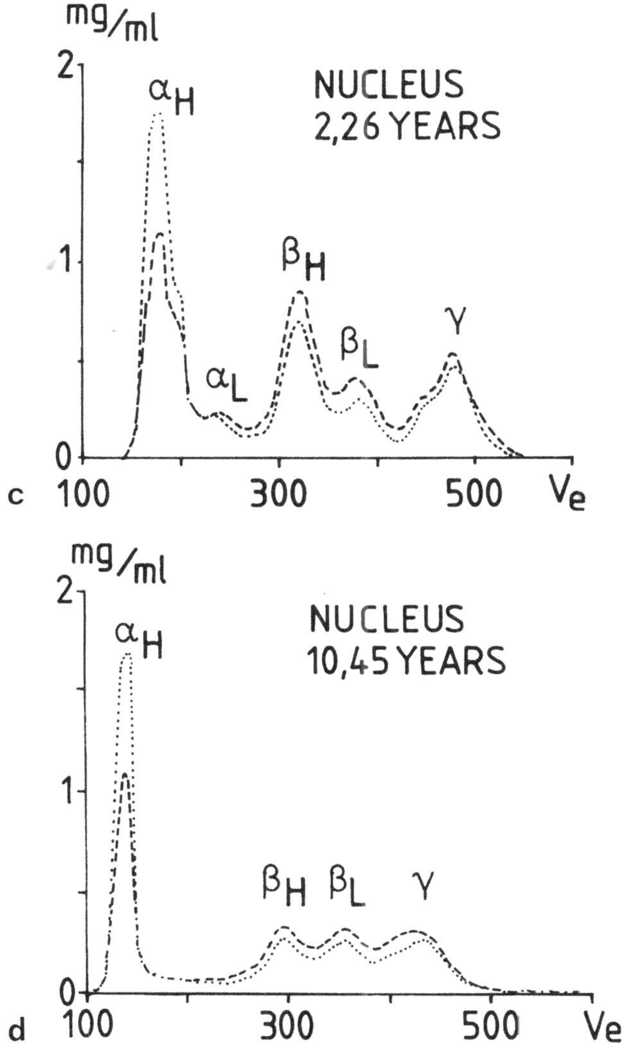

The water-insoluble protein is found in highest concentration in the nucleus compared with the equator. During aging, the concentration increases in the nucleus. This increase is correlated with a decrease of the high molecular weight α_H and β_H crystallin. The border between high molecular weight (HMW) protein and the water-insoluble (WI) fraction is vague and the definition of these fractions is operational and more or less arbitrary. A great similarity between urea-soluble (US) and HMW fractions with regard to their polypeptide chain composition has led to the assumption that the HMW aggregates form intermediates in the process of decreasing solubility, culminating in urea-insoluble (UI) protein

Crystallins → HMW protein → WI but US protein → UI protein

There are indications that glucose and calcium ions are involved in the formation of HMW protein; another factor causing superaggregation may be a relatively acidic polypeptide chain such as that isolated from calf lens nuclei (SIEZEN et al. 1979).

a) Deamidation and Degradation

Only two polypeptide chains of α crystallin, designated A_2 and B_2, are primary gene products and the other are produced from them by two distinct posttranslational processes, namely deamidation and specific limited cleavage at the COOH terminus. These events lead to a complex subunit composition of α crystallin in the older lens parts.

The proportion of shortened chains increases from cortex to nucleus, suggesting an age-dependent process since protein synthesis no longer takes place in the inner cortex and in the nucleus. The deamidation process, on the other hand, seems not to be related to the aging of the tissue. The reason for the stepwise breakdown at selective sites is still unclear; it is unlikely that the observed truncations are the result of enzymatic proteolysis (RINGENS et al. 1982).

b) Disulfide Bridges and Other Covalent Cross-Links

Definite changes in the distribution of protein sulfhydryl and disulfide groups were found to accompany aging: the first show a decline, the latter an increase in their level. Disulfide bridges could not be detected in young human lenses, whereas considerable amounts have been found in old ones. It is not yet sure, however, whether the sulfhydryl groups of the soluble proteins are oxidized before or after they become insoluble (ANDERSON et al. 1979) It has been clearly demonstrated that old human lenses, especially cataractous ones with dark-brown nuclei, contain nondisulfide, covalently cross-linked protein species of relatively high molecular weight (KRAMPS et al. 1978). Nontryptophan fluorescence is also associated with the cross-linked protein (AUGUSTEYN 1975).

Products with β-carboline structure, bityrosine, and anthranilic acid (TRUSCOTT et al. 1977) have been isolated from human lenses, but whether they serve as cross-linking structures is still an open question. Most recently, it has been demonstrated that in lenses of five different species, transglutaminase activity is present; moreover, it was shown that the cross-linked protein fraction of human cataracts indeed contains significant amounts of γ-glutamyl-ε-lysine cross-links or isopeptide bonds.

c) Racemization of Aspartic Acid

An interesting new aspect of lens protein aging, namely racemization of aspartyl residues, has also been discovered (MASTERS et al. 1978). D-Aspartyl residues were shown to accumulate in normal human lens nuclear proteins at a rate of 0.14%/year.

d) Nonenzymatic Glycosylation

Nonenzymatic glycosylation of hemoglobin is a well-established phenomenon (STEVENS et al. 1977). Crystallins of normal clear bovine lenses, 2–6 years old, have been investigated with relation to their reducibility by ^3H-labeled $NaBH_4$ and their content of sorbitol-lysine (MONNIER et al. 1980; CHION et al. 1981). It could be concluded from these experiments that there is an age-related increase in nonenzymatic glycosylation, particularly in high molecular weight α crystallin.

Although at least two important and current areas of lens protein aging have not been considered in this survey, namely photooxidative damage involving tryptophan residues (LERMAN 1980) and lipid peroxidation, including its deleterious influence on proteins (VARMA et al. 1982), it has to be kept in mind that quite a lot of posttranslational modifications take place in the protein of the aging lens and can account for most of their abnormalities. It cannot be excluded that they reflect only a transitional step in the normal catabolism of proteins (DREYFUS et al. 1977).

The real mechanisms are still hypothetical. Only one reaction is well defined: the deamidation of asparagine and glutamine residues. According to ROBINSON et al. (1970), controlled deamidation of proteins may serve as a general biologic clock. The longevity of a protein would be restricted by loss of amide groups via conformational change and increased susceptibility to proteolysis. Proteins with many unstable amide groups would therefore have short half-lives and vice versa.

2. Enzymes and Energy Metabolism

For the lens, glycolysis is of crucial importance with respect to energy metabolism.

The main functions of lens metabolism are evident if one considers the growth of the lens over the entire life span, and the necessity to maintain its transparency which depends on an intact protein structure. Except for the biosynthetic processes (protein and glutathione synthesis) most of the energy is necessary for two transport processes – uptake of amino acids and the Na^+, K^+-pump. It many be supposed that lens metabolism is an active factor in the process of accommodation (Sect. F.I.).

Extensive investigations of the lens metabolism in laboratory animals showed various changes which indicate an age-related decline of the energy metabolism (HOCKWIN 1971). Factor analysis of the results suggests that enzyme modifications might well be considered as one of the most important causes of the age-related metabolic changes (HOCKWIN et al. 1976a, b). Detailed investigations on young and old lens tissue with respect to the kinetic and physicochemical properties of the enzymes of carbohydrate metabolism involved studies on specific activity and substrate affinity, determination of heat lability, molecular weight and size, and electrophoretic mobility. The experiments were carried out with lenses from various species, such as rat and rabbit, but mostly with cattle lenses (OHRLOFF 1979). Findings on enzymes showed that their activity in the lens nucleus, that is, in old tissue, is lower than in the equator, i.e. in young tissue (Table 3). Experiments involving mixtures of old and young lens tissue showed that no influence of an age-dependent inhibitor need be taken into account (OHRLOFF 1978).

Investigating the substrate affinity of various enzymes, it could be demonstrated that in old tissue some enzymes, particularly hexokinase, phosphofructokinase, and enolase have formed certain enzyme forms of lesser substrate affin-

Table 3. Enzyme activities of bovine lenses after separation into lens nucleus (old tissue) and lens equator (young tissue)

Enzyme[a]	Specific activity (mU per milligram protein)			Age of animals (years)
	Equator (*E*)	Nucleus (*N*)	*E*/*N*	
GK	0.005	0		4
HK	0.3	0.02	15	5
KHK	0.3	0.06	5	2
ALD	0.6	0.03	20	5
G-6-PDH	0.7	0		4
SDH	1	0.2	5	4
Phosphorylase	3	0.1	30	5
AR	3	0.9	3.3	4
GD	3	0.5	6	6
PGluMu	4	2	2	4
PFK	8	0.5	16	4
MDH	8.3	2.8	3	5
GDH	8.4	0.15	56	6
LDH	8.5	4	2.1	5
UDPG-P	11	2	5.5	5
PGM	90	20	4.5	1
GAPDH	116	14	8.2	1
ENOL	204	47	4.3	11
PGI	300	120	2.5	4
PGK	314	150	2.1	1
TIM	360	170	2.1	6
GSH-red	1.5	0.7	2	5
GSH-Px	7.5	6.0	1.2	5

[a] Abbreviation according Enzyme Classification nomenclature

ity (Table 4). This age-related enzyme heterogeneity is most remarkable and gives rise to the following considerations:

1. Whether, with higher age, the native enzyme molecule is modified in a way that effects its catalytic properties.
2. Which of today's theories on aging, such as the genetic theory, the error–catastrophe theory or posttranslational changes might be responsible for such modifications.

In regard to the first question at issue, DREYFUS et al. (1977) reported that certain enzymes in old lenses show a higher electrophoretic mobility toward the anode, which might be due to deamidation. Investigations involving isoelectric focusing of lactate dehydrogenase showed that the enzyme forms 3, 4, and 5 could be determined (BOURS et al. 1977). Lactate dehydrogenase shows microheterogeneity and decline in old tissue where its anodic form can scarely be found any more.

With aging, an increase in the heat lability occurred in all enzymes investigated (BANROQUES et al. 1978; OHRLOFF et al. 1979a), as is demonstrated with aldolase and phosphofructokinase (Fig. 31). In the lens nucleus, however, not only is the heat lability significantly higher, increasing with aging, but some enzymes

Table 4. Substrate affinities (K_m) of enzymes in bovine lenses

Enzyme	Substrate	K_m for young lenses		K_m for old lenses	
		Equator	Nucleus	Equator	Nucleus
GAPDH-1	Glyc-3-P	1.6×10^{-3}	1.6×10^{-3}	2.0×10^{-3}	1.43×10^{-3}
-2		2.66×10^{-5}	2.7×10^{-5}	3.0×10^{-5}	2.82×10^{-5}
PGK	Glyc-3-P	1.18×10^{-4}	1.09×10^{-4}	1.05×10^{-4}	1.43×10^{-4}
PGM-1	Glyc-3-P	5.0×10^{-4}	5.0×10^{-4}	6.6×10^{-4}	5.0×10^{-4}
-2		0	0	0	3.0×10^{-5}
ENOL-1	Glyc-2-P	3.7×10^{-5}	3.7×10^{-5}	3.77×10^{-5}	4.26×10^{-5}
-2		0	0	0	1.6×10^{-4}
HK-1	Glucose	6.4×10^{-5} [b]			6.5×10^{-5}
-2		0			6.3×10^{-4}
PFK-1	F-6-P	7.0×10^{-5} [a]			5.0×10^{-5}
-2		0 [a]			5.0×10^{-4}
PGI	F-6-P	1.2×10^{-4} [a]		1.2×10^{-4} [a]	
PGluMu	G-1-P	3.5×10^{-5} [a]		3.5×10^{-5} [a]	
G-6-PDH	G-6-P	1.5×10^{-5} [a]		1.5×10^{-5} [a]	

[a] K_m values were obtained with crude extracts of total lenses
[b] Only anterior cortical layer

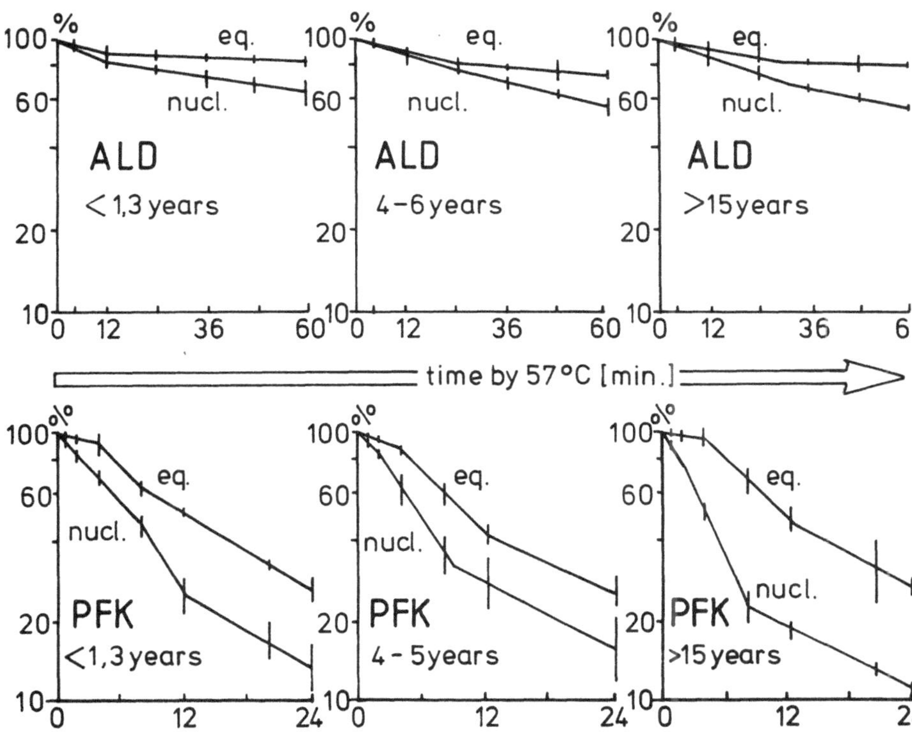

Fig. 31. Heat lability of fructose-1,6-diphosphate aldolase (*ALD*) and phosphofructokinase (*PFK*) in equator (*eq.*) and nucleus (*nucl.*) of bovine lenses, as a function of age

Table 5. Elution volume of maxima of activity of PGK, PGM, and ENOL after separation of the water-soluble protein of nucleus and equator (bovine lenses of 5.7 years) on Sepharose 6 B

	Elution volume with (ml) maximum activity	Protein content of fraction (mg/ml)	Enzyme activity (mU per milligram protein)	Molecular weight
Equator				
PGK	370	2.9	174	59,500
PGM	350	2.6	186	87,000
ENOL				
1st peak	340	1.65	364	105,000
2nd peak	360	3.25	162	72,000
Nucleus				
PGK	370	1.76	91	59,500
PGM				
1st peak	340	1.7	7	105,000
2nd peak	380	1.6	3	49,000
ENOL				
1st peak	340	1.7	129	105,000
2nd peak	370	1.76	43	59,500

even show variations in molecular size or weight, as demonstrated by gel filtration of the water-soluble lens proteins (Table 5). This is particularly the case with phosphofructokinase (BOUS et al. 1977), phosphoglyceromutase, and enolase (OHRLOFF et al. 1983). These findings indicate clearly that with advanced age the structure of the enzyme molecule is subjected to modifications and its conformation is no longer stable.

With respect to the second problem at issue, it should be called to mind that enzyme heterogeneity is mostly found in the lens nucleus where protein synthesis no longer takes place. Therefore the changes described must be considered as postsynthetic (posttranslational) molecular modifications leading to enzyme variations which differ in structure so that active as well as partially active and inactive molecules are present. By immunologic methods, even catalytically inactive forms of phosphofructokinase, aldose isoenzymes A and C, and superoxide dismutase can be determined in rabbit and rat lenses (OHRLOFF et al. 1979 b, 1980 a; DOVRAT and GERSHON 1981).

The immunologic precipitation of enzymes enables determination of inactive enzyme molecules as "cross-reacting material (CRM)", if these inactive enzymes still possess the immunologic properties of the originally active molecule (GERSHON and GERSHON 1970). The procedure involves quantitative titration of an isoenzyme in young and old tissue with monospecific antibodies, the activities in the test assay having been equilibrated previously. If inactive enzyme molecules are present in the old tissue, it is to be supposed that they react to the antibodies in the same way as the active enzyme, so that, for the precipitation of an equal degree of activity, more antibodies are necessary than is the case with young tissue.

All of these findings support the assumption that the decrease of enzyme activity in the aging tissue is closely related with the occurrence of inactive enzyme molecules. In recent years, the chemical nature of the postsynthetic modifications

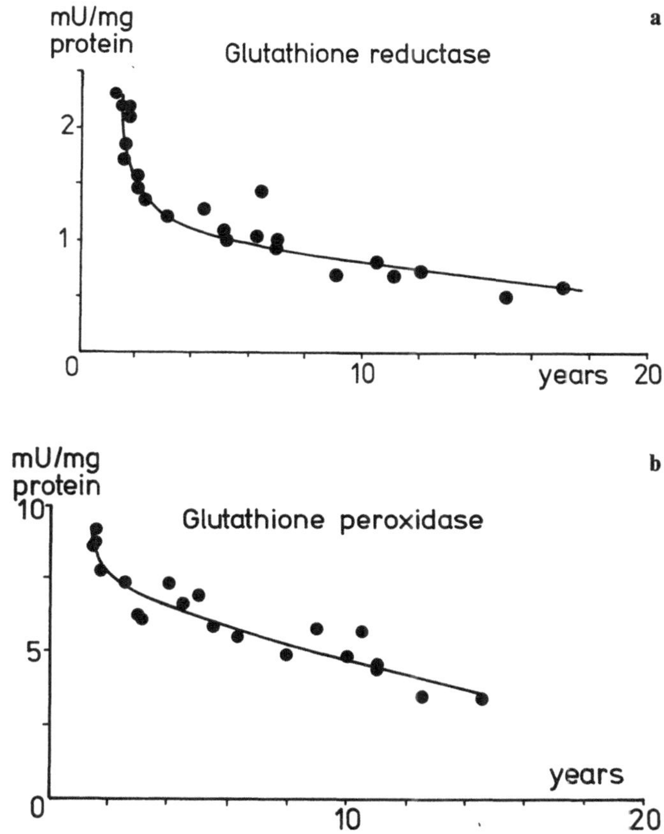

Fig. 32 a, b. Specific enzyme activities in bovine lenses as a function of age

responsible could be elucidated mainly with respect to the structural proteins of the lens, for instance, α crystallin (see Sect. F.III.1; HOENDERS et al. 1973; BOURS et al. 1978; HOENDERS and BLOEMENDAL 1983). In triggering these modifications, oxidative influences seem to play an important role (LERMAN 1980 a), the more so since, in old lens tissue, the functions of the antioxidative defence system (that is, a high level of glutathione) as well as those of the enzymes glutathione reductase and glutathione peroxidase (Fig. 32) are rather negligible (HARDING 1973; OHRLOFF et al. 1980 b).

Considering the age changes of lens biochemistry, there are several items which emphasize the importance of lens research within the scope of gerontology:

1. The lens is an ideal model for investigations on the age-induced posttranslational protein modifications of the enzyme and structural proteins since no other tissue is known where distinction between posttranslational modifications and neosynthesis is so easy. This also holds true for the elucidation and inhibition of factors leading to such changes.

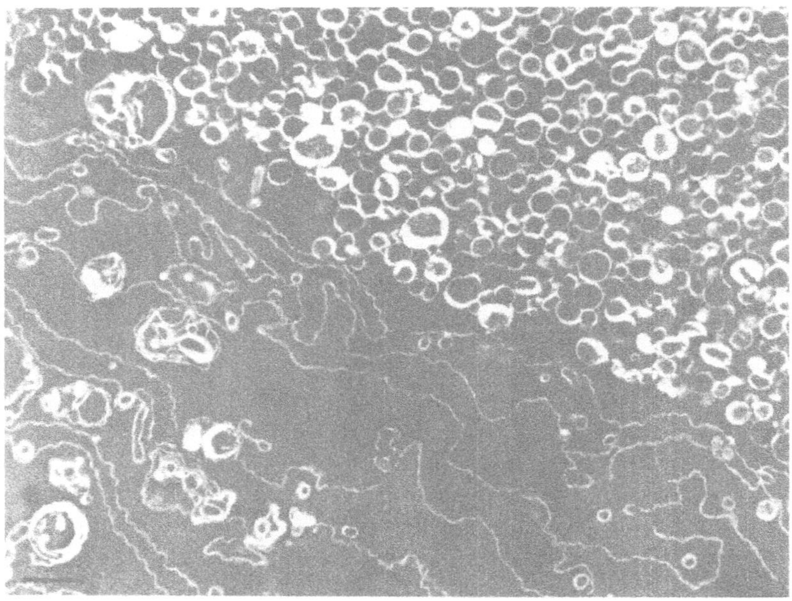

Fig. 33. Age changes of deeper cortex of a 76-year-old clear human lens, strong accumulation of globular bodies upper right and cell bodies in the fibers (lower left). (× 18,900) (KOBAYASHI and SUZUKI 1975)

2. The lens proteins have a longer life expectancy than any other protein in the human system. It is therefore of the utmost importance to study those properties which are responsible for such longevity.

3. The elucidation of the age-induced changes of the molecules of lens proteins is also a most important factor in our search for the mechanisms responsible for the incidence of senile lens opacities which are still one of the most frequent causes of blindness in people of advanced age.

IV. Age Changes of Lens Morphology

With aging, each lens fiber shows the morphological features of the underlying layer (KOBAYASHI and SUZUKI 1975). There is, further more, a close similarity between the morphological picture of the old, clear lens (Fig. 33) and the cataractous lens (Fig. 34). In some cases, deterioration of lens fibers happens in young lenses, this, however, is more frequent in older and most frequent in cataractous lenses. As a consequence of this event, small and large globular bodies appear (Morgagni's globules) which must be considered as protein aggregates (YANOFF and FINE 1975). Also, in intact fibers, cell bodies appear which are probably formed from cell protrusions of neighboring fibers. These morphological findings show that aging processes which finally lead to cell death are closely correlated

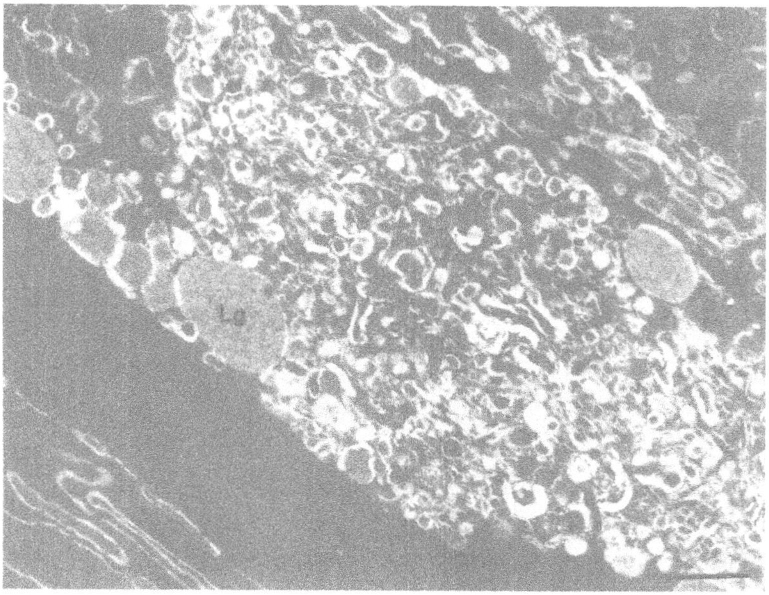

Fig. 34. Deeper cortex of a 62-year-old human lens with senile opacity. Strong accumulation of small and large (*Lg*) globular bodies occurring after fiber death. (× 17,556) (KOBAYASHI and SUZUKI 1975)

with the pathogenesis of senile lens opacities so that cataract must be regarded as lens aging in an advanced state.

It is also obvious that investigations of the biochemical interrelationships and modifications by aging should be performed on clear lenses where cell death has not yet occurred. The fact that even lenses of younger adults may, on electron microscopic examination, show the findings often see in later age points out that "aging" begins at a rather early date.

G. Senile Cataract as a Result of Multifactorial Origin

Today it is generally established that postsynthetic protein alterations are responsible for lens aging. However, to designate lens aging as senile cataract does not seem to be justified. With age, the lens is more susceptible to the formation of opacities, however, aging as such is not in itself cataractogenic. If that were the case, the modifications would only effect the nucleus, since it is only in the nucleus that faulty proteins are found. It is established beyond doubt that the development of lens opacities during aging, the so-called cataracta senilis, is due to a multifactorial process. Various clinical observations and numerous experimental findings support the assumption that this cataractogenic process runs either according to the mechanisms of cocataractogenesis or syncataractogenesis.

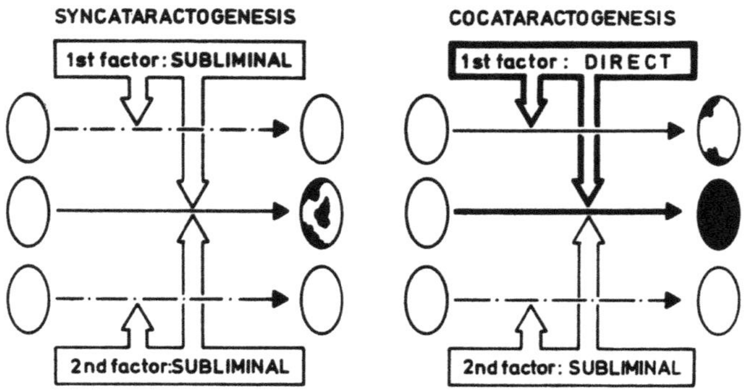

Fig. 35. Mechanisms of syn- and cocataractogenesis

Cocataractogenesis means that the influence of a directly cataractogenic factor is, with respect to time of onset and extent of cataract formation, increased by the simultaneous action of a second, subliminal cataractogenic factor (Fig. 35). Syncataractogenesis, on the other hand, means the coincidental action of two subliminal noxae, which in themselves are not liable to induce opacities (HOCKWIN and KOCH 1975). The question of which of the two mechanisms may be responsible for the individual case of senile cataract has not yet been elucidated, it may even be that both mechanisms are involved.

At any rate, age itself or the age-related alterations in lens biochemistry should not be considered as direct cataractogenic factors. A number of risk factors have already been detected which, within the interrelationship of aging processes, such as postsynthetic molecular transformation of the structural and functional (enzyme) proteins, may be regarded as being responsible for the formation of lens opacities. The course of action of the additive effects which are either cocataractogenic or syncataractogenic, determines the localization of the opacity known as cataracta senilis (Fig. 36). This is also important with a view to the fact that the onset of these opacities occurs at individually different times of life. The observed phenomena also explain why this disease, occurring at higher ages, is only found in a comparatively small part of the population.

Investigations of the epidemiology of lens opacities occurring in advanced age have seldom been performed. This may be due to the fact that the ophthalmologist accepts the diagnosis cataracta senilis or even presenilis as a matter of fact, and is able to apply the time-honored therapy of lens surgery. In recent years, however, a series of target investigations have been performed which elucidated in numerous cases the coincidence of cataract and additional factors, an event anticipated more than 100 years ago by BECKER (1877). It may be taken for granted that racial as well as climatic–geographic influences play a decisive role, while nutrition or metabolic disturbances also determine the age of onset (for instance with diabetics). As further factors, environmental influences and untoward side effects of drugs (drug abuse, barbiturates) must be considered. Investigations of PHILLIPS (1981, 1982) even indicated that certain forms of cataract may be associated with changes of the serum concentrations of urea and calcium. These problems should at any rate be investigated further.

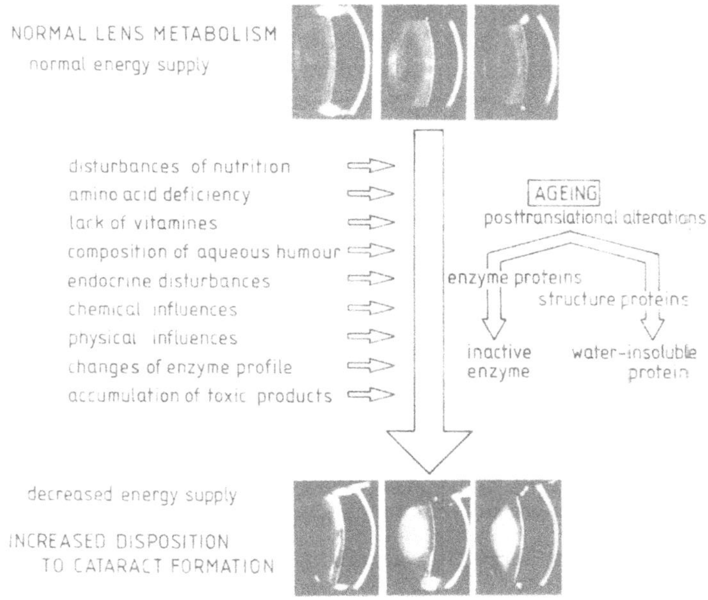

Fig. 36. Schematic representation of multifactorial cataractogenesis by interaction of risk factors with age changes of lens metabolism. This interaction probably leads to lens opacities

I. Surgical Therapy

It is undisputed that the surgical extraction of the opacified lens is still the only effective therapy for the disease. The technical development of the procedure has recently been considerably improved. However, one should not disregard the fact that visual acuity after cataract extraction is by no means as improved as the statistical data immediately after surgery show. Further, the patient's adaptability to the necessary aids to vision is individually different; in short, the visual faculty after surgery is certainly different from normal conditions, but first and foremost, the psychological attitude of the older patient toward surgery is a serious handicap of the method.

Among the complications of cataract surgery (BELLOWS 1975) bacterial endophthalmitis is the most serious, however, its incidence has greatly decreases recently. Today aphakia, glaucoma, loss or changes of vitreous body (weeks or months after surgery), flat anterior chamber with subsequent glaucoma, after cataract condition, edema of the macula, and retinal detachments still occur. Unfortunately, statistics on complications after cataract extraction are not very popular.

II. Drug Treatment of Lens Opacities

For these and other reasons, it is well worth making the attempt either to avoid the processes leading to opacification or to ameliorate the disease by drug treatment. Considering the mechanisms of co- and syncataractogenesis, this approach seems promising if one or several risk factors could be detected and their reactions inhibited (see Fig. 35). It should be pointed out, however, that such a procedure can never achieve reversal of an already existing opacity nor will it be possible to restore normal transparency since, according to biologic laws, the restoration of denatured proteins is impossible.

Another crucial point is the fact that we have to deal with a variety of risk factors which differ in their mode of action and therefore cause different types of opacities. It stands to reason that one special drug alone will never meet the requirements to act against all kinds of risk factors.

The goal of drug therapy should therefore be: (a) inhibition of the formation of opacities and/or delay of the progress of an already existing opacity; and (b) treatment appropriate to the different factors responsible.

There are already a great number of pharmaceutical preparations available which are said to have a favorable influence in cases of cataracta senilis. Chemically they belong to all classes of compounds, such as inorganic salts, substances to improve blood circulation, hormones, vitamins, enzyme inhibitors, inhibitors of quinone effects, substitutes for the sulfhydryl groups, etc. Experimental data on some of them indicate a possible effect; however, most of the preparations are only based on hypothesis. In most cases, not even the simplest tests such as distribution studies (penetration, concentration at the target zone, etc.) have been performed, to say nothing of controlled clinical double-blind studies. Although a lot of reports on clinical trials and successful treatments are found in the literature (KOCH et al. 1973), none of these stand the test of serious scientific verification, nor is the discussion of results in any way satisfactory.

In recent years, a few controlled clinical trials have been performed (MACLEAN 1978; HOCKWIN and WEIGELIN 1981; WEIGELIN and HOCKWIN 1982; WEIGELIN et al. 1982; HOCKWIN et al., to be published, b). The trials were conducted as double-blind studies with a parallel placebo group, both groups being homogeneous as to age, cataract type, visual acuity, and macular condition. Patients were randomly assigned to the two treatment groups. The assessment of drug efficacy was exclusively made by image analysis of Scheimpflug photographs taken at different time intervals at the follow-up examinations. Film blackening according to light scattering of the lens yielded quantitative data which permitted statistical comparisons of transparency changes with respect to the kind of treatment (HOCKWIN and DRAGOMIRESCU 1981 a, b, 1982). The authors were able to verify that opacifications in the cortical region of the lens can be delayed or even arrested by a certain preparation containing the precursors of the tripeptide glutathione besides pyridoxine hydrochloride and ascorbic acid. This was not the case with the placebo groups (WEIGELIN and HOCKWIN 1982; WEIGELIN et al. 1982; HOCKWIN 1982). Naturally these first positive results of drug treatment should not be interpreted as indicating that in the future cataract surgery will be superfluous.

The number of patients preferring drug therapy to surgery is naturally large. Development of effective preparations by means of clinically controlled trials involving Scheimpflug photography and image analysis presents (in contrast to the methods used up to now) the advantage of enabling one to prescribe preparations with a known delaying or arresting effect. Considering the still obscure problems of biologic tolerance of artificial lens implants it would be of advantage to perform this kind of surgery as late in life as possible. Adequate drug treatment of the affected eyes would probably postpone this moment.

References

Amsler M, Brückner A, Franceschetti A, Goldmann H, Streif EB (1961) Lehrbuch der Augenheilkunde, 3rd edn. Karger, Basel, p 325
Anderson EI, Wright D, Spector A (1979) The strate of sulfhydryl groups in normal and cataractous human lens proteins. II. Cortical and nuclear regions. Exp Eye Res 29:223–243
Augusteyn RC (1975) Distribution of fluorescence in the human cataractous lens. Ophthalmic Res 7:217–224
Augusteyn RC, Collin HB (1980) The eye, vol 2. Eden, St. Albans
Augusteyn RC, Collin HB, Rogers KM (1979) The eye, vol 1. Eden, St. Albans
Banroques J, Scala H, Schapira F, Dreyfus IC (1978) The aging of enzymes in eye lens Interdiscipl Top Gerontol 12:180–186
Barber GW (1973) Human cataractogenesis: a review. Exp Eye Res 16:85–94
Bargmann W (1962) Histologie und mikroskopische Anatomie des Menschen, 4th edn. Thieme, Stuttgart, p 725
Bartolić K (1982) Untersuchungen zur Zusammensetzung des sekundären Kammerwassers. Dissertation, Medizinische Fakultät der Universität Bonn
Becker O (1877) Pathologie und Therapie des Linsensystems. In: Graefe-Saemisch (ed) Hdb ges Augenheilk, vol 5. Engelmann, Leipzig
Bellows JG (1975) Cataract and abnormalities of the lens. Grune and Stratton, New York
Bellows JG (1981) Linse. In: François J, Hollwich F (eds) Augenheilkunde in Klinik und Praxis, vol 2. Thieme, Stuttgart
Benedek GB (1971) Theory of transparency of the eye. Appl Opt 10:459–473
Bernstein F, Bernstein M (1945) Law of physiologic aging as derived from long ranged data of refraction of the human eye. Arch Ophthalmol 34:378–388
Bettelheim FA, Balazs EH (1981) (eds) Biophysical properties of the lens. Exp Eye Res 586–630
Bito LZ, Petrinovic L, Salvador E (1973) The effects of the lens on the chemical composition of intraocular fluids, Abstr ARVO Meeting Sarasota, p 76/4
Bloemendal H (ed) (1981) Molecular and cellular biology of the lens. Wiley, New York
Borish JM (1970) Clinical refraction, 3rd edn. The Professional Press, Chicago, p 171
Bours J, Hockwin O (1977) Charakterisierung der wasserlöslichen Proteine der Linse mittels Immunologie und Isoelektrofokussierung und ihre Beziehung zum Alterungsprozeß. Klin Monatsbl Augenheilkd 170:51–59
Bours J, Neuhaus H, Hockwin O (1977) The thin-layer isoelectric focusing of lactate dehydrogenase isoenzymes in rabbit lens parts and in intraocular tissues. Albrecht von Graefes Arch Klin Exp Ophthalmol 203:9–19
Bours J, Wieck A, Hockwin O (1978) Gel filtration chromatography of crystallins, DNA and RNA from different parts of bovine lens in dependence on age. Interdiscip Top Gerontol 12:205–220
Bous F, Hockwin O, Ohrloff C, Bours J (1977) Investigation on phosphofructokinase (PFK, EC 2.7.1.11) in bovine lenses in dependence on age, topographic distribution and water soluble protein fractions. Exp Eye Res 24:383–389
Braus H (1960) Anatomie des Menschen, vol 3, 2nd edn. Springer, Berlin Göttingen Heidelberg, p 623
Brown N (1969) Slit-image photography. Trans Ophthalmol Soc UK 89:397–408
Brown N (1973a) Slit-image photography and measurement of the eye. Med Biol Illust 23:192–203
Brown N (1973b) Lens change with age and cataract; slit-image photography. In: The human lens in relation to cataract. Ciba Found Symp 19:65–78
Bruun-Laursen A, Lorentzen SR (1974) Glucose, pyruvate and citrate concentration in the aqueous humor of humans. Acta Ophthalmol (Copenh) 52:477–489
Chion SH, Chylack LT, Tung WH, Bunn HF (1981) Nonenzymatic glycosylation of bovine lens crystallins. J Biol Chem 256:5176–5180
Clark R, Zigman S, Lerman S (1969) Studies on the structural proteins of the human lens. Exp Eye Res 8:172–182

Cole DF (1970) The aqueous humor and ciliary body. In: Graymore CN (ed) Biochemistry of the eye. Academic, London, pp 105–181
Coleman DJ (1970) Unified model for accommodation mechanism. Am J Ophthalmol 69:1062–1079
Cordes FC (1957) Embryology of the lens. In: Haik GM (ed) Symposium on diseases and surgery of the lens. Mosby, St. Louis, pp 13–24
Dische Z, Borenfreund E, Zelmenis G (1956) Changes in lens proteins of rats during aging. Arch Ophthalmol 55:471–483
Dovrat A, Gershon G (1981) Rat lens superoxide dismutase and glucose-6-phosphate dehydrogenase: Studies on the catalytic activity and the fate of enzyme antigen as a function of age. Exp Eye Res 33:651–661
Dragomirescu V, Hockwin O, Koch HR, Sasaki K (1978) Development of a new equipment for rotating slit image photography according to Scheimpflug's principle. Interdiscip Top Gerontol 13:118–130
Dreyfus JC, Rubinson H, Schapira F, Weber H, Marie J, Kahn H (1977) Possible molecular mechanisms of ageing. Gerontology 23:211–218
Duke-Elder S (1963) System of ophthalmology, vol 2, pt 1, Kimton, London, pp 127–131
Duncan G (ed) (1981) Mechanisms of cataract formation in the human eye. Academic, London
Duverger C, Velter E (1930) Biomicroscopie du cristallin. Masson, Paris
Fischer FP (1931) Ernährung und Stoffwechsel von Augengeweben. Ergebn Physiol 31:507–591
Fischer FP (1938) Topographie der embryonalen Linse. Ber Zusammenkunft Dtsch Ophthalmol Ges 52:374–385
François J, Rabaey M (1956) De l'existence d'une proteine cristallienne embryonaire. Ann Ocul 189–836–854
Gershon H, Gershon D (1970) Detection of inactive enzyme molecules in aging organisms. Nature 227:1214–1217
Graeber W (1966) Die Gewichts- und Volumenzunahme der menschlichen Linsen in Abhängigkeit vom Alter. Acta XX Congress Ophthalmol Germania 1:493–495
Gullstrand A (1911) In: Von Helmholtz, Gullstrand A, Kries J, Nagel W (eds) Handbuch der physiologischen Optik, vol 1, 3rd edn. Voss, Leipzig
Harding CV, Susan S, Murphy H (1976) Scanning electron microscopy of the adult rabbit lens. Ophthalmol Res 8:443–455
Harding JJ (1973) Altered heat lability of a fraction of glutathione reductase in aging human lens. Biochem J 134:995–1000
Harding JJ, Dilley KJ (1976) Structural protein of the mammalian lens: A review with emphasis on changes in development, aging and cataract. Exp Eye Res 22:1–73
Harding JJ, Rixon KC, Marriot FHC (1977) Man have heavier lenses than woman of the same age. Exp Eye Res 25:651
Hart WM, Peckham RH (1953) Changes in specific gravity of the growing crystalline lens. Arch Ophthalmol 50:174–176
Hendrickson P, Koch HR (1977) Photographische Dokumentationsverfahren. In: Hockwin O, Koch HR (eds) Arzneimittelnebenwirkungen am Auge. Fischer, Stuttgart, pp 387–411
Herbrink P, Bloemendal H (1974) Studies on β-crystallin. I. Isolation and partial characterization of the principle polypeptide chain. Biochim Biophys Acta 336:370–382
Hockwin O (1961) Experimenteller Beitrag zur Wirkung von Röntgenstrahlen auf Stoffwechselabläufe der Augenlinse in Abhängigkeit vom Lebensalter. Habilitationsschrift, Universität Bonn
Hockwin O (1962) Early changes of lens metabolism after X-irradiation. Exp Eye Res 1:422–426
Hockwin O (1969) Klinische Bedeutung der Erzeugung experimenteller Katarakte durch Addition unterschwelliger Schädigungsereignisse. Ophthalmologica 158:481–487
Hockwin O (1971) Age changes of lens metabolism. In: Bredt H, Rohen JW (eds) Altern und Entwicklung, vol 1: Age changes in the eye. Schattauer, Stuttgart, pp 95–129

Hockwin O (1979) Aging of the lens and cataract. Paris INSERM Symp. Lens: development and aging, vol 60, pp 263–280
Hockwin O (ed) (1978 a) Lens ageing and development of senile cataract. Interdiscip Top Gerontol 12
Hockwin O (ed) (1978 b) Gerontological aspects of eye research. Interdiscip Top Gerontol 13
Hockwin O (1978 c) Experimental design in the longevity project on eye changes in Wistar rats. Interdiscip Top Gerontol 13:88–94
Hockwin O (1980) Linsenveränderungen nach Kammerwasserverlust. In: Naumann GOH, Gloor B (eds) Wundheilung des Auges und ihre Komplikationen. Bergmann, München, pp 97–102
Hockwin O (1981) Zur Pathogenese und Therapie der Alterskatarakt. Historische Aspekte und neue Vorstellungen. Hist Ophthalmol Intern 2:115–131
Hockwin O (1982 a) Veränderungen des Kohlenhydratstoffwechsels beim Altern. In: Hockwin O (ed) Altern der Linse, Symposium Strasbourg 1982, Mayr, Miesbach, pp 33–44
Hockwin O (1982 b) Multifaktorielle Genese von Linsentrübungen im Alter und medikamentöses Vorgehen. In: Hockwin O (ed) Altern der Linse. Symposium Strasbourg 1982, Mayr, Miesbach, pp 81–85
Hockwin O (1982 c) Gibt es eine medikamentöse Behandlung des grauen Stars? Fortschr Med 29:1355–1360
Hockwin O (to be published, a) Relevanz neuer Erkenntnisse aus der Grundlagenforschung für Pathogenese und Therapie der Katarakt. Nova Acta Leopold
Hockwin O, Dragomirescu V (1981 a) Die Scheimpflug-Photographie des vorderen Augenabschnittes. Eine Methode zur Messung der Linsentransparenz im Rahmen einer Verlaufsbeobachtung. Z Prakt Augenheilkd 2:129–136
Hockwin O, Dragomirescu V (1981 b) Scheimpflug-Photographie des vorderen Augenabschnittes. Eine Methode zur Messung der Linsentransparenz im Rahmen einer Verlaufsbeobachtung. In: Regnault F (ed) Symposium über die Augenlinse. Excerpta Medica, Amsterdam, pp 65–81
Hockwin O, Dragomirescu V (1982) Verlaufsbeobachtungen von Linsentrübungen mit der Scheimpflug-Photographie und densitometrischer Bildanalyse. In: Hockwin O (ed) Altern der Linse. Symposium Strasbourg 1982. Mayr, Miesbach pp 125–138
Hockwin O, Kleifeld O (1965) Das Verhalten von Fermentaktivitäten in einzelnen Linsenteilen unterschiedlich alter Rinder und ihre Beziehung zur Zusammensetzung des wasserlöslichen Eiweißes. In: Rohen JW (ed) Die Struktur des Auges. II. Symposium. Schattauer, Stuttgart, pp 395–401
Hockwin O, Koch HR (1975) Combination effects on noxious influences on the crystalline lens. In: Bellows JG (ed) Cataract and abnormalities of the lens. Grune and Stratton, New York, pp 243–254
Hockwin O, Koch HR (1976) Fortschritte auf dem Gebiet der experimentellen Kataraktforschung. Ihre Bedeutung für die praktische Augenheilkunde. In: Küchle H (ed) Aktuelle Ophthalmologie, Fachalmanach für die Augenheilkunde. Lehmann, München, pp 77–100
Hockwin O, Lerman S (1982) Clinical evaluation of direct and photosensitized UV radiation damage to the lens. Ann Ophthalmol 14:220–223
Hockwin O, Weigelin E (1981) Arzneimittelbehandlung der menschlichen Alterskatarakt. Kontrollierte Studie zur Prüfung der Wirksamkeit eines Präparates. In: Regnault F (ed) Symposium über die Augenlinse. Excerpta Medica, Amsterdam, pp 65–81
Hockwin O, Klein W, Korte I (1972) Beiträge zur ökologischen Chemie. 80. Veränderungen der Enzymaktivitäten der Linse des Auges durch Umweltchemikalien. Chemosphere 6:261–266
Hockwin O, Fink H, Glasmacher M (1976 a) Carbohydrate metabolism of the lens depending on age. II. Factoranalysis on changes of different enzyme activities and on changes in the concentration of glycolytic metabolism in bovine lenses. Z Alternsforsch 31:521–535

Hockwin O, Fink H, Ohrloff C (1976b) Carbohydrate metabolism of the lens depending on age. Evaluation of factor analysis. 5th European Symposium Basic Research in Gerontology, Weimar, GDR, 1976. Straube, Erlangen, pp 632–645

Hockwin O, Koch HR, Ohrloff C, Bours J (1976c) Altern der Linse und Kataraktentstehung. Klin Monatsbl Augenheilkd 169:165–181

Hockwin O, Kaskel D, Weigelin E (1978a) The importance of the lens in intraocular fluid exchange – demonstrated by biochemical interrelations in the system aqueous humor/lens. Doc Ophthalmol Proc Ser 16:129–136

Hockwin O, Rast F, Rink H, Münninghoff J, Twenhoeven H (1978b) Watercontent of lenses of different species. Interdiscip Top Gerontol 13:102–108

Hockwin O, Dragomirescu V, Koch HR (1979a) Photographic documentation of disturbances of the lens transparency during ageing with a Scheimpflug camera system. Ophthalmic Res 11:405–410

Hockwin O, Rast-Czyborra F, Schnitzlein W, Müller HJ (1979b) Age dependence of wet weight and water content of the Beagle dog Lens. Ophthalmol Res 11:136–142

Hockwin O, Dragomirescu V, Laser H (1983) Measurement of lens transparency or its disturbances by densitometrie image analysis of Scheimpflugphotographs. Graefes Arch Clin Ophthalmol 219:255–262

Hockwin O, Weigelin E, Kleifeld O (to be published, b)

Hoenders HJ, Bloemendal H (1982) Veränderungen des Proteinstoffwechsel beim Altern. In: Hockwin O (ed) Altern der Linse. Symposium Strasbourg 1982. Mayr, Miesbach, pp 45–58

Hoenders HJ, Bloemendal H (1983) lens protein und aging. Symposium the ocular lens as a model for studying aging parameters. Gerontol 38:278–286

Hoenders HJ, Van Kamp GJ, Liem-The K, Van Kleef FSM (1973) Heterogeneity, aging and polypeptide composition of α-crystallin from calf lens. Exp Eye Res 15:193–200

Ismail RM, Edelbi AH, Rösinger N (1977) Chemical composition of the aqueous humor of bovine eyes dependent on predetermined time upon removal. Albrecht von Graefes Arch Klin Ophthalmol 207:55–62

Jess A (1920) Die Monoaminosäuren der Linsenproteine. Z Physiol Chem 110:266–276

Johansen EV (1947) Studies on the inter-relation in size between the cornea and the crystalline lens in man, with special references to its significance for intercapsular cataract extraction (in Danish). Munksgaard, Copenhagen

Kabasawa I, Kinoshita JH (1974) Aging effects on the bovine lens γ-crystallins. Exp Eye Res 18:457–466

Kaskel D, Scholz D, Hockwin O, Ziesmer W (1975) Composition of the aqueous humor/lens after carotid ligation. Ophthalmic Res 9:409–415

Kern HL, Ho CK (1973) Transport of L-glutamic-acid and L-glutamine and their incorporation into lenticular glutathione. Exp Eye Res 17:455–462

Kibbelaar MA, Ramaekers FCS (1980) Is actin in eye lens a possible factor in visual accommodation? Nature 285:506–508

Kinsey VE (1957) Comparative chemistry of aqueous humor in posterior and anterior chamber of rabbit eye. Arch Ophthalmol 50:401–417

Kinsey VE, Reddy VN (1973) Studies on the crystalline lens. X. Transport of amino acids. Invest Ophthalmol Vis Sci 2:229–236

Kleifeld O (1954) Experimentelle Beiträge zum intrakapsulären Akkommodationsmechanismus. Habilitationsschrift, Universität Bonn

Kleifeld O (1956) Beiträge zum intrakapsulären Akkommodationsmechanismus. Doc Ophthalmol 10:132–173

Kleifeld O, Hockwin O, Fuchs R (1956) Untersuchungen über die wasserlöslichen Eiweiße in Kern und Rinde der Linsen alter und junger Tiere und menschlicher klarer und getrübter Linsen. Ber Zusammenkunft Dtsch Ophthalmol Ges 60:108–112

Klethi J, Mandel P (1965) Eye lens nucleotides of different species of vertebrates. Nature 205:1114–1115

Kobayashi Y, Susuki T (1975) The aging lens: ultrastructural changes in cataract. In: Bellows JG (ed) Cataract and abnormalities of the lens. Grune and Stratton, New York, pp 313–343

Koby FE (1924) Microscopie de l'oeil vivant. Masson, Paris
Koch HR (1976) Klinische und experimentelle Untersuchungen über den Einfluß von Corticosteroiden auf die Augenlinse. Habilitationsschrift, Medizinische Fakultät der Universität Bonn
Koch HR, Ebertz KH, Hockwin O (1973) Konservative Kataraktherapie in Klinik und Experiment. Doc Ophthalmol 35:85–286
Koch HR, Kremer E, Linnér E, Hockwin O, Kaufmann H, Breull W, Dahners HW (1974) On the influence of a monolateral carotid ligation upon formation of radiation cataracts in rats. Ophthalmic Res 6:175–181
Koch HR, Ohrloff C, Bours J, Riemann G, Dragomirescu V, Hockwin O (1982) Separation of lens proteins in rats with tryptophan deficiency cataracts. Exp Eye Res 34:479–486
Kramps JA, Hoenders HJ, Wollensak J (1978) Increase of non-disulphide cross links during progress of nuclear cataract. Exp Eye Res 27:731–735
Krause AC (1934) The biochemistry of the eye. John Hopkins, Baltimore
Kretzberg W (1982) Die Veränderungen im Stoffwechsel der Linse nach Punktion der Vorderkammer bei Kaninchen. Dissertation, Medizinische Fakultät der Universität Bonn
Kuck JFR (1975) Composition of the lens. In: Bellows JG (ed) Cataract and abnormalities of the lens. Grune and Stratton, New York, pp 69–96
Kuck JFR, Crosswell HH (1974) Lens as a chief source of fructose in aqueous humor. Ophthalmic Res 6:189–196
Kuwabara T (1975) The maturation of the lens cell: a morphologic study. Exp Eye Res 20:427–443
Larsen JS (1971) The sagittal growth of the eye. II: Ultrasonic measurement of the axial diameter of the lens and the anterior segment from birth to puberty. Acta Ophthalmol 49:427–435
Lepper RD, Trier HG, Reuter R (1980) Neuartige Ultraschallbiometrie. Klin Monatsbl Augenheilkd 177:101–106
Lerman S (1980a) Lens transparency and ageing. In: Regnault F, Hockwin O, Courtois Y (eds) Symposium ageing of the lens, 1979. Elsevier/North Holland Biomedical, Amsterdam, pp 263–279
Lerman S (ed) (1980b) Radiant energy and the eye. Macmillan, New York
Lerman S, Borkman RF (1976) Spectroscopic evaluation and classification of the normal, ageing and cataractous lens. Ophthalmol Res 8:335–353
Lerman S, Hockwin O (1981) UV-visible slit lamp densitography of the human eye. Exp Eye Res 33:587–596
Lerman S, Hockwin O, Dragomirescu V (1981) In vivo lens fluorescence photography. Ophthalmol Res 13:224–228
Maclean H (1978) A controlled trial of Catalin in senile cortical cataract. Acta XXIII. Concil Ophthalmol Japonica. 2:1357–1361
Masters PM, Bader JL, Zigler JS Jr (1978) Aspartic acid racemization in heavy molecular weight crystallins and water insoluble protein from normal human lenses and cataracts. Proc Natl Acad Sci USA 75:1204–1208
Meesmann A (1927) Die Mikroskopie des lebenden Auges an der Gullstrandschen Spaltlampe mit Atlas typischer Befunde. Urban und Schwarzenberg, Berlin
Miller D, Benedek G (1973) Intraocular light scattering. Thomas, Springfield, Ill
Monnier VM, Stevens VJ, Cerami A (1980) Nonenzymatic glycosylation of hemoglobin and lens crystallins. In: Srivastava (ed) Red blood cell and lens metabolism. Elsevier North-Holland, New York
Müller HK (1938) Über den Linsenstoffwechsel. Enke, Stuttgart, pp 205–218
Müller HK (1939) Kohlenhydratstoffwechsel der Linse. Albrecht von Graefes Arch Klin Exp Ophthalmol 140:171–190
Newsom WA, Hockwin O (1967) Chromatographic separation of calf and ox lens proteins. Albrecht vn Graefes Arch Klin Exp Ophthalmol 171:318–328
Niesel P (1966a) Spaltlampenphotographie mit der Haag-Streit Spaltlampe 900. Opthalmologica 151:489–504

Niesel P (1966 b) Spaltlampenphotographie der Linse für Meßzwecke. Opthalmologica 152:387–395

Niesel P (1982) Scheimpflug-Photographie des vorderen Augenabschnittes als Methode zur Beurteilung (und Messung) der Linsentransparenz. In: Hockwin O (ed) Altern der Linse. Symposium Strasbourg 1982. Mayr, Miesbach, pp 121–124

Niesel P, Bachmann E (1974) Beobachtungen am Abspaltungsstreifen der Linse bei Glaukomkranken. Albrecht von Graefes Arch Klin Ophthalmol 189:211–217

Niesel P, Rokos L (1976) Der Abspaltungsstreifen in der Spaltlampenphotographie der Linse bei Augenerkrankungen. Albrecht von Graefes Arch Klin Ophthalmol 199:21–29

Niesel P, Kräuchi H, Bachmann E (1976) Der Abspaltungsstreifen in der Spaltlampenphotographie der alternden Linse. Albrecht von Graefes Arch Klin Ophthalmol 199:11–20

Norby A (1958) On the growth of the crystallin lens, the eyeball and the cornea in the rat. Acta Ophthalmol (Copenh) [Suppl] 49

Nordmann J (1954) Biologie du cristallin. Masson, Paris

Nordmann J (1962) Acquisitions récentes dans le domaine de la biologie du cristallin. Fortschr Augenheilkd 12:1–264

Nordmann J (1972) Problems in cataract research. Ophthalmol Res 3:329–359

Nordmann J (1977) Au sujet du vieillissement du cristallin humain et de la pathogénie de la cataracte sénile. Adv Ophthalmol 34:1–73

Nordmann J, Fink H, Hockwin O (1974) Die Wachstumskurve der menschlichen Linse. Albrecht von Graefes Arch Klin Ophthalmol 191:165–175

Ohrloff C (1978) Age changes of enzyme properties in crystalline lens. Interdiscip Top Gerontol 12:158–179

Ohrloff C (1979) Altern der Augenlinse. Untersuchungen über molekulare und funktionelle Veränderungen von Enzymen des Kohlenhydratstoffwechsels während des Alterungsprozesses, die Anlaß zur Entwicklung seniler Linsentrübungen sein können. Habilitationsschrift, Universität Bonn

Ohrloff C, Stoffel C, Koch HR, Wefers U, Bours J, Hockwin O (1978) Experimental cataracts in rats due to tryptophanfree diet. Albrecht von Graefes Arch Klin Exp Ophthalmol 205:73–79

Ohrloff C, Teimann U, Hockwin O (1979 a) Post-synthetic alterations of bovine lens enzymes demonstrated by heat lability measurements. Doc Ophthalmol Proc Ser 18:205–217

Ohrloff C, Güntert A, Braun W, Hockwin O (1979 b) Untersuchungen des Verteilungsmusters der Aldolase Isoenzyme A, B und C und Bestimmung inaktiver Enzymmoleküle in Linsen verschiedenen Alters durch quantitative immunologische Präzipitation. Z Gerontol 12:40–45

Ohrloff C, Bensch J, Jaeger M, Hockwin O (1980 a) Immunologic detection of inactive enzyme molecules in the ageing lens. Exp Eye Res 31:573–579

Ohrloff C, Lange G, Hockwin O (1980 b) Postsynthetic changes of glutathione peroxidase and glutathione reductase in the ageing bovine lens. Mechanisms of ageing and development 14:453–458

Ohrloff C, Berdjis H, Hockwin O, Bours J (1983) Age related changes of glyceraldehyde-3-phosphate dehydrogenase E.C. 1.2.1.12),3-phosphoglyceratekinase (E.C. 2.7.2.3), phosphoglyceratemutase (E.C. 2.7.5.3), and enolase (E.C. 4.2.1.11) in bovine lenses. Ophthalmic Res 15:293–299

Phillips CI, Bartholomew RS, Clayton R, Duffy J, Seth J, Reid JM, Cuthbert J, Alexander M (1981) Katarakte: Ursächliche Faktoren und Zusammenhänge. In: Regnault F (ed) Symposium über die Augenlinse. Excerpta Medica, Amsterdam, pp 19–24

Phillips CI, Bartholomew RS, Clayton R, Duffy J, Seth J, Cuthbert J (1982) Untersuchungen zur Frage nach ursächlichen und assoziierten Einflüssen bei der Alterskatarakt. In: Hockwin O (ed) Altern der Linse. Symposium Strasbourg 1982. Mayr, Miesbach, pp 25–30

Pohjola S (1966) The glucose content of aqueous humor in man. Acta Ophthalmol (Copenh) [Suppl] 88

Regnauld J (1858) Sur la fluorescence des milieux de l'oeil chez hommes et quelques mammifers. L'Institut 26:410
Ringens JP, Hoenders HJ, Bloemendal H (1982) Protein distribution and characterization in the prenatal and postnatal human lens. Exp Eye Res 34:815–823
Robinson AB, McKerrow JH, Cary P (1970) Controlled deamidation of peptides and proteins: an experimental hazard and biological timer. Proc Natl Acad Sci USA 66:753–757
Sasaki K, Shibata T, Fukada M, Hockwin O (1980) Changes of lens transparency with ageing: A clinical study with human volunteers using a Scheimpflug camera. In: Regnault F, Hockwin O, Courtois Y (eds) Ageing of the lens. Elsevier/North-Holland Biomedical, Amsterdam, pp 195–206
Saunte OH (1905) Linse maalinger. Odense
Sauter H (1951) Die Trübungsformen der menschlichen Linse. Thieme, Stuttgart
Scammon RE, Hesdorffer MB (1937) Growth in mass and volume of human lens in postnatal life. Arch Ophthalmol 17:104–112
Scheimpflug T (1906) Der Photoperspektograph und seine Anwendung. Photogr Korresp 43:516–531
Schmutter J (1961) Untersuchungen über die Altersabhängigkeit des Gewichtes und Volumens von Rinderlinsen. Dissertation, Universität Bonn
Scholz R, Kaskel D, Hockwin O (1976) The effect of unilateral pressure ischemia on the carbohydrate metabolism in some ocular tissues. Ophthalmol Res 8:195–201
Siezen RJ, Bindels JG, Hoenders HJ (1979) The interrelationship between monomeric, oligomeric and polymeric α-crystallin in the calf lens nucleus. Exp Eye Res 28:551–567
Spector A, Li LH, Augusteyn RC, Schneider A, Freund T (1971) α-crystallin. The isolation and characterization of distinct macromolecular fractions. Biochem J 124:337–343
Sprenger U (1966) Ultraschallbiometrie des menschlichen Auges in Abhängigkeit vom Lebensalter. Dissertation, Universität Bonn
Srivastava SK (ed) (1980) Red blood cell and lens metabolism. Development biochemistry, vol 9. Elsevier/North Holland, New York
Stein AH, Slatt BJ (1968) The ophthalmic assistent; fundamentals and clinical practice. Mosby, St. Louis, p 3
Stevens VJ, Vlassara H, Abati A, Cerami A (1977) Nonenzymatic glycosylation of hemoglobin. J Biol Chem 252:2998–3002
Trayhurn P, Van Heyningen R (1973) The metabolism of glutamine in the bovine lens. Exp Eye Res 17:149–154
Truscott RJW, Faull K, Augusteyn RC (1977) The identification of anthranilic acid in proteolytic digests of cataractous lens proteins. Ophthalmol Res 9:263–268
Van Kamp GJ, Hoenders HJ (1973) The distribution of the soluble proteins in the calf lens. Exp Eye Res 17:417–426
Varma SD, Reddy VN (1972) Phospholipid composition of aqueous humor, plasma and lens in normal and alloxan diabetic rabbits. Exp Eye Res 13:120–125
Varma SD, Srivastava SK, Richards RD (1982) Photoperoxidation in lens and cataract formation: Preventive role of superoxide dismutase, catalase and vitamin C. Ophthalmol Res 14:167–175
Vogt A (1921) Atlas der Spaltlampenmikroskopie des lebenden Auges. Springer, Berlin
Vogt A (1922) Weitere Ergebnisse der Spaltlampenmikroskopie des vorderen Bulbusabschnittes. Albrecht von Graefes Arch Klin Ophthalmol 109:154–204
Vogt A (1931) Linse und Zonula. Springer, Berlin (Lehrbuch und Atlas der Spaltlampenmikroskopie des lebenden Auges, vol 2)
Von Helmholtz H (1855) Über die Accommodation des Auges. Albrecht von Graefes Arch Ophthalmol 1:1–74
Von Helmholtz H (1896) Handbuch der physiologischen Optik, 2nd edn. Voss, Hamburg
Weale RA (1963) The aging lens. Lewis, London
Weber D (1961) Über die mittlere Lebensdauer von Linseneiweißen, untersucht am lebendigen Kaninchen. Ber Zusammenkunft Dtsch Ophthalmol Ges 64:196–299

Weekers R, Delmarcelle Y, Luyckx JB, Collignon J (1973) Morphological changes of the lens with age and cataract. CIBA Found Symp 19:25–43

Weigelin E, Hockwin O (1982) Bericht über eine zufallsverteilte, kontrollierte klinische Studie mit PHAKAN®/PHAKOLEN®. In: Hockwin O (ed) Altern der Linse. Symposium Strasbourg 1982. Mayr, Miesbach, pp 183–199

Weigelin E, Boutros G, Hockwin O (1982) Konservative Kataraktbehandlung. Prüfung von Medikamenten. Diagn Intensivmed 7:48–54

Winter E (1981) Geometrische und densitometrische Vermessung des vorderen Augenabschnittes an Spaltlampenphotographien, die mit einer neuartigen, nach dem Scheimpflug-Prinzip arbeitenden Kamera erhalten werden. Dissertation, Universität Bonn

Yanoff M, Fine B (1975) Ocular pathology. Harper and Row, New York

The Aging Retina

R. A. WEALE

A. Introduction

There are two approaches that have been used in the assessment of the senescence of the retina, namely the direct and the indirect. The former involves anatomical, histological and ultrastructural studies, whereas the latter is based on retinal physiology: the senescence of the tissue is inferred from that of its function. In man, the physiological approach can be subdivided; e.g. retinal function can be gauged from the properties of the electro-retinogram (ERG) or the electro-oculogram (EOG), two potentials associated with the neural retina and the pigment epithelium respectively, and recorded when the illumination of the retina is changed. However, retinal function and its senescence are sometimes assessed more presumptively from quantitative sensory experiments, the subjective nature of which occasionally leaves one in doubt as regards the anatomical stage (or stages) wherein senescent changes are believed to occur.

B. A Dilemma

The retina is influenced by an individual's photic environment: after all, its function is to act as a recorder of the changes that occur in the outside world and to initiate a response to them. One therefore faces the question of whether senescent changes, characteristic of the retina, are due to age or, alternatively, manifestations of prolonged environmental abuse. In man, intense illumination can produce transient changes in the fundus oculi (e.g. BUSACCA 1957; WEALE 1962a; NOELL et al. 1966; LAWWILL et al. 1977). SEITZ et al. (1977) showed that light adversely affects the retina of the rat. Is it the case, then, that prolonged photic stimulation within normal "physiological" limits may, in the end, be more than the retina can repair (YOUNG 1982) and that a gradual loss in visual capacity, e.g. owing to cell loss (ORDY et al. 1980; WEALE 1975, 1982), should be the ineluctable result?

SEITZ et al. (1977) address themselves to this dilemma in connection with the eye of the rat though they are well aware of the need to avoid reaching trans-species conclusions. They compared the retinal histology of a rat population (A) consisting in equal numbers of males and females kept in a 12 h : 12 h light régime of less than 20 lx with that of similar ones (L) kept at higher levels of up to about ten times this light level. Having shown earlier (STÖTZER et al. 1970) that phototoxic effects are not observed in rat retinas exposed to less than 30 lx (which is equivalent to low but adequate artificial room-lighting), they assumed that changes observed over some 3 years in group *A* were due to senescence while those in group *L* were photogenic.

The cardinal result to emerge is that senescence affects the rat retina mainly in the outer and the inner nuclear layers, losses amounting to some 30%. The former thins more than the latter, and both suffer marked depredations, notably in the retinal periphery, perhaps on account of the concurrent changes in both the superficial and the deep capillaries of the retinal vasculature, readily stained with periodic acid–Schiff reagent (PAS). An increase in the area of the inner nuclei was highly significant: however, this is hard to interpret as no datum on their volume is given.

While age has not denuded the retina of its rods, light has emphatically achieved this after 3 years. No behavioural information as regards blindness is, however, presented. Moreover, both nuclear layers have vanished, with the external limiting membrane abutting such remnants of the inner nuclear layer as may be preserved. It is possible that the destruction of the inner nuclear layer occurred because the "photic" group is also likely to show changes due to senescence. The central areas suffer more than is true of the retinal periphery. This is significant in view of YOUNG's demonstration (1981) that the retinal illumination (in the albino rabbit) is maximal near the optical axis of the eye. SEITZ et al. (1977) note that intermediate retinal sections reveal marked neovascular transretinal capillary features which are accompanied by a thickening of the retinal pigment epithelium. Frequently this is manifested by hypertrophic epithelial cells lining the neocapillaries. Cystoid vacuoles are observed in atrophic retinas, hyalinoid deposits being seen in some cases. It is to be noted that all these changes occur in the layers between the pigment epithelium and the internal limiting membrane with Bruch's membrane remaining intact. The choroid and choriocapillaris also appear to be normal.

Whereas the changes due to senescence seem to be fairly universal, some 30% of the "photic" group failed to reveal the characteristic deteriorations, with only those due to senescence being noted. No information is available on whether their retinal illumination was reduced, say, owing to mitosed pupils or perhaps cataract. The loss of photoreceptors is linked empirically with the vascular changes associated with phototoxicity.

C. Structural Changes in *Homo sapiens*

We have to remain on our guard not to argue from rat to man. However, the results already mentioned alert us to several possibilities that have to be borne in mind when one tries to understand human retinal senescence. If we confine ourselves to just two theories of aging (LAUGHREA 1982), then one can hypothesize that phototoxic effects may be likened to "wear and tear" whereas the more typically senescent changes could be manifestations of programme failures or even error catastrophes (ORGEL 1963; MEDVEDEV 1972). However, one cannot rule out the possibility that changes here or elsewhere are secondary to antecedents, perhaps linked with the senescene of the blood supply. It is true that the retina ap-

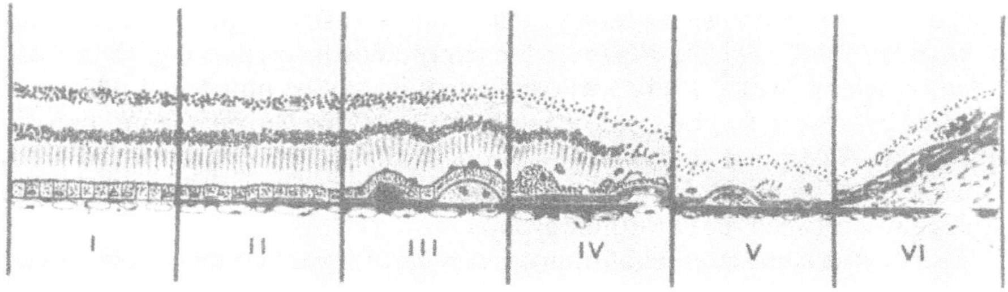

Fig. 1. The histological classification based on the development of the basal linear deposit below the retinal pigment epithelium. (SARKS 1976)

pears to be, if anything, tougher in its resistance to anoxia than is true of the brain (HUERKAMP and RITTINGHAUS 1950), but, as suggested by LERCHE (1967), capillary closure and retinal degeneration may interact, so producing a snowball effect wherein cause and effect are hard to disentangle.

Confining herself mainly to the central retinal region, SARKS (1976) has produced a study which is a model in more senses than one. Clinical observations were in many cases (378 eyes) linked with microscopic and ultrastructural observations on post-mortem material and the picture to emerge is set against a framework consisting of six stages. These are characterised histologically by the progressive development of a basal lamina below the retinal pigment epithelium (Fig. 1).

Group I revealed no trace basal lamina although Bruch's membrane (see later in this section) exhibited senescent changes such as hyalinisation. The visual acuity of this group peaked at 1.0, even though the mean age was as high as 67 years. The basal lamina first appeared in group II (mean age ~75 years, visual acuity peaking et ~0,75): hyalinisation of Bruch's membrane was more extensive, and the pigment epithelium showed degenerative traces. In group III (mean age 82 years, visual acuity peaking at ~0.6), the basal lamina have become continuous and the more severe hyalinisation of Bruch's membrane is topographically more extensive.

At this stage the situation is considered to be definitely pathological: in group IV (mean age 84 years, visual acuity peaking at 0.3), the basal lamina shows marked thickening, depigmentation is noticed clinically, but pigmentary clumping also appears. This group also shows neovascularisation (see Sect. C.I.) with capillary membranes growing beneath the pigment epithelium: the capillaries have by now penetrated the basal lamina. No datum for visual acuity is given for groups V mean age ~86 years) and VI (mean age ~82 years). Macular degeneration is more advanced, the basal lamina is hyalinised and stains similarly to hyalinised Bruch's membrane. Group VI is in fact, characterised by disciform degeneration, with the basal lamina located in a scar as a fragmented hyalinised layer. Drusen (see Sect. C.II) or choroidal atrophy were also observed.

A parallel study done on Japanese eyes (HOSHINO and MIZUNO 1982) revealed a similar correlation between group and age for the first three groups. However, only 3 (of 176) eyes could be placed into group IV and no example was found for groups V or VI. Astonishing though this result is at first sight, it becomes more so when we recall that the Japanese life expectancy is greater, e.g. than that in Australia where SARKS' study was conducted: it may be noted that 36% of the Japanese eyes were 80 years old or more, whereas this percentage amounted to 44% in the Australian study. Since 12% of Sarks' population occupied groups V and VI, it is highly likely, but not absolutely certain, that retinal aging differs significantly between the two ethnic groups.

There exists some conflict of opinion as regards the intactness or otherwise of Bruch's membrane as the years advance. WEALE (1982) has reviewed some of the evidence in support of the view that both Bruch's membrane and the choriocapillaris are affected by senescence, at least nonpathologically. The membrane thickens; vesicles accumulate (HOGAN 1967); and the hyalinisation observed by SARKS (1976) leads to obstructions in Bruch's membrane which GRINDLE and MARSHALL (1978) believe to reduce the metabolic exchange facilities between the retina and the pigment epithelium. The choriocapillaris shows a thickening (LANDOLT 1966) and its vessels reveal a systematic reduction in laminar diameter from 3.7 to 2.3 μm between the seventh and ninth decades of life (SARKS 1976); FRIEDMAN and TS'O (1968) consider that alterations in this tissue may, in some unspecified way, account for the presence of drusen, e.g. in Bruch's membrane.

By contrast, GARTNER and HENKIND (1981) found these tissues intact.

There is no question that with aging a variety of changes occur in the retinal pigment epithelium, Bruch's membrane, and the choroidal vasculature. These structures are all so closely interrelated that it has been difficult to ascertain the site of a primary defect. However, the present study [on the macular region of 104 human eyes in the age range 3–96 years] indicates that a progressive degeneration of cells in the outer nuclear layer and their photoreceptors may occur without significant changes in the adjacent layers.

We recall that this type of pattern was associated by SEITZ et al. (1977) with a history of photic exposure rather than with senescence (in the rat).

I. Vasculature

As may be imagined, vascular changes are as considerable as are the difficulties met in their quantitative evaluation. LERCHE (1967) obtained data on capillary volumes and numbers of the retinal vasculature (which supplies the inner retinal layers as distinct from the outer ones which are within metabolic reach of the choroid). Although the material consisted of central areas of only three patients, 58, 64, and 76 years old, useful information emerged. LERCHE confirms an earlier opinion to the effect that the retinal vasculature is not subdivided just into a superficial and a deep layer, but that there is, additionally, a layer of capillary loops to be seen in the layer of ganglion cells. Accordingly, there were observed senescent changes in this layer: not only was there atrophy of neurones to be seen, but, as between the 64- and the 76-year-old eyes, the percentage capillary volume (for vessels <8 μm in diameter) dropped from 1.8% to 1.3%. Both this, and a smaller change (1.4%–1.2%) in the inner nuclear layer are attributed to cell loss, which, judging by the sections shown, seems atypically severe. The mean intercapillary distance rises in these examples from 68 to 79 μm in the central area.

Table 1. Variation of entopically visualised number (N/mm^2) of leucocytes with age

Age (years)	< 20	20–29	30–39	40–49	50–59	≧ 60
N/mm^2	0.22	0.20	0.19	0.20	0.15	0.14

This linear rise of 16% implies a 57% rarefaction by volume, which can present an interesting situation as regards retinal performance (but see Sect. E).

Baurmann (1960) used the well-known method in which we can visualise individual blood corpuscles (Dartnall and Thomson 1949) and vessels (Bird and Weale 1974) and obtained comparable values on 69 patients in six age groups. Briefly, when one views a surface illuminated with short wavelength light (even the blue sky is suitable), the radiation absorbed in individual blood corpuscles allows their shadows to be detected by the underlying photoreceptors. Baurmann found that the number of corpuscles per unit area varied with age as shown in Table 1. More recently, Baurmann et al. (1974) showed that the entoptic assessment varies both with age ($P = 0.0015$) and with leucocyte counts ($P = 0.002$). It would seem, then, that the retinal vasculature becomes partly anaemic during the sixth decade of life. Note, however, that Baurmann's age range terminates roughly where Lerche's begins. It is, therefore, impossible at the present time to point at any functional change in retinal performance as being directly due to normal vascular insufficiency arising from senescence.

On purely structural grounds, the decrease in blood flow is unexpected, at least insofar as the capillary system is concerned. Leuenberger (1973) showed that the basement membrane thickness of the retinal capillaries of rodents increases with age. This also appears to be true of *Homo*. But the increase in capillary *diameter* is greater so that one has to infer an increase in the diameter of the lumen, which Leuenberger's ultrastructural photographs indeed show. However, this apparent facilitation has to be juxtaposed with Lerche's view which implies a progressive loss in the number of capillaries. Leuenberger also draws attention to the similarity between the senescent thickening of the basement membrane in retinal capillaries and in other structures such as glomerular capillaries where arteriolosclerotic changes are unlikely. However, the nature of the enlarging inclusions is undetermined. Kuwabara and Cogan (1965) noted vacuoles appearing in the elderly human endothelium (Fig. 2).

The geometry of the capillaries is unlikely to be the dominant factor. It may reflect little more than the result of a reduced elasticity combined with stretching, but this problem is more contentious than nearing resolution. The diameter of the larger vessels also increases with age, and when one considers the numerous ramifications and arborisations of the retinal vascular system a bulk approach to haemodynamics, not to mention its senile variation, may be devoid of validity. Local variations in the properties of the vascular wall which give rise to the knotted appearance of elderly vessels may play a role far greater than one might expect from their extent.

The idea of progressive capillary rarefaction has received objective confirmation at the hands of Laatikainen and Larinkari (1977) who used

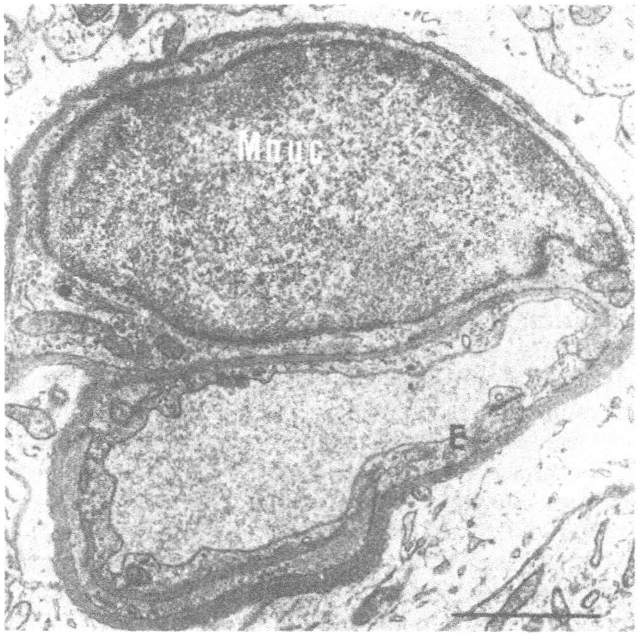

a

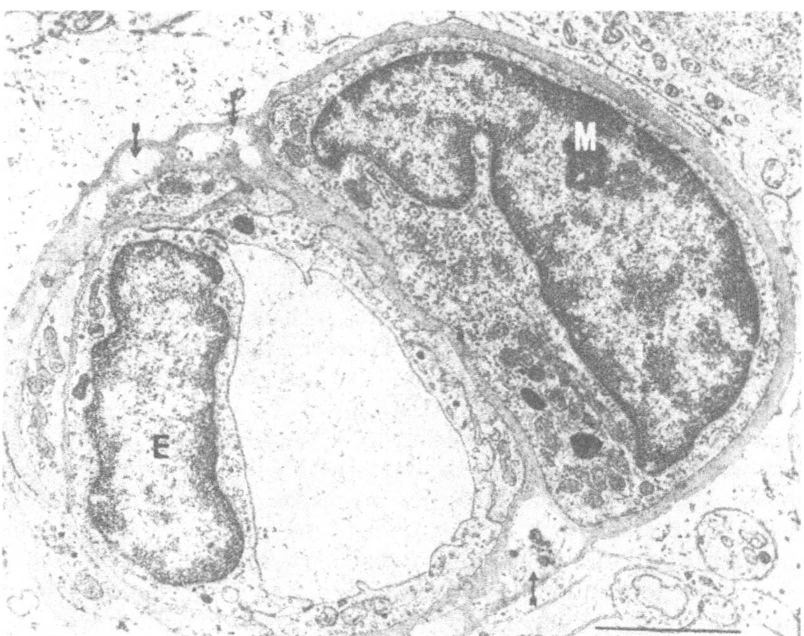

b

Fig. 2, a, b. Normal retinal capillary **a** young, **b** elderly *Arrows* indicate vacuoles in basement membrane on the endothelial side. *E* endothelium; *M* mural cell. *Bar.* 1.0 μm. (KUWABARA and COGAN 1965) fluorescein angiography on 167 eyes in 158 subjects under conditions facilitating the visualisation of macular capillaries. The broad picture to emerge is complicated, but if four children under the age of 10 years are excluded, then the mean diameter of the capillary-free zone of persons aged less than 40 years is 0.53 mm as compared with 0.61 mm for an older group, the result being significant with $P<0.001$. The situation relating to the children (two of whom were 12 and 22 months old, respectively) is not explained, and remains to be confirmed. As regards the question of senescence, the increase in the size of the avascular area (which ceases after the fifth decade) may be due to the atrophy of noncentral capillaries, and the age of onset of the latter (COGAN 1963) happens to coincide with the termination of the increase in the avascular zone, clearly also a matter that needs resolving. In the light of these results, one also wonders whether the senescent increase in capillary lumen may not be also the result of the sort of compensation that occurs in other parts of the vascular system as a response to haemodynamic changes.

As regards the macrovasculature, FANTA (1967) reviewed the role of arteriosclerosis, in particular the question of whether one is concerned with a universal physiological, i.e. gerontological, phenomenon or with a basically pathological problem. He specifically draws attention to the fact that fundal changes have to be viewed in the light not only of hypotonic influences on the aetiology of arteriosclerosis, but also on senile changes in lipid metabolism; these are, of course, not specific to the eye. The correlation, if any, between the appearance of the retinal vessels and the serum cholesterol balance is contentious. But it has to be said that FANTA will have been familiar largely with Austrian fundi the appearance of which may have been conditioned by a lifelong consumption of whipped cream, much as the incidence of diabetic retinopathy in Cuba may be greatly augmented by the extensive intake of sugar by the inhabitants of that island. These remarks are intended not to be final in any sense, but rather to alert the reader to the need for a careful sifting of the evidence before a possibly environmental influence is invested with gerontological significance simply on account of a local ubiquity.

Insofar as the choroid is concerned, LANDOLT (1966) sees it as subject to the same aging processes as the rest of the body (cf. Sect. B). However, its structure causes the appearance of choriospecific lesions, e.g. as regards the loss of cells and of pigment (this is also observed, e.g. in the iris; WEALE 1982). The arterial walls thicken, notably in the larger vessels, hyalin appears, but the lumina constrict. The choriocapillaris which is hard to identify in the young becomes well defined, and the formation of drusen observed in the retinal pigment epithelium is linked by LANDOLT with epithelial function although an influence of the choriocapillaris is not excluded in view of the initial absence of drusen in intercapillary spaces.

II. Changes in the Pigment Epithelium

WOLTER (1957) stresses that drusen replacing cells of the pigment epithelium which, when fully developed adhere firmly to Bruch's membrane of the choroid, contain hyalin, and that there are two developmental types (cf. SARKS 1976). One set is derived from the accumulation of hyalin within gradually degenerating cells of the retinal pigment epithelium, whereas the other results from the extracellular

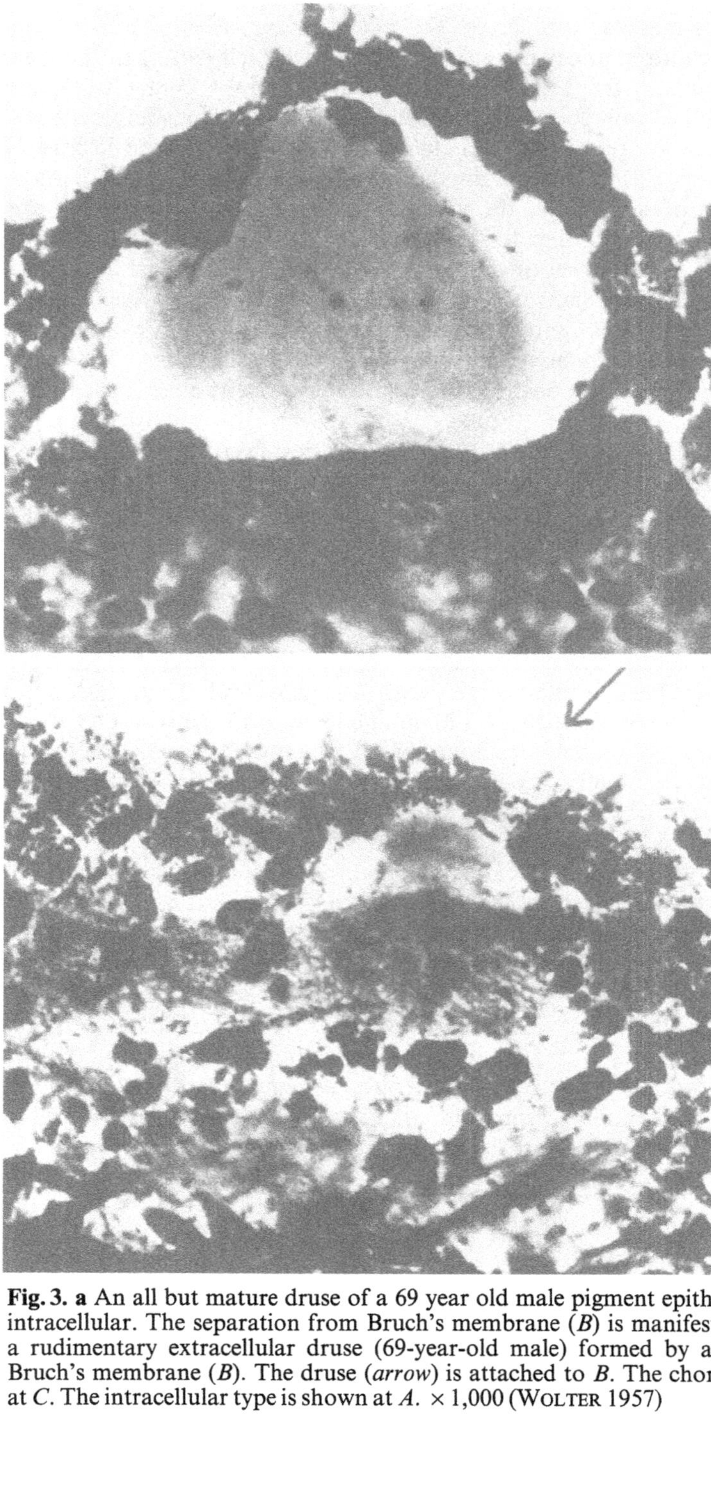

Fig. 3. a An all but mature druse of a 69 year old male pigment epithelium. Its origin *A* is intracellular. The separation from Bruch's membrane (*B*) is manifest. 1,000. **b** Section of a rudimentary extracellular druse (69-year-old male) formed by a hyaloid deposit on Bruch's membrane (*B*). The druse (*arrow*) is attached to *B*. The choriocapillaris is shown at *C*. The intracellular type is shown at *A*. × 1,000 (WOLTER 1957)

deposition between the epithelium and Bruch's membrane (Fig. 3). WOLTER observes that the old dispute as to whether drusen are the result of a transformation of cells or of the deposition of material in them, missed the point: both mechanisms of drusen formation occur. The newer dilemma concerns the question of whether inclusion is due to secretion (KORNZWEIG 1979) or to deteriorating phagocytosis of discarded photoreceptor lamellae (BOK and YOUNG 1979). As is now well known, there is a finite turnover of the protein constituting receptor outer limbs (for review, see YOUNG 1982) and the débris is normally digested by the cells of the pigment epithelium engulfing it. If senescent cells suffer from indigestion a buildup of broken pieces of lamellae may occur. The hypothesis is amenable to an experimental test in species that exhibit senile drusen. YOUNG (1982) has demonstrated the turnover of receptor material by means of autoradiography. If drusen contain undigested photoreceptor detritus then they should be detectable by the same technique. One would expect them to contain a higher concentration of radioactive material than does their environment.

FRIEDMAN and TS'O (1968) studied the histology of the senescent pigment epithelium in bleached flat mounts (cf. later in this section). The largely mononucleate units (~97%) become progressively more pleomorphic as regards both size and shape of the single-layered cells (Fig. 4). Old epithelia also exhibit a large number of basophilic nuclei. The size gradient as between the posterior pole and the ora serrata is reversed between childhood and old age. In the young eye, the cells at the retinal centre are broad and low, and vice versa at the equator and beyond. However, in the old eye, the macular cells tend to be longer and narrower, with the periphery showing the reverse. The equatorial cells appear to be invariant.

Pigmentation, too, reveals systematic senescent changes. In the young, the central area is pale in comparison with the periphery, and vice versa in the older eye. This observation of FRIEDMAN and TS'O can be juxtaposed to the observations due to WING et al. (1978) who determined the topographic and senile variation of lipofuscin in the retinal pigment epithelium (Fig. 5) by autofluorescence. According to GLEES and SPOERRI (1977) the accumulation of lipofuscin results from mitochondrial degeneration. With age, there is a monotonic rise in pigment, following not primarily the distribution of any particular anatomical retinal structure, but more nearly the distribution of light as estimated by YOUNG (1981). In a microhistological study of isolated cells, BÜLOW (1968) found subtle but nonsystematic changes in pigment colour. He states categorically that "the results were independent of the age of the eye [in a range of 0.17–88 years], the site of the retina from which the material was obtained and the age of cultures of living cells".

STREETEN (1961) carefully distinguishes between sudanophilic and melaniferous cells and considers an earlier hypothesis to the effect that there was a link with "wear and tear" pigments such as lipofuscin (cf. WING et al. 1978) and ipso facto with melanin. STREETEN herself noted the increase in size and number of sudanophilic granules with age and, though they resist fat solvents, lipid is present. No conclusive proof for the link with melanin could be obtained and, although the weight of evidence was against it, it was not ruled out. But unequivocal melanin granules are not sudanophilic. The fact that pale granules react positively

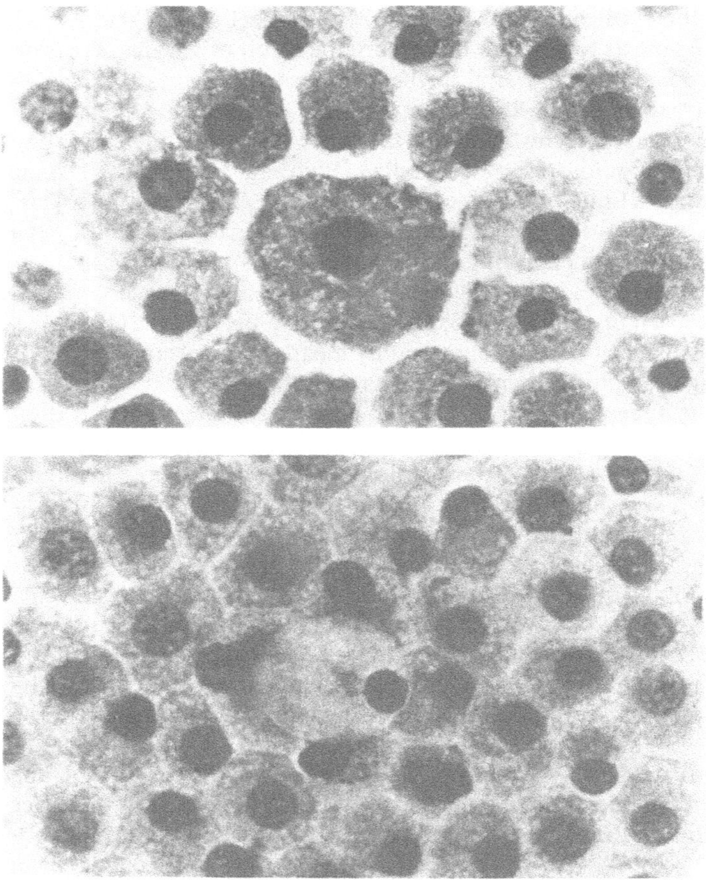

a

b

Fig. 4. a Cell from the retinal pigment epithelium from the ocular equator (23-year-old). Note the large nucleated cell and abundance of cytoplam. × 300 **b** Cell from the retinal pigment epithelium from the ocular equator (60-year-old). The large cell has a small nucleus and pale cytoplasm. × 300 (FRIEDMANN and TS'O 1968)

in performic acid reactions and that rod outer limbs react similarly suggests that these granules contain digests of rod detritus. FEENEY et al. (1965) found a similar age distribution and readily distinguished lipofuscin from melanin granules following bleaching with potassium permanganate: the melanin granules lose their density in this procedure whereas those containing lipofuscin appear to remain unchanged. Figure 6 indicates a brief survey of the changes that take place. FEENEY et al. (1966) have shown that both melanin and lipofuscin can occur in the same adult cell: the former pigment occupying the apical, the latter the basal segment. This seems to be peculiar to *Homo* as GLEES and SPOERRI (1977) failed to find lipofuscin in melaniferous cells of the *Cynomolgus* retinal pigment epithelium.

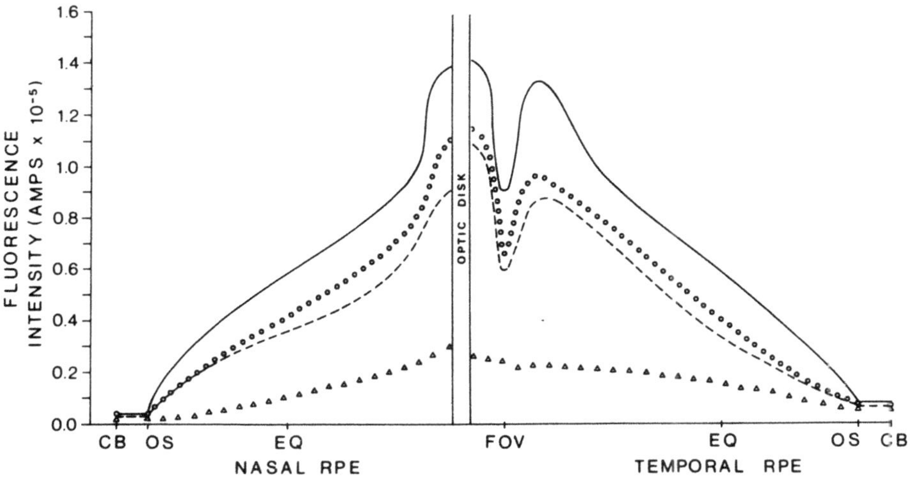

Fig. 5. Lipofuscin in the retinal pigment epithelium as a function of retinal location and age. *CB* ciliary body; *OS* ora serrata; *EQ* equator; *FOV* fovea; *triangles* premature birth to 12 months; *broken curve* 17 months to 30 years; *circles* 31–60 years; *full curve* 61–88 years. (WING et al. 1968)

a 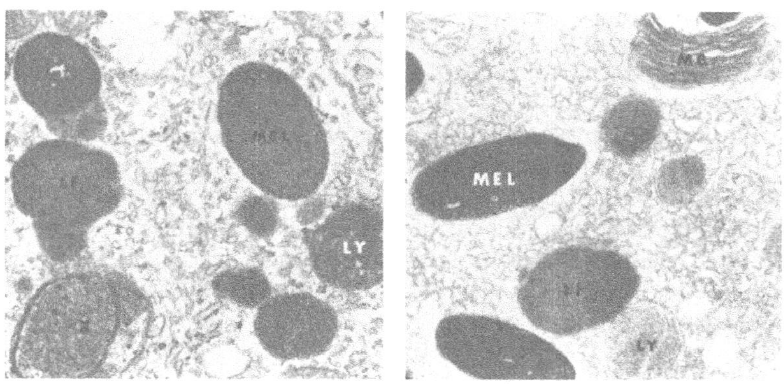 b

Fig. 6, a, b. Typical ultrathin sections of human retinal pigment epithelium **a** 26-year-old eye. In the young adult retinal pigment epithelium granules other than melanin are present. In this micrograph granules of lipofuscin, bodies resembling lysosomes, and an unidentified lamellated body are seen;
b 67-year-old eye. Granules of melanin, lipofuscin, and a body resembling a lysosome are seen. A myeloid body, consisting of several stacked membranes, appears to be in continuity with the smooth endoplasmic reticulum of the epithelial cell. *LF* lipofuscin; *LY* lysosome; *MB* myeloid body; *MEL* melanin granule; *X* unclassified granule. × 1,400 (FEENEY et al. 1965)

FRIEDMAN and TS'O's observations (1968) on the reversal of the pigment gradients need explaining. In principle, a progressive pigmentation of the macula and the concomitant depigmentation of the periphery need not cause us much surprise if we view the former as a pseudosenescent, and the latter as a truly senescent phenomenon. The senile depigmentation of the iris (cf. WEALE 1982)

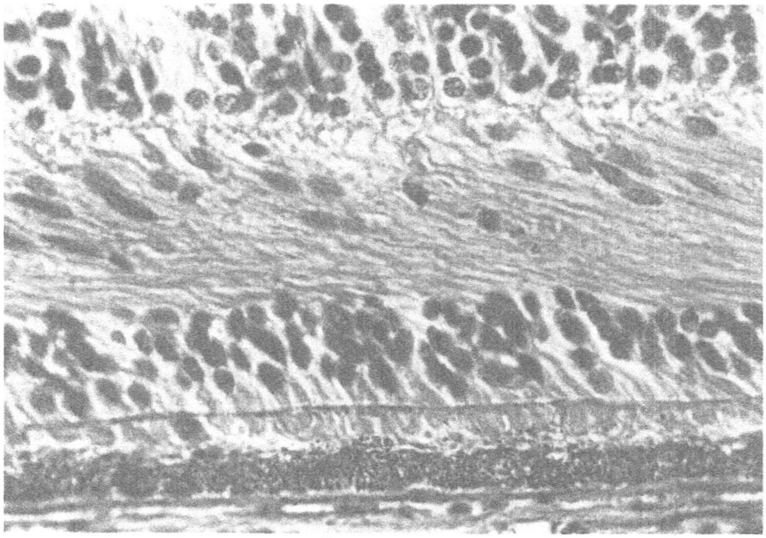

Fig. 7. Section through parafoveal zone of retina (63-year-old male). Note the displaced nuclei including the dark and pale ones. ×440 (GARTNER and HENKIND 1981)

provides a model for the latter. The former may reflect a result of the distribution of retinal illumination.

The changes in pleomorphism are harder to fathom. According to KOKOTT (1948), the accommodative mechanism exerts a "milking" action on the choroid, and MEESMANN (1952) has demonstrated choroidal movement following ciliary action. It is, therefore, conceivable that mechanical stress could change the shape of the epithelial cells. A crucial test would be provided by the histology of the epithelium derived from a congenitally blind eye wherein this type of stress is probably absent.

III. Outer Nuclear Layer and Photoreceptors

A nonspecific feature of retinal senescence has been described by GARTNER and HENKIND (1981) who studied the macular areas of 104 human eyes in an age spectrum extending from 3 to 96 years: they noticed nuclear displacement from nuclear layers into neighbouring ones (Fig. 7) resulting from forces that are unexplained. The authors speculate that displacement from the outer nuclear layer may be due to traction and draw attention to the change in shape of senescent human rods described later in this section. Such migrations are also observed in abnormal (pathological) retinas in younger years.

The translocation of nuclei from the outer nuclear into the outer plexiform (synaptic) layer starts earlier in life than is true of the reverse movement into the layer of rods and cones. One can rule out a mechanical artifact resulting from the production of the 14-µm sections because the displacement is bidirectional and, even in the higher age groups, there is marked directional asymmetry. GARTNER

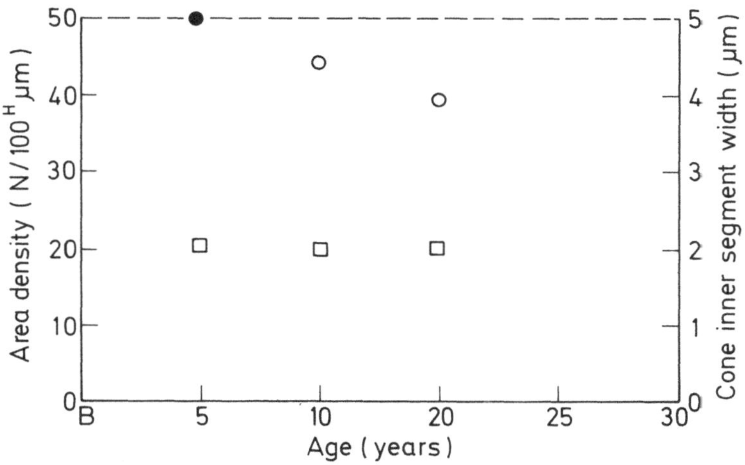

Fig. 8. Morphometric evaluations of age differences in macaque foveal cone density, estimated by area densities of cone nuclei (*full circles*) in young adult, and cone inner segments (*open circles*) for middle-aged human and aged foveal cones in macaque fovea. Age differences in cone inner segment width (*squares*) were not significant among the three age groups, whereas the density of cone inner segment decreased significantly ($p<0.05$) from middle age to aged. (ORDY et al. 1980)

and HENKIND (1981) comment on the considerable but unquantified receptor loss and it remains to be decided whether the stray nuclei are those belonging to vanished outer segments. Separation from the latter would obviously enhance the mobility of the former.

The fovea of the aging rhesus monkey was studied by ORDY et al. (1980), and we may note that the life span of this animals is 0.2–0.25 that of *Homo*. Hence their material from a range of 5- to 20-year-old animals can be compared with human adult and senescent retinas. While the size of the cone inner segments showed a nonsignificant variation, their number decreased from 50 to 39 per 100 (Fig. 8), a loss of 22%. In six decades, *Homo* loses about 16% of the cells in some parts of the central nervous system (see Sect. E), and, if allowance is made for a phototoxic component, the rhesus monkey data do not seem surprising (see Sect. E).

Very little information, comparative or otherwise, is available on the state of the inner neural layers of the retina. RADNÓT (1978) has produced some extraordinary scanning electronmicrographs from 57- and 75-year-old retinas, but, since each is used to illustrate different points, no comparison can be attempted at present. It is, nevertheless, possible to identify objects such as intact amacrine cells, but it remains to be established what fraction of the total they represent.

Whereas GARTNER and HENKIND's observations (1981) on the losses of photoreceptor outer limbs were obtained with the light microscope, ultrastructural studies were needed for the elucidation of the underlying mechanism. The story of its unravelling is typical of visual science in that early work is forgotten or overlooked. Some 20 years ago, there appeared a Japanese study which contained electron micrographs of human rod outer segments which were twisted into loops (YAMADA 1958; TOKUYASU and YAMADA 1960). These "whorls" were dismissed by electron microscopy *cognoscenti* as artifacts, with the implication that it needs really astonishing histological techniques for rod outer limbs to be bent into such shapes. Now, however, the whorls have become respectable.

MARSHALL et al. (1979) surveyed 73 human retinas within an age range of 19–90 years, and noted that nodular knots increased in frequency with advancing years. This could be seen in both sagittal and transverse sections not only on cones, but also on rods. The whorl, now called a convolution, is explained ultrastructurally in Fig. 9, with recourse to sagittal and transverse sections. The implication is that senescent outer limbs continue to grow beyond their juvenile limit either because the rate of differentiation $\dot{D}$ has become greater than that of phagocytosis $\dot{P}$, or, more probably, because senescent processes in the retinal pigment epithelium cause a reduction in $\dot{P}$. Evidently the rate at which the outer segment grows is given by

$$\dot{D}-\dot{P}=\dot{L}.$$

When $\dot{D}=\dot{P}$, $\dot{L}=0$ and therefore the length L is constant. It is clear that a cumulatively negative value of L (as in retinitis pigmentosa) or cumulatively positive one (as in senescent convolutions) can be brought about by extremely subtle changes in the underlying metabolism.

Let us assume that the turnover period of a primate receptor outer limb is of the order of 2 weeks (YOUNG 1982). Let us assume further that there are some 1,000 lamellae per segment. This means that one lamella is formed on average every 20 min if circadian variations are ignored. Since the segments are constant in length one lamella is also phagocytosed on average every 20 min (but see the following paragraphs). Further, let both differentiation D and phagocytosis P follow a linear time course so that $\dot{D}=m$ and $\dot{P}=n$ where m and n are rate constants. It follows that the rate at which the length of the segment changes depends on m and n and that the change in length L after a time t is proportional to $m-n$; when $m=n$ there is no change. These figures fix this equilibrium value at $2.98\ h^{-1}$, i.e. $t\sim 20$ min. Now assume that a convolution is identified when the length L has increased by, say, 30%. We ask: given that phagocytosis slows down by 0.1%, how long will it take for such a convolution to be formed? If we assume that one of the rate constants, say n, changes by 0.1% then the 30% increase in outer limb length is achieved in over 11 years. Similarly, a 26% reduction in the length of the outer segment produces that sort of suprathreshold rise noted in retinitis pigmentosa (HIGHMAN and WEALE 1973) in 10 years after the onset of the postulated reduction in m of 0.1% (see Appendix).

There is no magic in these partly arbitrary numbers. What they are intended to illustrate is the exceedingly small change in some biogenic factor which may suffice to produce marked changes after a very long time. The outlined mechanisms, namely reductions in the rate constants of differentiation and phagocytosis in retinitis pigmentosa and senescence, respectively, are hypothetical. Although STEINBERG et al. (1977) used human retinas between the ages of 5 and 60 years in order to advance our understanding of the ensheathing and phagocytosis of nonfoveal cones, they stress that the major part of their observations was done

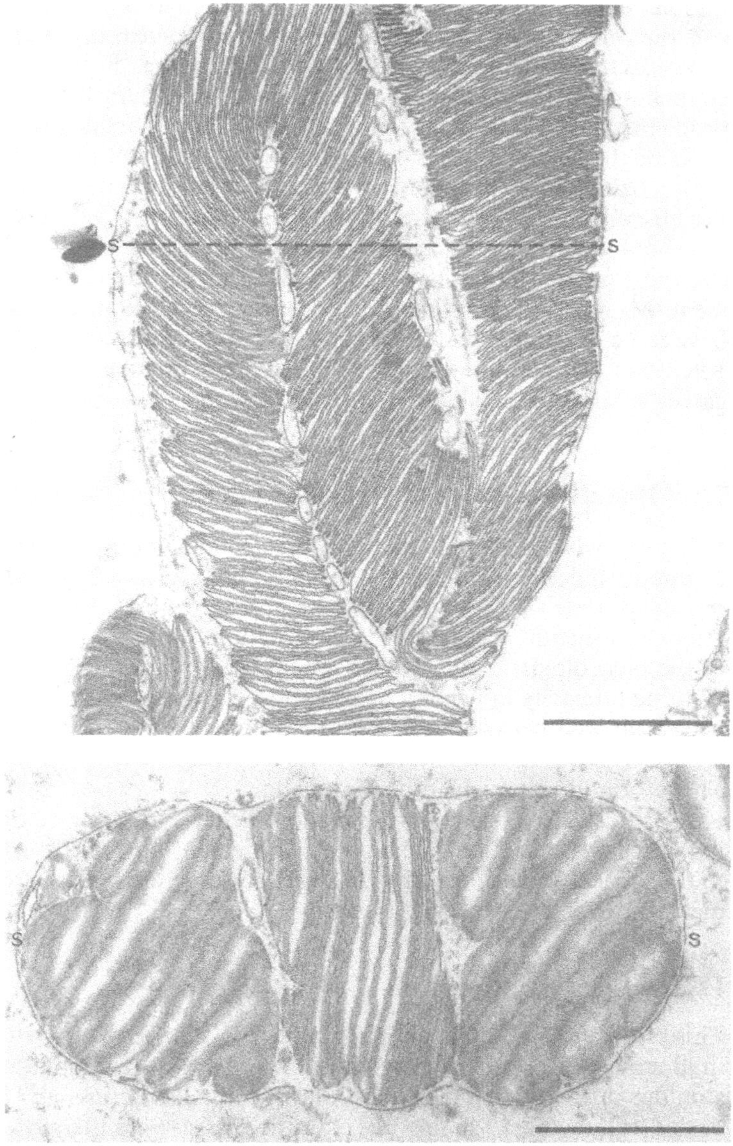

a

b

Fig. 9 a, b. Sections through convoluted rods **a** axial; **b** radial. *Bar* 1 μm. (MARSHALL et al. 1979)

on the youngest retina and that "additional evidence, obtained in the 45-year-old and 60-year-old retinas corroborated the major findings on the 5-year-old". Their results put into relief a major simplification in the calculation, namely that the number of lamellae in a cone phagosome range from 9 to 62, and averages 29. Hence, circadian considerations apart, while differentiation is more nearly continuous, ensheathing involves an aspect of a catastrophe: a breakaway of lamellae and their subsequent phagocytosis occurs only when it is economical for these processes to be set into motion. Perhaps, as they age, the processes of the pigment epithelium lose their appetite for, or recognition of, lamellar clumps: but the basic problem appears to lie in the failure of the clumps to break away in the first place.

It might be argued that a lengthening of the outer limbs favours vision; the reason being that light travelling along the outer limb has a greater chance of being absorbed in a longer than in a shorter segment; and, therefore, the visual threshold would drop as age advances. This supposition is unlikely to be valid: clumping frequently involves fractures (cf. MARSHALL et al. 1979) in the outer segment. Moreover, for optimum absorption, the molecules of the visual pigment have to be orientated with their dipoles at right angles to the receptor axis (DENTON 1954): this condition may be fulfilled in an intact photoreceptor that is elongated, but no longer holds in a convoluted one.

D. Objective Indices of Retinal Function

Evidently, what matters to the individual is not a morphological change as much as one in function. Indeed, the visual system is subject to continuing changes throughout life (WEALE 1982), but we are unaware of them unless ensuing alterations in function exceed a specific threshold. Speaking from the point of view of the physiologist or the doctor, one is aware that the study of morphology is of value primarily in helping one to understand senescent changes in perception, behaviour and performance. Information on these depends on the individual's consciousness and will. It is, therefore, subject to the ego, and can be distorted. The information may therefore be invalid.

For this reason, attempts are made, whenever possible, to obtain information untainted by the self, i.e. to use objective means. Some of these have been adapted to the clinical scene where they are used for diagnosis for the reasons already indicated.

I. The Electro-retinogram

This bioelectric potential, abbreviated as ERG, arises in the retina when a change in illumination occurs (for review see RIPPS 1978). Its amplitude is a function of stimulus intensity, its time course one of retinal structure, and, ipso facto, an index of its intactness. On the face of it, the ERG would therefore provide an index of retinal performance and of the senescence of the tissue. This line was pursued by LEHNERT and WÜNSCHE (1966) and more recently by WELEBER (1981). The former authors report that the amplitudes of both the a-wave and the b-wave decrease with advancing age. The former is an early part of the ERG and associated specifically with receptor activity. By contrast, the later b-wave is thought to arise in the inner nuclear layer (DAVSON 1976). It may be deduced that these decreases in response amplitude are signs of a senescent, not to say moribund, tissue, perhaps due to tissue anoxia, or to metabolic inadequacy. And these are the sorts of conclusion drawn by these and other authors.

Unfortunately, they are not the only conlusions to be drawn. The amplitudes also vary, as indicated, with stimulus intensity. It is frequently overlooked that, even though the stimulus may be constant for a variety of eyes at the level of the cornea where it enters the eye, this is no longer true by the time it arrives at the retina (cf. WEALE 1982). Usually there can be two causes for this. The pupil area may be different, as may the light transmission of the lens. Since the senescent pupil is contracted, the older retina receives less light than does the young one: hence, other things being equal, the retinal stimulus and therefore the amplitude of the ERG are likely to decrease. The lens acts similarly as it manifests a senescent decrease of light transmissivity, notably for short wavelengths. WELEBER (1981) therefore stimulated the retina with red and blue stimuli in turn, and, indeed, the latter caused a sharper decrease in the older ERG than did the former. However, he failed to control the pupil diameter, and an unexceptionable study of the relation between the amplitude of the human ERG and senescence still remains to be published. This is not an academic point. Unless we have a reliable standard with which to compare clinical ERGs, the latter will remain a cruder diagnostic index than modern technology allows one to expect.

II. The Electro-oculogram

A similar argument applies to the electro-oculogram (EOG) which is considered to be an index of the state of the retinal pigment epithelium. Being photogenic, the EOG could be expected to vary with age (cf. ZONNEVELDT and VAN LITH 1980), but preretinal factors affect its amplitude. However, it is much less sensitive to light than is the ERG, and, as currently used, it is unlikely to provide any significant information on epithelial senescence.

III. The Early Receptor Potential

The early receptor potential (ERP) which was much investigated almost 20 years ago, and is the one potential to give direct information on receptor function, has apparently not been used in ocular gerontology. This is strange since GOLDSTEIN and BERSON (1970), among others, found it useful in connection with retinitis pigmentosa. However, the technique involved is unpleasant as it involves the use of such high light intensities that the retinal visual pigments are temporarily bleached (cf. WEALE 1962b).

E. Subjective Information on the Senescent Retina

As is well known, a great deal of useful information on the state of the visual system can be obtained merely by asking a patient questions, or by the presentation of variable stimuli on the perception of which the patient is asked to pronounce. The determination of visual acuity by means of Snellen chart is one good example, and the differential diagnosis afforded by the use of a pinhole which helps to distinguish between neural and optical defects is another. Although measurement is implicit in such tests, the patient has to understand their nature, has to ask private questions about them, and has to be willing and able to respond.

The difficulty with such tests is that, while they may inform, and inform satisfactorily, on the performance of the visual system as a whole, the information specifically relating to retinal capability is not always easy to extract. Take the example of visual acuity. There is universal agreement that it deteriorates with age, generally during the second half of the normal human life span (WEALE 1982). It is reasonable to place visual resolution at retinal level, since it involves the retinal image. There is less certainty as regards contrast differentiation which is not part and parcel of the process of just visual resolution. Therefore it does not follow that the retina is senescent just because visual acuity deteriorates. Such a result can moreover also be obtained from the clouding of the preretinal media, and this is why most ocular gerontologists studying the senescent eye select observers free from pathologically turbid media, notably crystalline lenses. The amount of light scattered by the latter systematically increases with age quite normally (cf. WEALE 1982) so that this has to be viewed as part of gerontological physiology rather than geriatric pathology. However, studies on artifically clouded media (ZUCKERMAN et al. 1973) show that, under normal conditions, the changes in the quality of the retinal image are too small to account even for the relatively small drop in visual acuity with age that is observed.

I. Visual Resolution

With the preretinal media thus, one hopes, exonerated, what else could cause a senile reduction in visual acuity? There could be central problems. Alcohol is known to cause a deterioration in visual acuity, as do schizophrenia and, probably, β-blockers. In each of these there is a restriction in sensory differentiation, but no one has been able to demonstrate the presence (or absence) of the active agent in the retina. It follows that visual acuity is merely a presumptive index of retinal activity.

WEALE (1975, 1978) hypothesized that the decrease in visual acuity with age is to be sought in stochastic cell death (Sect. B). Cell loss is not confined just to the retina but, as shown by MARSHALL (1978), occurs also there. In principle, a visual response may be vitiated by a defect in a primary neurone, in a secondary one, or more centrally. A final defective or senile response, therefore, cannot help to locate the lesion. Nevertheless, if one assumes that the rate of cell death is much the same in the various stages of the visual light path, then one is led to the possibility that there are about half a dozen synaptic stages between the absorption of light by the rods and cones and the locus of decision making.

Such types of hypothesis emphasise the importance of information on the cumulative effects of light on the retina. While there is some controversy on its alleged influence on the more central retinal layers, the phototoxicity of even normal light is not greatly in dispute as regards the photoreceptors (cf. Sect. B). It is not clear how receptor senescence would manifest itself in the absence of light, and, conversely, whether receptors age at all. It must be remembered that impermanence is one of the attributes that distinguish receptors from most of the rest of the central nervous system. Whereas the latter is laid down for life, the turnover

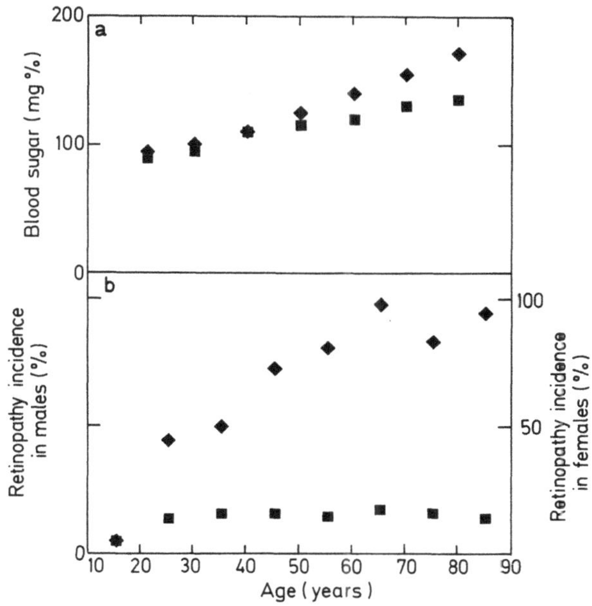

Fig. 10. a Blood sugar (mg%) as a function of age in years (females *lozenges*; males *squares*) **b** Distribution of retinopathy amongst diabetic patients as a function of age (females *lozenges*; males *squares*). Note that graph **b** is based on two different scales so that the different time courses may be emphasised

of the receptors is such that the component material lasts only for a few weeks. They need no memory: like the wind they come and like the wind they go, because their function is one of transduction rather than nervous activity.

There is one aspect of alleged visual aging which has received hardly any notice but which is probably retinal in nature. Careful analysis of the FRAMINGHAM REPORT (1980) shows that, in later life, the visual acuity of women is somewhat poorer than that of men, and this is statistically significant ($P<0.01$). With hindsight such a result is not altogether surprising. The origin of the retina is ectodermal, and there are many ectodermal tissues which show sex differences as regards senescence, hormonal differences not being implicated in every case. We need only remind ourselves of the different forms of aging found in skin (BLACK 1969), in hair and in the crystalline lens (WEALE 1982, 1983). Such differences extend to retinal pathology; e.g. the incidence of diabetic retinopathy shows a higher incidence amongst American women than amongst men in later life although only 5% of diabetic teenage girls are affected as compared with 12% of diabetic teenage boys (Fig. 10). Note that the time course of the retinal condition amongst women appears to be exponential with a half-life of about 35 years whereas diabetes itself progresses almost linearly with age. Moreover, the time course of the prevalence of the systemic disease differs less between the sexes than is true of the retinopathy.

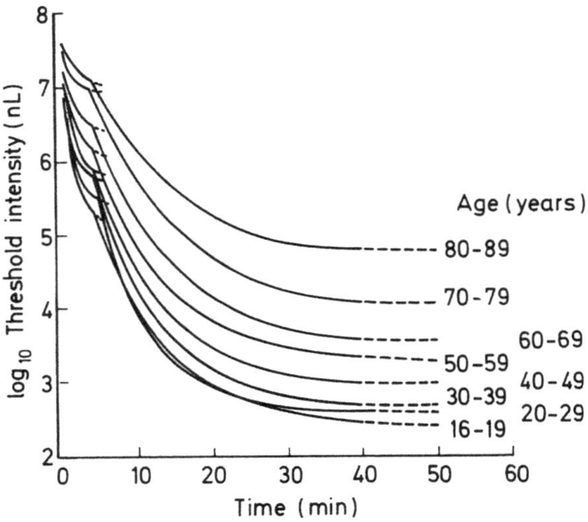

Fig. 11. Dark adaptation as a function of age. (DOMEY and MCFARLAND, 1961)

II. Dark Adaptation

Our final example of what weight can be placed on indirect assessments of senescent retinal activity is provided by dark adaptation. When our eyes have been adapted to light and we are then plunged into darkness, the minimum amount of radiation needed to evoke a visual sensation progressively decreases for about 45 min. This is known as dark adaptation. The underlying mechanism is still not fully understood (cf. DOWLING 1967), but most workers in the field associate it with retinal processes. There are several reasons for this. Vision is impossible without visual pigments the concentration of which is reduced following exposure to light. However, left in the dark, their concentration regenerates in suitable conditions, and HECHT (1938), DOWLING and WALD (1958) and RUSHTON (1961) were amongst those to see a significant link between dark adaptation and pigment regeneration (but see DOWLING and RIPPS 1970). Other workers (e.g. ARDEN and WEALE 1954; RUSHTON and COHEN 1954) clearly demonstrated the involvement of neural, i.e. postreceptoral, components, and, as already indicated, the problem is still incompletely grasped (cf. RIPPS 1976).

As regards the question of senescence and dark adaptation, there is no doubt that DOMEY and MCFARLAND (1961) have given us the most detailed answer of all. They found that, in all age groups between the teens and the nineties, the course of dark adaptation is similar: it is bipartite, reflecting the more rapid restoration of the cone threshold than that of the rods. At all ages, the final (absolute) threshold is reached after 30–40 min. However, the actual dark adaptation curves for each age group are displaced in relation to each other (Fig. 11). At each moment of dark adaptation, the older the retina the larger the stimulus needed for light to be seen. The explanation for this was obvious to the American workers. Similar rises in threshold being observed at simulated high altitudes when the

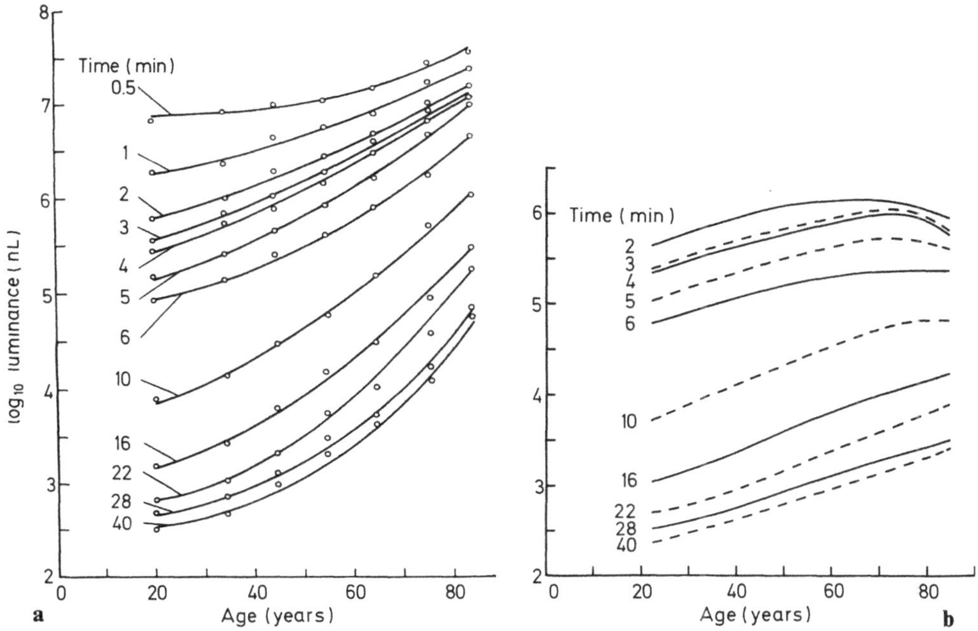

Fig. 12. a Thresholds (measured with violet light) as a function of age with the time of dark adaptation as a parameter. (DOMEY and McFARLAND 1961)
b The same functions corrected for lenticular absorption. (WEALE 1982)

oxygen tension is reduced, they concluded that the threshold is raised because of a progressively accentuated retinal oxygen deficiency with advancing age.

This highly plausible explanation turns out, however, to be an over-simplification. It has the hallmark of the principal bugbear of visual reseach, namely an attempt to convert a correlation into a causative explanation. The test stimulus used by DOMEY and McFARLAND (1961) was violet light of wavelength 405 nm. This was used to maximise the stimulation of rods as compared with that of cones. Unfortunately the very use of this wavelength stamped another mark of senescence onto the threshold data. Before reaching the retina, the stimulus has to traverse the ocular optical media. From our point of view the crystalline lens is the most important of them. Its ability to transmit light decreases systematically and significantly with age, notably in the violet part of the spectrum. The implicit loss of light has to be made good experimentally with an increase in stimulus strength so that the threshold is raised no matter whether the retina ages or not. When thresholds are plotted against age, the time of dark adaptation serving as parameter (Fig. 12a), and a correction is applied for lenticular senescence (WEALE 1978), the rise in threshold is much reduced (Fig. 12b). A similar conclusion has been drawn by GUNKEL and GOURAS (1963) who compared thresholds in normal observers with those obtained for aphakic coeval ones.

Attention has to be drawn to the decrease in threshold, notably shortly after the onset of dark adaptation, when the higher age groups are considered (Fig. 12b).

It is unlikely that there should be an improvement in the sensitivity of cone vision as we approach the highest ages. Suppose, however, that, when the threshold is high and a high stimulus intensity is therefore entering the eye, the retina is stimulated by radiation that is not measured because it is not part of the stimulus delivered by the experimental apparatus. Both the retina and the crystalline lens are known to fluoresce when exposed to short wavelength radiation. The situation is particularly well authenticated in the lens (LERMAN and BORKMAN 1978): after the age of 40 years, the lens accumulates a fluorogen sensitive to violet radiation and fluorescing with blue-green light. Immediately after the initial light adaptation that always precedes measurements of dark adaptation, the rods are held to be inactive, or saturated, leaving the cones to mediate the visual response. The suggestion is that the cones do not respond to the violet stimulus, but to the fluorescent light to which they are, in any case, much more sensitive.

Unfortunately, not even allowance for this additional source of error will make it unnecessary to repeat DOMEY and MCFARLAND's exhaustive study if we are to obtain indirect information on retinal senescence. The reason for this is to be sought in the level of the intensity of the initial light adaptation, which determines the time course of dark adaptation.

This was kept fixed at a luminance of 1,600 mL for all observers. However, we see from Fig. 12 that, between the ages of 20 and 80 years, the rod threshold rises approximately by 1 logarithmic unit or a factor of 10. This would apply to the aphakic situation. To compensate for the changes occurring in the crystalline lens, the phakic eye needs another factor of 10. But this means that the adapting light (which was white) was less of an effective stimulus for the old than for the young. The error cannot have amounted to a factor of 100 since the lens ages less as regards the transmission of radiation of long wavelengths than of short ones, and white light is made up of a mixture of the whole spectrum. The error must nevertheless have lain between the factors of 10 and 100, and one of 25 would be a reasonable guess.

The implication is that, for the curves in Figs. 11 and 12 to be comparable, the level of initial light adaptation has to be related to the sensitivity of the retina under test. On the basis of present-day evidence, its intensity should have been raised in proportion to the final threshold. This would involve a tiresome trial and error approach, but seems inevitable if unexceptionable information is to be obtained. One cannot postulate that such a correction would apply also to the early (cone) part, since the senescence of the rod and cone mechanisms need not follow similar courses. But one would expect that the results in Fig. 12 represent a lower limit: it is probable that the real rise in retinal threshold as between the ages of 20 and 80 years is in excess of the factor of 10 there indicated.

Scant though the information on retinal senescence appears to be, it has to be realised that, from many points of view, the relevant research is still in its infancy. The results that are reliable are more often than not first generation work. The expected rise in visual problems in our aging world seems to me to demand more support than we are receiving in our quest to understand normal retinal senescence if we are to find a badly needed yardstick with which to assess the pathology that awaits many of us.

Appendix

To show that changes in the retinal pigment epithelium, if due to changes in concentration of a metabolite amounting to 1 in 1,000, may take a decade or two to become manifest.

Assume that both the differentiation D, and detachment (and phagocytosis P) of receptor lamellae are linear functions of the time t. Then

$$D = mt + a,$$

$$P = nt + b.$$

Consequently, the length of the outer segment

$$L = D - P = (m - n)t + a - b.$$

In the equilibrium condition, when $m = n$

$$L_e = a - b.$$

Therefore

$$L = (m - n)t + L_e.$$

If $m \neq n$, then $(m-n)t$ represents the difference between L and L_e so that $100(m-n)t/L_e$ gives the percentage change C from the equilibrium value. If m and n differ by 1 in 1,000, i.e. $m - n = 0.001m$, then

$$t = 10CL_e/m$$

If L_e is measured in lamellar units and t in hours, then $t \sim 11.4$ years for $C = 30$. In point of fact it is unlikely that $m - n$, though finite, remains constant, but a similar result will still be obtained if its mean value is of the order of $0.001m$ between the time of onset of its change and the time at which C is being considered. This argument offers an explanation of why the metabolic changes underlying slowly developing modifications of the so-called norm are hard to unravel.

References

Arden GB, Weale RA (1954) Nervous mechanisms and dark-adaptation. J Physiol (Lond) 125:417–426

Baurmann H (1960) Über das Phänomen der entoptisch sichtbaren Blutbewegung. Klin Monatsbl Augenheilkd 137:621–630

Baurmann H, Fink H, Brockmann F (1974) Die entoptisch sichtbare Blutbewegung in verschiedenen Kreislaufsituationen. Klin Monatsbl Augenheilkd 164:220–224

Bird AC, Weale RA (1974) On the retinal vasculature of the human fovea. Exp Eye Res 19:409–417

Black MM (1969) A modified radiographic method for measuring skin thickness. Br J Dermatol 81:661–666

Bok D, Young RW (1979 Phagocytic properties of the retinal pigment epithelium. In: Zinn KM, Marmor MF (eds) *The retinal pigment epithelium*, part 1. Harvard University Press, Cambridge Mass, pp 148–174

Bülow N (1968) Light scattering by pigment epithelium granules in the human retina. Acta Ophthalmol 46:1048–1053

Busacca A (1957) La biomicroscopie de la partie centrale du fond de l'oeil. In: Busacca A, Goldmann H, Schiff-Wertheimer S (eds) Biomicroscopie du corps vitré et du fond de l'oeil. Masson, Paris, p 187
Cogan DG (1963) Development and senescence of the human retinal vasculature. Doyne memorial lecture 1963. Trans Ophthalmol Soc UK 83:465–489
Dartnall HJA, Thomson LC (1949) Retinal oxygen supply and macular pigmentation. Nature 164:876
Davson H (ed) 1976) The eye, vol 2A. Visual function in man, 2nd edn. Academic Press, New York
Denton EJ (1954) Une nouvelle méthode pour déterminer la courbe d' absorption du pourpre rétinien. CR Séances Acad Sci [III] 239:1 315–1 316
Domey RG, McFarland RA (1961) Dark-adaptation as a function of age: Individual prediction. Am J Ophthalmol 51:1262–1268
Dowling JE (1976) The site of visual adaptation. Science 155:273–279
Dowling JE, Ripps H (1970) Visual adaptation in the retina of the skate. J Gen Physiol 56:491–520
Dowling JE, Wald G (1958) Vitamin A deficiency and night blindness. Proc Nat Acad Sci (USA) 44:648–661
Fanta H (1976) Netzhautgefäßveränderungen im höheren Lebensalter. Wien Klin Wochenschr 79:713–716
Feeney L, Grieshaber JA, Hogan MJ (1965) The structure of the eye. II. Symposium. Rohen JW (ed) Studies on ocular pigment. Schattauer, Stuttgart, pp 535–548
Feeney L, Grieshaber J, Alvarado J (1966) New observations on human retinal pigment epithelium. Invest Ophthal Vis Sci 5:111
The Framingham Eye Study Monograph (1980) Surv Ophthalmol 24 [Suppl]:472–479
Friedman E, Ts'o MOM (1968) The retinal pigment epithelium. Arch Ophthalmol 79:315–320
Gartner S, Henkind P (1981) Aging and degeneration of the human macula. 1. Outer nuclear layer and photoreceptors. Br J Ophthalmol 65:23–28
Glees P, Spoerri PE (1977) Ultrastructure of Cynomologus retina with special emphasis on possible age related changes. J Physiol (Lond) 266:15 P.
Goldstein EB, Berson EL (1970) Rod and cone contributions to the human early receptor potential. Vision Res 10:207–218
Grindle CFJ, Marshall J (1978) Aging changes in Bruch's membrane and their implications. Trans Ophthalmol Soc UK 98:172–175
Gunkel RD, Gouras P (1963) Changes in scotopic visibility thresholds with age. Arch Ophthalmol 69:4–9
Hecht S (1938) The photochemical basis of vision. J Appl Physics 9:156–164
Highman VN, Weale RA (1973) Rhodopsin density and visual threshold in retinitis pigmentosa. Am J Ophthalmol 75:822–832
Hogan MJ (1967) Bruch's membrane and disease of the macula – Role of elastic tissue and collagen. Trans Ophthalmol Soc UK 87:113–161
Hoshino M, Mizuno K (1982) Aging of the retina and choroid in the macular region. A light microscopic study an 176 eyes. Acta Soc Ophthalmol Jpn 86:1616–1632
Huerkamp B, Rittinghaus FW (1950) Über die Blutversorgung der menschlichen Retina unter der Einwirkung veränderter Sauerstoffspannung, von Kohlensäure, Hyperventilation und Adrenalin. Pflügers Arch 252:312–330
Kokott W (1948) Über die funktionelle Struktur der Aderhaut. Albrecht von Graefes Arch Klin Ophthalmol 148:706–724
Kornzweig AL (1979) Aging of the retinal pigment epithelium. In: Zinn KM, Marmor MF (eds) The retinal pigment epithelium, part 2. Harvard University Press, Cambridge Mass, pp 478–495
Kuwabara T, Cogan DG (1965) Retinal vascular patterns, VII. A-cellular change. Invest Ophthalmol vis Sci 4:1049–1058
Laatikainen L, Larinkari J (1977) Capillary-free area of the fovea with advancing age. Invest Ophthalmol Vis Sci 16:1154–1157

Landolt E (1966) Zur Histologie der Altersveränderungen der Aderhaut. Fortschr Augenheilkd 17:138–145
Laughrea M (1982) On the error theories of aging. Exp Gerontol 17:305–317
Lawwill T, Crockett S, Currier G (1977) Retinal damage secondary to chronic light exposure. Doc Ophthalmol 44:379–402
Lehnert W, Wünsche H (1966) Das Elektroretinogramm in verschiedenen Lebensaltern. Albrecht von Graefes Arch Klin Ophthalmol 170:147–155
Lerche W (1967) Die Capillardichte in der menschlichen Retina unter Berücksichtigung altersbedingter Veränderungen. Albrecht von Graefes Arch Klin Ophthalmol 172:57–68
Lerman S, Borkman R (1978) Ultraviolet radiation in the aging and cataractous lens. A survey. Acta Ophthalmol 56:139–149
L'Esperance FA, James WA (1981) Diabetic retinopathy, Chap 2. Epidemiology. Mosby, St Louis
Leuenberger PM (1973) Ultrastructure of the aging retinal vascular system, with special reference to quantitative and qualitative changes of capillary basement membranes. Gerontologia 19:1–15
Marshall J (1978) Retinal injury from chronic exposure to light and the delayed effects from chronic exposure to intense light sources. In: Tengroth B (ed) Ergophthalmology. Karolinska Institut, Stockholm, pp 81–104
Marshall J, Grindle CFJ, Ansell PL, Borwein B (1979) Convolution in human rods: an aging process: Br J Ophthalmol 63:181–187
Medvedev ZA (1972) Repetition of molecular-genetic information as a possible factor in evolutionary changes of life span. Exp Gerontol 7:227–228
Meesmann A (1952) Experimentelle Untersuchungen über die antagonistische Innervation der Ciliarmuskulatur. Albrecht von Graefes Arch Klin Ophthalmol 152:335–356
Noell WK, Walker VS, Kang BS, Berman S (1966) Retinal damage by light in rats. Invest Ophthalmol Vis Sci 5:450–473
Ordy JM, Brizzee KR, Hansche J (1980) Visual acuity and foveal cone density in the retina of the aged rhesus monkey. Neurobiol Aging 1:133–140
Orgel LE (1963) The maintenance of the accuracy of protein synthesis and its relevance to ageing. Proc Nat Acad Sci USA 49:517–521
Radnót Magda (1978) Scanning electron microscopic study of the human retina. Ophthalmologica 176:308–312
Ripps H (1976) Night blindness and the retinal mechanisms of visual adaptation. Ann R Coll Surg Engl 58:222–232
Ripps H (1978) Electrophysiology of the visual system (1928–1978). Invest Ophthalmol Vis Sci [Suppl] 17:46–54
Rushton WAH (1961) Rhodopsin measurement and dark-adaptation in a subject deficient in cone vision. J Physiol (Lond) 156:193–205
Rushton WAH, Cohen RD (1954) Visual purple level and the course of dark-adaptation. Nature 173:301–302
Sarks SH (1976) Ageing and degeneration in the macular region: a clinico-pathological study. Br J Ophthalmol 60:324–341
Seitz R, Weisse I, Stötzer H (1977) Altersbedingte und lichtabhängige Netzhautveränderungen. Klin Monatsbl Augenheilkd 171:431–422
Steinberg RH, Wood I, Hogan MJ (1977) Pigment epithelial ensheathment and phagocytosis of extrafoveal cones in human retina. Philos Trans R Soc Lond [Biol] 277:459–471
Stötzer H, Weisse I, Knappen F, Seitz R (1970) Die Retina-Degeneration der Ratte. Arzneimittelforsch 20:811–817
Streeten BW (1961) The sudanophilic granules of the human retinal pigment epithelium. Arch Ophthalmol 66:391–398
Tokuyasu K, Yamada E (1960) The fine structure of the retina. V. Abnormal retinal rods and their morphogenesis. J Biophys Biochem Cytol 7:187–191
Weale RA (1962a) An early stage in the pathology of photocoagulation. Am J Ophthalmol 53:665–669
Weale RA (1962b) Further studies of photo-chemical reactions in living human eyes. Vision Res 1:354–378

Weale RA (1975) Senile changes in visual acuity. Trans Ophthalmol Soc UK 95:36–38
Weale RA (1978) The eye and aging. Interdiscip Top Gerontol 13:1–13
Weale RA (1982) A biography of the eye–development–growth–age. Lewis, London
Weale RA (1983) Transparency and power of post-mortem human lenses: variation with age and sex. Exp Eye Res 36:731–741
Weleber RG (1981) The effect of age on human cone and rod ganzfeld electroretinograms. Invest Ophthalmol Vis Sci 20:392–399
Wing GL, Blanchard GC, Weiter JJ (1978) The topography and age relationship of lipofuscin concentration in the retinal pigment epithelium. Invest Ophthalmol Vis Sci 17:601–607
Wolter JR (1957) Die Histogenese der Drüsen im Pigmentepithel der Netzhaut des menschlichen Auges. Klin Monatsbl. Augenheilkd 130:86–95
Yamada E (1958) A peculiar lamellated body observed in the cells of the pigment epithelium of the retina of the bat, *Pipistrellus abramus*. J Biophys Biochem Cytol 4:329–331
Young RW (1981) A theory of central retinal disease. In: Sears ML (ed) *New directions in ophthalmic research*. Yale University Press, New Haven, pp 237–270
Young RW (1982) The Bowman lecture (1982). Biological renewal. Applications to the eye. Trans Ophthalmol Soc UK 102:42–75
Zonneveldt A, Van Lith G (1980) The electro-oculogram and its interindividual and intraindividual variability. Ophthalmologica 181:165–169
Zuckermann JL, Miller D, Dyes W, Keller M (1973) Degradation of vision through a simulated cataract. Invest Ophthalmol Vis Sci 12:213–224

Dermatology

Physiologic and Pathologic Alterations in Old Skin

BARBARA A. GILCHREST

A. Overview

Few statistics are available concerning the burden of dermatologic disorders in the elderly. However, an estimated 40% of Americans aged 65–74 years suffer from a skin disease sufficiently severe to warrant at least one physician visit and the average affected individual had 1.5 such disorders (JOHNSON and ROBERTS 1977). Although hospitalization is infrequently required for dermatologic disease alone, decubitus ulcers, drug rashes, and other cutaneous disorders may greatly complicate and prolong other hospitalizations for the elderly. In addition to the medical and surgical disorders conventionally included in calculations of disease burden, one must consider the omnipresent "normal" changes in aging skin which may have devastating psychological effects and which may predispose the elderly to certain infections and inflammatory diseases.

B. Age-Associated Changes in Normal Skin

Early histologic, physiologic, and biochemical studies of aging human skin, emphasizing its gradual physiologic decline and increasing individual variability, are well summarized in the 1964 Symposium on the Biology of the Skin (MONTAGNA 1965). Detailed, extensively reference discussions of subsequent work are available in recent texts (BALIN et al. in press; GILCHREST 1984). In most individuals, sun damage is in fact responsible for the majority of clinically evident age-associated cutaneous changes, and this "dermatoheliosis" is discussed separately. This section concerns only intrinsic aging unless otherwise specified.

I. Morphologic and Histologic Changes

The major aging changes in gross morphology of the skin include "dryness" (by which is meant roughness), wrinkling, laxity, uneven pigmentation, and a variety of proliferative lesions. Appendageal changes include diffuse thinning and depigmentation of all body hair as well as conversion of coarse terminal hairs to fine vellous hairs on the scalp ("baldness").

Of the histologic features associated with aging in human skin, the most striking and consistent is flattening of the dermo-epidermal junction, shown schematically in Fig. 1. The number of interdigitating papillae and rete pegs per unit skin surface length also declines with age, further reducing the surface area between

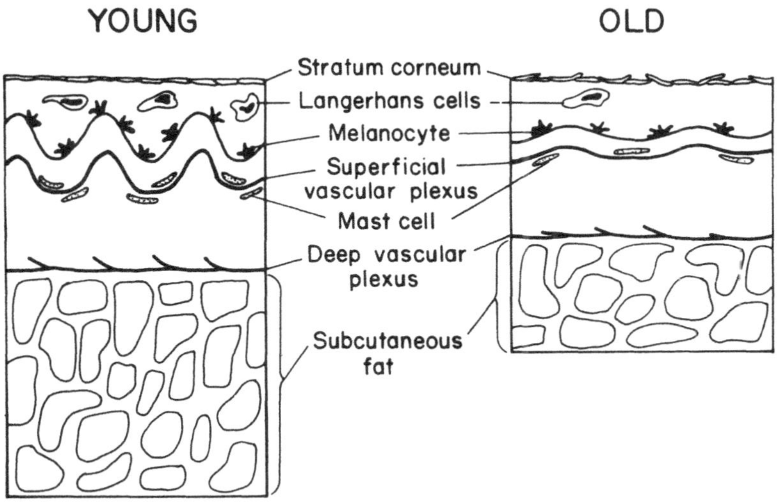

Fig. 1. Histologic changes in aging normal skin. Schematic drawings emphasize the age-associated flattening of the dermo-epidermal junction, indicated by an undulating line at the base of the epidermis, immediately below the melanocytes (pigment cells). Loss of dermal and subcutaneous mass; shortened capillary loops; and reduced numbers of melanocytes, Langerhans cells, and mast cells are also apparent. In most body areas, epidermal thickness is approximately 0.1 mm; dermal thickness ranges from 1.0 to 4.0 mm, depending on body site. (Reproduced with permission, GILCHREST 1982)

the two compartments, impairing "communication" and nutrient transfer, and decreasing resistance to shearing forces. Epidermal thickness, number of corneocyte layers, and degree of compaction of the stratum corneum appear constant with age.

A decrease in the number of enzymatically active melanocytes per unit surface area of the skin, 10%–20% of the remaining cell population each decade, progressively reduces the body's protective barrier against sunlight. A nearly 50% reduction in the number of morphologically identifiable epidermal Langerhans cells between early and late adulthood may account in part for the age-associated decrease in immune responsiveness observed in the skin.

Loss of dermal thickness approaches 20% in elderly individuals, and the remaining tissue is relatively acellular and avascular. Precise histologic concomitants of wrinkling, if any, are unknown, although age-related loss of normal elastin fibers may be contributory.

The striking age-associated loss of vascular bed and especially of the vertical capillary loops which occupy dermal papillae in young skin is felt to underlie many of the physiologic alterations in old skin. In one study, an approximately 50% reduction in mast cells and 30% reduction in venular cross-sections were noted in the papillary dermis of buttock skin from old adults compared to young adult controls, associated with a reduction in histamine release and other manifestations of the inflammatory response following a standardized ultraviolet (UV) light exposure. The marked reduction in the vascular network surrounding hair bulbs, eccrine, apocrine, and sebaceous glands may be responsible for their gradual atrophy and fibrosis with age.

Eccrine glands decrease approximately 15% in average number during adulthood in most body sites, and lipofuscin ("age pigment") gradually accumulates with age in the secretory cells of both eccrine and apocrine sweat glands. Sebaceous (oil) gland size and number appear not to change with age, despite evidence of decreased function.

Pacinian and Meissner's corpuscles, the cutaneous end organs responsible for pressure perception and light touch, progressively decrease to approximately one-third their initial average density between the second and ninth decades of life as determined histochemically in two body sites and display greater variation in size and irregularities in structure.

II. Physiologic Changes

Although the data in several instances are best considered preliminary, virtually all the major functions of human skin have been shown to decline with age (Table 1). Desquamation rates for corneocytes as well as thymidine labeling index of the epidermis in vivo, measures of epidermal turnover rate, have been reported to decline nearly 50% with age. Other investigators have reported a corresponding 100% prolongation in stratum corneum replacement rate in old vs. young men. Repair rate in the skin likewise declines with age, whether measured as development of wound tensile strength or collagen deposition, regeneration of excised blister roofs, or excision of thymine dimers in UV-irradiated DNA of cultured dermal fibroblasts.

Abnormalities of increased as well as decreased proliferation are common. Neoplasia, associated with aging in virtually all organ systems, is especially characteristic of skin. Acrochordons, cherry angiomas, seborrheic keratoses, and lentigenes are evident in nearly every adult beyond age 65 years, and most individuals have dozens of these benign lesions.

There appears to be an age-related increase in percutaneous absorption of at least some substances, although the presumably kindred barrier phenomenon of transepidermal water loss does not vary with age for normal adult skin. Aging is also accompanied by a decreased clearance of transepidermally absorbed materials from the dermis, probably due to alterations in the vascular bed and extracellular matrix, and resorption of intradermally injected saline in young and old subjects requires approximately twice as long in the elderly as in young adults. Such aging effects are well illustrated by experiments utilizing topical application of a 50% ammonium hydroxide solution (GROVE et al. 1982). The initial response, characterized by minute perifollicular vesicles, appears earlier in the old adults, consistent with either a reduced stratum corneum barrier or an increased shunting of the irritant material through appendageal orifices, while the time required after vesiculation for development of a tense blister averaged nearly twice as long in the old as in young adult skin, suggesting a decreased transudation rate with age in injured skin.

Decreased sensory perception was documented in old skin more than three decades ago, using several techniques; optimal stimulus in grams for light touch,

Table 1. Functions of human skin that decline with age. Modified and reproduced with permission (GILCHREST 1984)

Cell replacement	Immune responsiveness
Injury response	Vascular responsiveness
Barrier function	Thermoregulation
Chemical clearance	Sweat production
Sensory perception	Sebum production
Mechanical protection	Vitamin D production

vibratory sensation, and corneal sensation. Cutaneous pain threshold has also been reported to increase up to 20% with advancing adult age.

Spontaneous eccrine sweating and sebum production are reduced more than 70% in healthy old subjects as compared to young control subjects. There is no direct relation to xerosis or seborrheic dermatitis.

Decreased vascular responsiveness in the skin of older individuals has been documented by clinically assessing vasodilation and transudation after application of standardized irritants, histamine, and the mast cell degranulating agent 48/80, to young and old skin. Compromised thermoregulation, which predisposes the eldery to hypothermia and possibly to heat stroke, may be due in part to reduced reflex vasodilation or vasoconstriction of dermal arterioles, in part to decreased eccrine sweat production, and in part to loss of subcutaneous fat, all of which occur with advancing age.

Dermo-epidermal separation occurs more readily in the elderly under experimental conditions (GROVE et al. 1982; KIISTALA 1972), as might be anticipated from the histologic finding of reduced interdigitation between the dermis and epidermis. The poor adhesion between these two cutaneous compartments in the elderly undoubtedly explains their propensity to "torn" skin following minor trauma and to bulla formation in edematous sites. It may also contribute to the increased prevalence of bullous pemphigoid in the elderly.

Healthy older subjects are more difficult to sensitize to dinitrochlorobenzene and have a lower rate of positivity for standard test antigens compared to young adult controls. The decrease undoubtedly reflects the well-documented decrease in total number of circulating thymus-derived lymphocytes and in their responsiveness to standard mitogens, as well as the above-mentioned local cutaneous changes. The decrease with age in cutaneous manifestations of immediate hypersensitivity, manifest by positive wheal-and-flare reactions to standard allergens, is equally pronounced.

An endocrine function of human skin suspected to decline with age is vitamin D production. The level of epidermal 7-dehydrocholesterol, converted by sun exposure to previtamin D_3, decreases linearly by approximately 75% during adulthood, suggesting that lack of the immediate biosynthetic precursor may limit vitamin D production. Although avoidance of dairy products, the principal dietary source of vitamin D, and insufficient sun exposure undoubtedly contribute to vitamin D deficiency in the elderly, this possible age-associated functional deficiency of human skin warrants careful investigation, since bone fractures, a major cause of morbidity and mortality in the elderly, are now believed to be associated with osteomalacia ("adult rickets") in 25%–40% of cases.

III. Biochemical and Biophysical Changes

There is a slight but progressive age-associated increase in the force of contraction for collagen, consistent with increasing cross-linkage of the molecule (BENTLEY 1979), and a progressive decrease in the ratio of soluble to insoluble collagen (MIYAHARA et al. 1982; SCHNIDER and KOHN 1981). The increasing mechanical stability of old collagen appears to result from progressive cross-links which are then reduced or oxidized in vivo, rendering them unmeasureable by conventional techniques. Elastin fibers in skin are less well studied, but have been reported to show progressive cross-linkage and calcification with age in adult skin.

There are few data concerning possible postmaturational age-associated changes in mucopolysaccharides or other molecules of the ground substances in which collagen and elastic fibers are embedded. There appears to be a slight decrease with age in mucopolysaccharide content relative to dry weight or collagen content of the skin, especially for hyaluronic acid (FLEISHMAJER et al. 1972), which may adversely influence skin turgor, as proteolycans bind water in the dermis.

Mechanical properties of the skin also change during adulthood. Uniaxial and biaxial tension tests performed on excised abdominal skin strips demonstrate progressive loss of elastic recovery, consistent with gradual destruction of the dermal elastin network, and the time required for excised skin to return to its original thickness after 50% compression is markedly prolonged in elderly vs. young adults.

C. Age-Associated Pathologic Processes in the Skin

No skin disease occurs exclusively in the elderly, but some disorders do occur more commonly in this age group. Moreover, conditions may evolve differently in older patients and treatment regimes derived from experience with young adults may require modification to ensure optimal efficacy and safety.

I. Decubitus Ulcers

The decubitus ulcer or pressure sore is a systemic rather than cutaneous disorder, as major illness involving at least one and usually several organ systems is invariably present.

The ulcers occur over bony prominences where external pressures produce tissue anoxia with necrosis of epidermis and superficial dermis. Since pressures up to 70 mmHg at the sacrum and 45 mmHg at the heels may be sustained when the body is supine (AGRIS and SPIRA 1979), it is not surprising that decubitus ulcers may arise after as little as an hour of total immobility.

In the first study to actually obtain pressure readings in frail elderly as well as healthy young adults, external pressure in the ischial area necessary for complete blood flow cessation exceeded 120 mmHg in all the young subjects, but ranged from less than 20 mmHg in two elderly subjects to 150 mmHg in one, with a much reduced average value for the elderly group (BENNETT et al. 1981). Older patients also manifested much greater variation in pressure over the sitting surface. This implies that an older individual experiences foci of greater pressure when seated or lying on a firm surface than does a younger individual of the same size and weight, possibly due to loss of skin "tone," that property of the dermis responsible for conducting forces away from local maxima in young adult skin. Shear forces, generated largely by folding and lateral displacement of lax skin, were three times greater in the elderly than in the young. Not surprisingly, at any given external pressure, the elderly were far more likely to experience vascular occlusion.

Prevention, although difficult in high risk patients, is much easier than cure. All effective measures redistribute pressure from bony prominences. The simplest is frequent turning of the bedridden patient, at least every 2 h. Air-space or fluid-filled mattresses tend to equalize pressure over the entire area of contact and are thus a major improvement over conventional mattresses. Strategically placed pillows are theoretically helpful, but in practice rarely remain in place. The best currently available support surface is the ripple mattress, which repeatedly inflates and deflates horizontally aligned tubes in an alternating pattern, so that the patient is supported first by the even-numbered tubes, then by the odd-numbered tubes, and no area is continuously weight bearing for more than the 5- to 10-min pump cycle time.

Healing of a decubitus ulcer may be retarded by general inanition, by incontinence with secondary chemical irritation and bacterial contamination of the ulcer base, or by inadequate vascular supply of the involved area. Surgical debridement of necrotic tissue and eschar speeds reepithelialization. Wet-to-dry saline dressings provide gentle debridement and reduce bacterial counts. Routine use of systemic antibiotics is ill-advised, since tissue levels are often subtherapeutic in the ulcer bed when sufficient elsewhere to dangerously alter bowel and skin flora. Topical antibiotics also penetrate granulation tissue poorly, may have a direct adverse effect on wound healing, and occasionally induce marked allergic sensitization with its attendant discomfort and risk of cross-reaction to subsequently administered systemic drugs. Acetic acid 0.25%–1.0% solution applied as a wet-to-dry dressing is helpful for pseudomonas organisms, but other agents are usually best given by the intramuscular or intravenous route and in preparation for definitive surgical treatment of a decubitus ulcer.

Mixtures of trypsin, streptokinase, vitamin E, dextran polymers, estrogens, and androgens are among the other agents intended to speed healing of decubitus ulcers, but the experience with them is almost entirely anecdotal. Maintaining a positive nitrogen balance is undeniably beneficial and may require supplementary feedings via naso-gastric tube or intravenous hyperalimentation line. Deficiencies of ascorbic acid and zinc, both implicated in wound healing, should be corrected if present.

II. Xerosis

Xerosis, the term used to describe the "dry" or rough quality of skin that is almost universal among the elderly, is a misnomer. The condition probably reflects minor abnormalities in the epidermal maturation process that in turn result in an irregular surface for the stratum corneum; to date it has not been investigated experimentally. The initial assumption that the disorder resulted from a lack of water in the skin appears incorrect, although recent data obtained from a single sun-exposed site do suggest an age-associated decrease in water content for the stratum corneum (POTTS et al. 1984).

Frequent regular use of a topical emollient makes dry skin more attractive and less pruritic. Water loss from the stratum corneum can be slowed markedly by application of a greasy (hydrophobic) substance to the surface. Emollients are most effective when applied to already moistened skin, e.g., immediately after the bath or shower. Emollients applied to nonhydrated skin act by trapping within the stratum corneum the water constantly entering it from below, but transepidermal water loss is a slow process and emollients have frequently worn off before hydration is complete.

III. Pruritus

Among all patients seeking medical attention for pruritus, the prevalence of underlying systemic disease has been reported as 10%–50%, the percentage depending on patient selection, diagnostic evaluation, and period of follow-up. The great majority of these suffer from chronic renal failure or cholestasis, a hematopoietic malignancy, or hyperthyroidism, mandating that these disorders be excluded in elderly patients presenting with pruritus in the absence of a causative dermatitis.

For the many patients without an identifiable etiology for their pruritus, nonspecific therapies must be employed. Often it is worthwhile to prescribe an emollient even in the absence of clinical xerosis, as minimal or intermittent dryness, present in virtually all elderly individuals, may notably exacerbate pruritus of another cause. Topical application of menthol or the anesthetic phenol in an appropriate vehicle also may provide considerable temporary relief; other topical anesthetics can be used only at the risk of allergic sensitization. Oral antihistamines are widely prescribed for pruritus of all causes, although their efficacy is slight in most instances, even when combinations of H_1 and H_2 blockers are used. Antihistamines may have the additional problems in the elderly of pardoxical restlessness or significantly impaired psychomotor function (VESTAL 1978).

IV. Herpes Zoster

Herpes zoster or "shingles" is a vesicular dermatomal eruption due to reactivation of latent varicella virus in the dorsal sensory ganglia of a partially immune host. More than two-thirds of cases occur in patients older than 50 years with age-adjusted annual incidence rate per 1000 population less than 1 at age 0 to 10 years, approximately 2.5 at age 20–50 years, and more than 10 at age 80 years. It has been estimated that by age 85, an individual has a 50% risk of having had at least one attack of herpes zoster and a 10% risk of having had two attacks.

Dysesthesia or paresthesia of the involved dermatome usually begins days before the appearance of vesicles and may mimic angina, spinal cord compression, renal or biliary colic, muscle sprains, or many other disorders. Rarely, preherpetic neuralgia resolves without the development of a cutaneous eruption (JUEL-JENSEN and MACCALLUM 1973), but in most cases pathognominic clusters of vesicles erupt in a dermatomonal distribution, do not cross the midline, and remain unilateral in at least 98% of patients, although occasional individual "disseminated" vesicles occur in up to one-third. The diagnosis of herpes virus infection may be confirmed by Tzanck stain of material scraped from the base of an intact vesicle. The initially clear vesicles may become pustular or, especially in the elderly, hemorrhagic within a few days. Vesicle fluid is contagious. New lesions continue to appear for several days, often progressing distally along the dermatome. Dissemination, if it is to occur, usually does so during this period. Pain, sometimes requiring narcotic analgesics, is frequently prominent during the first days of the eruption. Vesicles usually begin to crust in the second week and resolve within 4 weeks in most patients, but the eruption tends to persist longer and to be more severe in the elderly.

Herpes zoster infections in young and old adults differ primarily in the incidence and severity of postherpetic neuralgia. This problem occurs in approximately 10% of cases overall, but is uncommon in patients less than 40 years old; in one large survey, more than half of those above 60 years old experienced pain lasting at least 1 year (DE MORAGAS and KIERLAND 1957). The increase in severity and duration of postherpetic neuralgia with age is even more marked than the increase in incidence. Persistent pain is especially common in these patients with trigeminal involvement or immunosuppression. Persistent hyperpigmentation or true scarring of involved skin are also more common in the elderly.

Fortunately, patients with herpes zoster appear not to be at increased risk for the subsequent development of malignancy compared to age-matched controls (RAGOZZINO et al. 1982).

Early skin lesions are best treated with local compresses of Burow's solution (1 : 20 in cool water) or other hypertonic soaks for 10 min 3 or 4 times daily, followed by gentle washing with Hibiclens or other antibacterial soap, to hasten drying and prevent bacterial superinfection. Topical antibiotic ointment may be applied twice daily to already crusted lesions.

Several forms of treatment have been proposed for the devastating problem of postherpetic neuralgia. In patients at least 50 years old with early severe herpes zoster, oral steroids equivalent to prednisone 40 mg/day for 10 days, then tapered over 3 weeks, accelerate healing of skin lesions and reduce the incidence of postherpetic neuralgia from 65% to 15% (KECZKES and BASHEER 1980). In Europe, pain associated with herpes zoster has been successfully treated with levodopa, previously demonstrated effective in relieving the pain associated with bony metastases. Among elderly patients average healing time and pain intensity were significantly reduced in one study (KERNBAUM and HAUCHERCORNE 1981) and the data suggested a possible reduction in the incidence and/or duration of postherpetic neuralgia. More rapid healing and decreased pain during herpes zoster infection have also been reported for nonimmunocompromised patients treated with the guanine derivative acyclovir (PETERSLUND et al. 1981).

V. Bullous Pemphigoid

Bullous pemphigoid (BP) is an idiopathic disease in which an autoantibody directed against a basement membrane component produces dermal-epidermal separation. The elderly are affected most commonly, and conversely, BP is almost certainly the most common blistering disease affecting older patients. Untreated, BP varies in severity from mild to disabling and may be fatal. The disease is self-limited, lasting months to years (LEVER 1979), with recurrences following disease-free periods in a substantial minority of patients (AHMED et al. 1977).

BP is characterized clinically by large, tense bullae arising on either erythematous or normal appearing skin, most often on the trunk and proximal extremities. Preceeding or accompanying pruritus is common and may be intense. Approximately one-third of patients have oral lesions, although unlike pemphigus vulgaris, the mouth is rarely the initial site of involvement. In some patients, bullae remain localized to one area for several months, and in a small group, the lesions never become widespread. Crusted erosions and urticarial wheals may coexist with intact bullae; hemorrhagic bullae are not unusual. The diagnosis of BP is confirmed by routine skin biopsy; occasionally immunofluorescent sections of an early lesion are necessary. Corticosteroids are the mainstay of therapy. In mild or localized cases, topical application of a potent steroid cream once or twice daily may control the lesions, but most patients require prednisone or its equivalent. Dosage and schedule of administration are determined by the extent, severity, and rate of progression of the disease as well as by patient age and the presence or absence of relative contraindications, such as hypertension, diabetes, osteoporosis, or infection (JORDON 1979; LEVER 1979). Patients should be reevaluated at weekly intervals, and the prednisone reduced rapidly as new blisters cease forming and clinical remission is achieved. An immunosuppressant such as daily azothioprine or cyclophosphamide may reduce the eventual maintenance level of prednisone, and sulfapyridine or sulfones may be valuable alternative therapies for patients with major contraindications to systemic steroids. Most patients achieve prolonged remissions and at least half can ultimately discontinue treatment without recurrence of lesions (JORDON 1979).

Concern that BP might be a marker for concurrent or subsequent development of malignancy has not been substantiated by controlled studies (LEVER 1979). Malignant neoplasms appear to occur in approximately 10%–11% of both patients with BP and their elderly, age-matched controls (STONE and SCHROETER 1975).

VI. Skin Cancer

1. Epidemiology

Like other "adult" malignancies (in contrast to "childhood" leukemias, neuroblastoma, etc.), skin cancers demonstrate an increasing incidence (diagnosis rate) with age (SCOTTO and FEARS 1978), with very little increase in cancer rate during the third to fifth decades, and a very steep increase during the next 3 decades. The most reliable data suggest that the point prevalence approximately doubles every 9 years until age 80, then increases only slightly thereafter. The increasing incidence throughout adulthood for all three major cutaneous malignancies – basal cell carcinoma, squamous cell carcinoma, and melanoma – requires emphasis, as absolute incidence figures, uncorrected for the size of each age cohort in the population, peak during middle age and decline in the elderly.

Nonmelanoma skin cancers are the most common malignancies of man. Approximately 80% are basal cell carcinomas, and virtually all the remainder are squamous cell carcinomas. Incidences rose from 1972 to 1978, according to statistics compiled by the National Cancer Institute (SCOTTO et al. 1981), probably due in part to the increasing proportion of elderly Americans, the group at highest risk, in part to changing lifestyles with increased sun exposure over recent decades, and perhaps in part to depletion of the ozone layer of the earth with the resultant increase in midrange UV intensity of sunlight. Although cure rates exceed 95% for virtually all treatment modalities in all large series, the actual number of deaths in the U.S. annually ascribed to nonmelanoma skin cancer exceeds that for melanoma (SCOTTO et al. 1981), which has itself increased approximately sixfold in incidence over the past 4 decades and is now more common than either Hodgkin's disease or thyroid carcinoma (SOBER et al. 1980).

2. Possible Age-Associated Risk Factors

Factors which have been postulated to contribute to the development of skin cancer in the elderly include cumulative exposure to carcinogens, especially UV; increased induction times after exposure; decreased DNA repair capacity; decreased immunosurveillance (Langerhans cell and T-cell factors); decreased melanocytes (UV barrier); disturbed regulation of keratinocyte proliferation;[79] and altered dermal matrix. In the cases of DNA repair capacity, immunosurveillance, and dermal matrix composition, habitual sun exposure is believed or known to exacerbate the separate age-associated changes, rendering sun-exposed skin of the elderly at especially high risk for carcinogenesis on theoretic grounds.

3. Prevention and Treatment of Skin Cancer in the Elderly

Because UV irradiation is known to be a major etiologic factor in basal cell carcinoma and squamous cell carcinoma and is strongly suspected to contribute to the development of malignant melanoma, it is not surprising that prevention of skin cancer is virtually synonymous with sun avoidance. Currently available sunscreens are capable of blocking 90%–95% of the erythemogenic UVB spectrum (PATHAK 1981), and tumor formation itself in experimental animals (KLIGMAN et al. 1980). Unfortunately, no study has investigated the benefit of beginning sunscreen protection later in life, after tumor initiation has already occurred.

The average American male who was 65 years old in 1980 will live another 14 years; the average women, more than 18 years. Mean life expectency at

90 years of age now approaches 5 years in the U.S. (Health Care Financing Administration, 1981). Increased physician awareness of this long life expectancy for the elderly has helped to avoid the often disastrous decision not to treat skin cancer on the grounds that death from other causes will supervene before the lesion becomes clinically significant.

Basal cell carcinomas and squamous cell carcinomas are usually treated with one or more of the following: electrosurgery (curettage and electrodesiccation); excision with primary closure, tissue flap rotation, or split-thickness grafting; radiation therapy with external beam or radium implants; liquid nitrogen cryotherapy or microscopically controlled (Mohs') chemosurgery (ALBRIGHT 1982). Cure rates for primary (nonrecurrent) nonmelanoma skin cancer exceed 90% in all large series and approach 100% for small lesions, regardless of treatment modality. Approach to a specific lesion is therefore based on multiple criteria including cell type, tumor size and location, cosmesis, patient comfort and convenience, and cost, in addition to anticipated success rate. For elderly patients, general health and mental acuity, presence of specific systemic diseases, ambulatory status, and home environment are frequently important factors in the physician's choice of therapy. Issues directly related to cutaneous aging have not yet been addressed in the literature, but include rate of healing for various types of wounds, character of the resulting scar, intensity of the inflammatory reaction during and after certain procedures, and risk of superinfection. Premalignant lesions such as actinic keratoses and the much less common keratoacanthoma and lentigo maligna present similar management decisions.

VII. Dermatoheliosis (Sun-Induced Aging)

Dermatoheliosis is the array of clinical and histological findings which characterize chronically sun-exposed skin in middle-aged and elderly adults. Initially due to ignorance of its true pathophysiology and more recently due to lack of appropriate word, dermatoheliosis has been widely mislabeled as "aging," "premature aging," or "accelerated aging."

Clinical features of actinically damaged skin include "dryness" or roughness, actinic keratoses, irregular pigmentation, wrinkling, stellate pseudo-scars, elastosis, ineslaticity, telangiectasia, purpura (easy bruising), comedones (Maladie de Favre et Racouchot), and sebaceous hyperplasia. The relative severity of these changes varies considerably among individuals, undoubtedly reflecting inherent differences in vulnerability and repair capacity for the solar insult. All occur predominantly in fair-skinned Caucasians with a history of ample past sun-exposure and usually involve the face, neck, or extensor surface of the upper extremities most severely. Genetic determinants beyond those for melanin synthetic capacity are undoubtedly operative.

In the epidermis, injury to basal keratinocytes is presumed to result in an altered morphology and a defective maturation program for the terminally differentiated daughter cells, with the clinical and histologic consequences of an irregular, "scaly" stratum corneum, atrophy, and multiple actinic keratoses. In the dermis, fibroblast injury appears to underlie most or all of the clinical changes of dermatoheliosis. Both fine "surface lines" and deep furrows in sites of frequent skin flexure are widely presumed to result from changes in elastin and/or collagen fibers and possibly from changes in the dermal ground substance.

References

Agris J, Spira M (1979) Pressure ulcers: prevention and treatment. Ciba Clin Symposia Little, Brown, and Co., Boston, 31 p
Ahmed AR, Maize JC, Provost TT (1977) Bullous pemphigoid. Clinical and immunologic follow-up after successful therapy. Arch Dermatol 112:185–189
Balin AR, Grove GL, Kligman AM (eds) Aging and the skin. Raven Press, New York, in press
Bennett L, Kavner D, Lee BY, Trainor FS, Lewis JM (1981) Skin blood flow in seated geriatric patients. Arch Phys Med Rehabil 62:392–398
Bentley JP (1979) Aging of collagen. J Invest Dermatol 73:80–83
deMoragas JM, Kierland RR (1957) The outcome of patients with herpes zoster. Arch Dermatol 75:193–196
Fleishmajer R, et al. (1972) Human dermal glycosaminoglycans and aging. Biochim Biophys Acta 279:165-269
Gilchrest BA (1982) Age-associated changes in the skin. J Am Geriatr Soc 30:139–143
Gilchrest BA (1984) Skin and aging processes. CRC Press, Boca Raton, FL, 120 pp
Grove GL, Duncan S, Kligman AM (1982) Effect of aging on the blistering of human skin with ammonium hydroxide. Br J Dermatol 107:393–400
Health Care Financing Administration (1981) Discussion paper: Long-term-care: Background and future directions. U.S. Government Publication No (HFCA) 81-20047
Johnson MLT, Roberts J (1977) Prevalence of dermatological disease among persons 1–74 years of age. United States Advance Data No 4, US DHEW, Washington, DC
Jordon RE (1979) Bullous pemphigoid, cicatricial pemphigoid, and chronic bullous dermatosis of childhood. In: Fitzpatric TB, Eisen AZ, Wolff K, Freedberg IM, Austen KF (eds) Dermatology in general medicine. McGraw-Hill, New York, p 318–323
Juel-Jensen BE, Maccallum FO (1972) Herpes simplex, varicella and zoster. Lippincott, Philadelphia
Keczkes K, Basheer AM (1980) Do corticosteroids prevent post-herpetic neuralgia? Br J Dermatol 102:551–555
Kernbaum S, Hauchecorne J (1981) Administration of Levodopa for relief of herpes zoster pain. JAMA 246:132–134
Kiistala U (1972) Dermal-epidermal separation. I. The influence of age, sex, and body region on suction blister formation in human skin. Ann Clin Res 4:10–22
Kligman LH, Akin F, Kligman AM (1980) Sunscreens prevent ultraviolet photocarcinogenesis. J Am Acad Dermatol 3:30–34
Lever WF (1979) Pemphigus and pemphigoid. J Am Acad Dermatol 1:2–11
Miyahara T, Murai A, Tanaka T, Shiozawa S, Kameyama M (1982) Age-related differences in human skin collagen: solubility in solvent, susceptibility to pepsin digestion, and the spectrum of the solubilized polymeric collagen molecules. J Gerontol 37:651–656
Pathak MA (1982) Sunscreens: topical and systemic approaches for protective of human skin against harmful effects of solar radiation. J Am Acad Dermatol 7:285–292
Peterslund NA, Ipsen J, Schonheyder H, Seyer-Hansen K, Esmann V, Juhl H (1981) Acyclovir in herpes zoster. Lancet 2:827–830
Potts RO, Buras EM, Chrisman DA (1984) Changes with age in the moisture content of human skin. J Invest Dermatol 82:97–100
Ragozzino MW, Melton LJ, Kurland LT, Chu CP, Perry HO (1982) Risk of cancer after herpes zoster: a population-based study. N Engl J Med 307:393–395
Schnider SL, Kohn RR (1981) Effects of age and diabetes mellitus on the solubility and nonenzymatic glycosylation of human skin collagen. J Clin Invest 67:1630–1635

Scotto J, Fears TR (1978) Skin cancer epidemiology: research needs. Natl Cancer Inst Monogr 50:169–177

Scotto J, Fears TR, Fraumeni JF Jr (1981) Incidence of nonmelanoma skin cancer in the United States, U.S. Dept of Health and Human Services Publication No (NIH) 82-2433

Sober AJ, Fitzpatrick TB, Mihm MC Jr (1980) Primary melanoma of the skin: recognition and management. J Am Acad Dermatol 2:179–186

Stone SP, Schroeter AL (1975) Bullous pemphigoid and associated malignant neoplasms. Arch Dermatol 11:991–994

Vestal RE (1978) Drug use in the elderly: a review of problems and special considerations. Drugs 16:358–382

Subject Index

acetabular erosion
  "soft top" endoprothesis 184, 185
  surgery, Hastings hip 79
achalasia
  esophagus, diagnosis, treatment 263, 264
adenocarcinoma
  prostate, clinical picture 202, 203
age distribution
  anovular cycles, shortened luteal phase, normal cycles 54
  biological (menstrual) age groups, menopause 58
  bronchial carcinoma 231
  cholelithiasis, choledocholithiasis 159
  diverticular disease, colon 168
  female genitalia tumors 17
  fertility statistics 55
  lung cancer 231
  malignant tumors of female genitalia 17
  menopause, epidemiology 49, 52
  ovarial tumors 32
  population over 65 177
  postoperative deaths 120, 121
  preexisting diseases, surgical patients 105
  surgical patients 102, 103
aging changes
  accomodation, ciliary muscles 395
  anomalies in position of the eyelids 301
  anterior eye chamber, dephth 352, 353
  anterior eye segment, Scheimpflug photographs 393, 394
  blood sugar, serum levels 443
  brain 113, 114
  cardovascular system 106, 107
  ciliary body 342, 343
  collagen concentration, vitreous gel of the eye 362
  cornea, arcus sinilis 311, 312, 321, 322
  cornea, biochemical changes 319, 320
  cornea, cornea guttata 312, 313
  cornea, Descemet's membrane 318
  cornea, endothel cell count 315
  cornea, glycosaminoglycans 320, 321
  cornea, hexosamine, sulfate, hydroxyproline 320
  cornea, increased Shagreen 312
  cornea, line of Stähli 312
  cornea, regenerative power of epithelium 316, 317
  cornea, sensitivity, relation 314
  cornea, swelling properties of stroma 316
  cornea, thickness 313
  cornea, white limbus girdle of Vogt 312, 313
  dark adaptation 444
  dermatoheliosis 462
  ectropion, entropion 300, 302
  electroretinogram, electro-oculogram 440
  epidural anesthesia, dose requirements 117
  eye lens 374, 375
  eyelids 298–309
  foveal cone density 437
  glaucoma 336, 337
  intraocular pressure 354
  iris structure 346
  lens, specific enzyme activities 411
  lens weight 374
  lenticular leight absorption 445
  leucocytes, entopically visualised, variation of number 429
  liquid vitreous volume 362
  local anesthesia, age-related efficacy 116
  lung function parameters 109
  muscle relaxants, dose-related efficacy 116
  pain intensity 116
  pharmacokinetics, pharmacodynamics 114, 115
  pars plana cysts of the eye 343
  respiratory system 108, 109, 237
  retinal pigment epithelium 427, 431, 433

aging changes
  retinal senescence, measurement 444, 445, 446
  retinopathy, diabetes mellitus 443
  senile ptosis 302
  skin, physiologic and pathologic alterations 452–463
  sodium hyaluronate concentration, vitreous gel of the eye 362
  thiopental, half life elimination 115
  total lung capacity 109
  violet light thresholds, time of dark adaptation 445
  vitreous gel volume 362
  zonular apparatus 344
allergic reactions
  estrogen therapy, contraindication 5
Alzheimer's disease
  anesthesiologic problems 113, 114
amenorrhoea
  climacteric woman, age distribution 55
anal tumors
  treatment 168
analgesic agents
  postoperative period, indications, contraindications 140, 141
anatomy
  eye lens 377, 378
anesthesiology
  age distribution of surgical patients 102, 103
  analgetic agents, postoperative period, indications, contraindications 140, 141
  anesthetic agents, pharmacologic effects, lung function 112, 113, 132
  anesthetic procedures, geriatric patients 122
  anesthetic risk, quantification 117, 118
  arterial pressure, cardiac output, effect of various anesthetics 132, 133
  cardiovascular system, changes with increasing age 107, 108
  cardovascular and pulmonary risks, quantification 118, 119
  central respiratory depression, contributing factors 139
  changes of aging, brain 113, 114
  changes of aging, cardovascular system 106, 107
  changes of aging, pharmacokinetics, pharmacodynamics 114, 115, 116
  changes of aging, respiratory system 108, 109
  complications, postoperative deaths, age groupes 120, 121
  controlled respiration, lung function parameters 112
  duration of anesthesia and surgery 121
  elective vs emergency surgery 121
  epidural anesthesia, age-related dose requirements 117
  epidural and systemic postoperative analgesia 140
  fluid and electrolyte balance 127
  fractures near the hip 73
  geriatric patients, preexisting disorders of organ systems 104, 105
  general anesthesia, management 131, 132
  general, regional anesthesia, comparative studies, indications 122, 123
  geriatric patiens, history 102, 103, 122
  hasards, quantification 117, 118
  inhalation narcotic agents 132
  local anesthetic agents, age-related efficacy 116
  lung function parameters, respiratory therapy maneuvers 110, 112, 113, 128
  metabolic disorders, monitoring 134
  mortality, elderly surgical patients 102, 103
  peri-, postoperative complications, incidence, nature of operation 119, 120
  physical status, classification 118
  postoperation care 135, 136
  postoperative deaths, nature of the operation 120, 121
  premedication 128, 129
  preoperative management, preexisting disease, diagnosis, treatment 123
  regional anesthesia, indications 116, 130, 131
  respiratory depression, contributing factors 139
  respiratory disorders, pathophysiology, pathogenesis 133, 138, 139
  surgery, fractures near the hip 73
  surgical procedures 120–122
  vital functions, monitoring 134
angle fractures
  treatment 86
anti-inflammatory agents
  arthritis, peptic ulcerations 156
aorta
  anuloaortic ectasia, aneurysms 226
  coarctation, pathophysiology, surgery 220, 221
  dissections, techniques of repair 226, 227

intraaortic balloon counter pulsation 227
surgery, in the elderly 217, 218
aqueous humor
aging changes 352–360
arrhenoblastoma
ovarian, malignant transformation 33, 34
arteriosclerosis
retinal vessels, gerontological phenomenon 431
arthroplasty
femoral neck fracture, steoporosis 182
operative technique 97, 98
practical management 91, 92
arthrosis deformans
hip-joint, Hastings hip 75, 82
aspirin
peptic ulceration, complications 156
assessment clinic
general management 93, 94
atrial septal defect
pathophysiology, surgery 219
^{198}Au
prostatic carcinoma, interstitial irradiation 206
audiogram
bresbycusis 273, 276
Austin-Moore-prothesis
hip joint, acetabular protrusion 185

basal cell carcinoma
eyelids 307, 308
skin, treatment 462
benign prostatic hyperplasia
clinical picture, diagnosis, treatment 194–199
biological age groups
frequency, calendar age groups, criteria 58
biopsy
bronchial carcinoma 235
bladder incontinence
treatment 78, 79
blepharochalasis
eyelids 299, 300
blepharophimosis
senile 300
blood sugar
serum levels, function of age 443
body-section radiography
bronchial carcinoma 234
bone
menopause, metacarpal cortical width index, estrogen-, calcium therapy 10
scintigraphy, pathological fractures 89
bone fractures
incidence, osteoporosis 11
bradyarrhythmies
preoperative diagnosis, treatment 125, 126
bradycardia
diagnosis, algorithm 138
brain
changes of aging 113, 114
metabolism, bronchial carcinoma 239
breathing exercises
preoperative management 127
Brenner tumor
ovarian, malignant transformation 33
bronchial carcinoma
age distribution 231
biopsy 235, 236
bronchoscopy 234, 235
carcinomatous neuromyopathy 233
chemotherapy 242
chest radiography, asymptomatic 233
choise of operation 240, 241
clinical picture 232, 233
cytology 234
histologic types 231
hypertrophic pulmonary osteoarthropathy 233
incidence of types 231
lung function, limits for pneumonectomy 238
lymphangitic dissemination 231
malignancy staging, histologic 231
mediastinoscopy 235
operability, evaluation 236
osteoarthropathy, differential diagnosis 233
palliative treatment 242
pathology 230
pre-, postoperative treatment 240, 241
prognosis, histologic types 231
radiology 234
staging, treatment 232
surgery, indications, contraindications 236, 237, 239
symptomatology 232, 233
thoracotomy, exploratory 236
unusual manifestations 233
bronchoscopy
bronchial carcinoma 234
bullous pemphigoid
clinical picture, treatment 460

cancer
adenocarcinoma of endometrium 14
basal cell carcinoma eyelids 305, 307
bronchus, surgery in elderly people 230–242

cancer
  cervical stump 26, 27
  cervix uteri 21–26
  colon, diagnosis, treatment 166
  corpus uteri 27–31
  deaths, 1966–1979 153
  ear 289, 290
  endometrium, clinical features 28
  endometrium, estrogen induced increase 13
  esophageal, surgery 153, 154, 252, 254
  estrogen-dependent, estrogen therapy 5
  eyelids, diagnosis, differential diagnosis, treatment 302, 304, 305
  Fallopian tubes 31, 32
  female genitalia, age dependent frequency 17
  gallbladder, surgery 162, 163
  granulosa cell tumors, ovarian 33, 34
  ileocecal tumors, differential diagnosis 38
  incidence in older people 16
  large bowel, diagnosis, treatment 163–168
  mammary glands 41–43
  meibomian, eyelids 305, 306
  morphea-like basal cell carcinoma 308
  nose 289, 290
  older patients, incidence 16
  ovarian, clinical features 32, 33
  ovarian, metastatic 35, 36
  pancreas, surgery 162, 163
  periampullary region, surgery 163
  postericord, resection 255
  precancerous lesions, eyelids 304, 305
  prostatic 195, 201, 202
  rectal, diagnosis, treatment 166, 167
  rectal, differential diagnosis 38
  stomach, surgery 155, 156
  sebaceous gland carcinoma, eyelids 305
  skin 460–462
  squamous cell carcinoma, eyelids 305
  synchronous tumors, carcinoma of large bowel 166
  throat 289, 290
  vagina 19–21
  vulva 16–19
cardia
  antireflux fundoplication operation 260
  carcinoma, surgical treatment 253, 254
  ulcerative stenosis, reflux esophagitis 259
cardiac arrhythmias
  preoperative diagnosis and treatment 125, 126
cardiac edema
  estrogen therapy, contraindication 5
cardiac effects
  commonly used anesthetics 133
cardiac failure
  postoperative, diagnosis, treatment 137
  risk, perioperative complications 119
cardiac surgery
  principles 213
cardiogenic shock
  diagnosis, treatment 136
cardiopulmonary system
  bronchial carcinoma, assessment 237
cerebrovascular accidents
  hypertension, risk in old age 108
cardiovascular disorders
  preexisting, surgical patients, different ages 105, 106
cardiovascular homeostasis
  postoperative disorders 136
cardiovascular risk
  preoperative prediction 118, 119
cardiovascular system
  changes of aging 106, 107
  preexisting disease, preoperative management 124
cataracta senilis
  biochemistry 399, 402
  densitometry, Scheimpflug photographs 398
  development 399
  enzymes, energy metabolism 407
  multifactorial origin 413, 415
  optic sections 400, 401
  protein metabolism 402, 403
  surgical therapy 415, 416
catheterization
  benign prostatic hyperplasia, indications 199
cervical carcinoma
  age dependent frequency, peak incidence 17
  diagnosis, staging, treatment, prognosis 21–25
  radiotherapy, results of treatment 26, 27
cervical stump carcinoma
  results of treatment 26
chemotherapy
  ovarian cancer 39, 40
  prostatic carcinoma 208
chest trauma
  diagnosis, treatment 247

chest X-ray
bronchial carcinoma, asymptomatic 233
preoperative, functional evaluation 126
cholelithiasis
choledocholithiasis, surgery 159, 160
classification
basal linear deposit, retina 427
bronchial carcinoma 232
endometrial carcinoma 30
mammary cancer 43
osteoporosis, trabecular pattern 180
ovarian tumors 37, 39
physical status, elderly patients 118
prostatic adenocarcinoma 204
trochanteric fractions 186, 187
vulva cancer, International Federation of Gynecology and Obstetrics 18, 19
climacteric period
international definitions 47, 48
climacteric woman
adenocarcinoma of endometrium 14
age, methods of study 49, 50
biological age groups 58
epidemiology 45
extragenital symptoms, complaints 57, 58
fertility 55, 56
hormonel status 59
hypothalamic regulation, estrogen production 59, 60
international definitions 47, 48
menstrual patterns 52, 53, 55
metacarpal certical width index, calcium-, estrogen therapy 10
metrorhagia, incidence 56
mortality, long-term estrogen therapy 14
steoporosis, diagnosis, treatment 179, 180
postmenopausal period 56, 57
reproductive stage, duration 52, 53
clinical picture
anesthesia procedures, indications 123
benign prostatic hyperplasia 195, 196
bronchial carcinoma 232
bullous pemphigoid 460
cancer of esophagus 250, 251
cancer of Fallopian tubes 31
cancer of large intestine 164, 165
cancer of mammary glands 41, 42
cancer of vagina 19, 20
cervical carcinoma 21–24
circulatory complications, general anesthesia 136
climacteric woman, Blatt's menopausal index 58, 59, 60
dysplasia of endometrium 27, 28
early menopause 60
endometrial carcinoma 28, 29, 30
femoral neck fractures 74, 75
fractures near the hip 67
fractures of lower limb 85, 86
gastro-esophageal reflux 250, 258
hiatus hernia 258
malignant tumors of female genitalia 17
metastatic ovarian tumors 35, 36
osteoporosis 178–181
ovarian tumors 32, 33, 34
prostatism 193
shoulder-, arm fractures 87, 88
spinal stenosis 90, 91
trochanteric fracture 70, 71
vulva cancer 18
colitis ulcerosa
Crohn's disease, diagnosis, differential diagnosis, treatment 171, 172
malignant transformation 164
colon
adenomatosis, clinical picture, treatment 165, 166
anal tumors, surgery 168
benign villous tumors, treatment 155
carcinoma, prophylaxis, treatment 166
carcinoma, synchronous tumors 166
colitis in the elderly 171, 172
diverticular disease 168–171
massive bleeding, diverticular disease, treatment 170, 171
polyposis, malignancy, incidence 164
rectal carcinoma, diagnosis, treatment 166, 167
rectal prolapse, incontinence, diagnosis, treatment 172, 173
colonoscopy
annual, colonic lesions, malignant transformation 164
colovesical fistules
diverticular disease surgery 170
complications
acute urinary retention 193
anti-convulsant therapy, osteomalacia 184
anti-inflammatory agents, peptic ulcerations, treatment 156, 157
bleeding, peptic ulcerations, mortality 156, 157
cardiac, perioperative, criteria 119
cardiovascular, old age, anesthesia, hypertension 107, 108

complications
  carotid endarteriectomy 120
  cataract surgery 415
  central respiratory depression, pathogenesis 138, 139
  cholelithiasis, choledocholithiasis 160, 161
  circulatory, postoperative 136, 137
  deaths, postoperative, age groupes 120, 121
  diverticular disease, colon 168, 169
  estrogen therapy 12, 13, 14
  femoral head necrosis, neck fracture 184
  gallstones, pancreatitis 161, 162
  gastro-esophageal reflux 258
  haemorrhage, heart surgery 216
  hip joint sugery 84, 85
  infective, diverticular disease 169
  intraoperative, geriatric patients 122, 123
  mortality rate, nature of operation 119, 120
  ovarian cancer 37
  perforation, gastric ulceration 158
  perioperative, anesthesiologic risks 107, 108, 119
  postoperative, abnormal lung function 111
  postoperative period, anesthesiologic monitoring 136, 137
  prostatic adenocascinoma, radiotherapy 206
  respiratory, postoperative 137–141
  respiratory depression, contributing factors 139
  "soft top" endoprothesis, acetabular erosion 184, 185
  surgical, elderly patients 102, 103
computer assisted tomography
  stenosis of lumber spine 90, 91
congestive heart failure
  risks, old age, anesthesia 107, 108
contraindications
  analgetic agents, postoperative period 140, 141
  bronchial carcinoma, operability 237, 239
  estrogen therapy, climacteric woman 4, 5
cornea
  anatomy, histology, physiology 326, 327
  Descemet's membrane, histology, pathophysiology 330
  endothelium, architecture of the trabecular meshwork 331
  ultrastructure 332
coronary heart disease
  preoperative diagnosis, treatment 125
cor pulmonale
  bronchial carcinoma, operability 237
corpus uteri
  carcinoma, age dependent 17
  endometrial dysplasia, malignant neoplasms 27, 28
Crohn's disease
  clinical picture, treatment 171, 172
Cushing's syndrome
  bronchial carcinoma 233
cystadenoma ovarii
  potential malignancy, incidence 32, 33
cytodiagnosis
  adenocarcinoma of prostate 202, 203
cytologic examination
  cervical carcinoma 21
cytology
  bronchial carcinoma 234
  retinal pigment epithelium 434, 435

deaths
  cancer, 1966–1970 153
  postoperative, age groupes 120
decubitus ulcer
  pathophysiology, treatment 456, 457
definition
  climacteric period 47
  elderly patients, physiologic rather temporal age 213
  empyema 242
  osteoporosis 179
dermatology
  basal cell carcinoma 461
  biochemical, biophysical changes 456
  bullous pemphigoid 460
  decubitus ulcers 456
  dermatoheliosis (sun induced aging) 462
  endocrine function of skin 455
  functions of skin, age-related 455
  herpes zoster 458
  histologic changes 453
  melanoma, nonmelanoma 461
  normal skin, age assoziated changes 452
  pruritus 458
  skin cancer 460–462
  squamous cell carcinoma 461
  xerosis 458
dermoid cyst
  ovarian, malignant transformation 33
Descement's membrane
  cornea, aging changes 318, 319
diabetes mellitus
  estrogen therapy, contraindication 5

preexisting, surgical patients, age 105
retinopathy, function of age 443
diagnosis
achalasia, esophageal 263
adenocarcinoma of prostate 202
benign prostatic hyperplasia 194, 195
bradycardia, algorithm 138
breast cancer 42
bronchial carcinoma 233, 234
carcinoma of the large bowel 164
carcinoma of the pancreas 162, 163
cataracta senilis 399, 400
chest trauma 247
colitis ulcerative, elderly patients 171
colonic adenomas 165
Crohn's disase 171
empyema 243
endometrial carcinoma 29, 30
esophageal diverticula 261, 262
Fallopian tubes, cancer 31
fistules, large bowel 170
fractures near the hip 72
gastro-esophageal reflux 258, 259
herpes zoster 458, 459
hiatus hernia 258
neuromuscular disorders of esophagus 261, 262
osteoporosis 179
pathological fractures 89, 90
postoperative circulatory complications 136
postoperative respiratory disorders 137, 138
preexisting disease, anesthetic procedures 123, 124
rectal carcinoma 166, 167
spontaneous pneumothorax 245
stress fractures 89, 90
tachycardia, algorithm 138
urinary retention, indications for treatment 195, 196
vulva cancer 18
differential diagnosis
cataracta senilis 389
colonic bleeding 165, 170, 171
diabetic retinopathy 431
herpes zoster 459
obstructive jaundice 163
osteomalacia 181
squamous cell carcinoma, eyelids 303
ovarian tumors 38, 39
vertigo in the aged 277
digitalis
prophylactic use, elderly patient 125
diverticula
esophageal, diagnosis, operation 261, 262
diverticular disease
diagnosis, treatment 168, 169
dose
oral estrogens 6, 7
drugs
premedication, anesthesia 128, 129, 130
ductus arteriosus
persistent, pathyphysiology, surgery 219, 220
ear
helix, modular chondrodermatitis 278
presbycusis, morphology, physiology, treatment 270
tympanic membrane, auditory ossicles, changes in the elderly 277
"early gastric cancer"
incidence, prognosis 155
ECG
abnormalities, old age, risks of cardiovasular complications 107, 108
postoperative disorders, monitoring 136
ECG lead programm
postoperative period, anesthesiologic monitoring 136, 137
ectropion, entropion
senile 300, 301, 302
electroretinogram
advancing age 440
emboly
estrogen therapy, contraindication 5
embryology
lens structure 375, 376
emergency cholecystectomy
indications, prognosis 159, 160
emergency surgery
mortality rate 121
emphysematous cysts
surgery 246
empyema
diagnosis, treatment 242, 243
endarteriectomy
carotid, postoperative complications 119, 120
endocrine disturbances
bronchial carcinoma 233
endocrine function
human skin 455
endocrinium
biomorphosis, menstrual pattern 56
endocrinology
control of prostatic growth 193, 194
endometrial cancer
clinical features, diagnosis, treatment 28, 29

endometrial cancer
estrogen therapy, risk 13, 14
endometrial dysplasia
precancerosis 27
endoscopy
esophagus 249, 251
enterocutaneous fistulas
diverticular disease, surgery 170
epidemiology
climacteric period 45–62
epidural anesthesia
elderly patients 131
epilepsy
estrogen therapy, contraindication 5
epistaxis
age distribution, causes 280
esophagus
achalasia, diagnosis, treatment 263, 264
diffuse spasm, myotomy 265
diverticula, diagnosis, operation 261, 262
neuromuscular disorders 261
scleroderma 265
strictures, treatment 260, 261
esophagectomy
transhiatal, without thoracotomy 255
esophagitis
reflux, diagnosis, treatment 258, 259
esophago-jejunostomy
carcinoma of esophagus 253
esophagus
carcinoma, clinical picture 251
carcinoma, nonresectable 257
carcinoma, pathology 250, 251
carcinoma, radiotherapy 257, 258
carcinoma, surgery 252, 254
endoscopy 249, 251
functional anatomy 250
manometry 249
pH studies 249
radiographic examination 248
surgery 248–265
estrogen
producing ovarian tumors 33
estrogen production
hypothalamic regulation, climacteric woman 59, 60
estrogens
preparations, dose, results of treatment 7, 8
estrogen therapy
bone fractures incidence, osteoporesis 11
double-blind crossover-study 7
indications, contraindications, results of treatment 4, 5, 7
kraurosis vulvae, results of treatment 8
osteoporosis 9, 10
psychotropic effects 8, 9
risks 13, 14
treatment recommendations, summary 16
side effects 11, 12
vascular complications 12, 13, 14
eye
see ophthalmology

Fallopian tubes
carcinoma 28, 31, 32
femoral head necrosis
surgical management 184
femoral head prosthesis
acetabular erosion, causes 80, 81
femoral neck fractures
osteoporosis, surgical, technique 182, 184
femoral shaft fractures
treatment 85, 86, 183, 186, 188, 190
femur
diaphysical fractures, internal fixation 186, 188
fertility
age distribution 55
fibrosis dysplasia
metabolic disorders of bone, fractures in the elderly 177
fistula
bronchopleural, spontaneous pneumothorax 245
fistulas
enterocutaneous, diverticular disease 170
fluid, electrolyte balance
preoperative management 126, 127
foot fractures
treatment 86, 87
fractures
diaphyseal femoral, surgical procedures 186, 188
femoral neck, surgical technique 67, 182, 184
femoral shaft 85, 86
foot, treatment 86, 87
general management 85
hip joint, survival rates, anesthesia procedure 122, 123
humerus, shoulder 87, 88
near the hip 69, 70
old age 177–192
Paget's disease, tibia, internal fixation 183
patella 86

pathological, in the elderly 177
pathological, metastatic paraplegia 88
pelvis 87
spine 87
stress-, diagnosis, treatment 90
tibia, treatment 86, 190, 191
trochanteric, stable and unstable types 186
trochanteric, surgery 76
upper limb 190

fundoplication
carcinoma of esophagus 253

gallbladder
cancer, surgery 162

gallstones
complications 161, 162
surgery 159, 160

gastrectomy
esophago-jejunostomy, carcinoma of esophagus 253
postoperative lung function 112

gastro-esophageal reflux
diagnosis, preoperative 249
symtomatology 250, 258

gastrointestinal symptoms
menopause, estrogen therapy 11

genital atrophy
estrogen therapy, results 7, 8

glaucoma
anterior chamber volume, aging changes 352
"Gitterkollagen", ultrastructure 335
histologic findings 359

goiter
retrosternal, surgery 246

grading
osteoporosis, trabecular pattern 180

granulosa cell tumors
ovarian, estrogen-producing 33, 34

gynecology
anovular cycles, shortened luteal phases, age distribution 54
breast cancer 41–43
cancer, incidence in the older 16
cervical carcinoma 21–25
cervical stump carcinoma 26
climacteric, causes 2, 3
climacteric, epidemiology 45–62
climacteric, mortality 14, 15
climacteric, osteoporosis 9, 10
climacteric, psychotropic effects 8, 9
climacteric, treatment 4, 5
corpus uteri neoplasms 27, 28
endometrial cancer, clinical features 28, 29, 30
endometrial cancer, estrogens risk 13
estrogen decrease, consequences 3, 4
estrogen therapy, indications, contraindications 5
estrogen therapy, recommendations 16
estrogen therapy, results of treatment 7, 8
Fallopian tubes, cancer 31, 32
genital atrophy, estrogen therapy 7, 8
hypothalamopituitary ovarian feedback system, pre-, postmenopause 3, 4
menopause, symptomatology 2
menstrual pattern, climacteric, epidemiology 52, 54
metastases, mammary, ovarian cancer 36
ovarial tumors 32
premenopause 2
sarcoma of the uterus 31
vaginal cancer 19–21
vulva cancer 16, 17

Hamilton rating scale
estrogen therapy, results 9

Hastings hip
radiography 82, 83

heart
acquired lesions 221, 222
arrhythmics, anesthesia 134
bronchial carcinoma, operability 237
complications, perioperative, multivariate discriminante function coefficients 119
congenital lesions 218, 219
left ventricular assist devices 228
surgery, in the elderly 213–228

heart function
old age 106, 107

hemoccult test
colonic tumors, screening population 166

hepatic diseases
preexisting, surgical patients, different ages 105

herpes zoster
diagnosis, treatment 458, 459

hiatus hernia
clinical picture, treatment 258, 259

hip fractures
surgery, survival rates after anesthesia 122, 123

hip joint
arthroplasty, acetabular protrusion 184, 185

hip joint
Hastings hip 75, 82
Thomson prosthesis, causes of acetabular erosion 79

histology
  bronchial carcinoma 230, 231
  eye, archetecture of trabecular meshwork 331, 332
  lens, age changes 378, 412, 413
  morphea-like basal cell carcinoma 308
  meibomian carcinoma, eyelid 306
  ovarian tumors 33
  perifocal zone of retina 436
  retinal pigment epithelium, druse formation 427, 432
  retinal pigment epithelium, senescent 433
  skin, normal, aging 452
hormonal therapy
  prostatic carcinoma 207, 208
hormones
  climacteric woman 59
  control of prostatic growth 193, 194
humerus
  fractures 87, 178
hypertension
  cardiovascular complications, risk in old age 108
  estrogen therapy, contraindication 5
  perioperative complications, risk 120
  preexisting, old age, risks of cardiovascular complications 108
  preoperative diagnosis, treatment 125
hypothalamic-pituitary-gonadal axis
  testosterone metabolism in the aged 193, 194
hypothalamic pituitaryovarian feedback system
  estrogen decrease, pre-, postmenopause 3
hypoxemia
  postoperative, pathogenesis 138, 139

icterus
  estrogen therapy, contraindication 5
ileocecal tumors
  differential diagnosis 38
incidence
  abnormal lung function, preoperative 111
  bone fractures, menopause, estrogen-, calcium therapy 11
  bone fractures, osteoporosis 179
  bronchial carcinoma 230, 231
  cancers, older patients 16
  carcinoma of the esophagus 153
  carcinoma of the pancreas 162
  cardiovascular disturbances, elderly patients 107, 108
  climacteric complaints 3
  cervical carcinoma 21–25
  complications, nature of operation, mortality rate 119, 120
  complications, postoperative deaths, age groupes 120, 121
  diabetic retinopathy 443
  diverticular disease, colon 168
  gastric carcinoma 155
  large bowel carcinoma 164
  last pregnancy, postmenopausal group 53
  metastases, ovarian carcinoma 36
  metrorrhagia, climacteric period 56
  myocardial infarction, postoperative, nature of operation 119, 120
  osteomalacia 184
  ovarial tumors 32
  preexisting diseases, surgical patients 105, 106
  reflux esophagitis 259
  skin diseases, in the elderly 452
  skin cancer 460, 461
  analgetic agents, postoperative period 140, 141
  benign prostatic hyperplasia, treatment 195
  brachial plexus block 131
  bronchial carcinoma, operability 237, 239
  climacteric, estrogen therapy 4
  emergency cholecystectomy 159, 160
  gastric surgery, anti-inflammatory treatment: Arthritis 158
  gastric ulceration, surgery 157
  general, regional anesthesia, geriatric patients 122, 123, 130, 131, 132
  polyposis of large bowel, surgical excision 164
  regional anesthesia 130, 131
  surgery, diverticular disease, colon 169
  thoracotomy in the elderly, operative mortality 154
intensive care unit
  postoperative circulatory complications, diagnosis, treatment 136, 137
intermittend positive pressure breathing (IPPB)
  pre-, postoperative management 127
intraocular pressure
  function of age 353, 354

jaundice
  obstructive, differential diagnosis 162, 163

keratoacanthoma
  eyelid, differential diagnosis 303, 304

kidney
function limits, bronchial carcinoma 238
knee arthroplasty
operative technique 97, 98
kraurosis vulvae
estrogen therapy, results of treatment 8
kyphoscoliosis
osteoporosis, diagnosis 179

laparotomy
survival, gastric cancer 156
large bowel
anal carcinoma 168
cancer, surgery in the elder 163–168
colitis in the elderly 171–172
diverticular disease 168, 169
fistulas 170
infective complications 169
rectal carcinoma 166, 167
larynx
morphologic, functional changes in aging 283, 284
voice in old age 285, 286
leucocytes
entopically visualised, variation with age 429
lobectomy
indication, bronchial carcinoma 240
lumbar spine stenosis
computer assisted tomography 90, 91
lung function
abnormal, preoperative, frequency 111
parameters, effect of age 109
preoperative evaluation 126
lymphatics
adenocarcinoma of prostate 203, 204
cervical carcinoma 22
endometrial cancer 29
esophagus 249

mastopathia fibrosa cystica
estrogen therapy, contraindication 5
estrogen therapy, side effects 11
mediastinoscopy
bronchial carcinoma 235
melanoma
estrogen therapy, contraindication 5
risk factors 461
menopause
age, methods of study 49
Blatt's index, symptomatology 59
estimated median ages 49, 51
see climacteric woman
menstrual pattern
climacteric, epidemiology 52, 54
metabolic disorders
anesthesia, monitoring 134
fractures in the elderly 177
metastases
bronchial carcinoma 231
ovarian carcinoma 35, 36
pathological fractures, treatment 88, 89, 90
prostatic adenocarcinoma 203, 204, 205
metrorrhagia
menopauseal women, age distribution 56
migraine
estrogen therapy, contraindication 5
monoamine oxidase levels
estrogen treatment, results 8
mortality
bleeding, peptic ulerations 156, 157
carcinoma of the stomach 155
elderly surgical patients 102, 103
fractures in the elderly 177
long-term estrogen-trated patients 14
operative, carcinoma of esophagus 154, 252
operative, carcinoma of the pancreas 163
operative, elderly patients 102, 103
thoractomy in the elderly 153
mortality rate
complications, nature of operation 119, 120
emergency surgery 121
myocardial infarction
hypertension, risk in old age 108
postoperative, complete ECG lead program 136
postoperative, incidence, nature of operation 119, 120

nephrogenic edema
estrogen therapy, contraindication 5
neuromuscular disorders
esophageal, diagnosis, treatment 261, 262
neuromyopathy
bronchial carcinoma 233
nose
epistaxis 280
external, aging changes 278
mucosa, paranasal sinus 278, 279
nasal polyps 279
olfactory impairment 280
rhinophyma 279
sinusitis frontalis, maxillaris 279, 280

obstructive ventilation disorders
  preoperative management 127
operability
  bronchial carcinoma, assessment 236
operations
  see surgery
opthalmology
  anterior eye segment, age related changes 326–351
  anterior eye segment, Scheimpflug photographs 393
  aphakic eyes, aqueous composition 383
  aqueous humor, aging changes 352–360
  chorioid, Bruch's membrane, changes in pigment epithelium 431, 433, 435
  ciliary body, age-related changes 338, 342
  ciliary body, anatomy, histology 327, 331, 338, 339
  ciliary body, histologic changes, aqueous humor formation 357
  ciliary epithelium 341
  ciliary processes 340, 341
  clinical changes in the elderly 313–318
  cornea, arcus senilis 311, 312, 321, 322
  cornea, biochemical changes, old age 319, 320
  cornea, cell density, different age groups 331
  cornea, Descemet's membrane, aging changes 318, 328, 329
  cornea, electron micrographs 332, 334, 335, 337
  cornea, endothelium, aging changes 315, 330, 331
  cornea, hexosamine sulfate, hydroxyproline, aging changes 320
  cornea, horizontal section 327
  cornea, increased Shagreen 312
  cornea, lipid spectra, lipoproteins, aging changes 321, 322
  cornea, microscopic changes, old age 318–320
  cornea, physiology, metabolism 311
  cornea, regenerative popwer of epithelium 316, 317
  cornea, sensitivity, age related 314
  cornea, swelling properties of stroma 315
  cornea, ulcerations 323
  cornea, white limbus girdle of Vogt 312, 313
  dark adaptation, function of age 444
  densitograms 390, 391, 393
  eye, ultrastructures 332, 334, 335, 337
  eyelids, aging changes 298, 299
  eyelids, bags 300
  eyelids, basal cell carcinoma 306, 307
  eyelids, blepharochalasis 299, 300
  eyelids, blepharophimosis 300
  eyelids, covering defects 300
  eyelids, ectropion 300, 301
  eyelids, fat hernia 300
  eyelids, motor disorders 302, 303
  eyelids, precancerous lesions 304, 305
  eyelids, seborrhoic dermatitis 301
  eyelids, seborrhoic keratosis 303
  eyelids, senile atrophy 298, 299
  eyelids, senile ectropion, entropion 300, 301
  eyelids, senile pigment abnormalities 299
  eyelids, significance in vision 298
  eyelids, tumors 302, 303
  foveal cone density, morphometric evaluations 437
  glaucoma, incidence, age-related 337
  glaucoma, ultrastructures 336
  human eye, cross section 374
  iris, age-related changes 345, 346
  intraocular pressure, increase with age 354
  iris, arm-iris circulation time 357
  iris, topography 327, 345
  lens, accomodation, function of age 395
  lens, anatomy, topography 374, 377
  lens, aqueous humor composition 382, 383
  lens, biochemistry, age related changes 399, 400
  lens, cataracta cuneiformis, coronaria 389
  lens, cataracta senilis, development 399, 400
  lens, cataracta senilis, surgery 415, 416
  lens, chemical composition 353
  lens, densitograms, cataract 398, 400
  lens, densitometric image analysis 387
  lens, elastic properties, loss of accomodation 396
  lens, electrolyte dynamics 384
  lens, embryology 375, 376
  lens, fine structure 378, 379
  lens, fluorescence 386
  lens, histology 378, 379
  lens, light absorption, function of age 445
  lens, light scattering 397
  lens, light transmission 385

lens, morphology, age changes 412, 413
lens, nuclear cataract 389
lens, opacities, different mechanisms 397, 398
lens, opacities, epidemiology 414
lens, opacities, optic sections 400, 401
lens, photography 386, 387, 389
lens, planimetry, methodological errors 392
lens, presbyopia 394, 395
lens, refraction mechanism 374, 375
lens, Scheimpflug photography, applications 386, 387, 389, 398
lens, slit lamp microscopy 387
lens, specific weight 380, 381
lens, thickness, diameter of equator 381
lens, transparency, age changes 396
lens, transparency disturbances 385
lens, ultrastructure 379
lens, ultraviolet and visible light transmission 386
lens, volume in relation to age 380
lens, weight as a function of age 374
photoreceptors, retinal senescence 436, 437
pigment abnormalities 299
retina, arterial filling, intraocular pressure 357
retina, basal linear deposit, classification 427
retina, Bruch's membrane, senescent changes 431, 433
retina, dark adaptation, function of age 444
retina, diabetes mellitus, retinopathy 443
retina, early receptor potential 441
retina, electroretinogram, electro-oculogram 440, 441
retina, function indices 440, 441
retina, lipofuscin, function of location and age 435
retina, photoreceptors 436
retina, pigment epithelium, histology 427, 431
retina, pigment regeneration, dark adaptation 444
retina, structural changes 426, 427
retina, subjective information of the senescent 441, 442
retina, ultrastructures of capillaries 430
retina, vasculature, ultrastructure 426, 428
senile atrophy 298, 299
senile ptosis 303
Sondermann's channel 331
sclera, topography 327
tonometry 354
trabecular meshwork, architecture 331
vitreous body, structure, composition, aging changes 360, 362
zonular apparatus, internal limiting membrane 344
organ disorders
preexisting, elderly surgical patients 103, 104, 105
osteoarthropathy
pulmonary, bronchial carcinoma 233
orthopaedics
arthroplasty in the elderly 91, 92
assessment clinic 93
femoral head prosthesis, acetabular erosion, causes 80, 84
femoral neck fractures, operative technique 74
fractures, arm, pelvis, spine 87, 88
fractures, general management 85
fractures near the hip 67, 68
fractures of the neck, of the femur 67
geriatric orthopaedic team 69
geriatric population 66, 67
Hastings hip 79–84
pathological fractures 88, 89
trochanteric fractures 76
osteomalacia
clinical picture, treatment 181
osteoporosis
bone fractures incidence, androgen-, estrogen prophylaxis 11
crush fracture of spine 87
diagnosis, treatment 179, 180
estrogen therapy 9, 10
fractures near the hip 67
grading, trabecular pattern 180
trochanteric fracture 70
vertebral fractures 178, 179
otolaryngology
conservative treatment 287
ear, in the elderly 270–277
larynx, changes in the elderly 283, 284
nose, paranasal sinuses 278–280
pharynx 280
salivary glands 281, 282
surgical therapy 288, 290
ovarial cancer
age dependent frequency, peak incidence 17
ovarial tumors
frequency, clinical features 32–40

Paget's disease
bone fractures in the elderly 177, 183
clinical picture, therapeutic aspects 181, 182
pain intensity
age related 116
pancreas
surgery, epidural, systemic postoperative analgesia 140
carcinoma, incidence, clinical picture, surgical procedures 162, 163
pancreatitis
complication: Gallstones 161, 162
estrogen therarpy, contraindication 5
PaO_2
lung volume, age changes 110, 113
paroxysmal tadycardia
preoperative diagnosis, treatment 125, 126
patellar fractures
treatment 86
Paterson-Brown-Kelly syndrome
carcinoma of esophagus 250
pathogenesis
central respiratory depression 138, 139
pathology
bronchial carcinoma 230
esophageal cancer 250, 251
pelvis
fractures, treatment 87
pemphigoid
bullous, clinical picture, treatment 460
periampullary region
carcinoma, surgery 163
pharmacokinetics
changes with age 114, 115
pharynx
loss of taste with aging, pathophysiology 284
mucosal changes 280, 281
pH studies
esophagus, gastroesophageal reflux 249
physiotherapy
assessment clinic 94
pigment abnormalities
eyelids 299
Plummer-Vinson syndrome
carcinoma of esophagus 250
pneumonectomy
indication, bronchial carcinoma 240
pneumothorax
diagnosis, treatment 245, 246
postmenopause
complaints, symptoms, hormonal status 59, 60
genital changes 56, 57
postoperative care
anesthesiologic, monitoring 136, 137
postoperative disorders
cardiovascular homeostasis 136
postoperative management
esophageal carcinoma, surgery 256
postoperative respiratory failure
factors contributing 139
precancerosis
polyposis, large bowel 164
pregnancy
age, postmenopausal group 53
menopausal, postmenopausal complaints, symptoms 61
premenopause
hormonal status 2
preoperative anesthetic risk
quantification 117, 118
presbycusis
morphology, physiology, contributory fractures, treatment 270–275
prognosis
cancer of vulva 17
early gastric cancer 155
fractures in the elderly 177
lung cancer 231
mammary cancer 43
ovarian tumors, histologic thypes 40
peptic ulceration, in the older patient 156
tumour situation, surgical staging 232
prophylaxis
annual colonoscopy, lesions of large bowel, malignant transformation 164, 166
prostate
adenocarcinoma, diagnosis, clinical staging, treatment 201–209
benign prostatic hyperplasia 194, 195
examination, expressed secretions 201
growth, hormonal control 193, 194
perineal prostatectomy 194
prostatitis, clinical picture 199–201
prostatodynia 201
suprapubic prostatectomy 197
transperineal, transrectal needle biopsy 202, 203
transurethral resection 196
prostatism
clinical picture 193
pruritus
causes, treatment 458
pseudo-fractures
osteomalacia 181
psychotropic effects
estrogen therapy 8
pulmonary disease
preoperative management 126, 127

pulmonary risks
preoperative, prediction 118, 119
pulmonary surgery
elderly people 224–247

radiotherapy
anal tumors 168
carcinoma of the esophagus 153, 154
cervical cancer 25, 26, 27
ovarial cancer 39, 40
prostatic adenocarcinoma 206, 207
rectal carcinoma 167
rectal carcinoma
diagnosis, treatment 166, 167
rectal polyposis
malignant transformation, diagnosis, treatment 164, 165
rectal prolapse
treatment 172, 173
recurrence
endometrial carcinoma 30, 31
reflux esophagitis
diagnosis, incidence, treatment 259, 260
regional lymph nodes
cervix uteri, parametria, pelvic wall 22
corpus uteri, endometrial carcinoma 29
vulva 18
renal diseases
preexisting, surgical patients, different ages 105
respiratory disorders
preexisting, surgical patients, different ages 105, 108, 109
respiratory system
functional investigation, preoperative 126
preexisting disease, preoperative management 126, 127
rheumatoid arthritis
bone fractures in the elderly 177
risks
anesthesia, quantification 117, 118
long-term estrogen therapy 14, 15
perioperative, cardiac complications 119

salivary glands
senile atrophy, pathophysiology 281, 282
scintigraphy
bone, pathologic fractures 89
scleroderma
esophagus, diagnosis, symptoms 265
Scheimpflug photography
technique, applications 386, 388, 389, 392
seborrheic dermatitis
eyelids 301
seborrheic keratosis
eyelids 303
senile atrophy
eyelids 298, 299
senile dementia
Alzheimer's disease, anesthesiologic problems 113, 114
shoulder
fractures, treatment 87, 88
side effects
estrogen therapy 11,12
sigmoidoscopy
colonic lesions, diagnosis 164
skeletal scintigraphy
pathological fractures, diagnosis 89, 90
skin
aging changes, physiologic and pathologic alterations 452–463
skin alterations
menopause, estrogen effect 11
specular microscopy
cornea, aging changes 314
spine
fractures, old age, osteoporosis 178, 179
fractures, treatment 87, 88
squamous cell carcinoma
skin, treatment 462
staging
adenocarcinoma of prostate 203, 204
bronchial carcinoma 232
cervical carcinoma 23
endometrial carcinoma 30
mammary cancer 43
ovarian cancer 37
vulva cancer 18, 19
steroids
peptic ulceration, complications 156
stress fractures
diagnosis, treatment 90
strictures
esophageal, treatment 260, 261
supracondylar fractures
femur, osteoporose, surgical management 188, 189
surgery
abnormal lung function, preoperative, frequency 111
acetabular erosion, Thompson prothesis 79
achalasia, esophageal 264, 265
age distribution of patients 102, 103
anal tumors 168

surgery
  analgetic agents, postoperative period, indications, contraindications 140, 141
  anesthetic management 122–129
  anesthetic risks, quantifikation 117, 118
  antireflux fundoplication operation 260
  benign prostatic hyperplasia 196, 198
  bronchial carcinoma 230–242
  carcinoma of the oesophagus 153, 154, 251, 252
  carcinoma of large intestine 163–168
  carcinoma of the pancreas 162, 163
  carcinoma of the periampullar region 163
  carcinoma of the stomach 155, 156
  cardiac, principles 213
  cardiovascular, pulmonary risk, prediction 118
  castration, prostatectomy 198
  cervical cancer, results 25, 26
  cholelithiasis, choledocholithiasis 159, 160
  colonic adenomas 165
  complications, circulatory 136
  deaths, postoperative, age groupes 120, 121
  diffuse esophageal spasm 265
  duodenal ulceration 158, 159
  elderly patients, mortality 102, 103
  elective vs emergency 121, 122
  emergency, mortality rate 121
  emphysematous cysts 246
  empyema 242, 243
  enterocutaneous fistulas, diverticular disease 170
  epidural anesthesia 131
  esophageal cancer 252
  esophageal diverticula 262
  esophagectomy, transhiatal 255
  esophago-jejunostomy 253
  femoral neck fracture, osteoporosis 74, 184, 186
  fractures near the hip 69, 70
  fractures, old age 177–192
  gastrointestinal, in the elderly 152–176
  gastro-oesophageal reflux 258, 259
  gallstones 159, 160
  gastric ulceration 157, 158
  general anesthesia 131–134
  geriatric patients, preexisting disorders of organ systems 104
  goiter, retrosternal 246
  heart, aneurysms 221
  heart, atrial septal defect 219
  heart, cardiopulmonary bypass 213
  heart, cold paraplegia 215
  heart, congenital lesions 218, 219
  heart, haemostasis 216
  heart, intraaortic balloon counterpulsation 227
  heart, left-to-right shunts 219, 220
  heart, left ventricular assist devices 228
  heart, mitral regurgitation 222
  heart, myocardial revascularisation 218
  heart, persistent ductus arteriosus 219, 220
  heart, protection 214, 215
  heart, ruptured chordae 225
  heart, technique 217, 218
  heart, valve defects 224, 225
  heart, ventricular septal defect 222
  Hastings hip 75, 82
  hiatus hernia 152, 258, 259
  hip fracture, survival rates after anesthesia 122, 123
  infective complications, diverticular disease, large bowel 169
  inhalation narcotic agents, selection 132
  lung, preoperative preparation 224
  lung function, influence of age 112
  lung function, risks in the elderly 126
  mortality, elderly patients 102, 103
  mortality rate, nature of operation 119, 120
  oesophageal 248–258
  old age fractures 177–192
  operative mortality, esophagectomy 154
  ovarian tumors 39, 40
  Paget's discase, tibia, fractures, internal fixation 183
  pancreas resection, epidural and systemic postoperative analgesia 140
  peptic ulceration 156, 157
  perioperative complications, multivariate discriminante function coefficients 119, 120
  polyposis of large bowel, malignant transformation 164
  postericoid cancer 255
  postoperative care, anesthesiologic monitoring 136, 137
  postoperative disorders, cardiovascular homeostasis, monitoring 136
  postoperative respiratory failure, contributing factors 139
  premedication 128, 129
  preoperative anesthetic risk, quantification 117, 118

preoperative cardio-pulmonary risks, prediction 118, 119
preparation of patient 95
prostate, adenocarcinoma 201–207
prostaste, perineal prostatectomy 198
prostate, retro-, suprapubic prostataectomy 197
prostate, transperineal, transrectal needle biopsy 202, 203
prostate, transurethral resection 196
pulmonary 224–247
rectal carcinoma 166, 167
rectal fistulas 170
rectal prolapse, incontinence 172, 173
reflux oesophagitis 152
regional anesthesia 130, 131
respiratory disorders, postoperative, treatment 137, 138
senile cataract, complications 415
strictures of oesophagus 260
suprapubic prostatectomy 197
thoracic, in the elderly 213–228
vital functions, monitoring 134

survival rates
carcinoma of esophagus, esophagectomy 154
cervical cancer 27
hip joint fractures, anesthesia procedure 122, 123
ovarian cancer 40
prostatic adenocarcinoma 205, 206

survival times
laparotomy for gastric cancer 156

symptomatology
benign prostatic hyperplasia 195
Blatt's menopausal index 58, 59, 60
breast cancer 42
bronchial carcinoma 232
cervical cancer 22
estrogen-producing ovarian tumors 33, 34
estrogen therapy, side effects 11, 12
extragenital, climacteric women 57, 58
gastro-esophageal reflux 250, 258
gastrointestinal, estrogen therapy, side effects 11
menopause, estrogen therapy, double blind cross-over study 7
ovarian tumors 33, 36
postoperative circulatory disorders 136

synchronous tumors
large bowel carcinoma 166

tachyarrhythmias
preoperative diagnosis, treatment 125, 126

tachycardia
diagnosis, treatment, algorithm 138

technique
aortic dissection 226, 227
arthroplasty 97, 98
cold cardioplegia 215
mitral regurgitation, myocardial infarct 223
perineal prostatectomy 198
retropubic prostatectomy 197
surgical, esophagectomy, palliative procedures 153, 154
surgical, femoral neck fractures, osteoporosis 182, 184
surgical, gastric cancer 155
transurethral resection of prostate 196
ventricular septal defect 222

teratoma
malignant, ovarian tumors 33

testosterone
hormonal metabolism in the aged 193, 194

Thompson prosthesis
causes of acetabular erosion 80, 84

thoracic surgers
heart and great vessels 213–228

thoracotomy
bronchial carcinoma 236

thrombosis
venous, estrogen therapy 5

tibia
fractures, treatment 86

TNM system
mammary cancer 43
ovarian cancer 37
vulva cancer 18, 19

total lung capacity
age changes 109

treatment
acute empyema 243, 244
anal tumors 168
basal cell carcinoma of skin 462
benign prostatic hyperplasia 196, 198
bladder incontinence 78, 79
brady-, tachycardia, algorithms 138
breast cancer 42
bresbycusis 275, 276
cataracta senilis 415, 416
cervical cancer 23–25
cervical stump carcinoma 26, 27
chest trauma 247
climacteric, indications, contraindications 4, 5
colonic adenomas 165
colitis ulcerative 171, 172
Crohn's discase 171, 172

treatment
  decubitus ulcer of skin 457
  diverticular disease, large bowel 168, 169
  ear, nose, throat diseases 287, 288
  endometrial cancer 30, 31, 32
  enterocutaneous fistulas, diverticular disease 170
  esophageal carcinoma, surgical 252
  estrogen therapy, double-blind crossover-study, estriol, placebo 7
  estrogen therapy, Hamilton rating scale 9
  Fallopian tubes, cancer 31, 32
  femoral shaft fractures 85, 86
  fistulas, diverticular disease 170
  fractures near the hip 69, 70
  fractures of patella, tibia, ankle and food 86, 87
  gasto-esophageal reflux 259, 260
  herpes zoster 459, 460
  hiatus hernia 259, 260
  long-term estrogen therapy, relative risk 14
  neuromuscular disorders of esophagus 261, 262
  osteomalacia 184
  osteoporosis 179, 180
  pruritus 458
  reflux esophagitis 259, 260
  scleroderma, esophageal 265
  skin cancer 461, 462
  squamous cell carcinoma of skin 462
  structures of esophagus 260, 261
  supracondylar fractures of femur 188, 189
  ovarian cancer 39, 40
  pathological fractures 88, 89
  physiotherapy, assessment clinic 94
  polyposis of large bowel 164, 165
  postoperative respiratory disorders 137, 138
  preexisting disease, anesthesia 123, 124
  preoperative cardiac 124
  rectal carcinoma 166, 167
  rectal prolapse 172, 173
  spontaneous pneumothorax 245
  stress fractures 90
  tachycardia, algorithm 138
  vulva cancer 19
trochanteric fracture
  radiogram 70
tryptophan
  Hamilton rating scale, estrogen treatment, menopause 9

ulceration
  peptic, surgery 156, 158
ultrastructures
  cornea 332, 334, 337
  corneo-scleral meshwork membrane 357
  eye lens fibers 379
  glaucoma, "Gitterkollagen" 335
  retina, capillaries 430
  retina, convoluted rods 439
urinary retention
  partial, complete, indications for treatment 195
urogenital system
  atrophic changes, estrogen treatment 8
uterine bleeding
  menopausal, postmenopausal, histologic findings 13

vaginal cancer
  clinical features, treatment 19, 20
vagotomy
  gastric ulceration 157
vertigo
  in the elderly, differential diagnosis 277
visual acuity
  advancing age 442
vitamin D
  calcium, estrogen therapy, menopause 10
vitreous production
  aging changes 360–367
vulva
  kraurosis, estrogen therapy, results 8
vulva cancer
  incidence, symptoms, treatment, prognosis 16–19

wedge resection
  indications, bronchial carcinoma 240, 241
Whipple's procedure
  epidural and systemic postoperative analgesia 140
  postoperative lung function 112

Xerosis
  aging skin 458

Zenker's diverticulum
  esophagus, diagnosis, operation 261, 262

Geriatric Medicine

Volume 1

Medical, Psychiatric and Pharmacological Topics

Editors: **C.K. Cassel, J.R. Walsh**
1984. 136 figures. Approx. 590 pages
ISBN 3-540-90944-3

Volume 2

Fundamentals of Geriatric Care

Editors: **C.K. Cassel, J.R. Walsh**
1984. 50 figures. Approx. 410 pages
ISBN 3-540-90958-3

Written by acknowledged American authorities in the fields that make up geriatric medicine, this extraordinary work delivers in-depth-coverage of the entire spectrum of medical care for elderly patients. *Geriatric Medicine* is a two-volume tour de force that not only brings you extensive information on the most important advances being made in this emerging discipline, but also provides you with a deeper understanding of the social, economic, legal and ethical issues involved in treating the aged in the United States.
Volume 1: *Medical, Psychiatric and Pharmacological Topics* is designed to expand your understanding of geriatric itself. Its content ranges from the cell biology of aging to careful scrutinies of each of the organ system, diseases affecting them and their treatments. Therapy recommendations emphasize the practical interventions currently available. Pharmacological chapters include an examination of drug interactions and how elderly metabolism differs in its responses to treatment.
Volume II: *Fundamentals of Geriatric Care* covers social, legal, ethical and economic aspects of geriatric care, plus the management of chronic pain and the spiritual care of the hospitalized elderly. All of these topics are discussed by experts in a practical and focused way, supplying clincians and gerontologists with information not available elsewhere. Volume II expands your perception of the interdisciplinary needs of the elderly. It helps you to understand the complex demographic, social and philosophical perspectives that are often forgotten when concentrating on the medical side of a problem. It provides reliable information about the intricate relationship that exists between health care payment systems and geriatric medicine. This unique volume also brings a clearer idea of the directions research is leading as well names and addresses of health care resources, making it a reference you will use over and over again.

Springer-Verlag
Berlin
Heidelberg
New York
Tokyo

GPSR Compliance
The European Union's (EU) General Product Safety Regulation (GPSR) is a set of rules that requires consumer products to be safe and our obligations to ensure this.

If you have any concerns about our products, you can contact us on

ProductSafety@springernature.com

In case Publisher is established outside the EU, the EU authorized representative is:

Springer Nature Customer Service Center GmbH
Europaplatz 3
69115 Heidelberg, Germany

www.ingramcontent.com/pod-product-compliance
Lightning Source LLC
Chambersburg PA
CBHW080535250926
51846CB00016B/982
* 9 7 8 3 6 4 2 6 8 9 7 8 9 *